Pediatric Neurovascular Disorders

Editors

PRAKASH MUTHUSAMI
TODD ABRUZZO

NEUROIMAGING CLINICS
OF NORTH AMERICA

www.neuroimaging.theclinics.com

Consulting Editor
SURESH K. MUKHERJI

November 2024 • Volume 34 • Number 4

ELSEVIER

1600 John F. Kennedy Boulevard • Suite 1800 • Philadelphia, Pennsylvania, 19103-2899

http://www.neuroimaging.theclinics.com

NEUROIMAGING CLINICS OF NORTH AMERICA Volume 34, Number 4
November 2024 ISSN 1052-5149, ISBN 13: 978-0-443-29408-2

Editor: John Vassallo (j.vassallo@elsevier.com)
Developmental Editor: Anirban Mukherjee

Neuroimaging Clinics of North America (ISSN 1052-5149) is published quarterly by Elsevier Inc., 360 Park Avenue South, New York, NY 10010-1710. Months of issue are February, May, August, and November. Business and editorial offices: 1600 John F. Kennedy Blvd., Suite 1800, Philadelphia, PA 19103-2899. Business and editorial offices: 6277 Sea Harbor Drive, Orlando, FL 32887-4800. Periodicals postage paid at New York, NY, and additional mailing offices. Subscription prices are USD 430 per year for US individuals, USD 100 per year for US students and residents, USD 493 per year for Canadian individuals, USD 573 per year for international individuals, USD 100 per year for Canadian students and residents and USD 260 per year for foreign students and residents. For institutional access pricing please contact Customer Service via the contact information below. To receive student/resident rate, orders must be accompanied by name of affiliated institution, date of term, and the *signature* of program/residency coordinator on institution letterhead. Orders will be billed at individual rate until proof of status is received. Foreign air speed delivery is included in all *Clinics* subscription prices. All prices are subject to change without notice. Orders, claims, and journal inquiries: Please visit our Support Hub page https://service.elsevier.com for assistance.

Reprints. For copies of 100 or more of articles in this publication, please contact the Commercial Reprints Department, Elsevier Inc., 360 Park Avenue South, New York, NY 10010-1710. Tel.: 212-633-3874; Fax: 212-633-3820; E-mail: reprints@elsevier.com.

Neuroimaging Clinics of North America is covered by *Excerpta Medical/EMBASE,* the RSNA Index of Imaging Literature, *MEDLINE/PubMed (Index Medicus),* MEDLINE/MEDLARS, SciSearch, Research Alert, and Neuroscience Citation Index.

JOURNAL TITLE: Neuroimaging Clinics of North America
ISSUE: 34.4

PROGRAM OBJECTIVE

The goal of *Neuroimaging Clinics of North America* is to keep practicing radiologists and radiology residents up to date with current clinical practice in radiology by providing timely articles reviewing the state of the art in patient care.

TARGET AUDIENCE

Practicing radiologists, radiology residents, and other healthcare professionals who utilize neuroimaging findings to provide patient care.

LEARNING OBJECTIVES

Upon completion of this activity, participants will be able to:

1. Review neurovascular malformations in the fetus and neonate.
2. Discuss foundational principles of pediatric neuroimaging and technological advances that significantly improved the diagnostic and treatment.
3. Recognize arterial ischemic stroke (AIS) in children has a high mortality and life-long disability rate.

ACCREDITATION

The Elsevier Office of Continuing Medical Education (EOCME) is accredited by the Accreditation Council for Continuing Medical Education (ACCME) to provide continuing medical education for physicians.

The EOCME designates this journal-based CME activity for a maximum of 10 *AMA PRA Category 1 Credit*(s)™. Physicians should claim only the credit commensurate with the extent of their participation in the activity.

All other healthcare professionals requesting continuing education credit for this enduring material will be issued a certificate of participation.

DISCLOSURE OF RELEVANT FINANCIAL RELATIONSHIPS

The EOCME assesses conflict of interest with its instructors, faculty, planners, and other individuals who are in a position to control the content of CME activities. All relevant conflicts of interest that are identified are thoroughly vetted by EOCME for fair balance, scientific objectivity, and patient care recommendations. EOCME is committed to providing its learners with CME activities that promote improvements or quality in healthcare and not a specific proprietary business or a commercial interest.

The authors and editors listed below have identified no financial relationships or relationships to products or devices they have with ineligible companies related to the content of this CME activity:
Todd Abruzzo, MD, FAHA, FACR, FSNIS; Khalid Al-Dasuqi, MD; Anas Al-Smadi, MD; Timothy J. Bernard, MD; Marta Bertamino, MD, PhD; Kartik D. Bhatia, MBBS, PhD, FRANZCR; Karen Chen, MD; Betul E. Derinkuyu, MD; Nevena Fileva, MD, PhD; Samagra Jain, BS; Sulaiman Karim, BS; Katherine S. Kelson; Pradeep Krishnan, MD; James L. Leach, MD; Prakash Muthusami, MD; Darren B. Orbach, MD, PhD; Vivek Pai, MD; Carmen Parra-Farinas, MD; Ayman M. Qureshi, MBChB, MMed, FRCR; Karen I. Ramirez-Suarez, MD; Adam Rennie, MBBS, BMSc, FRCR; Joanne M. Rispoli, MD; Fergus Robertson, MD, MA, MRCP, FRCR; Mariasavina Severino, MD; Ali Shaibani, MD; Manohar Shroff, MD, FRCPC, DABR, DMRD; Nicholas V. Stence, MD; J. Michael Taylor, MD; Luis O. Tierradentro-Garcia, MD; Domenico Tortora, MD, PhD; Sudhakar Vadivelu, DO

The authors and editors listed below have identified financial relationships or relationships to products or devices they have with ineligible companies related to the content of this CME activity:
Mesha L. Martinez, MD: *Consultant*: Vizai, RapidAI, Siemens, Guerbet, Cerenovus; *Speaker*: Cerenovus

The Clinics staff listed below have identified no financial relationships or relationships to products or devices they have with ineligible companies related to the content of this CME activity:
Kothainayaki Kulanthaivelu; Michelle Littlejohn; Patrick J. Manley; Anirban Mukherjee; John Vassallo

UNAPPROVED/OFF-LABEL USE DISCLOSURE

The EOCME requires CME faculty to disclose to the participants:

1. When products or procedures being discussed are off-label, unlabelled, experimental, and/or investigational (not US Food and Drug Administration [FDA] approved); and
2. Any limitations on the information presented, such as data that are preliminary or that represent ongoing research, interim analyses, and/or unsupported opinions. Faculty may discuss information about pharmaceutical agents that is outside of FDA-approved labelling. This information is intended solely for CME and is not intended to promote off-label use of these medications. If you have any questions, contact the medical affairs department of the manufacturer for the most recent prescribing information.

TO ENROLL

To enroll in the *Neuroimaging Clinics of North America* Continuing Medical Education program, call customer service at 1-800-654-2452 or sign up online at http://www.theclinics.com/home/cme. The CME program is available to subscribers for an additional annual fee of USD 254.00.

METHOD OF PARTICIPATION

In order to claim credit, participants must complete the following:

1. Complete enrolment as indicated above.
2. Read the activity.
3. Complete the CME Test and Evaluation. Participants must achieve a score of 70% on the test. All CME Tests and Evaluations must be completed online.

CME INQUIRIES/SPECIAL NEEDS

For all CME inquiries or special needs, please contact elsevierCME@elsevier.com.

NEUROIMAGING CLINICS OF NORTH AMERICA

SERIES OF RELATED INTEREST

Advances in Clinical Radiology
Available at: https://www.advancesinclinicalradiology.com/
MRI Clinics of North America
Available at: https://www.mri.theclinics.com/
Neuroimaging Clinics
Available at: https://www.neuroimaging.theclinics.com/
PET Clinics
Available at: https://www.pet.theclinics.com/

THE CLINICS ARE AVAILABLE ONLINE!
Access your subscription at:
www.theclinics.com

Contributors

CONSULTING EDITOR

SURESH K. MUKHERJI, MD, MBA, FACR
Professor of Radiology and Radiation
Oncology, University of Illinois, Peoria, Illinois;
Robert Wood Johnson Medical School,
Rutgers University, New Brunswick, New

Jersey; Faculty, Otolaryngology Head Neck
Surgery, Michigan State University,
Farmington Hills, Michigan, USA; National
Director of Head and Neck Radiology, ProScan
Imaging, Carmel, Indiana, USA

EDITORS

PRAKASH MUTHUSAMI, MD
Associate Professor, Interventional
Neuroradiology, Department of Diagnostic
Imaging and Image Guided Therapy, The
Hospital for Sick Children, University of
Toronto, Toronto, Ontario, Canada

TODD ABRUZZO, MD, FAHA, FACR, FSNIS
NeuroInterventional Radiologist, Professor,
Departments of Child Health and Radiology,
University of Arizona, Creighton University, and
Mayo Clinic; Co-Director, Section of Vascular
Disorders and Therapeutics, Barrow
Neurological Institute at Phoenix Children's
Hospital, Phoenix, Arizona, USA

AUTHORS

KHALID AL-DASUQI, MD
Fellow, Department of Radiology, Boston
Children's Hospital, Boston, Massachusetts,
USA

ANAS S. AL-SMADI, MD
Fellow, Department of Radiology, Neurology
and Neurosurgery, Northwestern University
Feinberg School of Medicine, Section of
Interventional Neuroradiology, Department of
Radiology, Northwestern Memorial Hospital,
Chicago, Illinois, USA

TIMOTHY J. BERNARD, MD
Professor, Department of Pediatrics, Section of
Child Neurology, University of Colorado
Anschutz School of Medicine, Aurora,
Colorado, USA

MARTA BERTAMINO, MD, PhD
Medical Director, Physical Medicine and
Rehabilitation Unit, IRCCS Instituto Giannina
Gaslini, Genoa, Italy

KARTIK D. BHATIA, MBBS, PhD, FRANZCR
Paediatric Interventional Neuroradiologist,
Department of Medical Imaging, Sydney
Children's Hospital Network, Clinical
Associate Professor, Children's Hospital at
Westmead Clinical School, University of
Sydney, Westmead, New South Wales,
Australia

KAREN CHEN, MD
Director, Edward B. Singleton Department of
Radiology, Texas Children's Hospital,
Assistant Professor, Departments of Radiology
and Neurosurgery, Baylor College of Medicine,
Houston, Texas, USA

BETUL E. DERINKUYU, MD
Pediatric Radiology Fellow, Division of
Pediatric Neuroradiology, Department of
Radiology, Cincinnati Children's Hospital
Medical Center, University of
Cincinnati College of Medicine, Cincinnati,
Ohio, USA

NEVENA FILEVA, MD, PhD
Neuroradiology Unit, IRCCS Istituto Giannina Gaslini, Genova, Italy; Chief Assistant Professor, Department of Diagnostic Imaging, UMHAT Aleksandrovska, Sofia, Bulgaria

SAMAGRA JAIN, BS
Baylor College of Medicine, Houston, Texas, USA

SULAIMAN KARIM, BS
Texas Tech University Health Science Center School of Medicine, Lubbock, Texas, USA; Edward B. Singleton Department of Radiology, Texas Children's Hospital, Houston, Texas, USA

KATHERINE S. KELSON
University of Colorado Anschutz School of Medicine, Aurora, Colorado, USA

PRADEEP KRISHNAN, MD
Staff Neuroradiologist, Division of Neuroradiology, Department of Diagnostic and Interventional Radiology, The Hospital for Sick Children, Department of Medical Imaging, University of Toronto, Toronto, Ontario, Canada

JAMES L. LEACH, MD
Professor, Division of Pediatric Neuroradiology, Department of Radiology, Cincinnati Children's Hospital Medical Center, University of Cincinnati College of Medicine, Cincinnati, Ohio, USA

MESHA L. MARTINEZ, MD
The Edward B. Singleton Department of Radiology, Texas Children's Hospital, Associate Professor of Radiology, Baylor College of Medicine, Austin, Texas, USA

DARREN B. ORBACH, MD, PhD
Division Chief, Division of Neurointerventional Radiology, Boston Children's Hospital, Boston, Massachusetts, USA

VIVEK PAI, MD
Clinical Associate, Division of Neuroradiology, Department of Diagnostic and Interventional Radiology, The Hospital for Sick Children, Department of Medical Imaging, University of Toronto, Toronto, Ontario, Canada

CARMEN PARRA-FARINAS, MD
Pediatric Interventional Neuroradiologist, Division of Pediatric Interventional Neuroradiology, Hospital for Sick Children, Toronto, Ontario, Canada

AYMAN M. QURESHI, MBCHB, MMED, FRCR
Consultant, Lysholm Department of Neuroradiology, National Hospital for Neurology and Neurosurgery, UCLH NHS Foundation Trust, Queen Square, London

KAREN I. RAMIREZ-SUAREZ, MD
Postdoctoral Research Fellow, Department of Radiology, Children's Hospital of Philadelphia, University of Pennsylvania, Philadelphia, Pennsylvania, USA

ADAM RENNIE, MBBS, BMSC, FRCR
Consultant Interventional Neuroradiologist Lysholm Department of Neuroradiology, National Hospital for Neurology and Neurosurgery, UCLH NHS Foundation Trust, Great Ormond Street Hospital for Children NHS Foundation Trust, London, United Kingdom

JOANNE M. RISPOLI, MD
Staff Neuroradiologist, Department of Radiology, Boston Children's Hospital, Boston, Massachusetts, USA

FERGUS ROBERTSON, MD, MA, MRCP, FRCR
Consultant, Lysholm Department of Neuroradiology, National Hospital for Neurology and Neurosurgery, UCLH NHS Foundation Trust, Great Ormond Street Hospital for Children NHS Foundation Trust, London, United Kingdom

MARIASAVINA SEVERINO, MD
Pediatric Neuroradiologists, Neuroradiology Unit, IRCCS Istituto Giannina Gaslini, Genova, Italy

ALI SHAIBANI, MD
Professor, Department of Radiology, Neurology and Neurosurgery, Northwestern University Feinberg School of Medicine, Chicago, Illinois, USA

MANOHAR SHROFF, MD, FRCPC, DABR, DMRD
Staff Neuroradiologist, Division of Neuroradiology, Department of Diagnostic and Interventional Radiology, The Hospital for Sick Children, Department of Medical Imaging, University of Toronto, Toronto, Ontario, Canada

NICHOLAS V. STENCE, MD
Professor, Department of Radiology, Section of Pediatric Radiology, University of Colorado Anschutz School of Medicine, Aurora, Colorado, USA

JOHN MICHAEL TAYLOR, MD
Pediatric Stroke and Neurocritical Care Specialist, Division of Neurology, Department of Pediatrics, Cincinnati Children's Hospital Medical Center, University of Cincinnati College of Medicine, Cincinnati, Ohio, USA

LUIS O. TIERRADENTRO-GARCIA, MD
Resident Physician, Department of Radiology, Hospital of the University of Pennsylvania, University of Pennsylvania, Philadelphia USA

DOMENICO TORTORA, MD, PhD
Neuroradiology Unit, IRCCS Istituto Giannina Gaslini, Genova, Italy

SUDHAKAR VADIVELU, DO
Associate Professor, Division of Pediatric Neurosurgery, Department of Neurosurgery, Cincinnati Children's Hospital Medical Center, University of Cincinnati College of Medicine, Cincinnati, Ohio, USA

Contents

Pediatric cerebrovascular diseases have distinct clinical presentations, pathophysiology, and management compared to the adult counterparts. This introductory article discusses the imaging techniques and neurovascular conditions unique to each age group from the fetal stages through childhood, including vascular malformations, arteriopathy, and strokes. The article also underscores the importance of genetic factors and the need for a multidisciplinary approach in the diagnosis and treatment of pediatric neurovascular disorders.

Pediatric neurovascular diseases are a complex group of disorders associated with significant morbidity and mortality. Given their heterogeneous clinical manifestations, ranging from emergent presentations (eg, acute neurologic deficits) to chronic neurocognitive or developmental issues, cross-sectional imaging modalities play a key role in accurate diagnosis and direct further management. However, imaging pediatric patients is associated with logistical and technical issues. This article provides an overview of the cross-sectional findings of common pediatric neurovascular diseases and discusses the imaging techniques used for their diagnosis.

Catheter-directed angiography (CDA) remains the gold standard for diagnosing neurovascular conditions in both the brain and spinal cord in adults and children. This chapter explores the evolution of CDA in children, highlighting advancements in technology that have refined technique and improved safety. This chapter will discuss the CDA's essential role in the evaluation of complex neurovascular diseases, outlining specific indications, procedural considerations, and potential complications unique to pediatric patients. Through a comprehensive review, this chapter aims to equip clinicians with the knowledge needed to navigate the challenges of performing CDA in younger populations.

Vein of Galen malformations are the most common congenital neurovascular malformation and are a type of choroidal arteriovenous fistula involving the midline primitive choroidal venous circulation. The arteriovenous shunt zone of a VOGM may directly involve the embryonic precursor of the vein of Galen and/or its tributaries within the 3rd ventricle tela choroidea. Dural sinus malformations are characterized by dilated intracranial dural venous sinuses, some of which acquire multifocal arteriovenous shunts within the dural walls of these overgrown venous sinuses.Pial arteriovenous fistulae are high-flow shunts representing direct arterial to venous communication of pial blood vessels, with no definable nidus.

Intracranial vascular malformations (IVMs) represent a significant challenge in pediatric medicine due to their diagnostic and therapeutic complexity. Despite their rarity, the severity of potential neurologic outcomes necessitates a comprehensive understanding and approach to management. This article aims to provide an overview of pediatric IVMs, specifically nidal arteriovenous malformations, cavernous malformations, capillary telangiectasias, and developmental venous anomalies, and highlight the importance of advanced diagnostic imaging and therapeutic strategies in improving outcomes. Vein of Galen malformations, pial arteriovenous fistulas, dural sinus malformations, and intracranial venous malformations will be addressed in other articles. Following a discussion of imaging and clinical considerations within the field, novel imaging techniques will be discussed.

Intracranial arterial aneurysms in children are rare. They differ from adult aneurysms in their etiology, natural history, and management approach. Unruptured asymptomatic aneurysms in children can often be observed for growth over time. Endovascular treatment has become the primary interventional modality in children with intracranial aneurysms. The authors discuss the management approach to pediatric intracranial aneurysms.

Arterial ischemic stroke (AIS) in children has a high mortality and life-long disability rate in surviving patients. Diagnostic delays are longer and risk factors are different compared with AIS in the adult population. Congenital heart disease, cervical arterial dissection, and intracranial arteriopathies are the main causes of AIS in children. New revascularization time windows in children require the definition of diagnostic protocols for stroke in each referral center. In this article, we discuss the neuroimaging techniques and protocols, describe the main underlying causes, and review the current treatment options for pediatric and perinatal AIS.

Intracranial steno-occlusive large vessel arteriopathies refer to abnormalities of the arterial wall that typically express luminal stenosis. Notably, some entities that can find themselves within this category may also express luminal dilation, and/or aneurysm formation as an alternative phenotype. Intracranial steno-occlusive large vessel arteriopathies are a leading cause of arterial ischemic stroke (AIS) in children, often progress, and can predispose to recurrent brain infarction. Intracranial arterial dissections account for a subset of cases expressing the focal cerebral arteriopathy (FCA) phenotype because the affected arterial segment, clinical presentation, and AIS patterns are very similar to the inflammatory subtype of FCA.

Hemorrhagic stroke (HS) is an important cause of neurologic morbidity and mortality in children and is more common than ischemic stroke between the ages of 1 and 14 years, a notable contradistinction relative to adult stroke epidemiology. Rapid neuroimaging is of the utmost importance in making the diagnosis of HS, identifying a likely etiology, and directing acute care. Computed tomography and MR imaging with flow-sensitive MR imaging and other noninvasive vascular imaging studies play a primary role in the initial diagnostic evaluation. Catheter-directed digital subtraction angiography is critical for definitive diagnosis and treatment planning.

Hemangioblastomas are true benign vascular neoplasms arising from pluripotent mesenchymal stem cells that give rise to vascular endothelial cells and are most commonly found in the cerebellum, spinal cord, brainstem, and retina. These tumors may be isolated sporadic lesions or may be associated with hereditary genetic factors in the case of von Hippel-Lindau (VHL) syndrome. Spinal cord haemangioblastomas constitute 1.1% to 2.4% of all central nervous system tumors105, with the majority being single tumors that present in the fourth decade of life 106. In the pediatric population, sporadic spinal cord hemangioblastomas are exceedingly rare. The prevalence of spinal cord hemangioblastomas in children is increased among those with VHL syndrome. The thoracic cord is the most common site for spinal cord hemangioblastomas, followed by the cervical cord. Although these tumors are benign, they cause disabling symptoms due to spinal cord compression, syringomyelia, or hemorrhage from the tumor itself or from aneurysms that form on tumor-feeding arteries or intra-tumoral vessels.

Foreword
Pediatric Neurovascular Disorders

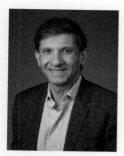

Suresh K. Mukherji, MD, MBA, FACR
Consulting Editor

Pediatric neurovascular diseases is one of the most challenging topics that we have covered in *Neuroimaging Clinics* over the past 25 years. This combines both pediatric neuroradiology and neurovascular radiology, which are areas not routinely interpreted by most neuroradiologists. Most patients with these complex disorders are seen in dedicated pediatric hospitals. However, the initial imaging diagnosis in children is often made in the community. Neuroradiologists need to be familiar with the spectrum of pediatric neurovascular disorders to make the correct diagnosis and ensure these children are seen by the correct specialists.

We decided to take on this challenging topic and were delighted when Drs Prakash Muthusami and Todd Abruzzo agreed to edit this unique issue. Both are gifted pediatric neurointerventional radiologists with many years of experience in both diagnosing and treating children with neurovascular conditions. They have created a very organized and comprehensive issue that can be used by radiologists and clinicians alike for their daily practice. The articles systematically and succinctly cover the complete range of vascular diseases and pathologies, at various stages of human development from fetal life to young adulthood. There are specific articles devoted to neurovascular malformations, aneurysms, pediatric stroke, and arteriopathies. There are also specific articles devoted to ordering of appropriate imaging studies in children with suspected various neurovascular disorders.

We would like to thank Drs Muthusami and Abruzzo for their tireless efforts in creating such a comprehensive and state-of-the-art issue of *Neuroimaging Clinics* on such a challenging topic. We would also like to thank and congratulate all the article authors on their wonderful contributions. Drs Muthusami and Abruzzo elegantly refer to the authors as "doyens" in their respective fields, and I could not agree more! This is truly a unique issue and one that will serve as a gold-standard reference on this important and complex topic for many years to come. Thank you again to all for making such a special issue!

Suresh K. Mukherji, MD, MBA, FACR
University of Louisville &
University of Illinois
ProScan Imaging
Carmel, IN 46032, USA

E-mail address:
sureshmukherji@hotmail.com

neuroimaging.theclinics.com

Foreword

Pediatric Neurovascular Disorders

Suresh K. Mukherji, MD, MBA, FACR
Consulting Editor

Preface
Pediatric Neurovascular Disorders

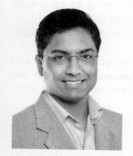

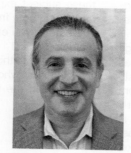

Prakash Muthusami, MD   Todd Abruzzo, MD, FAHA, FACR, FSNIS
Editors

We are excited to present this compendium, which spans the spectrum of pediatric neurovascular diseases from fetal life to young adulthood. Once considered rare and nebulous, neurovascular diseases of childhood are increasingly recognized, and their pathomechanisms are more completely understood owing to tremendous advances in neuroimaging, neurointervention, neuropediatrics as well as molecular, cellular, and developmental biology. While these conditions have historically been discovered on neuroimaging performed to evaluate a catastrophic clinical presentation, it is now routine to uncover pediatric neurovascular disorders on screening studies, or examinations requested to evaluate minor and sometimes unrelated symptoms. The imaging diagnosis of neurovascular diseases in children is no longer solely within the purview of large academic tertiary care medical centers. With this issue, we hope to disseminate important foundational concepts upon which modern neuroimaging diagnosis of childhood neurovascular disease is based. This issue is meant for radiologists and clinicians in all manner of practice who find themselves confronted with the complex and challenging task of neuroimaging study analysis.

The main drivers of neurovascular pathology in adults (ie, hypertension, smoking, and dyslipidemia) are conspicuously absent in children. Neurovascular diseases afflicting children stem from diverse causes, which uniquely interact with specific age-related physiologic changes to produce distinct natural histories and neuroimaging manifestations that profoundly vary across different stages of development. Neurovascular diseases in children do not respond to treatment as in adults with homologous conditions. Progress in our understanding of neurovascular development and pathophysiology, the introduction of innovative surgical and interventional techniques, and advances in neuroimaging have expanded indications for treatment in recent decades to include conditions once thought untreatable in children. The advent of artificial intelligence, modern cell-based therapies, immunotherapeutics, and gene therapy promise to usher in a new era of hope for children suffering from neurovascular disease. Neuroimaging will play an essential role in that future, serving as a tool for diagnosis, screening, staging, prognostication, treatment planning, treatment guidance, treatment assessment, and treatment target delineation.

The last two decades have also seen a transfer of reliance from gold-standard catheter-directed angiography to cross-sectional imaging as a means to interrogate pediatric neurovascular

Neuroimag Clin N Am 34 (2024) xvii–xviii
https://doi.org/10.1016/j.nic.2024.08.018
1052-5149/24/© 2024 Published by Elsevier Inc.

disease. The continuous and considerable advances in neuroimaging techniques have revolutionized the evaluation and understanding of these conditions. Several advanced clinical imaging sequences (eg, arterial spin-labeling perfusion, phase contrast flow imaging, and black blood vessel wall imaging) have enabled precise diagnostic characterization and disease monitoring using objective, quantifiable imaging biomarkers.

Whereas progress in MR imaging technology has reduced the need for invasive testing, it has increased the demand on diagnostic radiologists to make sense of imaging data across a plethora of conditions. In addition, the field of pediatric neurovascular medicine continues to burgeon in previously unforeseeable directions (eg, endovascular thrombectomy for arterial ischemic stroke, venous sinus stenting for idiopathic intracranial hypertension, and intra-arterial chemotherapy for retinoblastoma).

The nature of pediatric neurovascular disease necessitates a multidisciplinary approach to patient management, involving experts from pediatric radiology, pediatric neurosurgery, child neurology, diagnostic and interventional neuroradiology, neurocritical care, pediatric hematology, neurogenetics, and anesthesiology. In this collection, we aim to provide a comprehensive and up-to-date body of knowledge that can be used by radiologists and clinicians alike for their daily practice. The articles have been organized to systematically and succinctly cover the complete range of vascular diseases and pathologies, at various stages of human development from fetal life to young adulthood, accounting for disparate manifestations in a variety of settings. The outstanding contributions of the distinguished senior authors in this issue, each of whom is a doyen of neuropediatrics, provide readers with a contemporary understanding of neuroimaging as a practical tool for the diagnostic evaluation of children with known or suspected neurovascular disease.

We wish to thank Dr Suresh K. Mukerji, MD, MBA, FACR, Consulting Editor, for inviting us to guest edit this special issue. We would also like to thank Mr John Vassallo and Ms Saswoti Nath for their unwavering support throughout the editing and publication process.

We extend special thanks to all the authors, without whose contributions this issue would not have been possible. We are sincerely grateful to these subject experts for agreeing to contribute and taking time from their busy schedules.

We hope you enjoy this special issue of *Neuroimaging Clinics*!

We dedicate this work to our young patients and their families, who show unwavering courage and resilience in the face of overwhelming adversity each day.

DISCLOSURES

The authors have no conflicts of interest to disclose.

Prakash Muthusami, MD
Interventional Neuroradiology
Department of Diagnostic Imaging and
Image Guided Therapy
The Hospital for Sick Children
University of Toronto
Toronto, Canada

Todd Abruzzo, MD, FAHA, FACR, FSNIS
Departments of Child Health and Radiology
University of Arizona
Creighton University, Mayo Clinic
Section of Vascular Disorders and Therapeutics
Barrow Neurological Institute at
Phoenix Children's Hospital
Phoenix, AZ, USA

School of Biological &
Health Systems Engineering
Ira A. Fulton School of Engineering
Arizona State University
Tempe, AZ, USA

E-mail addresses:
Prakash.muthusami@sickkids.ca (P. Muthusami)
tabruzzo@phoenixchildrens.com (T. Abruzzo)

Introduction
Neurovascular Diseases across the Pediatric Age Spectrum

Khalid Al-Dasuqi, MD[a],*, Darren B. Orbach, MD, PhD[b],
Joanne M. Rispoli, MD[a]

KEYWORDS

- Pediatric cerebrovascular disease • Cerebral arteriopathy • Arteriovenous malformations
- Aneurysms • Pediatric neurovascular interventions

KEY POINTS

- Advancements in neuroimaging techniques and improved clinical understanding of pediatric neurovascular disorders have led to increased recognition and diagnosis of these conditions.
- The etiology of cerebrovascular diseases in children differs significantly from adults, often involving unique genetic and developmental factors.
- Effective management of pediatric cerebrovascular disease requires a coordinated, multidisciplinary approach, involving pediatric neuroradiologists, neurosurgeons, neurologists, geneticists, and other specialists to ensure optimal care and intervention.

BACKGROUND

Pediatric cerebrovascular diseases represent a unique group of conditions that differ from adult homologs in presentation, pathophysiology, and management. In addition, pediatric neurovascular pathologies not infrequently occur in the context of multisystem disorders that are important to recognize and address. Although pediatric cerebrovascular disease is rare, morbidity can be high, effects can be lifelong, and knowledge of disease entities is imperative for early diagnosis and optimal treatment. Diagnosis and management require an interdisciplinary approach that includes neuroradiologists, neurologists, neurosurgeons, and neurointerventionalists. This special edition of Neuroimaging Clinics of North America focuses on the neuroimaging aspects of commonly encountered pediatric neurovascular disorders, emphasizing key concepts that are relevant to clinical radiologists interpreting diagnostic neuroimaging studies. The study by Schroff M and colleagues provides an in-depth consideration of practical issues involved in the neuroimaging of children, emphasizing cross-sectional imaging modalities, while the study by Tierradentro-Garcia and colleagues' article, "Catheter-directed Cerebral and Spinal Angiography in Children," in this issue covers practical issues involved in the conduct of catheter-directed neuroangiography in children. Commonly encountered neuroimaging presentations of pediatric neurovascular disorders and age-oriented differential diagnoses are covered in the study on hemorrhagic stroke by Leach and colleagues' article, "Imaging of Hemorrhagic Stroke in Children," in this issue; the study on arterial ischemic stroke by Fileva and colleagues' article, "Arterial Ischemic Stroke in Children," in this issue; and the study on neurovascular trauma by Lee SK and colleagues. Given the fundamental role of cerebral arteriopathies as a cause of childhood arterial ischemic stroke, a study covering the neuroimaging features of commonly encountered

[a] Department of Radiology, Boston Children's Hospital, 300 Longwood Avenue, Boston, MA 02115, USA;
[b] Neurointerventional Radiology, Boston Children's Hospital, 300 Longwood Avenue, Boston, MA 02115, USA
* Corresponding author.
E-mail address: k.aldasuqi@gmail.com

Neuroimag Clin N Am 34 (2024) 481–490
https://doi.org/10.1016/j.nic.2024.08.024
1052-5149/24/© 2024 Elsevier Inc. All rights are reserved, including those for text and data mining, AI training, and similar technologies.

pediatric cerebral arteriopathies by Kelson and colleagues' article, "Steno-occlusive Intracranial Large Vessel Arteriopathies in Childhood: A Pattern Oriented Approach to Neuroimaging Diagnosis," in this issue is included. Since vascular malformations are among the most common causes of neurologic symptoms in children presenting for diagnostic neuroimaging, a series of studies are dedicated to fetal neurovascular malformations (Qureshi and colleagues' article, "Neurovascular Malformations in the Fetus and Neonate," in this issue), intracranial vascular malformations of childhood (Karim S and colleagues), and spinal vascular malformations of childhood (Shaibani A and colleagues). In this introduction, the authors provide a brief general overview of pediatric neurovascular disorders, from the perspective of imaging approaches, and pathomechanisms, emphasizing specific entities and presentations within distinct age groups, from fetal life through childhood.

FETAL PERIOD
Imaging Considerations

According to the American College of Radiology-American College of Obstetricians and Gynecologists-American Institute of Ultrasound in Medicine-Society for Maternal-Fetal Medicine-Society of Radiologists in Ultrasound, practice parameter guidelines, imaging of the head, face, and neck is a required component of the second-trimester anatomic survey. Although second-trimester screening is typically performed, much fetal cerebrovascular disease is detected in the third trimester. Typically, utilizing an abdominal transducer greater than or equal to 3 MHz is appropriate, with 4 standard views of the fetal head including the transventricular, falx, cavum, and transcerebellar views.[1] Color Doppler can be utilized for evaluation of arterial and venous flow.

Fetal abnormalities identified on screening ultrasound are subsequently referred for MR imaging if a finding cannot be resolved on ultrasound, requires confirmation, or if additional findings are expected. MR imaging protocols include fast T2-weighted imaging with half Fourier single-shot turbo spin-echo and balanced steady-state free precession in 3 orthogonal planes for evaluation of brain parenchyma, T1W images to evaluate for hemorrhage, and echo-planar imaging to evaluate for hemorrhage or mineralization.[2] DWI can also be helpful to evaluate for destructive brain processes or infarction in the setting of cerebrovascular malformations.[3] Given that fetal movement is a frequent contributor to image degradation, quality control through image review of crucial sequences relevant to the clinical question at hand, before the imaging session is ended, is critical.

Pathomechanisms

Development of the cerebrovascular system is a complex process, genetically driven but subject to environmental and epigenetic demands of embryogenesis. Soon after the neural tube can no longer be nourished by simple diffusion, during the first step of vasculogenesis, multipotent mesodermal cells are differentiated into endothelial cell precursor angioblasts. These angioblasts form primitive longitudinal vessels and a plexus of non-differentiated endothelial cells that proliferate on the surface of the neural tube to form a vascular network, which is soon fixed to the surface by a fibrous stroma called the meninx primitiva.[4] Invagination into the monoventricle of the closed neural tube carries an island of vascularized meninx primitive into each of what will become the 2 cerebral hemispheres, allowing for oxygenation and nutrient transfer from both the surface and from within the ventricle; these vascularized islands are the precursors of the choroid plexus.[4]

With increasing metabolic demands of the growing embryo, the vascular supply becomes insufficient and the process of sprouting (also known as [A.K.A.] proliferative) angiogenesis occurs. In contrast to intussceptive (A.K.A. nonproliferative) angiogenesis that occurs in the later stages of central nervous system (CNS) vascular development, sprouting angiogenesis is initiated by the extension of endothelial tubes from existing vessels as directed by chemotactic angiogenic signals (ie, vascular endothelial growth factor A [VEGF-A]).[5] As the brain grows, VEGF-A produced by thickening, insufficiently perfused tissue stimulates sprouting angiogenesis. The formation of the surface brain arteries has been described as occurring in 7 stages in Padget's classic work,[6] with bifurcation of a primitive internal carotid artery and multiple fetal carotid-vertebrobasilar anastomoses in early stages progressing to the more classic circle of Willis anatomy and vascular territory formation by stage 7 at 52 days.

The embryonic choroid plexus serves as a focal point of CNS vascular development, with the earliest formed CNS arteries being choroidal and the early deep CNS venous drainage organized around the embryonic choroid plexus. As the deep venous system initially develops, radially oriented transcerebral medullary veins with ventriculofugal flow connect to the superficial venous vasculature. The anterior embryonic choroid plexus within the developing lateral ventricles drains to the primitive superior sagittal sinus through a single midline median prosencephalic vein (MPV) of Markowski, while embryonic choroid plexus more posteriorly drains through paired dorsal and ventral diencephalic veins (precursors to the system that forms the basal vein of Rosenthal) to the primitive marginal and primitive tentorial sinuses, respectively. As the cerebral mantle thickens, the subependymal venous system acquires an increasing flow demand, and the subependymal internal cerebral veins form. The internal cerebral veins annex radially oriented transcerebral medullary veins with ventriculopetal flow and drain the anterior embryonic choroid plexus to the posterior segment of the MPV (vein of Galen). Involution of the anterior segment of the MPV within the roof of the third ventricle occurs during the 11th week of gestation under ordinary circumstances. When aberrant embryonic choroidal vascular development results in arteriovenous shunting to the anterior segment of the MPV, the flow-loaded vein fails to involute resulting in the vein of Galen malformation (VOGM), one of several types of congenital arteriovenous lesions covered in the study on fetal neurovascular malformations by Qureshi and colleagues' article, "Neurovascular Malformations in the Fetus and Neonate," in this issue.

A "2 hit hypothesis" has been proposed as the etiology of aberrant vascular development leading to congenital arteriovenous lesions. In this model, a germ line loss-of-function mutation affecting all embryonic cells (asymptomatic in isolation), and a second, spatially restricted somatic loss-of-function mutation in the other allele, affecting only lesional tissue, occurs in response to a localized environmental trigger. Putative environmental triggers include ischemic, infectious, or inflammatory processes though other currently undefined events may be involved.[7] Homozygous loss-of-function in a gene required for normal vasculogenesis and arteriovenous differentiation results in the formation of a focal choroidal, pial, or dural arteriovenous lesion depending on the location and timing of events.

Some loss-of-function mutations associated with pediatric arteriovenous lesions, such as Ephrin-B2 mutations and ALK1 mutations, contribute to pathologically increased sprouting of the vascular bed (proliferative angiogenesis).[5] Conversely, other loss-of-function mutations associated with pediatric arteriovenous lesions, such as RASA1 mutations and Ephrin receptor B4 mutations, have been implicated in failed intussusception (nonproliferative angiogenesis). Hereditary vascular malformation syndromes such as hereditary hemorrhagic telangiectasia (HHT) and capillary malformation-arteriovenous malformation (CM-AVM) syndrome typically involve staged homozygous loss-of-function mutations (one germ line mutation plus one somatic mutation). In contrast, sporadic arteriovenous malformations (AVMs) are typically associated with heterozygous somatic gain-of-function mutations of KRAS and BRAF superfamily genes isolated to lesional tissue. Genetic mutations associated with VOGM have been the subject of multiple studies over the past decade, with recent studies employing whole exome sequencing and single-cell transcriptomics to identify mutations in 6 genes as associated with VOGM: RASA1, EPHB4, ACVRL1, NOTCH1, ITGB1, and PTPN11.[8]

It has been hypothesized that in dural sinus malformations (DSMs), aberrant overgrowth of the dural venous sinuses, potentially as a result of aberrant intussceptive angiogenesis, promotes varying degrees of intraluminal thrombus formation that can lead to the generation of large amounts of VEGF-A during a period of rapid vascular growth. In this setting, disruption of the normal VEGF-A gradient can affect the rate of endothelial cell proliferation and can potentially result in arteriovenous fistulae and maladaptive remodeling of the dural venous sinuses. The postnatal phenotype expressed by DSM includes a range of lesions that variably express different degrees of sinus overgrowth, luminal thrombosis, and arteriovenous shunting as covered in detail by Qureshi and colleagues' article, "Neurovascular Malformations in the Fetus and Neonate," in this issue in the study on fetal vascular malformations.[9,10]

Pial arteriovenous fistulae, also covered in the study by Qureshi and colleagues' article, "Neurovascular Malformations in the Fetus and Neonate," in this issue, have primarily been described in association with RASA1 and HHT-related germ line mutations, but there is significant overlap with other mutations that have been linked to VOGM. The possibility that a 2 hit model is operative in the pathogenesis of pial AVF is likely but has not yet been thoroughly investigated.

Specific Entities and Presentation

Fetal arteriovenous fistulae such as VOGM may be detected in the third trimester, first by ultrasound (particularly with the use of color Doppler) and then with fetal MR imaging to elaborate the findings. While the malformations themselves are readily discernible, nonvascular brain findings in the prenatal period potentially include brain parenchymal injury in the form of infarction or hemorrhage and ventriculomegaly.[11] Fetal imaging of VOGM has recently been shown to reliably predict the severity of clinical presentation at birth, based on the mediolateral width of the narrowest point of the falcine sinus draining the MPV. Notably, fetuses with a wider sinus are at high risk of an aggressive neonatal clinical course.[12]

Fetal DSMs often present prenatally and are initially detected on fetal ultrasound in the second or third trimester with subsequent evaluation on MR imaging examination. Potential associated findings include hydrocephalus, mass effect on adjacent brain parenchyma, and polyhydramnios.[13] DSM can occur with concomitant thrombosis, and decrease in size overtime during gestation is a strongly positive prognosticator.[9]

NEONATAL PERIOD
Imaging Considerations

There are many factors that may influence the choice of imaging modality in neonates, including availability of MR imaging and clinical stability of the patient. Ultrasound is often performed as a first-line imaging modality, given ready availability and lack of ionizing radiation; however, ultrasound is limited in field-of-view and evaluation of soft tissue contrast. Computed tomography (CT) may be used if the patient is unstable or if MR imaging is unavailable or contraindicated; however, MR imaging remains the diagnostic test of choice and can be performed within the neonatal intensive care unit in certain facilities.[14]

Pathomechanisms

In addition to the fetal vascular malformations previously discussed, hemorrhagic and arterial ischemic stroke are important causes of neonatal neurologic morbidity and mortality. While perinatal hemorrhagic stroke is covered extensively in the study by Leach and colleagues' article, "Imaging of Hemorrhagic Stroke in Children," in this issue, perinatal arterial ischemic stroke is detailed in the study by Fileva and colleagues' article, "Arterial Ischemic Stroke in Children," in this issue. The differential diagnosis of neonatal hemorrhagic stroke is greatly simplified by first considering whether the patient is full term or premature. In term neonates, hemorrhagic stroke is usually due to medullary venous thrombosis, subpial hemorrhage, and coagulopathy. In premature neonates, hemorrhagic stroke is most commonly related to venous thrombosis, coagulopathy, and the spectrum of hemorrhagic germinal matrix pathologies (germinal matrix-intraventricular hemorrhage and periventricular hemorrhagic infarction). All of these entities are covered in detail in the study by Leach and colleagues' article, "Imaging of Hemorrhagic Stroke in Children," in this issue. The pathomechanisms of perinatal arterial ischemic

stroke are multifactorial and are incompletely understood but are well covered in the study by Fileva and colleagues' article, "Arterial Ischemic Stroke in Children," in this issue. A perinatal-specific etiology that is thought to represent an important contributor is that of placental emboli that enter the fetal circulation and then cross a patent foramen ovale.[15] Perinatal changes in maternal hemostasis and thrombophilias likely plan an important role as well.[16]

Specific Entities and Presentation

Symptomatic neonates with VOGM most commonly present with high-output heart failure and medically refractory pulmonary hypertension in the setting of massive lesional flow. Severely affected patients demonstrate elevated ventricular output, right heart dilation, and diastolic reversal of flow in the descending aorta.[17] These phenomena can result in inadequate perfusion of host tissues in multiple organ systems including the brain and at best can be only somewhat mitigated with medical management in the majority of cases. In symptomatic neonates, definitive treatment frequently requires diminution of lesional flow via embolization.[18] Additional intracranial neuroimaging findings may include ventriculomegaly, parenchymal volume loss, and findings suggestive of intracranial venous hypertension.[19]

Unlike older children (adolescents and teenagers) or adults with VOGM who often present with focal neurologic deficits in the setting of hemorrhagic stroke, neonates typically present with nonspecific neurologic symptoms such as seizures and encephalopathy within hours to days of birth.

LATE INFANCY AND CHILDHOOD
Imaging Considerations

MR imaging is the modality of choice for evaluation of neurologic symptoms in late infancy and childhood, particularly if stroke is suspected, given the lack of ionizing radiation and the ability to more accurately make a definitive diagnosis. Nonetheless, CT/CT angiography (CTA) may be performed in the event of limited MR imaging availability, need for sedation, or presence of MR imaging incompatible devices. In patients who are suspected to have an acute arterial ischemic stroke due to intracranial large vessel occlusion, an abbreviated protocol can be performed with diffusion-weighted imaging (DWI), fluid-attenuated inversion recovery (FLAIR), gradient echo (GRE)/ susceptibility weighted imaging (SWI) and 3 dimensional time of flight MR angiography or magnetic resonance angiography (MRA) to make a diagnosis.[20] In patients with a high pretest probability of acute intracranial large vessel occlusion due to embolus (child with congenital heart disease, cardiomyopathy, or extracorporeal circulatory device), CT/CTA is preferred over MR imaging given its high sensitivity, specificity, and rapidity in a situation where treatment selection and neurologic outcomes are highly time sensitive. Neuroimaging considerations in the child with arterial ischemic stroke are covered in detail in the study by Fileva and colleagues' article, "Arterial Ischemic Stroke in Children," in this issue. Acute hemorrhagic presentations may also be better assessed with CT and CTA in the initial phase of care for rapid surgical decision-making, with subsequent catheter-directed angiography to fully characterize and/or treat underlying lesions such as aneurysms or AVMs. Additionally, long-term follow-up neuroimaging is required following treatment of these lesions due to the risk of recurrence. An in-depth consideration of neuroimaging for children with hemorrhagic stroke is presented in the study by Leach and colleagues' article, "Imaging of Hemorrhagic Stroke in Children," in this issue. A detailed presentation of neuroimaging considerations in children with intracranial aneurysms and intracranial AVMs is given in the studies by Kartik D. Bhatia and Carmen Parra-Farinas's article, "Intracranial Arterial Aneurysms in Childhood," in this issue and Karim S and colleagues, respectively.

Pathomechanisms

Beyond the neonatal period, infants with VOGM and DSM most often present with macrocephaly as a result of enlarging cerebral ventricles. Ventriculomegaly and symptomatic hydrocephalus in infants with VOGM and DSM is mostly related to hydrovenous dysfunction, though a component of aqueductal compression may be contributory in VOGM. Hydrovenous dysfunction is primarily due to the elevated venous pressures caused by arteriovenous shunting in the setting of arachnoid granulation immaturity. Hydrovenous dysfunction is most commonly expressed as ventriculomegaly, but vasogenic edema, deep white matter injury, and venous ischemia with sequelae of cystic encephalomalacia and parenchymal calcification may also occur.

Congenital arteriovenous lesions, such as VOGM and DSM with associated arteriovenous shunting, often become associated with venous outlet stenosis in late infancy (with a peak at 2–3 years of age), most commonly involving the lower sigmoid sinuses and jugular bulbs. This phenomenon, which has been called jugular bulb

dysplasia, does not appear to be strictly a function of lesional flow, as some infants with low residual lesional flow develop progressive severe stenosis, while others with high flow never develop venous stenosis. Jugular bulb dysplasia aggravates hydrovenous dysfunction and can be complicated by symptomatic cerebral venous hypertension and cerebral venous congestion if redirection of cerebral venous drainage to the anterior venous confluence of the cavernous sinuses is not enabled by postnatal cavernous capture of the superficial middle cerebral veins. In such cases, increasing pressure within the posterior venous confluence (torcular Herophili) caused by outlet stenosis produces reversal of flow in the superior sagittal sinus, straight sinus, and falcine sinus with retrograde cortical venous drainage. While this flow pattern can cause extensive brain injury, it may be transiently tolerated if the superior sagittal sinus can drain to the cavernous sinuses through the superior anastomotic vein of Trolard and superficial middle cerebral vein.

Nidal-type AVM and intracranial aneurysms in childhood typically present with hemorrhage, although there is an increasing trend toward incidental diagnosis secondary to increasing availability and improving accuracy of cross-sectional imaging modalities. Notably, hemorrhagic presentation of AVM in children can be associated with the presence of high-risk features that signal a higher probability of short-term rebleeding such as flow-related aneurysm, pseudoaneurysm, or draining vein stenosis on initial imaging. Such high-risk features should be recognized by radiologists as they strongly influence clinical decision-making. Flow-related aneurysms or pseudoaneurysms that are closely associated with hematomas, particularly those bearing daughter sacs or teats, should be considered a likely source of acute bleeding and prioritized for endovascular or microneurosurgical occlusion to prevent early rebleeding.

Pediatric nidal-type pial arteriovenous malformation

Nidal-type pial AVMs of the brain (A.K.A. cerebral AVM) are the most common cause of intracranial hemorrhage in children. Although it had been assumed for decades that many or most cerebral AVMs are congenital, these lesions are virtually never seen on fetal imaging and have been shown to develop postnatally in children aged between 5 and 10 years by sequential brain imaging studies. It is now thought that cerebral AVMs most commonly develop postnatally through early childhood. As noted previously, some nidal-type cerebral AVMs are associated with heritable germ line loss-of-function mutations, such as in HHT. The pathogenesis of AVMs in HHT involves genes related to the transforming growth factor-beta (TGF-beta) and vascular endothelial growth factor signaling pathways. Nevertheless, the great majority of cerebral AVMs in children and adults are sporadic and are characterized by heterozygous somatic activating (gain-of-function) mutations in *KRAS* and *BRAF* genes.[21,22]

Intracranial arterial aneurysms Pediatric intracranial arterial aneurysms differ from adult aneurysms in presentation, morphology, and underlying pathogenic mechanisms. Underlying arteriopathy resulting from trauma, infection, maladaptive immuno-inflammatory response, mural dysplasia, collagenopathy, elastinopathy, or other defect of arterial wall composition must be considered in approaches to management of these patients. Dissecting aneurysms are more commonly seen in children. Such aneurysms are often fusiform or circumferential and frequently feature a focal stenosis proximal and/or distal to the aneurysm-bearing arterial segment.[7,23]

Ischemic and hemorrhagic stroke Risk factors and pathomechanisms of arterial ischemic stroke in children differ from both adult and perinatal stroke. Beyond the perinatal period, children most often develop arterial ischemic stroke as a result of heart disease (congenital cardiac malformations and cardiomyopathy), or arteriopathy that is congenital or acquired. The spectrum of arteriopathy in childhood is diverse and includes arterial dissection (cervical and intracranial), inflammatory, and infectious forms of arteriopathy, a variety of moyamoya arteriopathies and arteriopathies caused by hematologic disease (sickle cell disease and other anemias). The Childhood acute ischemic stroke (AIS) Standardized Classification and Diagnostic Evaluation criteria offer a standardized approach and classification system to the various subtypes of childhood acute ischemic stroke.[24-27] The role of neuroimaging in the evaluation of childhood arterial ischemic stroke, including the differential diagnosis of the most common etiologies encountered in clinical practice, is covered extensively in the study by Severino M and colleagues. Given the importance of cerebral arteriopathy as a cause of arterial ischemic stroke in childhood, a study by Stence N and colleagues is dedicated to this topic. While arteriopathies in children presenting with arterial ischemic stroke in the anterior cerebral circulation usually have an intracranial distribution, arteriopathy in vertebrobasilar arterial ischemic stroke is extracranial in the vast majority of cases. Although new evidence indicates that focal

cerebral arteriopathy has a posterior circulation variant affecting intracranial arteries, nontraumatic vertebral artery dissections involving the atlanto-axial and atlanto-occipital segments of the extracranial vertebral artery are increasingly recognized as the dominant cause of childhood posterior circulation stroke. Moreover, the mechanistic importance of Bowhunter syndrome in such cases has been widely established. In contrast, with the exception of Takayasu's disease and fibromuscular dysplasia, the vast majority of arteriopathy responsible for anterior circulation arterial ischemic stroke has an intracranial distribution.

Hemorrhagic stroke, excluding conversion of arterial ischemic infarction, constitutes more than 50% of childhood stroke. The most common cause is intracranial vascular malformations, with AVM and cerebral cavernous malformation (CCM) accounting for the vast majority of these. A smaller number of hemorrhagic strokes are related to intracranial arterial aneurysms and vessel wall degeneration attributable to chronic progressive arteriopathy (ie, moyamoya arteriopathies). Additional and important causes of pediatric hemorrhagic stroke include tumor-related hemorrhage and congenital or acquired coagulopathy.[28-31] The central role of neuroimaging in the diagnostic evaluation of childhood hemorrhagic stroke, and the age-oriented neuroimaging differential diagnosis of specific hemorrhagic stroke patterns and pathologies, is elaborated in the study by Leach and colleagues' article, "Imaging of Hemorrhagic Stroke in Children," in this issue.

Specific Entities and Presentation

In the setting of VOGM, or DSM that features arteriovenous shunting, severe venous outlet stenosis at the skullbase (ie, jugular bulb dysplasia) results in pressurization of the entire cerebral venous system that is transmitted through the posterior venous confluence (torcular) to the superior sagittal sinus, petrosal sinuses, straight sinus, and falcine sinus. This results in parenchymal vasogenic edema that is manifested as thalamic, brainstem, or corona radiata T2 signal hyperintensity on MR imaging. This is followed by parenchymal calcification and cerebral atrophy. Clinical presentation is typically with headache, followed by seizures, speech and developmental regression, and extraocular movement and bulbar abnormalities. In the setting of chronic reflux into pial veins with advanced stages of venous hypertension, there is also a risk of subarachnoid and parenchymal hemorrhage.[19] In these cases, cortical venous ectasia and tortuosity (venopathy) are important neuroimaging features that may precede hemorrhagic presentation. While hemorrhage is a late-stage complication of VOGM resulting from parenchymal venous hypertension, typically in school-age children and teenagers, hemorrhage is not a rare complication of cerebral venous hypertension in younger children with DSM featuring arteriovenous shunting. Recurrent epistaxis is another frequent mode of presentation in older children with untreated VOGM and occlusion of the posterior venous outlets. This is a result of cavernous sinus engorgement that is transmitted into ophthalmic veins and submucosal veins of the nasal cavity and paranasal sinuses. Early recognition of venous outlet stenosis and findings of cerebral venopathy should be sought by radiologists evaluating neuroimaging studies because prompt intervention informed by these findings may preempt irreversible brain injury. While dural venous sinus and jugular bulb stenosis are highly resistant to angioplasty and stenting, treatment should therefore be focused on definitive closure of the arteriovenous shunt lesion. The neuroimaging evaluation of children with VOGM, DSM, and other types of congenital arteriovenous lesions is covered in the study by Qureshi and colleagues' article, "Neurovascular Malformations in the Fetus and Neonate," in this issue.

As in the neonatal population, in younger children, there is often lack of specificity of symptoms from arterial ischemic stroke. While older children may present with focal limb or facial weakness, sensory change, or aphasia similar to adults with stroke, younger children can present with a variety of symptoms including headache, neck pain, seizures, nausea/vomiting dizziness, speech alteration, and Horner's syndrome. In addition, a wide range of stroke-like mimics frequently occur in children, such as seizures, demyelinating disease, migraines; these often focus caregivers away from a diagnosis of stroke and delay diagnosis in cases of true stroke. The critical role of neuroimaging in directing the diagnostic evaluation and treatment of children with acute neurologic deficits is detailed in the studies by Fileva and colleagues' article, "Arterial Ischemic Stroke in Children," in this issue and Shrof M and colleagues.

The presentation of hemorrhagic stroke in children does not differ fundamentally from acute arterial ischemic stroke, other than in the case of large hemorrhage with mass effect, which frequently manifests sudden loss of consciousness and seizures. Although brain AVM occurs in adults and children, the presentation is distinct to some degree. Children far more often present with acute hemorrhage (as opposed to seizures). Notably, while acute hemorrhage is reported in up to 80% of pediatric cases,[32,33] hemorrhage-free survival is reportedly higher in pediatric patients.[34] Similar to AVMs, pediatric aneurysms have an increased incidence of hemorrhagic presentation as compared to adults.[35] More recent studies that have focused on longitudinal outcomes in children with small unruptured aneurysms have reported a relatively low cumulative incidence of hemorrhage, particularly for those aneurysms that are incidentally discovered in children with cerebral arteriopathies. The importance of cerebral aneurysms in children with hemorrhagic stroke is covered in the study by Leach JL, while the role of neuroimaging in the evaluation of children with aneurysmal disease is covered in the study by Kartik D. Bhatia and Carmen Parra-Farinas's article, "Intracranial Arterial Aneurysms in Childhood," in this issue.

SYNDROMIC CONSIDERATIONS

A subpopulation of children presenting with intracranial or spinal arteriovenous lesions (nidal-type AVM and/or AVF) have HHT or CM-AVM syndrome, which are the 2 most common monogenic conditions associated with arteriovenous pathology. Whole exome sequencing in unselected pediatric patients with cerebral AVM has revealed that novel variants in HHT genes may be found in children with isolated non-syndromic cerebral AVMs who do not meet standard diagnostic criteria for HHT. While HHT can present with typical nidal-type cerebral AVM angioarchitecture, pial AVF, micro-AVM, cerebral capillary malformation, and transitional forms may also occur. The study by Karim S and colleagues gives an in-depth overview of the different cerebral vascular malformation phenotypes found in HHT. Notably, micro-AVM and capillary malformation should be considered pathognomic for HHT as they are not typically found in isolation. Non-shunting arterial dysplasia has also been described in HHT. Some or all of the lesions listed earlier may be expressed simultaneously or develop asynchronously in individuals with HHT. The coexistence of multiple intracranial arteriovenous lesions should also be considered pathognomonic of HHT. The finding of pulmonary AVMs and/or gastrointestinal AVMs in a child with an intracranial or spinal arteriovenous lesion is strong corroborative evidence of HHT. Four major pathogenic gene variants have been described in HHT affecting the ALK1, SMAD4, growth differentiation factor 2, and endoglin (ENG) genes, with mutations in ALK1 being the most common.[36] Leading models of arteriovenous lesions in HHT are based on a 2 hit model involving sequential loss-of-function mutations affecting 2 alleles of these genes. CM-AVM syndrome presents with cutaneous capillary malformations and

AVMs (most commonly in the brain, spine, head, and neck but potentially in other organs as well). CM-AVM syndrome is an autosomal dominant disorder with germ line loss-of-function mutations in RASA1 (for CM-AVM1) or Ephrin Receptor B4 (for CM-AVM2). A second hit somatic mutation in the unaffected allele is thought to be necessary to reveal the AVM phenotype in affected tissues. As mentioned earlier, VOGM has also been associated with RASA1 and EPHB4 mutations. Mutations in the PTEN gene are associated with a predisposition to both hamartomas and malignant solid tumors (formerly known as Cowden syndrome), but patients also harbor AVM-like lesions of the soft tissues (frequently in the head and neck) that tend to be resistant to embolization therapy.

FUTURE DIRECTIONS

Progress in the understanding of disease pathophysiology and molecular genetics has unveiled numerous gene families and molecular pathways governing vasculogenesis and the development of vascular anomalies. These pathways are implicated in various pediatric neurovascular disorders. Several genetic variants in the RNF213 gene encoding for a Dynein-like protein have been described in moyamoya arteriopathy across patients with diverse ethnic backgrounds. Additionally, autosomal dominant multisystem disorders of vascular smooth muscle cell phenotype are associated with genetic variants in the ACTA2 and MYH11 genes. These monogenic disorders clinically manifest with intracranial arterial steno-occlusive disease. Consequently, genetic screening is now standard practice for childhood cerebral arteriopathy in many centers, especially in cases with a familial history of childhood stroke or suggestive MR imaging findings (eg, ACTA2 arteriopathy).[37,38] As our understanding of the biology underlying monogenic cerebral arteriopathy deepens, the promise of effective medical therapies is increasingly within reach. For example, recent advances in laboratory research have suggested that cerebrovascular abnormalities expressed in individuals with ACTA2 mutations may be at least partially reversed by augmenting the mitochondrial respiration of vascular smooth muscle cells with nicotinamide riboside supplementation.[39] Other monogenic causes of cerebral arteriopathy and childhood stroke include COL4A1/COL4A2-related disorders, Menke's disease (ATP7A mutation), arterial tortuosity syndrome (SLC2A10 mutation), and adenosine deaminase 2 deficiency. A comprehensive list of these conditions is provided in the study by Fileva and colleagues' article, "Arterial Ischemic Stroke in Children," in this issue. Notably, screening for cerebral arteriopathy is advised for children with these conditions as well as those with specific chromosomal abnormalities (trisomy 21), monogenic multisystem disorders (Neurofibromatosis type 1, Alagille syndrome, Loeys–Dietz syndrome, type 4 Ehlers–Danlos syndrome, Marfan's syndrome, and microcephalic osteodysplastic primordial dwarfism type 2), and metameric neurocristopathies (posterior fossa brain malformations, hemangiomas, arterial anomalies, cardiac defects, eye abnormalities).[40]

Disordered assembly of normal vessel wall architecture that is the basis of CCMs has been linked to somatic loss of function mutations in the CCM1, CCM2, and CCM3 genes. Mutations in one of those genes are found in the vast majority of familial cases of CCMs. Therefore, screening of first-degree relatives is recommended for patients with multiple CCMs or in those with established familial inheritance patterns.[37,38] Genetic alterations that interrupt the normal function of diverse cellular signaling pathways have been found to play an important role in the development of cerebral vascular malformations. Loss-of-function mutations affecting genes within the TGF-beta and BMP signaling pathways, most commonly ALK1 and ENG, play a central role in the development of vascular malformations in HHT, while loss-of-function mutations in RAS-MEK-ERK and RAS-AKT-mTORC1 pathways (eg, loss-of-function mutations of the RASA1 and EPHB4) are linked to the development of vascular malformations in CM-AVM syndrome.[37,38]

SUMMARY

Pediatric neurovascular diseases represent a unique group of entities that differ from their adult homologs in both pathomechanism and clinical presentation. Neuroimaging plays a central role in the evaluation of affected children, and important age-related differences in disease expression must be considered in the interpretation of diagnostic neuroimaging studies obtained for affected patients. This introduction provides a framework for the coming studies that individually delve into specific aspects of neurovascular disease across different segments of the pediatric population from fetal life to young adulthood. With deepening insight into the mechanisms of neurovascular disease in childhood, targeted medical and genetic therapies may soon offer effective and enduring remedies for affected children. Neuroimaging is a powerful tool that has illuminated neurovascular disease processes in the past and promises to advance our understanding even further in the future.

CLINICS CARE POINTS

- Six genes have been identified as associated with the development of vein of Galen Malformations: RASA1, EPHB4, ACVRL1, NOTCH1, ITGB1, and PTPN11.
- Screening of first degree relatives is advised in children with multiple cerebral cavernous malformations (CCMs) or in those with established familial inheritance patterns of CCMS owing to the high incidence of genetic alterations.
- Nidal-type pial AVMs are the most common vascular cause of spontaenous intracranial hemorrhage in children.

DISCLOSURE

The authors declare no conflicts of interest related to the content of this article.

REFERENCES

1. Cater SW, Boyd BK, Ghate SV. Abnormalities of the fetal central nervous system: prenatal US diagnosis with postnatal correlation. Radiographics 2020; 40(5):1458–72.
2. Shekdar K, Feygin T. Fetal neuroimaging. Neuroimaging Clinics 2011;21(3):677–703.
3. Masselli G, Notte MV, Zacharzewska-Gondek A, et al. Fetal MRI of CNS abnormalities. Clin Radiol 2020;75(8):640-e1.
4. Raybaud C. Normal and abnormal embryology and development of the intracranial vascular system. Neurosurgery Clinics 2010;21(3):399–426.
5. Klostranec JM, Krings T. Cerebral neurovascular embryology, anatomic variations, and congenital brain arteriovenous lesions. J Neurointerventional Surg 2022;14(9):910–9.
6. Padget DH. The development of the cranial arteries in the human embryo. Contribution to embryology. Carnegie Institution 1948;32:205–61.
7. Lasjaunias P. A revised concept of the congenital nature of cerebral arteriovenous malformations. Intervent Neuroradiol 1997;3(4):275–81.
8. Zhao S, Mekbib KY, van der Ent MA, et al. Mutation of key signaling regulators of cerebrovascular development in vein of Galen malformations. Nat Commun 2023;14(1):7452.
9. Yang E, Storey A, Olson HE, et al. Imaging features and prognostic factors in fetal and postnatal torcular dural sinus malformations, part II: synthesis of the literature and patient management. J Neurointerventional Surg 2018;10(5):471–5.
10. Goldman-Yassen AE, Shifrin A, Mirsky DM, et al. Torcular dural sinus malformation: fetal and postnatal imaging findings and their associations with clinical outcomes. Pediatr Neurol 2022;135:28–37.
11. Jaimes C, Machado-Rivas F, Chen K, et al. Brain injury in Fetuses with vein of Galen malformation and Nongalenic arteriovenous fistulas: static snapshot or a portent of more? Am J Neuroradiol 2022; 43(7):1036–41.
12. Arko L, Lambrych M, Montaser A, et al. Fetal and neonatal MRI predictors of aggressive early clinical course in vein of Galen malformation. Am J Neuroradiol 2020;41(6):1105–11.
13. Sacco A, Pannu D, Ushakov F, et al. Fetal dural sinus thrombosis: a systematic review. Prenat Diagn 2021; 41(2):248–57.
14. Goldman-Yassen AE, Dehkharghani S. Chapter 1: Neuroimaging in perinatal stroke and cerebrovascular disease. In: Dehkharghani S, editor. Stroke. Brisbane (AU): Exon Publications; 2021. p. 1–24.
15. Curry CJ, Bhullar S, Holmes J, et al. Risk factors for perinatal arterial stroke: a study of 60 mother-child pairs. Pediatr Neurol 2007;37(2):99–107.
16. Nelson KB. Perinatal ischemic stroke. Stroke 2007; 38(2):742–5.
17. Patel N, Mills JF, Cheung MMH, et al. Systemic haemodynamics in infants with vein of Galen malformation: assessment and basis for therapy. J Perinatol 2007;27(7):460–3.
18. Cory MJ, Durand P, Sillero R, et al. Vein of Galen aneurysmal malformation: rationalizing medical management of neonatal heart failure. Pediatr Res 2023;93(1):39–48.
19. Burch EA, Orbach DB. Pediatric central nervous system vascular malformations. Pediatr Radiol 2015;45(S3):463–72.
20. Jiang B, Mackay MT, Stence N, et al. Neuroimaging in pediatric stroke. Semin Pediatr Neurol 2022;43: 100989.
21. Hongo H, Miyawaki S, Teranishi Y, et al. Genetics of brain arteriovenous malformations and cerebral cavernous malformations. J Hum Genet 2023; 68(3):157–67.
22. Nikolaev SI, Vetiska S, Bonilla X, et al. Somatic activating KRAS mutations in arteriovenous malformations of the brain. N Engl J Med 2018;378(3): 250–61.
23. Gross BA, Smith ER, Scott RM, et al. Intracranial aneurysms in the youngest patients: characteristics and treatment challenges. Pediatr Neurosurg 2015; 50(1):18–25.
24. Bernard TJ, Manco-Johnson MJ, Lo W, et al. Towards a consensus-based classification of childhood arterial ischemic stroke. Stroke 2012;43(2): 371–7.
25. Wintermark M, Hills NK, deVeber GA, et al. Arteriopathy diagnosis in childhood arterial ischemic stroke:

results of the vascular effects of infection in pediatric stroke study. Stroke 2014;45(12):3597–605.

26. Oesch G, Perez FA, Wainwright MS, et al. Focal cerebral arteriopathy of childhood: clinical and imaging correlates. Stroke 2021;52(7):2258–65.

27. Mertens R, Graupera M, Gerhardt H, et al. The genetic basis of moyamoya disease. Transl Stroke Res 2022;13(1):25–45.

28. Boulouis G, Blauwblomme T, Hak JF, et al. Nontraumatic pediatric intracerebral hemorrhage. Stroke 2019;50(12):3654–61.

29. Nash M, Rafay MF. Craniocervical arterial dissection in children: pathophysiology and management. Pediatr Neurol 2019;95:9–18.

30. Debette S, Leys D. Cervical-artery dissections: predisposing factors, diagnosis, and outcome. Lancet Neurol 2009;8(7):668–78.

31. Wilseck ZM, Lin LY, Chaudhary N, et al. Newer updates in pediatric vascular diseases. Semin Roentgenol 2023;58:110–30.

32. Kondziolka D, Humphreys RP, Hoffman HJ, et al. Arteriovenous malformations of the brain in children: a forty year experience. Can J Neurol Sci 1992; 19(1):40–5.

33. El-Ghanem M, Kass-Hout T, Kass-Hout O, et al. Arteriovenous malformations in the pediatric population: review of the existing literature. Interv Neurol 2016; 5(3–4):218–25.

34. Fullerton HJ, Achrol AS, Johnston SC, et al. Long-term hemorrhage risk in children versus adults with brain arteriovenous malformations. Stroke 2005;36: 2099.

35. Requejo F, Teplisky D, Dutra MLG, et al. Pediatric interventional neuroradiology. Semin Neurol 2023; 43(03):408–18.

36. Schimmel K, Ali MK, Tan SY, et al. Arteriovenous malformations—current understanding of the pathogenesis with implications for treatment. Int J Mol Sci 2021;22(16):9037.

37. Kahle KT, Duran D, Smith ER. Increasing precision in the management of pediatric neurosurgical cerebrovascular diseases with molecular genetics. J Neurosurg Pediatr 2023;31(3):228–37.

38. Sporns PB, Fullerton HJ, Lee S, et al. Childhood stroke (primer). Nat Rev Dis Prim 2022;8(1):12.

39. Kaw A, Wu T, Starosolski Z, et al. Augmenting mitochondrial respiration in immature smooth muscle cells with an ACTA2 pathogenic variant mitigates moyamoya-like cerebrovascular disease. Res Sq 2023;rs.3:rs-3304679.

40. Sinha R, Ramji S. Neurovascular disorders in children: an updated practical guide. Transl Pediatr 2021;10(4):1100.

Special Considerations for Cross-Sectional Imaging in the Child with Neurovascular Disease

Vivek Pai, MD[a,b], Pradeep Krishnan, MD[a,b],
Manohar Shroff, MD, FRCPC, DABR[a,b,*]

KEYWORDS

- Pediatric stroke • Arteriovenous Malformation • Cerebral venous sinus thrombosis

KEY POINTS

- An individualized evaluation for the need and type of sedation or general anesthesia is the critical first step in acquisition of diagnostic-quality imaging.
- MR imaging is the preferred choice of evaluation of children with suspected stroke; however, despite its poor sensitivity, CT plays a major role if MR imaging is unavailable or contraindicated.
- Utilization of the full potential of MR imaging is necessary when evaluating intracranial arteriovenous shunts, such that angioarchitecture and high-risk features are delineated before endovascular treatment.
- Anatomic variants of the major intracranial arteries are common and seldom of clinical significance, although in certain conditions detection of these is imperative to make an informed decision before conventional angiography and neurointervention.
- Imaging of sinovenous thrombosis is riddled with pitfalls, which need to be systematically excluded when interpreting cross-sectional studies.

INTRODUCTION

Broadly, pediatric neurovascular diseases can be divided into vaso-occlusive lesions, hemorrhagic lesions, drivers of hydrovenous dysfunction, and drivers of neonatal cardiopulmonary failure.[1] Compared with adults, pediatric neurovascular diseases are uncommon with an annual incidence of 2.5 to 3.1 per 100,000 population in children aged less than 15 years.[1] These disorders have varied presentations often limiting accurate clinical evaluation.[2] This limitation is further confounded by the age of these patients, with some lesions presenting as early as the neonatal period.

Cross-sectional neuroimaging plays a central role in the noninvasive evaluation of patients with suspected and previously known neurovascular lesions. This review provides an overview of pediatric neurovascular diseases and currently available, commonly used diagnostic imaging techniques.

Sedation: A Radiological Perspective

A major consideration before neuroimaging is assessment of the need for and type of sedation (drug-induced central nervous system depression) or general anesthesia (drug-induced loss of

[a] Division of Neuroradiology, Department of Diagnostic and Interventional Radiology, The Hospital for Sick Children, 170 Elizabeth Street, Toronto, Ontario M5G 1E8, Canada; [b] Department of Medical Imaging, University of Toronto, 263 McCaul Street, 4th Floor, Toronto, Ontario M5T 1W7, Canada
* Corresponding author. Division of Neuroradiology, Department of Diagnostic and Interventional Radiology, The Hospital for Sick Children, 170 Elizabeth Street, Toronto, Ontario M5G 1E8, Canada.
E-mail address: manohar.shroff@sickkids.ca

Neuroimag Clin N Am 34 (2024) 491–515
https://doi.org/10.1016/j.nic.2024.08.021
1052-5149/24/© 2024 Elsevier Inc. All rights are reserved, including those for text and data mining, AI training, and similar technologies.

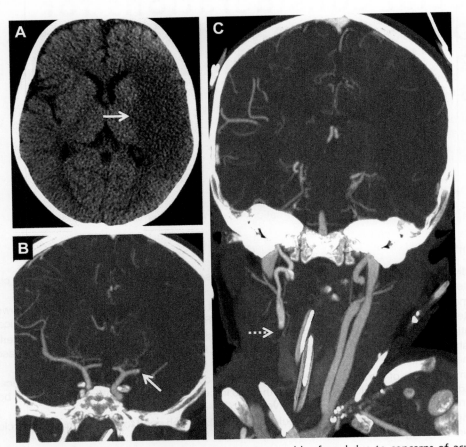

Fig. 1. Pediatric arterial ischemic stroke. CT imaging in a 1-year-old referred due to concerns of acute stroke following extracorporeal cardiopulmonary resuscitation. Axial CT image (*A*) reveals a large, wedge-shaped area of hypoattenuation (*arrow*), with loss of gray-white matter differentiation, involving the left middle cerebral artery (MCA) territory distribution, in keeping with an infarction. Coronal maximum intensity pixel projection (MIP) reconstruction of a CT angiography (CTA) (*B*) confirms the abrupt loss of contrast opacification along the left M1-MCA segment (*arrow*) in keeping with thrombo-occlusion. (*C*) Coronal MIP reconstruction of the CTA (including the neck vessels) demonstrates absent opacification of the proximal right common carotid artery (*dotted arrow*) secondary to ligation (commonly performed after extracorporeal membrane oxygenation).

consciousness, resulting in an unarousable state, even following noxious stimuli.[3,4] Achieving immobility during imaging is crucial because motion artifacts limit evaluation or obscure the pathologic condition. A nondiagnostic study may trigger patient and/or family anxiety as well as warrant repeat imaging, with consequent financial implications, loss of man-hours, and logistical issues.[5]

Decision for sedation or general anesthesia (S/GA) is made on a case-by-case basis, with age being the primary determinant. Generally, patients aged between 6 months and 6 years require some form of S/GA, depending on the imaging test.[5] The upper age limit may vary across institutions, some considering 5 years as the cutoff,[6] and also on the level of cooperation, comorbidities

present, and neurologic status of the child. Infants younger than 6 months may be imaged using a "feed-and-sleep" technique, although anesthesia may be indicated in clinically unstable patients.[6]

The need for S/GA is reduced in older children, but concomitant comorbidities (behavioral issues, involuntary movements) often necessitate S/GA.[5] In anxious patients, without comorbidities, nonpharmacologic methods may be useful (eg, familiarization with mock computed tomography [CT]/magnetic resonance [MR] imaging drills, allowing a family member into the imaging suite, application of soft restraints, and use of MR-compatible audiovisual projection goggles).[5,7] Desensitization with mock MR imaging drills is shown to reduce the need for GA by 16.8% in children

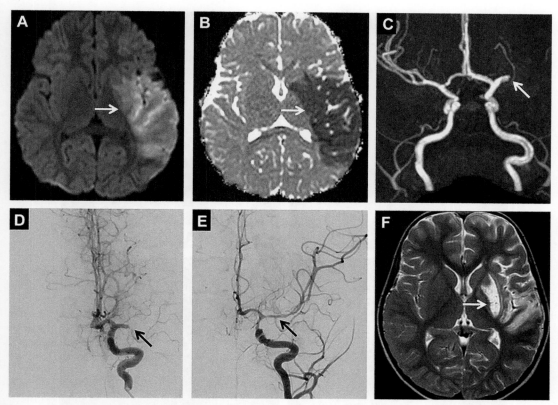

Fig. 2. Pediatric arterial ischemic stroke. MR imaging in a 3-year-old patient, with a complex cardiac anomaly, presenting with acute right-sided hemiplegia. Axial DWI (*A*) and apparent diffusion coefficient map (*B*) reveal a wedge-shaped area of restricted diffusion (*arrows* in *A, B*) involving the left MCA territory. MIP reconstruction of the TOF-MRA (circle of Willis) (*C*) confirms abrupt loss of flow signal in the left M1-MCA segment (*arrow*), in keeping with a thrombo-occlusion. TOF-MRA of the neck was also performed but did not demonstrate a tandem occlusion (not shown). anteroposterior (AP) projection of the left internal carotid artery (ICA) run before mechanical thrombectomy (*D*) confirms the left M1-MCA thrombo-occlusion (*arrow*). AP projection of the left ICA run following mechanical thrombectomy (*E*) demonstrates recanalization of the left MCA (*arrow*), with vasospasm that was treated with intra-arterial calcium channel blockers. Axial T2-weighted (T2W) image (*F*) obtained after 6 weeks reveals an area of encephalomalacia in the left MCA territory (*arrow*) in keeping with interval evolution of the presenting infarction.

aged between 3 and 8 years.[7] Psychological support provided by Child Life Specialists can also reduce the need for S/GA.[5,8]

The type of imaging is also another determinant when deciding if S/GA is warranted. With the advent of multidetector CT technology, multi-volume data collection for each complete gantry rotation is now possible with a resultant increase in table speeds and rate of data acquisition, the latter being 3-to 5-fold faster than the previous generations of CT scanners, thus reducing the need for S/GA.[9–11] On the other hand, MR imaging, which is more time and motion sensitive, may warrant imaging under GA, to reduce callback rates. Sammons and colleagues[12] reported a success rate of 100% among patients undergoing neuroimaging under GA (n = 111 children; 56% with neurodevelopmental disabilities).

Ensuring that fasting guidelines are met is of prime importance to eliminate aspiration of gastric contents and associated complications during GA. The reported incidence of aspiration among patients undergoing elective procedural sedation ranges between ~1 in 825 and ~1 in 30,037 cases, whereas single-institution data have shown that those undergoing emergency procedures under GA have an incidence of ~1 in 373 cases versus ~1 in 4544 for those undergoing elective GA.[4,13] The American Society of Anesthesiologists recommends a fasting period of 2 hours for clear fluids, 4 hours for human milk, 6 hours for nonhuman/formula milk, and 6 hours for a light meal.[4]

Under GA, patients undergo cardiorespiratory depression, therefore needing airway support and close monitoring.[5] Strict compliance with MR imaging safety protocols of all appliances

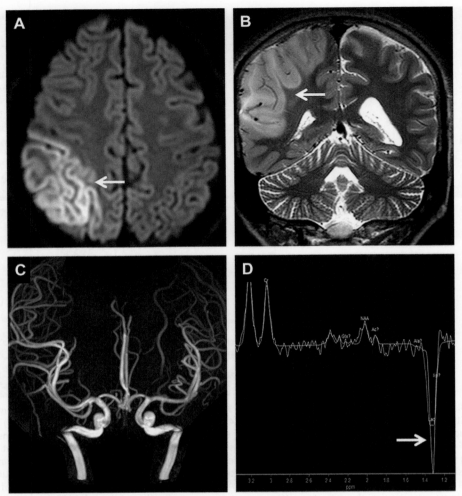

Fig. 3. Mitochondrial encephalomyopathy with lactic acidosis and strokelike episodes, an imaging and clinical mimic of stroke, diagnosed in a 9-year-old presenting with new onset of left-sided weakness. Axial DWI (*A*) reveals an area of restricted diffusion predominantly involving the right parietal lobe (*arrow*). Coronal T2W image (*B*) demonstrates corresponding gyriform T2-hyperintense swelling of the right parietal lobe (*arrow*), within the corresponding anterior circulation. Maximum intensity projection (MIP) of the TOF-MRA (*C*) reveals no large vessel occlusion or flow limiting stenosis along the anterior circulation. Single-voxel MR spectroscopy (TE 144; *D*) obtained from the affected right parietal lobe reveals a large lactate peak at 1.3 ppm (*arrow*).

used for monitoring patients under GA is critical, because the powerful pull of the magnetic field of the MR imaging machine can transform ferrous-containing appliances into a projectile object causing severe injury to the patient and personnel as well as hardware damage.[3]

Pediatric Arterial Ischemic Stroke Imaging: Computed Tomography versus Magnetic Resonance Imaging Considerations

Stroke accounts for 10% to 25% of all children presenting to the emergency department.[14] Pediatric stroke is differentiated into the broad categories of perinatal stroke (occurring between 20 weeks of intrauterine life and the 28th day of postnatal life) and childhood stroke (occurring beyond 29 days of life until 18 years of age).[14] In this section, only childhood stroke is discussed because perinatal stroke is best imaged only on MR imaging and hyperacute stroke therapies are not warranted in this age group.[15] The article by Flieva and colleagues in this issue provides a comprehensive overview of arterial ischemic stroke in children.

In pediatric stroke, CT as the initial line of imaging investigation is often reserved due to concerns of

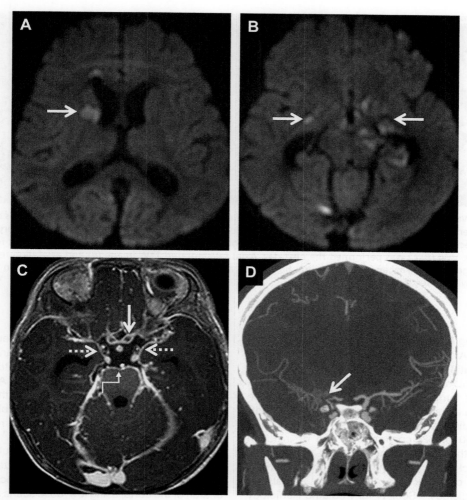

Fig. 4. Tuberculous vasculitis in an 8-year-old patient presenting with fever, seizures, and fluctuating levels of consciousness. Axial DWI (*A*, *B*) reveals multiple acute infarcts, predominantly in the perforator territories (*arrows* in *A*, *B*). Contrast-enhanced axial 3D T1 image (*C*) demonstrates extensive, thick, leptomeningeal enhancement/basal exudates coating the optic chiasm (*arrow*), mesial temporal lobes (*dotted arrows*), and the pial surface of the pons (*stepped arrow*). Follow-up CTA (*D*) reveals steno-occlusion of the right ICA with multiple lenticulostriate collaterals (*arrow*). Hydrocephalus was also noted on follow-up CT (not shown).

ionizing radiation.[14] CT has limited sensitivity and high false-negative rates in the detection of arterial ischemic stroke and may not detect as much as 47% of acute arterial ischemic strokes.[16–18] Despite these limitations, CT cannot be excluded from the armamentarium of pediatric stroke imaging. CT may be used in centers without MR imaging capabilities, if MR imaging is unavailable, if S/GA would substantially delay MR imaging, or if contraindications to MR imaging are identified (eg, cardiac devices)[14,16] (Fig. 1). In addition, CT is reasonable when the pretest probability of a large vessel occlusion is high (eg, following cardiac catheterization procedures or known cardiomyopathies) for thrombectomy candidature. Owing to

quick image acquisition, CT is often used to monitor expansion, evolution, and hemorrhagic transformation of infarction.[14] Hence, efforts must be made to ensure achieving doses as low as reasonably achievable, without compromise of diagnostic output. Techniques such as reduced rotation time, lowered kilovoltage and tube current, reducing unnecessary z-axis coverage, and dose modulation allow reduction in radiation dose without compromising image resolution.[14]

Craniocervical CT angiography (CTA) poses challenges with respect to accurate timing of contrast injection through a rather narrow intravenous line in children and dynamic changes in circulatory physiology related to age. In a study

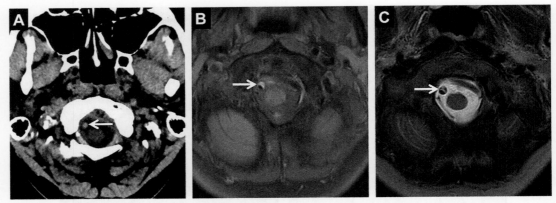

Fig. 5. VWI in a 17-year-old patient presenting with tearing neck pain. Axial unenhanced CT (A) reveals no acute brain parenchymal abnormality. However, a focal hyperdense attenuation of the right V4-vertebral artery (arrow) was suspected and MR imaging was suggested. MR imaging using the routine stroke protocol did not reveal an infarction. VWI (B, C) was performed the next day. Axial fat-saturated T1W image (B) and axial high-resolution T2W image (C) confirms an eccentric mural hematoma along the right V4-vertebral artery (arrows in B, C), in keeping with dissection.

evaluating image quality in pediatric cerebrovascular CTA, an objective improvement of contrast opacification was noted with higher flow rates (2.5–4 mL/s), thereby emphasizing the importance of larger-bore venous access (Poiseuille law).[19] In a survey conducted on Society of Pediatric Radiology (SPR) members, 44% of participants (30 of 68) confirmed a rate of injection greater than 3 mL/s for iodinated contrast for head/neck CTA examinations.[20] The American College of Radiology - American Society of Neuroradiology - Society for Pediatric Radiology (ACR-ASNR-SPR) consortium suggests dosing of contrast in children according to weight with a general guideline of 4 mL/s in any patient weighing 50 kg or more, reaching up to 6 mL/s for larger patients.[21] In infants, a 2-mL/s injection rate may be reasonable.[21]

Often patients may have venous access only via central lines. According to ACR guidelines, power injection of contrast media via a nonimplanted central venous catheter can be safely performed provided intravascular location of its tip is confirmed and venous backflow is tested.[20] Large-bore (9.5F–10F) central venous catheters can be injected using a flow rate of only up to 2.5 mL/s.[20] In the same survey by SPR, most responders preferred hand injection (54%) or a combination of hand and power injection (35%).[20] Although safe, a theoretic risk of catheter damage exists, especially during hand injections, which obviously is undesirable from a patient safety standpoint, particularly in the time-sensitive context of stroke.[20]

Substantial age- and physiology-dependent variations in circulation time mandate an appropriate delay following contrast injection, to ensure optimal arterial opacification for CTA. Accurate triggering of the scan can be achieved if the imaging is started as soon as contrast is visible in the region (artery) of interest, which in turn relies on the radiographer's skill and expertise.[19] Manual triggering has largely been replaced by automated triggering software based on real-time attenuation monitoring of vessels of interest (great neck vessel or arch of the aorta) using low-dose scans after the initiation of the contrast media injection; imaging is automatically triggered when enhancement reaches a predetermined attenuation.[21]

Last, CT contrast is associated with the potential risk of allergic and allergiclike reactions. In a study by Dillman and colleagues,[22] 11,306 pediatric intravenous administrations of low-osmolality nonionic iodinated contrast material revealed acute allergiclike reactions in 20 (0.18%) patients. Sixteen (80%) of these were categorized as mild, whereas 1 (5%) and 3 (15%) were categorized as moderate and severe, respectively.[22] Patients with known contrast allergies require premedication with steroids and antihistamines.

Accounting for these concerns and variables during CT imaging, better spatial resolution, and capability of vascular evaluation without injected contrast, MR imaging is the favored modality in the imaging workup of pediatric stroke.[14] MR imaging is also superior to CT scan in the diagnosis of alternate etiologies presenting with acute focal neurologic deficits.[14] MR imaging of a child with

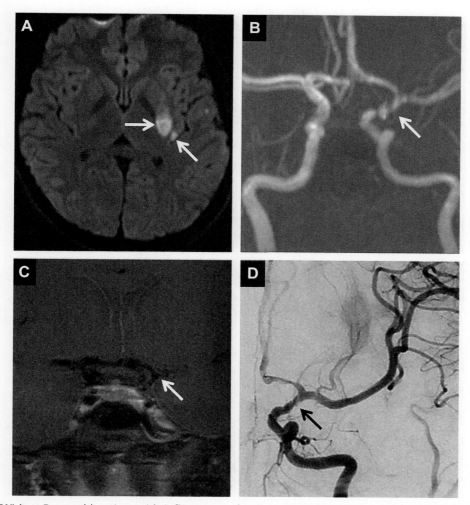

Fig. 6. VWI in a 5-year-old patient with inflammatory focal cerebral arteriopathy. Axial DWI (*A*) reveals focal striatocapsular acute infarcts (*arrows*) in the left MCA territory. MIP reconstruction of the TOF-MRA (*B*) reveals attenuation, and flow irregularity, involving the left supraclinoid ICA (*arrow*), extending into the left A1-anterior cerebral artery (ACA) and M1-MCA segments. Contrast-enhanced coronal black blood T1W VWI (*C*) reveals concentric wall enhancement along the affected left ICA (*arrow*) and the T-junction. Frontal projection of left ICA catheter-directed digital subtraction angiogram (*D*) reveals an irregular beaded appearance of the intradural left ICA (*arrow*).

suspected acute stroke comprises diffusion-weighted imaging (DWI) and apparent diffusion coefficient maps to detect acute parenchymal infarction, with susceptibility-weighted imaging (SWI) or gradient echo (GRE) sequences to assess for hemorrhage and intravascular thrombus and fluid-attenuated inversion recovery (FLAIR) imaging to assess subacute/chronic parenchymal changes.[16] Time-of-flight (TOF) MR angiography (MRA) of the craniocervical arteries is always performed to locate sites of arterial occlusion and identify evidence of arteriopathy[14] (**Fig. 2**). TOF-MRA uses short radio frequency pulses that

saturate (lose signal) stationary spins, whereas newly entering unsaturated spins within vessels impart a signal. Appropriate saturation bands are used to null out venous flow so that an angiogram depicting only arteries can be obtained.[23] In scenarios where hyperacute stroke therapy is not indicated, or where an imaging mimic of stroke is identified, a full-brain imaging protocol may be used for comprehensive characterization (**Figs. 3 and 4**).

Safe MR imaging relies on thorough knowledge of implanted hardware and medical devices, before the scan. These hardware and devices may interact

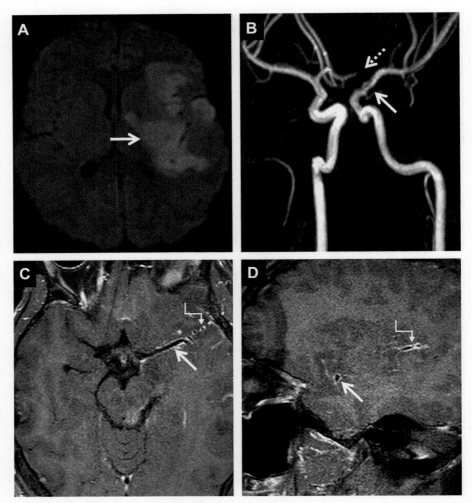

Fig. 7. Role of VWI in an 8-year-old patient presenting with acute right hemiplegia. Axial DWI (*A*) demonstrates acute infarction involving the left MCA territory (*arrow*). MIP reconstruction of the TOF-MRA (*B*) demonstrates mild attenuation, and flow irregularity, involving the left M1-MCA segment (*arrow*). Additionally, there is loss of flow signal in the proximal left A1-ACA (*dotted arrow*). Given that there was no thrombo-occlusion, VWI was performed. Contrast-enhanced axial (*C*) and sagittal (*D*) black blood T1W sequences reveal concentric enhancement of the left M1-MCA (*arrows* in *C, D*) and its cortical branches (*stepped arrows* in *C, D*) suggestive of an inflammatory arteriopathy.

with the magnetic fields causing susceptibility arti- facts that limit visualization of the anatomy, or even worse, these interactions can lead to device heat- ing, device movement, or device failure. Orthodon- tic hardware/dental braces are relevant in a pediatric setting, often distorting brain and MRA images.[24] Commercially available orthodontic braces may contain stainless steel (SS), ceramic, or titanium brackets.[24] As a consensus, SS brackets cause the most image distortion, requiring removal before MR imaging.[24] If needed, imaging on lower field strengths (1.5T), with signal-to- noise ratio (SNR) sacrifice, and use of sequences relatively less insensitive to susceptibility artifacts (turbo spin echo rather than GRE sequences) may be considered if braces cannot be removed.[14,24]

Perfusion-weighted imaging and flow-sensitive imaging in pediatric stroke

Although penumbral imaging in adults with arterial ischemic stroke is most often performed with CT or MR imaging-based contrast-enhanced perfusion-weighted imaging, flow-sensitive arterial spin labeling (ASL) technique is typically used to create cerebral blood flow maps in pediatric stroke imaging.[16] ASL uses endogenous flow tracers (magnetically labeled arterial blood water), without contrast agents. For ASL imaging, 2 sets of images are obtained: first a baseline brain image followed by imaging after labeling/tagging blood arterial water protons within the cervical arteries. The second set is obtained after a delay, allowing tagged protons to enter the imaging slice. Subsequent subtraction of the datasets allows quantification of the blood entering the brain.[23] Various types of tagging are available (continuous ASL, pulsed ASL, pseudocontinuous ASL), the discussion of which is beyond the scope of this article.

Vessel wall imaging in pediatric stroke

Black blood vessel wall imaging (VWI) is a technique in which high-resolution images of the intracranial or cervical arterial walls are obtained, distinct from the lumen.[23] Signals from blood are suppressed using long turbo spin echo readout or using an inversion recovery to null the longitudinal component of the blood-water magnetization.[17] VWI is often performed using a T1-weighted sequence due to the background cerebrospinal fluid suppression and the potential to perform contrast-enhanced imaging to detect vessel wall enhancement.[23] Owing to the need for high-resolution and thin-section

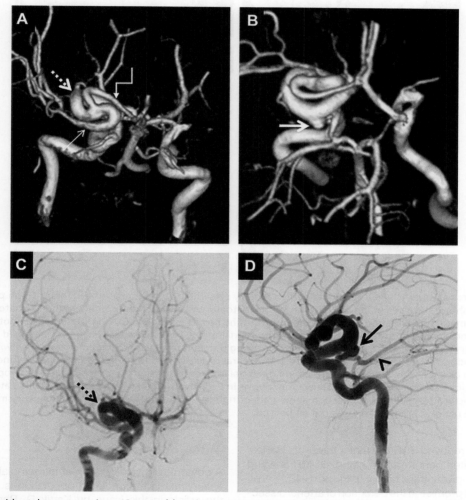

Fig. 8. Incidental aneurysm in a 12-year-old patient presenting with headache. 3D-volume reconstruction of a TOF-MRA (*A, B*) reveals marked dolichoectasia of the right supraclinoid ICA (*dotted arrow in A*). The right A1-ACA (*stepped arrow in A*) arises from the carotid terminus. The proximal right M1-MCA (*thin arrow in A*) demonstrates diffuse fusiform dilatation. Note the posteriorly directed saccular daughter aneurysm arising at the level of the right posterior communicating artery origin (*arrow in B*). Frontal (*C*) and lateral (*D*) projections of the right ICA catheter-directed digital subtraction angiogram confirms dolichoectasia of the intradural right ICA (*dotted arrow in C*) and associated posteriorly directed saccular daughter aneurysm (*arrow in D*); the latter is seen incorporating the right posterior communicating artery (*arrowhead*).

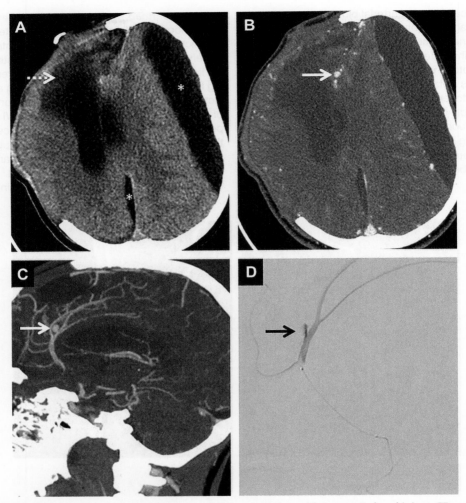

Fig. 9. Saccular aneurysm in a 9-year-old patient initially presenting with traumatic head injury. CT on presentation (not shown) revealed multifocal parenchymal hematomas and a large right frontal subdural hematoma warranting emergent evacuation and a decompressive right hemicraniectomy. CTA on presentation (not shown) revealed no significant intracranial or extracranial arterial injury. Unenhanced CT image (A) obtained 3 weeks postsurgery reveals extensive encephalomalacia involving the right frontal lobe (*dotted arrow*) along with hypodense subdural hygromas (*asterisk*) along the left cerebral convexity and the right posterior parafalcine region. Follow-up axial CTA image (B) and corresponding sagittal MIP reconstruction (C) reveals interval development of a traumatic saccular aneurysm/pseudoaneurysm (*arrows* in B, C) involving the right A2-ACA segment. Lateral projection microcatheter digital subtraction angiogram of right A2-ACA (D) showing the pseudoaneurysm (*arrow*) along the pericallosal ACA. This was coil embolized.

imaging, reduced SNR is a major trade-off. Hence, VWI is often performed on high-field MR imaging systems given their higher intrinsic SNR.[23] VWI has great promise in the detection of arterial dissections. In this setting, an unenhanced VWI sequence may depict a T1-hyperintense intramural hematoma[16,17] (Fig. 5). Contrast-enhanced VWI is also useful in the characterization of arteriopathies. Wall enhancement is presumed to reflect inflammation and increased flow within the vasa vasora of large arteries[16,17,25] (Figs. 6 and 7).

Pediatric Intracranial Aneurysms

A comprehensive overview of intracranial arterial aneurysms in the pediatric population is given in the article in this issue by Kartik D. Bhatia and Carmen Parra-Farinas's article, "Intracranial Arterial Aneurysms in Childhood," in this issue. For noninvasive imaging of intracranial arterial aneurysms in children, CTA, in conjunction with an unenhanced CT scan of the head, is widely used for initial workup. This approach is

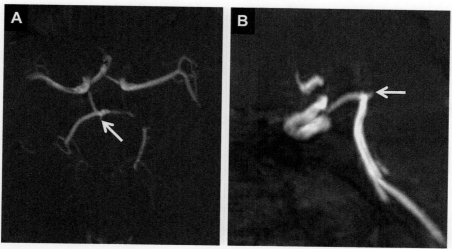

Fig. 10. MR appearance of an infundibulum in a 12-year-old presenting with focal seizures. Oblique axial (A) and oblique sagittal (B) MIP reconstructions of a TOF-MRA reveal an incidental conical, posteriorly directed outpouching (arrows) along the right P1-posterior cerebral artery segment in keeping with an infundibulum.

particularly favored in patients presenting with nontraumatic subarachnoid hemorrhage.[26,27] The sensitivity for detecting aneurysms less than 2 mm is 53%, improving to 95% for aneurysms larger than 7 mm.[28,29] CTA comes with the inherent limitations of calculating appropriate contrast dosage and timing of the CTA, but these are outweighed by the sensitivity and speed of imaging acquisition. MRA is often reserved only for follow-up imaging[28] Fig. 8.

Intracranial aneurysms may be encountered in children under specific clinical circumstances. Aneurysms following a traumatic brain injury account for approximately 5% to 10% of all pediatric intracranial aneurysms (PIAs) and often occur on the distal anterior cerebral artery (40%), on arteries crossing the skull base (35%), or on distal cortical branch arteries (25%)[30] (Fig. 9). Notably, traumatic aneurysms involving the petrocavernous internal carotid artery are frequently associated with direct carotid-cavernous sinus fistula. Nontraumatic dissecting aneurysms account for up to 50% of all aneurysms among neonates, infants, and young children.[30] These aneurysms are frequently circumferential or fusiform and may be associated with focal tortuosity or adjacent stenoses. Infectious (mycotic) aneurysms often involve distal cortical branch arteries.[30]

Infundibular dilations (also known as infundibula) are conical or funnel-shaped dilatations at arterial ostia, with the arterial mainstem seen extending from the apex[31] (Fig. 10). These structures mimic aneurysms but can be distinguished based on their morphology (ie, lack of neck or asymmetric outpouching).[32] In a study on pediatric infundibula, Dmytriw and colleagues[32] found infundibula are commonly located along the left P1-posterior cerebral artery (35%). Largely, infundibula are considered benign; however, adult literature has reported evolution into true aneurysms, attributed to flow-related wall shear stress, with histopathological studies confirming changes in the arterial media.[32] In the study by Dmytriw and colleagues,[32] none of the infundibula showed aneurysmal evolution over the pediatric age spectrum (total follow-up period of 86 patient-years; mean of 32.3 ± 35.7 months). Nevertheless, an increased incidence was noted in patients with sickle cell disease, which is a known association with PIAs.[32] Fenestration variants. which are commonly found at the vertebrobasilar junction and at the anterior communicating artery complex, can lead to unusual appearances that mimic aneurysms on cross-sectional imaging. In addition, arterial loops that are at the limit of cross-sectional imaging can mimic aneurysms, as can small arteries that turn out of the imaging plane in a TOF-MRA sequence.

Noninvasive Imaging of Intracranial Arteriovenous Shunts in Children

Numerous articles in this issue have content that address childhood hemorrhagic stroke and intracranial vascular malformations of childhood. To avoid redundancy, this article focuses specifically on principles of noninvasive cross-sectional imaging that are complementary to the other articles. A focused overview of intracranial vascular malformations of childhood including arteriovenous malformations

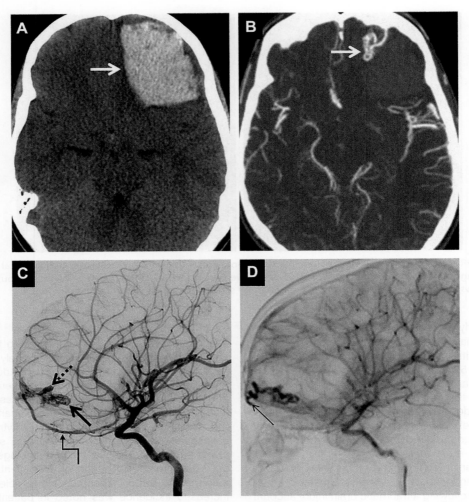

Fig. 11. Imaging appearances of a ruptured AVM with superficial venous drainage in a 16-year-old patient presenting with acute onset of headache. Axial unenhanced CT image (*A*) reveals a large, hyperdense, acute lobar hematoma in the left frontal lobe (*arrow*) exerting mass effect and a rightward midline shift. Axial MIP reconstruction of a CTA (*B*) reveals a small AVM nidus located along the anteromedial aspect of the hematoma (*arrow*). Lateral projections of the left ICA catheter-directed digital subtraction angiogram in early arterial (*C*) and capillary phases (*D*) confirm the AVM nidus in the basal left frontal lobe (*arrow* in *C*) supplied from the orbitofrontal branch of the left ACA (*stepped arrow* in *C*). A small superiorly directed pseudoaneurysm is also noted (*dotted arrow* in *C*). The AVM is drained via a superficial cortical vein (*thin arrow* in *D*) into the anterior aspect of the superior sagittal sinus.

(AVMs) is given Karim and colleagues' article, "Intracranial Vascular Malformations in Children," in this issue. Fetal vascular malformations (vein of Galen malformations, non-Galenic choroidal arteriovenous fistulae, pial arteriovenous fistulae, and dural sinus malformations) are covered in Qureshi and colleagues' article, "Neurovascular Malformations in the Fetus and Neonate," in this issue. Neuroimaging of childhood hemorrhagic stroke is presented in the Leach and colleagues' article, "Imaging of Hemorrhagic Stroke in Children," in this issue. The

initial imaging evaluation of hemorrhagic stroke in children is often done using CT/CTA[33,34] (**Figs. 11** and **12**). The lack of temporal resolution and the inability to detect micro-AVMs are a technical limitation of this technique. In patients with hereditary hemorrhagic telangiectasia, contrast-enhanced and ASL sequences are useful in detecting micro-AVMs and capillary malformations (**Fig. 13**). MR imaging/MRA is useful in the evaluation of both ruptured and unruptured AVM and arteriovenous fistula (AVF) (**Figs. 14–17**).

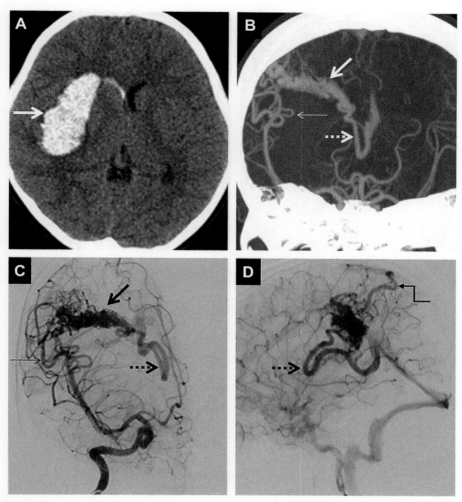

Fig. 12. Imaging appearances of a ruptured AVM with deep and superficial venous drainage in an 11-year-old patient presenting with left-sided weakness. Axial unenhanced CT image (*A*) reveals a large, hyperdense acute hematoma in the right external capsule (*arrow*). Note the marked mass effect exerted by the hematoma with resultant compression of the right lateral ventricle and a midline shift toward the left. A small amount of hemorrhage dissecting into the right frontal horn is also seen. Coronal oblique MIP reconstruction of a CTA (*B*) reveals a large AVM nidus located along the superior aspect of the hematoma (*arrow*), supplied by the distal cortical branches of the right MCA (*thin arrow*) and drained via the right thalamostriate vein into the right internal cerebral vein (*dotted arrow*). Frontal (*C*) and lateral (*D*) projections of the follow-up right ICA catheter-directed digital subtraction angiogram confirm a compact AVM nidus in the in the right frontoparietal lobe (*arrow* in *C*) supplied by arteries distributed by the right MCA (*thin arrow* in *C*) and drained by the right thalamostriate vein (*dotted arrows* in *C, D*) into the corresponding internal cerebral vein along with superficial drainage via a single cortical vein (*stepped arrow* in *D*) into the midportion of the superior sagittal sinus.

Catheter-directed digital subtraction angiography (DSA) is the gold-standard for imaging intracranial arteriovenous shunts. A detailed overview of catheter-directed neuroangiography in children is presented in the Tierradentro-Garcia and colleagues' article, "Catheter-directed Cerebral and Spinal Angiography in Children," in this issue. Exceptional spatial (0.08 mm × 0.08–0.2 mm × 0.2 mm) and temporal (up to 24 frames per second) resolution is achieved with DSA.[35] Superselective microcatheter angiography and 3D rotational reconstructions allow detailed evaluation of AVM angioarchitecture.[35] C-arm cone-beam CT (CBCT) imaging is performed with a C-arm-mounted flat-panel detector system and provides fast, high-resolution volumetric imaging. This

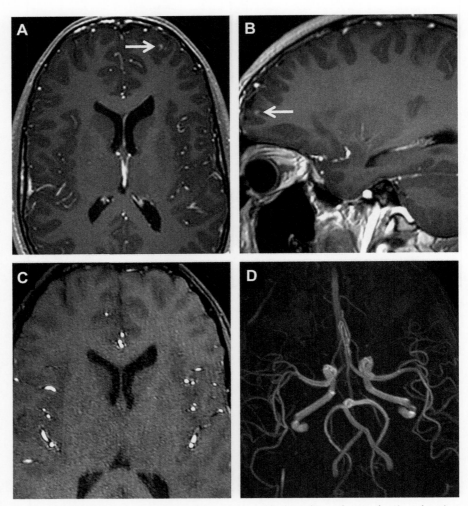

Fig. 13. Capillary malformation in a 5-year-old patient with hereditary hemorrhagic telangiectasia. Axial contrast-enhanced 3D T1 image (*A*) and its sagittal reconstruction (*B*) reveal a punctate focus of enhancement in the left frontal cortex (*arrows in A, B*). Axial TOF-MRA (*C*) and its MIP reconstruction (*D*) reveal no flow signal/nidus in this region or elsewhere intracranially. The findings favor capillary malformation over micro-AVM given the absence of discrete macrovascular structures forming a central nidus. No arteriovenous shunting was observed on catheter-directed digital subtraction angiography.

imaging has been found to provide morphologic characteristics and anatomic relations of contrast-injected vessels with excellent spatial resolution (0.1–0.2 mm voxels).[35] CBCT also permits multiplanar and 3D volume reconstructions using a single acquisition dataset. However, despite these advantages, CBCT increases radiation dosage. Data from adult literature suggest that a 20-second CBCT angiogram acquisition is associated with 0.2 Gy radiation dose versus a 5-second 3D rotational angiography, which provides an exposure of 0.065 Gy. In comparison, a standard catheter-directed DSA run is associated with 0.15 Gy of radiation exposure.[36] Doses for 3D rotational pediatric neuroangiography can be significantly reduced to about

15% of a standard DSA run by tailoring protocols for effectiveness and dose optimization.[36]

Although TOF-MRA is a flow-sensitive MR imaging sequence that conveys some information about flow, it lacks hemodynamic information needed for adequate characterization of intracranial arteriovenous shunts.[23] Contrast-enhanced time-resolved MR angiography (CE TR-MRA), a modification of bolus-chase MRA, enables rapid acquisition of vascular flow data. Along with short repetition time, low spatial resolution, parallel imaging, and partial Fourier acquisition, this technique performs multiple, sequential, rapid acquisitions of the entire imaging volume following intravenous contrast bolus administration. The

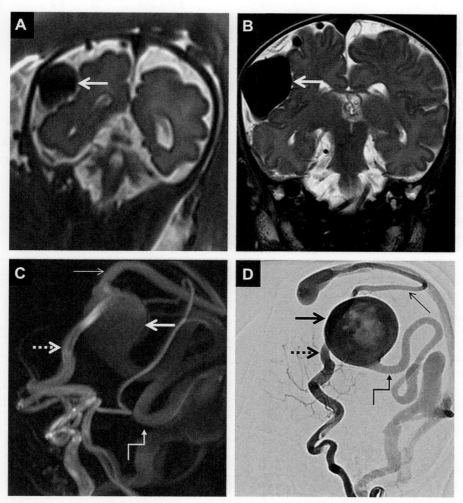

Fig. 14. Neonate with a single-hole pial arteriovenous fistula (PAVF). Coronal T2 image (*A*) obtained antenatally reveals a large venous pouch (*arrow*) along the right parietal lobe. Follow-up coronal T2 image (*B*) obtained a few hours following birth reveals an unchanged venous pouch (*arrow*) along the right parietal lobe. MIP reconstruction of a TOF-MRA (*C*) and lateral projection of the right ICA catheter-directed digital subtraction angiogram (*D*) confirm a PAVF supplied by a parietal branch of the right MCA (*dotted arrows* in *C, D*) with a large venous pouch (*arrows* in *C, D*). The arterialized venous pouch is drained via 2 venous structures, one draining superomedially toward the superior sagittal sinus (*thin arrows* in *C, D*) and the other via a posteriorly directed vein (*stepped arrows* in *C, D*) draining into the right transverse sinus.

acquisitions serve as snapshots of contrast transit and can be summed as maximum intensity pixel projections to be displayed as time-resolved "movies."[23] Temporal imaging enables assessment of intracranial hemodynamics and the venous drainage patterns for shunting lesions.[37] There is little literature on time-resolved MRA use in the pediatric age group, but experience from adult literature is encouraging. In a study by Machet and colleagues,[38] CE TR-MRA was able to detect 17 of 19 AVMs confirmed by catheter-directed DSA and found good agreement between the 2 techniques when evaluating

nidus size and venous drainage (k = 0.75, 0.77) along with moderate agreement (k = 0.44) when evaluating arterial feeders. Furthermore, Farb and colleagues[39] reported that CE TR-MRA accurately identified and assigned Borden classification for 93% of adult-type dural arteriovenous fistula.

Vascular Anatomy and Variants

Selective ophthalmic artery infusion chemotherapy

Retinoblastoma is the most common pediatric primary ocular malignancy, affecting 1 in 15,000

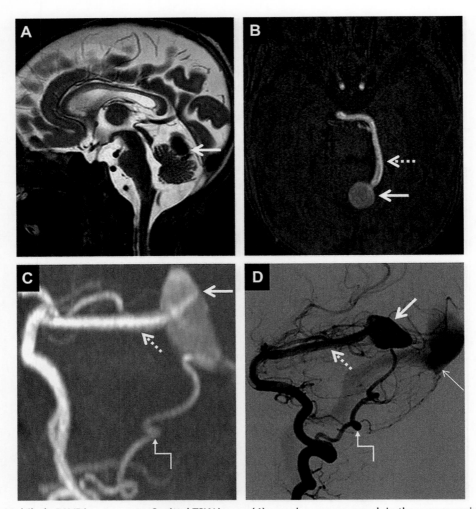

Fig. 15. Multihole PAVF in a neonate. Sagittal T2W image (*A*) reveals a venous pouch in the supravermian cistern (*arrow*). Axial TOF-MRA (*B*) reveals arterialized flow within the venous pouch (*arrow*) supplied by a hypertrophied left superior cerebellar artery (*dotted arrow*). MIP reconstruction of the TOF-MRA (*C*) and lateral projection of the left vertebral catheter-directed digital subtraction angiogram (*D*) confirm the multihole PAVF with a solitary venous pouch (*arrows* in *C, D*), supplied by the left superior cerebellar artery (*dotted arrows* in *C, D*) and left posterior inferior cerebellar artery (*stepped arrows* in *C, D*). The postfistulous venous drainage is noted via the torcula (*thin arrow* in *D*).

to 20,000 live births. Two-thirds of all cases are diagnosed before age 2 years and 95% before the age 5 years.[40,41] Treatment options in patients with retinoblastomas have evolved over the years from enucleation and external beam radiotherapy to more targeted chemotherapeutic drug delivery via the superselective catheterization of the ophthalmic artery (intra-arterial chemotherapy [IAC]).[42]

At our institution, all patients who are candidates for selective ophthalmic artery infusion chemotherapy undergo MR imaging of the brain and orbits, along with TOF-MRA to assess the OA. We use the results of TOF-MRA for

neuroendovascular surgical treatment planning to improve procedural workflow efficiency. When a small caliber of the OA, variant OA origin, or unfavorable angulation of the proximal OA stem suggests that direct catheterization of the OA will be difficult or impossible, an alternative approach is formulated in advance. In such cases, chemotherapy can be administered directly into the orbital branch of the middle meningeal artery or into the infraophthalmic internal carotid artery during concurrent balloon occlusion of the supra-ophthalmic internal carotid artery. Advanced planning of this nature can reduce the number of vessel catheterizations, reduce patient radiation

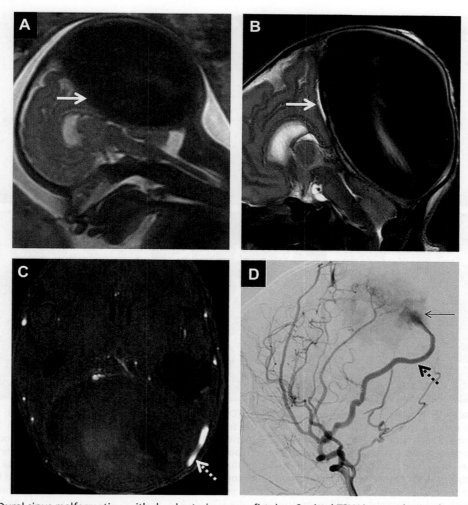

Fig. 16. Dural sinus malformation with dural arteriovenous fistulae. Sagittal T2W image obtained prenatally (*A*) and sagittal T2 image obtained within the first few hours postnatally (*B*) reveal a large venous pouch created by massive enlargement of the posterior segment of the superior sagittal sinus and contiguous torcula (*arrows in A, B*). Note the marked mass effect exerted over the posterior aspects of the cerebral hemispheres and the posterior fossa structures. Axial TOF-MRA (*C*) and lateral projection of the left external carotid artery (ECA) catheter-directed digital subtraction angiogram (*D*) reveal an arteriovenous macrofistula (*thin arrow in D*) between the venous pouch and the posterior division of the left middle meningeal artery (MMA) (*dotted arrows*). Arterial supply via the contralateral MMA and the dural branches of the posterior cerebral arteries was also noted (not shown).

exposure, reduce contrast load, and ensure that all necessary equipment is available at the time of neuroendovascular treatment.[43,44] (**Fig. 18**)

Wada test

Despite significant advances in functional brain MR imaging, the Wada test remains an important part of the preoperative evaluation of patients with medically refractory seizures who are under consideration for temporal lobectomy. This test typically entails slow injection of sodium amobarbital (100–500 mg) into the cervical ICA. This injection anesthetizes the ipsilateral cerebral hemisphere for almost 5 to 10 minutes, during which memory and language function can be evaluated in awake patients.[45] In patients with persistent primitive carotid-vertebrobasilar anastomoses (ie, trigeminal artery), a modified superselective Wada test involving microcatheter-directed infusion of amytal directly into the intracranial internal carotid artery is necessary to prevent amytal-induced respiratory depression and loss of consciousness[46] (**Fig. 19**). Recognition and reporting of persistent primitive carotid-vertebrobasilar anastomoses can

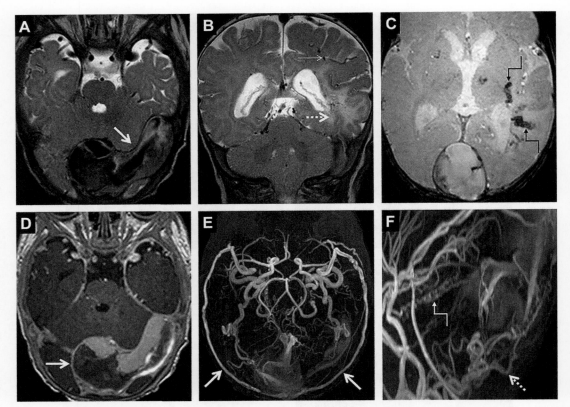

Fig. 17. Partially thrombosed dural sinus malformation (DSM) in a 3-month-old patient presenting with seizures. Axial T2W image (*A*) reveals marked ectasia of the left transverse sinus and torcula in keeping with a DSM (*arrow*). Coronal T2W image (*B*) reveals confluent T2 hyperintensity (*dotted arrow*) in the left temporal lobe along with distended cortical veins (*thin arrow*) in the left parietal region representing changes of chronic venous congestion. Axial multiplanar gradient recalled acquisition (MPGR) (*C*) demonstrates tubular foci of T2 hypointensity (*stepped arrows*) corresponding to thrombosed cortical veins and/or hemorrhage in the affected left temporal lobe. Axial contrast-enhanced 3D T1W image (*D*) reveals a large filling defect (*arrow*) within the DSM in keeping with partial thrombosis. MIP reconstructions of a TOF-MRA (*E, F*) reveal dominant arterial supply arising from the middle meningeal arteries (*arrows* in *E*), the occipital arteries (*dotted arrow* in *F*), and the meningohypophyseal arteries (*stepped arrow* in *F*).

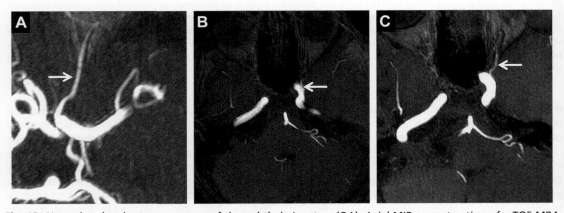

Fig. 18. Normal and variant appearances of the ophthalmic artery (OA). Axial MIP reconstruction of a TOF-MRA (*A*) reveals normal takeoff of the left OA (*arrow*) arising from the intradural paraclinoid segment of the left ICA (*A*). Axial (*B*) and oblique (*C*) 2D-MIP reconstructions of a TOF-MRA in another patient reveals dorsal variant anatomy of the left OA (*arrows* in *B, C*) arising from the lateral aspect of the cavernous left traversing the left superior orbital fissure.

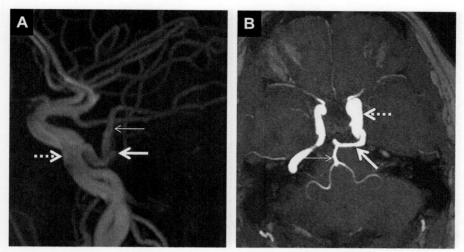

Fig. 19. Appearances of a persistent trigeminal artery. Lateral (*A*) and axial (*B*) MIP reconstructions reveal a persistent trigeminal artery (*arrows*) arising from the cavernous segment of the left ICA (*dotted arrows*) and supplying the distal basilar trunk (*thin arrows*). Note that the basilar artery caudad to the trigeminal artery is hypoplastic.

therefore improve procedural workflow efficiency for patients undergoing Wada testing. Although many such variants are well demonstrated on conventional brain MR imaging studies, TOF-MRA may be valuable for detection of less-conspicuous variants that influence the distribution of drug infused into the cervical internal carotid artery.

Cerebral Sinovenous Thrombosis: Pearls and Pitfalls

Cerebral sinovenous thrombosis (CSVT) refers to thrombo-occlusion of the dural venous sinuses, cortical veins, and/or deep cerebral veins. CSVT is a neurologic emergency with an incidence of 0.25 to 0.67 per 100,000 children per year and 0.82 to 12 per 100,000 neonates per year.[47] The associated mortality rate and risk of permanent neurologic damage range between 8% to 19% and 38% to 48.1%, respectively.[47] Patients may present with a wide spectrum of symptoms (headache, seizures, altered mentation, lethargy, and/or focal neurologic deficits).[48] Dehydration, infection, trauma, cancer, anticancer treatment, prothrombotic states (antiphospholipid syndrome, prothrombin G20210A mutation, antithrombin III deficiency, elevated homocysteine), lupus, and nephrotic syndrome are reported causes of CSVT in children.[48,49]

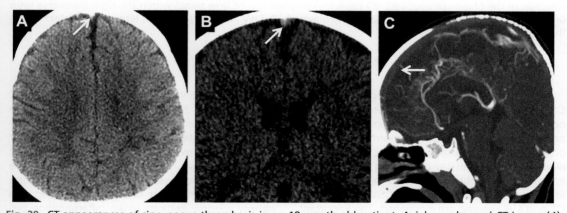

Fig. 20. CT appearances of sinovenous thrombosis in an 18-month-old patient. Axial unenhanced CT image (*A*) reveals hyperdensity within the superior sagittal sinus (*arrow*); however, this may be overlooked due to inadequate window settings. Axial unenhanced CT image viewed using a narrow window setting (*B*) accentuates the hyperdense attenuation of the superior sagittal sinus (*arrow*). CT venography (*C*) performed subsequently confirms the occlusive thrombus within the superior sagittal sinus (*arrow*).

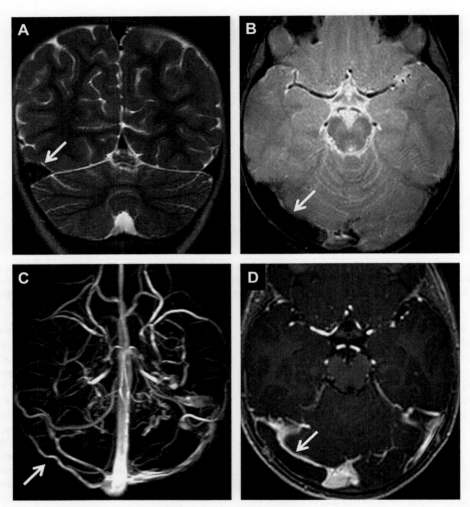

Fig. 21. Typical appearances of an acute CSVT in a 2-year-old patient. Coronal T2W image (*A*) reveals marked distention of the right transverse sinus (*arrow*), due to a T2-hypointense thrombus mimicking a flow void. Axial MPGR sequence (*B*) reveals abnormal susceptibility within the occluded right transverse sinus (*arrow*). MIP reconstruction of the phase contrast MRV (*C*) confirms complete loss of flow signal within the right transverse sinus (*arrow*) and the right sigmoid sinus. Contrast-enhanced 3D T1W image (*D*) reveals a large filling defect within the right transverse sinus (*arrow*).

Neuroimaging is essential to diagnose/confirm CSVT, identify the extent of cerebral venous compromise, and evaluate for secondary complications (venous ischemia, hemorrhage, and so on).[49] CT and MR imaging, with venographic techniques, are the mainstay of imaging a patient with known or suspected CSVT.[49] In this section the imaging features and pitfalls of CSVT imaging on CT and MR imaging are discussed. The important role of CSVT as a cause of pediatric hemorrhagic stroke and related neuroimaging issues is presented in Leach and colleagues' article, "Imaging of Hemorrhagic Stroke in Children," in this issue.

On CT imaging the intraluminal thrombus of CSVT appears hyperdense in the acute phase due to low water and high hemoglobin concentrations. This situation persists for 1 to 2 weeks, after which the clot evolves to become isodense and later hypodense. It is imperative to ensure adequate window settings when evaluating the dural venous sinuses on unenhanced CT because narrow window settings make differentiation between the sinus and the adjacent bone difficult. Beam-hardening artifacts at the skull base may obscure the venous system. Diffuse venous hyperdensity must also be evaluated with caution

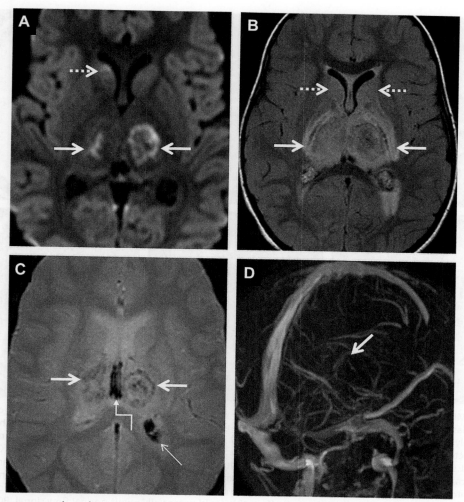

Fig. 22. Deep venous thrombosis in a 6-year-old patient presenting with altered mentation. Axial DWI (*A*) reveals bilateral, asymmetric areas of restricted diffusion in the thalami (*arrows*), more extensive on the left. Subtle restricted diffusion is also seen in the right caudate nucleus (*dotted arrow*). Axial FLAIR (*B*) reveals marked hyperintense swelling of the thalamocapsular regions (*arrows*). Subtle similar signal is also noted in the caudate nuclei (*dotted arrows*). Axial MPGR (*C*) reveals foci of hemorrhage within the involved thalami (*arrow*) along with abnormal susceptibility within the internal cerebral veins (*stepped arrow*). Some hemorrhage along the glomus of the left choroid plexus is also seen (*thin arrow*). Oblique MIP reconstruction of a TOF-MRV (*D*) reveals complete absence of flow signal within the deep cerebral venous system (*arrow*).

because this finding may be due to physiologic polycythemia (eg, in neonates).[47] On CT venography, intraluminal clot is seen as a filling defect within the sinus or vein[47] (**Fig. 20**).

The appearance of intraluminal venous clot on MR imaging varies with the stage of its evolution. In the acute phase, the clot is isointense on T1 but hypointense on T2/FLAIR sequences. As the clot evolves into the subacute phase, the degradation of deoxyhemoglobin to methemoglobin imparts a hyperintense signal on T1 sequences initially, with hyperintensity seen on T2/FLAIR sequences in the late subacute phase (extracellular methemoglobin).

SWI/GRE is reliable at these stages because the degradation of hemoglobin causes a blooming artifact (hypointense signal) (**Figs. 21** and **22**). A chronic thrombus may be variable in signal intensity but usually hypointense on T1 and T2 sequences. Flow voids within a partially recanalized thrombus may be noted. SWI in the chronic phase is not as reliable because ferritin and hemosiderin (superparamagnetic substances) are removed by macrophages.[47] In a study on 37 patients with CSVT, Wagner and colleagues[49] concluded that 96% of cases could be identified on T1 and T2 sequences (74 of 77) and 88% (68 of 77) were detected on

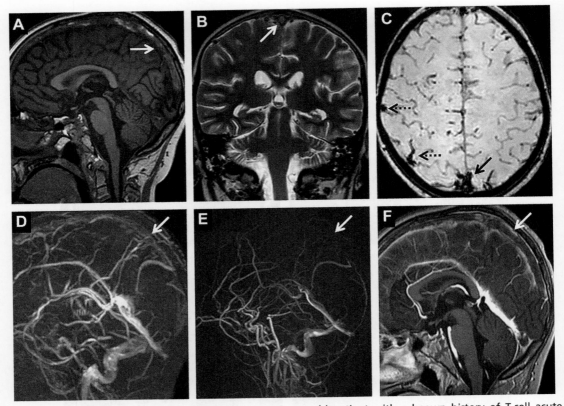

Fig. 23. MR imaging of sinovenous thrombosis in a 9-year-old patient with a known history of T-cell acute lymphoblastic leukemia on pegylated L-asparaginase. Sagittal T1W image (A) reveals hyperintense thrombosis extensively involving the superior sagittal sinus (arrow). Coronal T2W image (B) reveals corresponding loss of the expected flow void within the midportion of the superior sagittal sinus (arrow). Axial SWI (C) reveals abnormal susceptibility within the superior sagittal sinus (arrow). Also note, similar susceptibility artifacts in the cortical veins along the right frontoparietal convexity (dotted arrows), suggestive of concomitant cortical venous thrombosis. MIP reconstruction of a TOF-MRV (D) reveals apparent faint signal within the superior sagittal sinus (arrow), due to thrombus shine through effect; this could potentially mimic normal flow signal. PC-MRV (E) confirms absent flow in the superior sagittal sinus (arrow). Sagittal contrast-enhanced 3D T1W image (F) confirms a filling defect (arrow) extensively involving the superior sagittal sinus in keeping with thrombosis.

FLAIR images. Although 94% of thrombi within the dural venous sinuses were revealed by DWI/Diffusion tensor imaging (DTI) (72 of 77), only 40% showed restricted diffusion.[49]

Although these sequences help in the initial identification of CSVT, they are not enough to delineate the site and extent of the thrombus. TOF-MR venography (TOF-MRV) is useful in detecting defects in flow within the venous sinuses. Saturation of mobile spins, depicted as flow gaps, due to parallel orientation of the vessel and the imaging plane may mimic an occlusion. Thrombus shine through effect due to the native T1 hyperintensity of a clot, resulting in apparent flow signals in the lumen, is another important pitfall. This pitfall can be mitigated by correlating with spin echo sequences and phase contrast MRV (PC-MRV).[47,50]

PC-MRV uses bipolar gradients to induce a phase shift of mobile spins and restore it to generate a signal. A velocity-encoding gradient (VENC) is then applied to filter out the flow within the vascular structure of choice (veins in this case). Hence use of the correct VENC is critical to obtain robust intraluminal flow signals with PC-MRV. Flow velocity outside the VENC is not displayed and hence may erroneously be interpreted as occlusion. This phenomenon is more common at sites where flow is faster or turbulent, for example, around an arachnoid granulation or along the stenotic distal transverse sinuses in the setting of idiopathic intracranial hypertension.[47,50]

Contrast-enhanced MRV is a technique that uses intravenous gadolinium to cause intraluminal T1 shortening, thereby producing a lumenogram.

This technique provides better spatial resolution and is devoid of the effects of in-plane saturation or the need for application of a velocity-based gradient. Thrombi, including those with T1 hyperintensity, are seen as filling defects. (**Fig. 23**) However, chronic thrombi may enhance due to replacement of thrombus with organized connective tissue and capillary proliferation (granulation tissue).[47,50]

SUMMARY

Cross-sectional neuroimaging rests on 2 major pillars, that is, CT and MR imaging. These technologies have revolutionized the evaluation of children with neurovascular pathology, by improving the delineation of neurovascular lesions and illuminating diverse mechanisms of disease pathogenesis. The addition of catheter-directed angiographic techniques and hemodynamic imaging enables a deeper and complementary characterization of pediatric neurovascular pathologies. Expert interpretation of cross-sectional and catheter-directed neuroimaging data empowers neuropediatric specialists to formulate optimal patient-oriented treatment strategies across the full range of clinical neurovascular pathology. Despite the advantages that neuroimaging has brought to pediatrics, there are limitations and trade-offs that interpreting radiologists must be cognizant of to avoid erroneous diagnostic evaluations.

CLINICS CARE POINTS

- MRI with abbreviated stroke specific sequences is the modality of imaging modality of choice in patients presenting with clinical features of stroke. However, stroke mimics are frequent. Hence active monitoring during image acquisition is warranted so that further imaging sequences, as necessary, may be obtained.

- AV shunts in pediatric patients are different in terms of pathophysiology and angioarchitecture compared to adults. Most shunts which cause high output cardiac failure may be detected in utero. In those who present in the post-natal MRI and CT both play a complimentary role in evaluating the shunting lesion as well as its effects on the brain parenchyma.

- Sinovenous thrombosis in children may be due to underlying prothrombotic causes, complication of an intracranial pathology

(e.g., infection) or idiopathic. The dural venous sinuses are an important review area in clinical practice. Understanding the physics, advantages and limitations of the various imaging sequences available is extremely important in order to avoid a mis- or missed diagnosis.

DISCLOSURE

The authors have nothing to disclose.

REFERENCES

1. Hetts SW, Meyers PM, Halbach VV, et al. Anomalies of the cerebral vasculature: diagnostic and endovascular considerations. In: Barkovich AJ, Raybaud C, editors. Pediatric neuroimaging. 6th edition. Philadelphia: Wolters Kluwer; 2019.
2. Montaser A, Smith ER. Intracranial vascular abnormalities in children. Pediatr Clin 2021;68(4):825–43.
3. Choudhary P, Neha B. Sedation and general anesthesia in diagnostic pediatric imaging. Indographics 2022;01:101–9.
4. Coté CJ, Wilson S. Guidelines for monitoring and management of pediatric patients before, during, and after sedation for diagnostic and therapeutic procedures. Pediatrics 2019;143(6):e20191000.
5. Fawole C, Webber A. Approaches to sedation in pediatric neuroimaging: what the radiologist should know. J Pediatr Neurol 2017;16(02):056–60.
6. Barkovich MJ, Xu D, Desikan RS, et al. Pediatric neuro MRI: tricks to minimize sedation. Pediatr Radiol 2018;48(1):50–5.
7. Carter AJ, Greer MLC, Gray SE, et al. Mock MRI: reducing the need for anaesthesia in children. Pediatr Radiol 2010;40(8):1368–74.
8. Khan J, Donnelly L, Koch B. A program to decrease the need for pediatric sedation for CT and MRI. Appl Radiol 2007;36:30–3.
9. Pappas JN, Donnelly LF, Frush DP. Reduced frequency of sedation of young children with multisection helical CT. Radiology 2000;215(3):897–9.
10. Callahan MJ, Cravero JP. Should I irradiate with computed tomography or sedate for magnetic resonance imaging? Pediatr Radiol 2021;52(2):340–4.
11. Arlachov Y, Ganatra RH. Sedation/anaesthesia in paediatric radiology. Br J Radiol 2012;85(1019):e1018–31.
12. Sammons HM, Edwards J, Rushby R, et al. General anaesthesia or sedation for paediatric neuroimaging: current practice in a teaching hospital. Arch Dis Child 2010;96(1):114.
13. Warner MA, Warner ME, Warner DO, et al. Perioperative pulmonary aspiration in infants and children. Anesthesiology 1999;90(1):66–71.

14. Jiang B, Mackay MT, Stence NV, et al. Neuroimaging in pediatric stroke. Semin Pediatr Neurol 2022;43: 100989.

15. Ferriero DM, Fullerton HJ, Bernard TJ, et al. Management of stroke in neonates and children: a scientific statement from the American heart association/American stroke association. Stroke 2019;50(3). https://doi.org/10.1161/str.0000000000000183.

16. Mirsky DM, Beslow LA, Amlie-Lefond C, et al. Pathways for neuroimaging of childhood stroke. Pediatr Neurol 2017;69:11–23.

17. Donahue MJ, Dlamini N, Bhatia A, et al. Neuroimaging advances in pediatric stroke. Stroke 2019;50(2): 240–8.

18. McGlennan C, Ganesan V. Delays in investigation and management of acute arterial ischaemic stroke in children. Dev Med Child Neurol 2008;50(7): 537–40.

19. Thust SC, Chong WKK, Gunny R, et al. Paediatric cerebrovascular CT angiography-towards better image quality. Quant Imag Med Surg 2014;4(6):469–74.

20. Callahan MJ, Servaes S, Lee EY, et al. Practice patterns for the use of iodinated IV contrast media for pediatric CT studies: a survey of the society for pediatric radiology. Am J Roentgenol 2014;202(4): 872–9.

21. American College of Radiology. ACR-ASNR-SPR practice parameter for the performance and interpretation of cervicocerebral computed tomography angiography (CTA). Revised. 2020. Available at: acr.org/-/media/ACR/Files/Practice-Parameters/Cervico CerebralCTA.pdf?la=en. Accessed February 28, 2024.

22. Dillman JR, Strouse PJ, Ellis JH, et al. Incidence and severity of acute allergic-like reactions to IV nonionic iodinated contrast material in children. Am J Roentgenol 2007;188(6):1643–7.

23. Vossough A. Cerebrovascular diseases in infants and children: general imaging principles. Springer eBooks; 2016. p. 1–48.

24. Poorsattar-Bejeh Mir A, Rahmati-Kamel M. Should the orthodontic brackets always be removed prior to magnetic resonance imaging (MRI)? J Oral Biol Craniofac Res 2016;6(2):142–52.

25. Dlamini N, Yau I, Muthusami P, et al. Arterial wall imaging in pediatric stroke. Stroke 2018;49(4):891–8.

26. de Aguiar GB, Ozanne A, Elawady A, et al. Intracranial aneurysm in pediatric population: a single-center experience. Pediatr Neurosurg 2022;57(4): 270–8.

27. Xu R, Xie ME, Yang W, et al. Epidemiology and outcomes of pediatric intracranial aneurysms: comparison with an adult population in a 30-year, prospective database. J Neurosurg Pediatr 2021; 28(6):685–94.

28. Chung C, Peterson RB, Howard BM, et al. Imaging intracranial aneurysms in the endovascular era: surveillance and posttreatment follow-up. Radiographics 2022;42(3):789–805.

29. Sanchez S, Hickerson M, Patel RR, et al. Morphological characteristics of ruptured brain aneurysms: a systematic literature review and meta-analysis. Stroke 2023;3(2). https://doi.org/10.1161/svin.122.000707.

30. Krings T, Geibprasert S, terBrugge KG. Pathomechanisms and treatment of pediatric aneurysms. Child's Nerv Syst 2009;26(10):1309–18.

31. Kameda-Smith M, Plessis J, Bhattacharya JJ. First demonstration of resolution of an infundibulum by direct treatment of the arterial wall with Pipeline flow-diverting stent. Neuroradiology 2013;56(1):35–9.

32. Dmytriw AA, Bisson DA, Phan K, et al. Locations, associations and temporal evolution of intracranial arterial infundibular dilatations in children. J Neurointerventional Surg 2019;12(5):495–8.

33. El-Ghanem M, Kass-Hout T, Kass-Hout O, et al. Arteriovenous malformations in the pediatric population: review of the existing literature. Interv Neurol 2016;5(3–4):218–25.

34. Garzelli L, Shotar E, Blauwblomme T, et al. Risk factors for early brain AVM rupture: cohort study of pediatric and adult patients. Am J Neuroradiol 2020; 41(12):2358–63.

35. Mossa-Basha M, Chen J, Gandhi D. Imaging of cerebral arteriovenous malformations and dural arteriovenous fistulas. Neurosurgery Clinics of North America 2012;23(1):27–42.

36. Safain MG, Rahal JP, Raval A, et al. Use of cone-beam computed tomography angiography in planning for gamma knife radiosurgery for arteriovenous malformations. Neurosurgery 2014;74(6):682–96.

37. Grossberg JA, Howard BM, Saindane AM. The use of contrast-enhanced, time-resolved magnetic resonance angiography in cerebrovascular pathology. Neurosurg Focus 2019;47(6):E3.

38. Machet A, Portefaix C, Kadziolka K, et al. Brain arteriovenous malformation diagnosis: value of time-resolved contrast-enhanced MR angiography at 3.0T compared to DSA. Neuroradiology 2012; 54(10):1099–108.

39. Farb RI, Agid R, Willinsky RA, et al. Cranial dural arteriovenous fistula: diagnosis and classification with time-resolved MR angiography at 3T. Am J Neuroradiol 2009;30(8):1546–51.

40. Chen Q, Zhang B, Dong Y, et al. Comparison between intravenous chemotherapy and intra-arterial chemotherapy for retinoblastoma: a meta-analysis. BMC Cancer 2018;18(1). https://doi.org/10.1186/s12885-018-4406-6.

41. Rauschecker AM, Patel CV, Yeom KW, et al. High-resolution MR imaging of the orbit in patients with retinoblastoma. Radiographics 2012;32(5):1307–26.

42. Fabian ID, Onadim Z, Karaa E, et al. The management of retinoblastoma. Oncogene 2018;37(12): 1551–60.

43. Manjandavida FP, Stathopoulos C, Zhang J, et al. Intra-arterial chemotherapy in retinoblastoma – a paradigm change. Indian J Ophthalmol 2019;67(6): 740–54.

44. Klufas MA, Gobin YP, Marr B, et al. Intra-arterial chemotherapy as a treatment for intraocular retinoblastoma: alternatives to direct ophthalmic artery catheterization. Am J Neuroradiol 2012;33(8):1608–14.

45. Loring DW, Meador KJ, Westerveld M. The Wada test in the evaluation for epilepsy surgery. Neurosciences (Riyadh, Saudi Arabia) 2000;5(4):203–8.

46. Manraj KSH, Abruzzo T. Diagnostic cerebral angiography and the Wada test in pediatric patients. Tech Vasc Interv Radiol 2011;14(1):42–9.

47. Bracken J, Barnacle A, Ditchfield M. Potential pitfalls in imaging of paediatric cerebral sinovenous thrombosis. Pediatr Radiol 2012;43(2):219–31.

48. Heller C, Heinecke A, Junker R, et al. Cerebral venous thrombosis in children. Circulation 2003; 108(11):1362–7.

49. Wagner MW, Bosemani T, Oshmyansky A, et al. Neuroimaging findings in pediatric cerebral sinovenous thrombosis. Child's Nerv Syst 2015;31(5):705–12.

50. VP20. Pai V, Khan I, Sitoh YY, et al. Pearls and pitfalls in the magnetic resonance diagnosis of dural sinus thrombosis: a comprehensive guide for the trainee radiologist. J Clin Imaging Sci 2020;10:77.

Catheter-directed Cerebral and Spinal Angiography in Children

Luis O. Tierradentro-Garcia, MD[a], Karen I. Ramirez-Suarez, MD[b], Mesha L. Martinez, MD[c],*

KEYWORDS

- Catheter-directed angiography (CDA) • Diagnostic cerebral angiography
- Diagnostic spinal angiography conventional angiography • Neuroangiography
- Neurovascular conditions

KEY POINTS

- Catheter-guided angiography (CGA) remains the gold standard for diagnosing neurovascular conditions in pediatric patients, offering unmatched detail of vascular anatomy despite advancements in noninvasive imaging techniques.
- Pediatric spinal angiography (SA) is essential for diagnosing spinal vascular conditions and for preoperative vascular mapping, providing detailed insights into spinal vasculature to guide treatment and prevent surgical complications.
- Pediatric CDA is safe and effectuve for diagnosing neurovascular conditions, with low complication rates and rare adverse events, aided by ongoing advancements in techniques and radiation safety.

INTRODUCTION: NEUROANGIOGRAPHY IN CHILDREN

Catheter-directed angiography (CDA) is the gold standard neuroimaging study employed in the workup of most neurovascular conditions in both adults and children. When neuroangiography was first introduced in 1927 by Egas Moniz, it was performed by direct percutaneous injection of a contrast bolus into the cervical carotid arteries without catheters. This method was associated with a high risk of serious complications.[1–5] Though neuroangiography was performed in the pediatric population as early as in the 1940s, it was not until the 1950s that development of Seldinger technique and angiographic catheters enabled CDA to be performed as it is today. CDA served as the principal diagnostic modality to examine brain pathologies until the advent of CT technology in 1975.[6,7]

In the 1950s and 1960s, advancements in technique and catheter technologies allowed percutaneous catheterization of the cervicocerebral arteries using over-the-wire catheters advanced from peripheral arterial access sites, which proved simpler and safer than direct carotid or vertebral access.[8–10] These newer approaches enabled the evaluation of unique angiographic configurations in the pediatric population.[11–13] Takaku and Suzuki[14] conducted one of the earliest and most extensive studies, including 14 fetuses (postmortem angiograms) and 70 children of all ages, to

[a] Department of Radiology, Hospital of the University of Pennsylvania, University of Pennsylvania, 3400 Spruce Street 1, Silverstein - Radiology Administration, Suite 130, Philadelphia, PA 19104, USA; [b] Department of Radiology, Children's Hospital of Philadelphia, University of Pennsylvania, 3401 Civic Center Blvd, Philadelphia, PA 19104, USA; [c] The Edward B. Singleton Department of Radiology, Texas Children's Hospital, Baylor College of Medicine, 9835 N Lake Creek Parkway, Ste. PA120, Austin, Texas 78717, USA
* Corresponding author. The Edward B. Singleton Department of Radiology, Baylor College of Medicine, 9835 N Lake Creek Pkwy, Ste. PA120, Austin, Texas 78717.
E-mail address: MeshMart@IU.edu

Neuroimag Clin N Am 34 (2024) 517–529
https://doi.org/10.1016/j.nic.2024.08.019
1052-5149/24/© 2024 Elsevier Inc. All rights are reserved, including those for text and data mining, AI training, and similar technologies.

determine the normal appearances and development of the internal carotid artery, "carotid siphon," anterior cerebral artery, middle cerebral artery, and degree of arterial filling. They then compared these data to the cerebral angiograms of 108 children with low IQ and showed differences in artery length, angulation, and contralateral filling.[15] In their pictorial essay, Bentson and Wilson[16] depicted the cerebrovascular anatomy in both arterial and venous phases, providing a comprehensive atlas of normal pediatric angiograms.

Subsequently, transfemoral catheterization gained popularity for pediatric neuroangiography.[7,17-22] In 1971, Takahashi and Kawanami[23] reported their experience with 62 children (ages 0-14 years) who underwent transfemoral carotid and vertebral angiography; while similarly, in 1975, Numaguchi and colleagues[17] described the use of the 21 gauge needle and polyethylene catheter inserted transfemorally as a successful technique to perform selective cerebral angiography in infants and children. Pediatric indications of CDA began expanding to also include diagnosis of bacterial infections of the brain such as cerebritis and brain abscesses,[24] evaluation of hydrocephalus,[25] and for the diagnosis of brain death.[26]

In like manner, pediatric catheter-directed spinal angiography has evolved significantly since its inception in the 1950s.[27] Initially used to diagnose arteriovenous malformations (AVMs) and tumors, it has become an essential neuroradiological procedure for neuroimaging diagnosis of a wide spectrum of spinal vascular conditions.[28] CDA is now used for various spinal vascular diagnostic indications, including arterial ischemia, vascular malformations, tumors, and for preoperative treatment planning.[29,30] Modern studies have demonstrated its safety and efficacy in children, with low complication rates reported from high-volume pediatric centers.[31,32] Despite rapid advances in MRI and MRA technology, pediatric CDA remains an essential diagnostic tool, with ongoing advancements in angiographic imaging and neuroendvascular technique contributing to its continued development and application in pediatric neurovascular care.

Most of the literature concerning CDA presents studies conducted in adults, and there are few guidelines on the performance of pediatric CDA. For example, a comprehensive literature search in PubMed with the following keywords in the Title/Abstract ("Catheter-directed cerebral angiography" OR "catheter-directed spinal angiography" OR "Catheter-based cerebral angiography" OR "catheter-based spinal angiography" OR "diagnostic cerebral angiography" OR "diagnostic spinal angiography" OR "cerebral angiography" OR "spinal angiography") AND ("children" OR "pediatric" OR "child" OR "kid" OR "neonate" OR "toddler" OR "adolescent") yielded a total of 76 studies about cerebral and spinal angiography in the pediatric population. One of the main reasons for this paucity of literature is the heterogeneous and limited pediatric neuroangiographic training among practitioners. Nevertheless, it is paramount for providers to understand the particularities of performing CDA in children, including smaller-caliber vessels that are more prone to vasospasm and thrombosis, age-dependent changes in neurovascular anatomy including the wide range of normal anatomic variation, the natural history of pathologic conditions, variation of pathologic presentations as compared to adult homologue diseases, radiation exposure concerns, common pediatric-specific comorbidities (ie, sickle cell disease), age-dependent and physiology-dependent systemic manifestations and pediatric dosages of commonly used drugs. This study aims to present an up-to-date review of diagnostic cerebral and spinal CDA in children.

CATHETER-DIRECTED PEDIATRIC CEREBRAL ANGIOGRAPHY
Indications

CDA serves as the gold standard imaging modality for numerous neurovascular conditions in children, including hemorrhagic stroke, shunting vascular malformations, aneurysms, arteriopathies (including but not limited to vasculitis), venous outflow obstruction and as a planning or image-guidance tool for surgical or endovascular therapies.[33-38] In most cases, CDA is performed after detailed cross-sectional imaging studies have been obtained.[33] This allows better planning of the CDA examination so that it can be tailored to the important questions at hand.

The major advantages of CDA over computed tomography angiography (CTA) and MRA are far superior spatial and temporal resolutions, both of which are crucial for elucidating and interpreting neurovascular pathologies. For example, CDA is superior to MRA when evaluating children with central nervous system (CNS) vasculitis, as MRA fails to detect lesions beyond second order branches, especially in the posterior circulation. CTA techniques and most MRA techniques do not provide temporal information regarding blood flow patterns and their local alterations, and time-resolved MRA or flow-sensitive arterial spin labeling (ASL) techniques that do, end up trading temporal resolution for spatial resolution. This is unfavorable in children who have inherently small caliber vasculature, and for conditions like micro-AVM that are common in children. CDA performs better at informing about collateral blood supply and persistent embryologic anastomoses, which are common findings in children both in physiologic and disease states. CDA is also not limited by slow flow insensitivity that could lead to false assumptions of vessel stenosis or occlusion.[39,40] Consequently, despite considerable technological advances in cross-sectional modalities that have helped close the gap in diagnostic performance, catheter directed angiography (CDA) remains relevant for accurate diagnosis in most conditions.

Sawiris and colleagues[6] evaluated the added value of CDA in 111 patients, including adolescents, who underwent diagnostic CDA in a tertiary urban academic medical center. The authors sought "new anatomic cerebrovascular findings" in CDA studies that were not readily evident in noninvasive modalities (CTA or MRA) and which had a meaningful impact on patient management. Novel findings were seen in 43% of the cases, namely in patients with intracranial arterial stenosis, cerebral aneurysms, cerebral AVMs, cerebral vasculitis, brain tumors, intracerebral hemorrhage, subarachnoid hemorrhage, and arterial ischemic stroke. A clinically impactful anatomic description yielded by CDA was present in 23.4% of cases, characterized by a better depiction of anatomic relationships, evaluation of vascular diameter, degree of vascular stenosis, and extent of disease. Additionally, CDA detected false-positive and false-negative cases compared to CTA/MRA in 11.7% and 9.9% of cases, respectively.[6]

Several indications for CDA are specific to, or more common in the pediatric population. Some specific indications for CDA in neonates and infants include the work-up of hypervascular intracranial masses like choroid plexus tumors or teratomas, as a presurgical adjunct and to plan endovascular embolization. In infants and toddlers with complex cardiac/aortic arch pathologies that affect intracranial blood flow, CDA can provide crucial information about brain vascular physiology which can guide the formulation of treatment plans that preserve the intracranial circulation. CDA is also important to diagnose the cause of arterial ischemic stroke in children and adolescents, with or without large vessel occlusion. CDA is also performed as a part of the Wada test in older children with epilepsy,[41] to confirm the successful management of vascular lesions through intraoperative and postoperative angiography,[42] during balloon occlusion testing prior to undertaking vessel sacrifice, and for the evaluation of dynamic extracranial vertebral artery insufficiency in posterior fossa stroke (Bowhunter syndrome). Three dimensional (3D) and 4 dimensional (4D) rotational angiographic capabilities allow for detailed evaluation of micro-

AVMs and complex aneurysms from different projections, and reconstruction into high-resolution cross-sectional images for treatment planning. CDA is also useful for delineating relevant venous anatomy in children with dural sinus occlusion secondary to high-flow arteriovenous shunts, chronic venous thrombosis, or craniosynostosis, and to determine the direction of venous drainage in sinus pericranii associated with venous malformations prior to undertaking definitive treatment.

Despite the above, it is important to be cautious and selective when deciding to perform CDA in children, more so in infants and small children where benefit–risk ratios for CDA might be less favorable. Too often CDA is requested and performed for the evaluation of presumed neurovascular pathologies that could have been diagnosed or ruled out adequately using cross-sectional imaging modalities. For example, transcranial Doppler ultrasound is a valuable tool in neonates and young infants for the evaluation of abnormal vascularity associated with intracranial hemorrhage or tumors, especially given the low likelihood of nidal-type pial AVM in this age group and therefore resultant low yield of CDA. Transcranial Doppler techniques can also be used in the follow-up of treatments or disease evolution, for example, following staged endovascular embolization of dural arteriovenous fistula (AVF) or to monitor vasospasm following subarachnoid hemorrhage. Similarly, it is important to ensure that ultrasound, CT and MRI techniques have been exhausted before embarking on CDA for the elucidation of aberrant neurovascular anatomy or suspected pathology in older children. For example, duplex Doppler ultrasound studies with head maneuvers are a useful screening tool to evaluate older cooperative children with suspected Bowhunter syndrome. As another example, most cases of large vessel arteriopathy or vasculitis can be diagnosed accurately by a combination of a detailed clinical history and examination in conjunction with appropriate implementation of magnetic resonance angiography (MRA) and high-resolution vessel wall imaging, while arteriovenous shunts occult to routine MRI sequences can be detected by flow-weighted arterial spin labeling. Clearly, the pediatric neuroangiographer must have a keen sense of the neurovascular conditions that affect children, anatomic, or pathologic variants that can mimic these conditions, and alternative modalities to identify or exclude them.

Pre-procedural Workup

A comprehensive medical and surgical history must be obtained as a first step in planning any neuroendovascular procedure including CDA.

This critical knowledge enables providers to properly prepare the patient, to administer patient-centered intra-procedural care and to safely recover the patient with a focus on mitigating the risk of complications. Clinical history can shape the plan for procedural timing in a way that critically impacts patient safety. Beyond an accurate history, a baseline neurologic examination is essential. While a complete detailed neurologic examination is not always possible in critically ill children who are sedated out of necessity, the most recent neurologic status should be obtained by chart review and discussion with caregivers. Potential access sites, including downstream pulses and capillary refill should also be assessed. While most CDA procedures do not require routine blood tests, the decision to obtain certain laboratory tests should be tailored to the patient's medical needs. Preoperative anesthesia evaluation has to be considered in all children with preexisting comorbidities, especially those with a cardiopulmonary disease history or those with difficult airways.[43–45] Moreover, pediatric patients with a high risk for hematological, cardiopulmonary, vascular or renal complications (ie, sickle cell disease) may require additional precautions such as consultation with subspecialty pediatric services (eg, hematology or nephrology), overnight admission, blood transfusions, or supplemental hydration. Children with contrast allergies must receive premedication with steroids and antihistamines using age appropriate doses. Although gadolinium has been used for performing CDA in adults with allergies to iodinated contrast media, there is no rationale for a similar use in children, especially with recent reports of gadolinium deposition in brain tissue.[46,47]

A family-centered approach is key to performing CDA in children. Patients and families must understand the rationale, the risks and benefits of the planned procedure. The risks of pediatric CDA have been consistently shown to be low in high-volume centers with pediatric expertise.[48] Nonetheless, catastrophic events that could occur include arterial injury at the access site with threatened limb perfusion in small children, ischemic stroke from arterial wall injury or embolism (air, thrombus, polymer coating of catheters or guidewires), and hemorrhagic stroke from disruption of fragile pathologic vessels. It is therefore crucial that pediatric neuroangiography be performed in centers that are equipped to handle the consequences of these complications, with personnel that are trained to handle pediatric emergencies and imaging systems optimized for pediatric examinations.

Procedural Setup

For children under 2 years of age, or small in size, optimal leg positioning can help make vascular access easier. Placing a child's leg in the frog lateral position separates the overlapping common femoral artery and vein, allowing easier access with ultrasound guidance and decreasing the risk of iatrogenic AVF formation. Placing a roll under the hip can help to reduce anterior fat folds in small children and "fix" the femoral artery from excessive displacement by the needle tip. It is essential to pad the heels of both feet and other body parts that contact the table because children have less subcutaneous fat and more easily develop pressure sores. Ensuring that patient gowns are devoid of metal snaps, and that all metal containing objects are outside the field of imaging avoids time wasted on repositioning once the angiographic catheter is introduced into the patient and the procedure is underway. Rectal rather than esophageal temperature probes should be used to avoid interference with imaging of cervicocerebral vessels.

General endotracheal anesthesia with neuromuscular blockade is recommended for CDA in pediatric patients. Exceptions can be made in mature cooperative adolescents who could participate in the examination and comply with breath holds while under conscious sedation, when pediatric anesthesia services have limited availability or anesthetic risks are considered excessive. The decision for conscious sedation also depends on whether the neuroimaging goals can tolerate some diagnostic inaccuracy. Pediatric cerebral and spinal CDA using digital subtraction technology is uniquely sensitive to even very small degrees of motion. Since accurate pediatric neuroangiographic diagnosis often relies on detection of subtle irregularities involving very small vessels, or on differentiating numerous very closely spaced and overlapping tortuous vessels, the correct diagnosis can be obfuscated by misregistration artifact caused by minor degrees of motion. Vibration-related image degradation may be improved by temporarily pausing patient warming apparatuses during digital subtraction angiography (DSA) runs, and by triggering mask acquisition after the capnography trace has flattened. Peng and colleagues evaluated 62 children aged 6 to 15 years who underwent diagnostic angiography and compared the use of propofol versus dexmedetomidine for sedation. The authors found that the number of airway events and total adverse events were lower in the group using dexmedetomidine; also, diagnostic angiograms performed under the effect of dexmedetomidine took less time than those with propofol.[49–51] While endotracheal intubation is preferred, a laryngeal mask airway is an option. As noted, the use of paralytic agents, which are safer with endotracheal intubation, ensures decreased motion artifact, better image quality, shorter procedural duration, reduced radiation exposure, reduced contrast media dose and fewer diagnostic errors.

For patients with a history of hereditary hemorrhagic telangiectasia, patent foramen ovale, or pulmonary AVMs, venous line filters should be used to remove microbubbles that could be the cause of paradoxic embolus and microembolic stroke. An arterial line for continuous blood pressure monitoring is not usually required for CDA but may be preferred by the anesthesiologist for blood pressure control during induction and emergence in children with moyamoya arteriopathies or other disorders that severely limit cerebral perfusion. An indwelling urinary catheter is recommended to avoid bladder distension and patient distress in the anesthetized supine patient. The SNIS Pediatric Committee recommends a pre-procedure checklist to improve safety and outcomes for children undergoing CDA59 (**Fig. 1**).

Technique

Pediatric CDA should preferably be performed in a biplane neuroangiographic room equipped with means for radiation dose reduction. Biplane neuroangiography is important to reduce fluoroscopic and catheter indwelling time, number of DSA runs performed, and to maximize diagnostic information obtained from different 2 dimensional (2D) projections. The common femoral artery is the preferred access site for pediatric neuroangiography. Using a thin-walled vascular sheath with the smallest outer diameter necessary (most commonly 4 Fr thin-walled sheaths) to access the vasculature can significantly reduce access-site complications secondary to vasospasm and thrombosis. The femoral artery in a child is relatively more mobile due to an elastic femoral connective tissue sheath. Consequently, it responds to needle tip pressure with displacement and distortion. The pediatric femoral artery is more prone to and less tolerant of vasospasm than in adults. As such, real-time ultrasound guidance can aid in a nontraumatic vascular access in a small child, despite a superficial and easily palpable pulse. A digital pulse oximeter is placed on the distal toe ipsilateral to sheath placement to monitor limb perfusion. An audible Doppler probe placed over the dorsalis pedis or posterior tibial artery can be used to intermittently report pulse status to the operator. Direct intra-arterial

administration of a vasodilator (nitroglycerin and/or verapamil) can be considered prior to sheath insertion as a means of limiting access artery vasospasm, particularly in children less than 6 years of age. Vascular access complications are uncommon in children, occurring in less than 3% of cases.[44] Events are broad in severity and can span from subclinical temporary vasospasm and local hematoma to painful pseudoaneurysm formation or, rarely, development of iatrogenic arteriovenous fistulae. While unusual to occur following routine diagnostic neuroangiography, femoral arterial vasospasm in small children can progress to thrombosis and occlusion. The risk is increased in the setting of lengthy therapeutic procedures, particularly when larger diameter vascular access sheaths are used. Small intramural hematomas or dissections related to access vessel trauma may contribute to procedure-related access vessel occlusion. Femoral artery occlusion may lead to limb-threatening ischemia that requires further medical or surgical intervention. With early recognition and management, however, most children develop robust collaterals to the leg from abdomino-pelvic arteries, but occasionally severe ischemia can develop leading to limb length discrepancies or even limb loss.[52] Pediatric CDA is most commonly performed through 4 Fr diagnostic catheters. Given the small diameter and fragility of pediatric blood vessels, catheters, and guidewires must be advanced carefully under fluoroscopic guidance, ensuring the absence of any resistance as indicated by tactile or imaging feedback.

More recently, trans-radial catheter access (TRCA) has been shown to be feasible and safe in older children.[53] The main drivers for TRCA in adult populations, such as reduced femoral access-site complications and avoidance of challenging aortic arch anatomy are not present in children. Advantages of TRCA in children and adolescents include patient comfort, earlier mobilization, a quicker return to sports and school activities, and preservation of modesty during postprocedural access-site checks. Transradial access with a microcatheter-only technique has also been described for intra-arterial chemotherapy in small children with retinoblastoma, with an added advantage of faster and easier postprocedural immobilization as compared to femoral access in this age group.[54] Critics of this approach cite the inability to obtain adequate anatomic or hemodynamic data for safe and effective procedural conduct when angiograms can only be performed through a microcatheter. Lee and colleagues[45] evaluated 35 pediatric patients who underwent transradial neuroangiography with no cases of technical failure. The main differences between transfemoral and transradial CDA were increased radiation dose (mGy) and dose area product (μGy m^2) in the transradial group, as well as increased fluoroscopy time and total examination time. These disadvantages of TRCA are a major concern in the pediatric population, particularly in longer procedures that carry an expectation of high radiation exposure because of long fluoroscopy times and numerous DSA runs. Moreover, complications from the TRCA approach in children include radial artery stenosis, puncture-site hematoma, and thrombotic occlusion.[45] Another multicenter pediatric study showed that radial artery vasospasm can occur in up to 13% of cases and require femoral conversion in 8% of cases.[55] The distal trans-radial (snuffbox) approach was studied in a mixed population of teenagers and adults. Using this technique, selective catheterization was successful for 91% of vessels, with no radial artery occlusion reported. Although this technique seems promising, it lacks validation in younger children.[56–58] A general statement from the Task Force members of the Society of Neurointerventional Surgery Pediatric Committee, did not recommend radial access in children unless specific contraindications such as severe aortic coarctation or bilateral femoral artery occlusion are present.[59]

In the early neonatal period, umbilical arterial access can be employed. In these patients, who are usually being treated for high-flow intracranial arteriovenous shunts, the diameter of the femoral artery is further reduced by arterial steal from the systemic circulation, with a high risk of vasospasm and limb ischemia. An umbilical arterial catheter placed at birth can be exchanged for a vascular sheath and/or angiographic catheter, through which diagnostic and interventional procedures can be performed. In a recent study on 7 consecutive neonates, all neuroangiographic procedures performed through an umbilical arterial catheter were successful and without complications, including multiple procedures in 5 of the 7 patients.[60]

Pediatric neuroangiography is performed under systemic heparinization in most instances. This is more important for smaller children where the risks of access artery thrombosis and cerebral thromboembolic complications are higher. The operator might choose to give a reduced dose of systemic heparin in certain instances such as in the case of hyperacute intracranial hemorrhage or ongoing intracranial surgery, particularly in the setting of short diagnostic procedures. In children who are taking antiplatelet agents, it is usually preferable to continue those medications without interruption since these medications do not typically interfere with access-site management and protect against catheterization-related cerebral thromboembolism. Heparinized flush lines are required for all catheter systems. In infants, it is important to be cognizant of fluid volumes and heparin doses administered through flush lines.

Radiation dose-reducing techniques are an important aspect of pediatric CDA. Most modern clinical neuroangiography systems have reduced exposure settings for fluoroscopy and DSA. The benefits of radiation dose-reducing measures must be judiciously balanced against any tradeoffs in image quality that can lead to diagnostic errors or compromise image guidance during therapeutic neuroendovascular procedures.[61] The pediatric neurointerventionalist should do everything possible to decrease the patient's exposure to ionizing radiation during the procedure, including having the child as far away from the x-ray source (located below the table), placing the source to image distance (SID) detector as close to the patient as possible, maximizing collimation, minimizing fluoroscopy time, lowering the fluoroscopy dose settings when possible and using variable frame rates for DSA tailored to the pathology under investigation. Every center that performs pediatric neuroangiography must have an audit mechanism for assessing individual case radiation exposures, as well as trends over time.

In small children, particularly neonates with high output cardiac failure and renal insufficiency, specific efforts to limit the volume of contrast media administered during CDA should be made to mitigate risks of cardiac volume overload, pulmonary edema, and procedure-related renal injury. Total contrast volumes can be reduced by using 1:3 or 1:2 dilution of contrast media for test injections. Aspirating residual contrast media from the dead space of angiographic catheters after each DSA run may also help to reduce unnecessary contrast administration. Although early reports suggested a maximal contrast media to avoid nephropathy, there is limited evidence to support this practice and recent studies have confirmed the safety of using as much as 6 mL/kg of contrast media for pediatric catheterization procedures.[62] Nonetheless, it is important to keep track of total contrast volumes particularly in smaller children. Power injectors may be used for obtaining DSA runs, with age-modified rates and volumes, but many operators prefer hand syringe injections that allow real-time tactile and visual feedback. Moreover, there is a theoretic possibility that power injector use may increase the risk of cerebral microemboli due to air bubbles and other insoluble materials.[63]

Meticulous technique is the cornerstone of neuroangiography. This includes catheter and guidewire handling, but also ensuring that flush bags, lines, syringes, power injectors, and catheter dead spaces are clear of air, clot, cloth/gauze fibers, precipitated contrast media residue, and other foreign particulate matter. The outer surfaces of catheters and guidewires should be regularly wiped with moist sponges that have a fiber-free composition. Pressure bags to arterial systems should be carefully monitored to avoid air emboli, which can cause devastating strokes. Stagnant blood must be restricted from the interior and luer-lock recesses of syringes and catheters. While performing the CDA procedure, the operator should be attentive, and distractions should be limited. Brief lapses in attention can lead to serious and irreversible mishaps.

A typical neuroangiographic examination may include selective catheterization and multiprojection DSA interrogation of 5 or 6 distinct vessels. DSA series or sequences are usually obtained in standard projections for the internal carotid arteries, external carotid arteries, and vertebral arteries. In addition, specialized projections might be obtained depending on the angiographic findings and questions at hand. In some instances, such as postoperative angiography, the examination may be highly tailored to address the technical success of surgery and a 1 or 2 vessel examination might be sufficient. Superselective microcatheterization of high order branches, particularly intracranial branches, is not a routine part of diagnostic CDA, but in certain instances diagnostic value may be added. Superselective microcatheter angiography may be helpful to reveal elusive slow flow patterns in the setting of traumatic vessel injuries, or to render a discrete hemorrhagic focus within a complex AVM more conspicuous.

3D rotational angiography is increasingly becoming a valuable addition to pediatric neuroangiography. This technique brings together the superior spatial and temporal resolution of CDA and allows display of the image volume in infinite number projections which do not need to be specified prior to image acquisition. A time-resolved component is added to this in 4D rotational angiography, so that all angiographic phases can be evaluated at different chosen projections. Reconstruction of the image volume and fusion with MRI sequences enable detailed multi-modal cross-sectional evaluation of individual arterial territories.[64] Notably, factory settings for radiation dose from rotational angiographic sequences can be reduced several-fold for pediatric neuroangiography, while maintaining adequate image quality for interpretation.[65]

Postoperative Care

Hemostasis can be safely and effectively achieved by non-occlusive manual compression in most children. Recommendations after the procedure include bed rest with the access leg straight and head of bed flat for 4 hours once the sheath has been removed and hemostasis has been established.[43] During this time, the access site and distal circulation are monitored closely. Younger or developmentally delayed children usually require sedation to comply with the prescribed period of bedrest. The patient's neurologic status should be closely monitored to the extent that sedation permits, and a complete neurologic examination should be performed when sedation is discontinued. Elective CDA is most often performed on an outpatient basis with same day discharge. Most children undergoing outpatient CDA can return to activity the following day. Although unusual to occur, the access site and limb must be monitored for bleeding or swelling over the next few days. Pain at the site persisting for more than 24 to 48 hours, with or without swelling or bruising, must be investigated with Doppler sonography to exclude pseudoaneurysm formation.

SPINAL CATHETER-DIRECTED ANGIOGRAPHY
Indications

Spinal CDA involves a detailed evaluation of the vasculature of the spinal cord, vertebrae, and paraspinal soft tissues. Pediatric spinal CDA is the gold standard neuroimaging study for a wide range of spinal vascular abnormalities. It is also utilized for investigation of traumatic and nontraumatic spinal hemorrhage and to perform preoperative vascular mapping studies for children undergoing complex spinal, paraspinal, or mediastinal surgery.

Patients presenting with acute spinal cord infarction are typically diagnosed and followed with MRI. In most cases the diagnosis can be established by a combination of clinical and MRI findings however in some cases spinal CDA can be helpful for diagnosis and clinical decsion making. Spinal CDA is a powerful tool to diagnose spinal vascular malformations in children and to plan therapeutic strategies. Spinal vascular malformations are discussed in detail in a Ali Shaibani, MD and Anas Al-Smadi's article, "Pediatric Spinal Vascular Abnormalities: Overview, Diagnosis, and Management," in this issue. In addition, spinal vascular malformations, classified by location (i.e., intramedullary, perimedullary, radicular, and extradural) and flow pattern (i.e., high-flow AV

Airway management		Radiation protection	
▶ GA ▶ Paralytic ▶ Discuss frequent breath-holds		▶ Grids in or out ▶ Select pediatric protocol	
Non-invasive monitoring devices		**Heparin**	
▶ Blood pressure cuff ▶ O2 saturation probe ▶ EKG leads ▶ Temperature probe ▶ Twitch monitor	*Ensure devices are accessible and do not obscure catheter visualization	▶ Bolus IV dose after access ▶ Dose for saline flush bags ▶ Protamine availability	
Invasive monitoring devices		**Recovery plan**	
▶ Arterial line ▶ Foley	*Not routinely indicated for elective DCA	▶ Disposition ▶ Immobilization plan: for example, ▶ exmedetomidine	
▶ Antibiotics	*Not indicated	Any other special concerns	

DCA, diagnostic cerebral angiography ; EKG, electrocardiogram; GA, general anesthesia.

Fig. 1. SNIS Pediatric Committee pre-procedure checklist for DCA including airway management (e.g., general anesthesia, paralysis, discussion of frequent breath-holds), radiation protection (e.g., grids in or out), non-invasive monitoring devices (blood pressure cuff and telemetry monitors, ensuring that devices do not obscure visualization of catheter), heparin (e.g., bolus IV dose after access, dose for saline flush bags, protamine availability), invasive monitoring devices if needed, and recovery plan.

shunts, low-flow AV shunts, and no AV shunts), in recent and less ambiguous classification system proposed by Gailloud et, al. Three types of spinal vascular malformations occur in the pediatric population: 1) high-flow perimedullary fistulas, 2) spinal AVMs, and 3) spinal extradural AV fistulas. This corresponds to the commonly used Takai classification types IV, II/III, and V, respectively. Dural AV fistulas, a common vascular malformation in adults (acquired, not congenital), have not been described in the pediatric population to date.[53] Following treatment, spinal vascular malformations can be adequately followed up with MRI, although more complex and growing lesions could require spinal CDA for long-term follow up.

Spinal CDA can aid in vascular mapping for children undergoing surgery involving the posterior mediastinum (ie, neuroblastoma) or paraspinal masses. Historically, preoperative spinal CDA studies were performed to investigate the spinal cord circulation between T4 and L2 before corrective scoliosis surgery.[66] Nordin and colleagues[29] describe how arterial mapping before removing posterior mediastinal masses can help prevent damage to major radiculomedullary arteries (2013). Clark and colleagues suggested that routine preoperative spinal CDA may help prevent complications after resection of posterior paraspinal thoracic tumors in children. The authors performed

spinal CDA in 14 patients, which identified complicated anatomy that posed a risk of iatrogenic spinal vascular complications, such as Artery of Adamkiewicz.[67–70] For pediatric patients who are diagnosed with primary bone tumors, such as aneurysmal bone cysts, or secondary bone tumors that need to be resected, spinal CDA serves as a vascular mapping tool, and preoperative embolization can be performed at the same time.

Special Considerations for Pediatric Spinal Catheter-directed Angiography

Thorough knowledge of the anatomy of the spinal vasculature and common anatomic variants is needed to tailor a spinal angiographic examination to the indication, in order to avoid diagnostic failure by omission. Preoperative evaluation, procedural set-up, and intra-procedural precautions are largely similar to what has been discussed previously in this study for cerebral CDA. Some considerations specific to performing spinal CDA are addressed here:

- Use of a large monitor can help reduce radiation dose and increase visibility given the small size of the spinal vessels in children.
- Spinal angiography in small children is often limited by the small diameter of the descending thoracic aorta. As such, a number of catheter-

tip shapes should be available, including pigtail catheters, reverse curve catheters (eg, Mikaelsson, Sos Omni and Simmons 1), angled-tip catheters (eg, vertebral, multipurpose, DAV, and Berestein) and double angle catheters (eg, Cobra 2, Cobra 3, Renal double curve).

- There are no reports of TRCA or umbilical artery access for the performance of spinal angiography (SA) in the pediatric population.
- To definitively exclude vascular pathology, non-selective angiography is insufficient. A complete spinal angiographic examination includes selective angiography of all segmental arteries supplying the anatomic region of interest. If a discrete region of interest cannot be specified, a complete spinal angiogram may include selective angiograms of all posterior intercostal arteries, all lumbar arteries, the common iliac arteries, the internal iliac arteries, the median sacral artery, the vertebral arteries, the common carotid arteries, the external carotid arteries, the vertebral arteries, and the subclavian arteries. Selective angiograms of the thyrocervical and costocervical trunks may be needed depending on the findings of subclavian artery angiography.
- Weight based glucagon administration is recommended to decrease bowel peristalsis.
- Neuromuscular blockade (paralysis) monitored with a peripheral nerve stimulator and strict attention to flattening of the capnography trace is recommended.
- A radiopaque ruler should be placed under the patient to one side of the spine and secured to the table. This will allow for proper vessel identification, avoid redundant vessel injections, and ensure all vessels are injected to prevent missing vessels containing significant pathology.
- Single plane imaging in the frontal projection, with an angiographic frame rate of 1 to 2 frame per second should be used for each angiographic sequence. Lateral projection angiography and higher frame rates should be used selectively for angiographic characterization of significant pathology. In general, the use of a power injector should be avoided due to increased procedural duration and time under anesthesia, increased risk of nondiagnostic "bust" runs that cause unnecessary contrast administration and radiation exposure and increased risk of microemboli.
- Given the unusually large number of vessels catheterized and correspondingly large number of angiographic sequences obtained during spinal CDA, patient contrast dose and

exposure to radiation can be dangerously high. With proper training, adequate planning and good technique, radiation exposure, and contrast dose can be limited to a safe range. If necessary, spinal CDA can be staged to avoid excess radiation exposure and contrast administration. Good technique, to avoid extra GA session, is highly recommended. If pre-procedural outpatient hydration cannot be reliably ensured in children undergoing elective spinal CDA, advanced admission to the hospital for supplemental hydration with intravenous fluids should be considered.

Complications of Catheter-directed Angiography in Children

Historical studies on the safety of catheter angiography from the 1980s and 1990s showed that cerebral thromboembolic events and persistent neurologic deficits occurred in 0.5% of patients.[71,72] In one study that followed 3731 consecutive angiograms in infants and children, there were 14 cases of iatrogenic cerebral embolization (0.4% of all angiographic examinations).[71] In a cohort of 152 pediatric patients with moyamoya arteriopathies, only one patient had speech impairment after the procedure, which subsided within 12 hours.[73] Other subsequent studies reported very low[74] or no intra-procedural cerebral thromboembolic events or iatrogenic vessel injuries,[32,75,76] even in children younger than 3 years of age[75]; moreover, most neurologic events in more recent studies did not generate permanent sequelae.[77] Of note, an increased risk of neurologic complications was associated with emergency procedures and cases of intracerebral hemorrhage or subarachnoid hemorrhage.[77] While rare, fatal complications of pediatric cerebral angiography have been reported.[76] A lower incidence of adverse events in pediatric cerebral angiography compared to adults is explained by fewer risk factors for stroke in children and less tortuous blood vessels.[48] Nevertheless, subclinical complications such as silent infarctions detected by diffusion-weighted brain MRI after CDA have been reported, especially in patients with a history of arteriopathy.[78] Such infarctions vary in size but most are punctate and are likely related to microemboli (air bubbles or thrombus). Studies show that microembolic infarctions correlate with surrogate measures of catheter dwell time and the extent of catheter manipulation within the cervicocerebral vessels such as the amount of contrast media used and procedural fluoroscopy time.[79–81]

Lauzier and colleagues retrospectively assessed the rate of cerebral CDA complications in a sample of 390 children undergoing a total of 587 cerebral CDA procedures in a large academic medical center. They documented neurologic complications in 1.9% of the procedures and non-neurological complications in 4.8%, for a total complication rate of 6.5%. Significant complications included thalamic infarction in a 15 year old boy with a recent history of subarachnoid hemorrhage and contrast-related anaphylaxis; with only one patient developing permanent sequelae. Complications seemed to be associated with a history of ischemic stroke, hypertension, and female sex, and occurred less when the access site was femoral.[48]

A study involving 394 pediatric patients who underwent 697 neuroendovascular procedures between 2006 and 2013 (429 diagnostic cerebral CDA and 268 therapeutic embolizations) demonstrated only 3 non-neurological complications in the diagnostic group, including mild contrast allergy and hair loss. Interestingly, this cohort included more than 20 infants in the diagnostic subgroup, 179 children between 1 and 10 years of age, and 227 children older than 10 years. After multivariate logistic regression analysis, age was not considered a significant risk factor for periprocedural complications.[32]

Allergic reactions to intravenous contrast agents in children are uncommon and have been reported in less than 0.2% of procedures. Most of them are not severe, including skin manifestations such as hives and urticaria rash; bronchospasm and anaphylaxis are even rarer.

Contrast-induced nephropathy is usually dose dependent in children with renal disease. With adequate procedural planning and preparation, pediatric cerebral and spinal CDA can usually be achieved without excessive contrast media.

Children are susceptible to stochastic radiation effects. Therefore, the risk of long-term complications from radiation use must be acknowledged. There is wide variability in reported radiation doses for pediatric cerebral angiography, ranging between 350 and 4100 mGy.[82] This could be explained by differences in technique and operator dependency. Recommendations to reduce radiation dose in children include using biplane systems with direct flat-panel detectors, optimizing dose settings, removing scatter grids when possible, minimizing air gap and angulation, and monitoring radiation doses during and after the procedure. When available, 3D and 4D rotational angiography can enhance depiction of anatomic structures, especially their spatial relationships, but they generally utilize higher radiation doses than 2D angiography unless modified specifically for use in pediatric practice.

The concept of "radiation awareness" has reduced unnecessary radiation exposure without losing the quality of imaging studies. Schneider and colleagues implemented several strategies to minimize radiation exposure in a cohort of 31 pediatric patients undergoing DCA; the most common conditions in this cohort were moyamoya vasculopathy and AVMs. They focused on the proper recording of radiation parameters for each procedure, including angiography technique, fluoroscopy time, and measurements related to air kerma (reference air kerma in mGy and kerma-area product in $\mu Gym2$), comparing the methods over four years.[72] General improvements in protocols involved decreasing the DSA frame rate by using combined fixed and combined frame rates and decreasing the number of vessels catheterized. A significant achievement was to reduce the median total fluoroscopy time from 6.0 to 2.5 minutes per procedure; positive results were also related to the reduction of radiation dose with lower values or air kerma (by 78.6%) and kerma-area product (by 77.4%). Other approaches to radiation reduction include engaging in conversations with manufacturers and PACS systems to obtain systematic records of parameters of interest that can be easily analyzed in the future.[72]

Gautam and colleagues conducted a retrospective study to evaluate the safety of pediatric spinal CDA in 36 procedures (diagnostic and therapeutic) conducted in 27 children. They did not find any neurologic or non-neurological complications in their cohort. Additionally, they could perform such procedures with low radiation exposure.[29] In general, spinal CDA has shown fewer complications than cerebral CDA, as the spinal cord has more collateral flow networks and is less sensitive to ischemia than the brain.[83]

Goethe and colleagues[83] conducted a systematic review of studies describing pediatric spinal CDA. Of the 87 pediatric patients who underwent diagnostic or therapeutic spinal CDA, there were only 2 patients who had complications: one with scrotal swelling due to groin hematoma and one with procedure-related subarachnoid hemorrhage. The authors reported their experience with 6 cases at a tertiary pediatric hospital over 11 years. Indications included spontaneous thoracic epidural hematoma, AVM, AVF, AVF with concomitant flow-related aneurysm, spinal cord infarction, and lumbar spinal meningioma with associated subarachnoid hemorrhage and subdural hematoma. In that study, spinal CDA detected the presence and location of feeding and draining vessels and flow-related aneurysms initially missed by MRI.

CLINICS CARE POINTS

- Diagnostic cerebral angiography (DCA) is superior to non-invasive imaging methods for detecting small aneurysms and evaluating CNS vasculitis. Complications from pediatric catheter angiography are generally low, with studies reporting neurological complications in less than 2% of procedures.

- Allergic reactions to contrast agents are uncommon in pediatric patients, and measures like hydration and dilution can mitigate the risk of contrast-induced nephropathy.

- It is crucial to implement strategies to minimize radiation exposure in pediatric patients due to their increased sensitivity to stochastic effects.

- Use of pediatric-specific protocols and techniques, such as biplane systems and optimized dose settings, can significantly reduce radiation doses.

- Thromboembolic events are rare, with historical data showing rates as low as 0.4%.

REFERENCES

1. Poser CM, Taveras JM. Clinical aspects of cerebral angiography in children. Pediatrics 1955;16(1):73–80.
2. Gurdjian ES, Hardy WG, Lindner DW, et al. Four-vessel angiography: experiences with three hundred consecutive cases. Clin Neurosurg 1964;10:251–74.
3. Brandt S, Brunner S, Westergaard-Nielsen V. Arteriographic studies in children with cerebral palsy. Acta Paediatr 1961;50:586–94.
4. Frantzen E, Jacobsen HH, Therkelsen J. Cerebral artery occlusions in children due to trauma to the head and neck. A report of 6 cases verified by cerebral angiography. Neurology 1961;11:695–700.
5. Picaza JA. Cerebral angiography in children; an anatomoclinical evaluation. J Neurosurg 1952;9(3):235–44.
6. Nader S, Alexander V, Ouyang B, et al. Current utility of diagnostic catheter cerebral angiography. J Stroke Cerebrovasc Dis 2014;23(3):e145–50.
7. Tadanori T. Pediatric neuroimaging in pre-CT era: back to the future. Childs Nerv Syst 2023;39(10):2595–604.
8. Scott M, Murtagh F, Lapayowker M, et al. Vertebral basilar and carotid angiography by injection of brachial artery. Am J Roentgenol Radium Ther Nucl Med 1963;90:546–53.
9. Boulos RS, Gilroy J, Meyer JS. Technique of cerebral angiography in children. Am J Roentgenol Radium Ther Nucl Med 1967;101(1):121–7.
10. Carrea R, Schuster G. Observations about retrograde brachial cerebral angiography in children

(analysis of 100 aortographies and 28 cerebral angiographies via the brachial artery). Acta Neurochir 1961;9:456–67.
11. Siqueira EB, Amador LV. Normal angiographic configuration of carotid siphon in the pediatric patient. J Neurosurg 1964;21:216–8.
12. Faris AA, Guth C, Youmans RA, et al. Internal carotid artery occlusion in children; diagnosis by arteriography. Am J Dis Child 1964;107:188–92.
13. Francisco CB, Davidson KC, Youngstrom KA, et al. Transfemoral cervicocephalic angiography in children. Pediatrics 1964;33:119–22.
14. Takaku A, Suzuki J. Cerebral angiography in children and adults with mental retardation. I. Control series. Dev Med Child Neurol 1972;14(6):756–65.
15. Takaku A, Suzuki J. Cerebral angiography in children and adults with mental retardation. II. Mentally retarded group. Dev Med Child Neurol 1972;14(6):766–82.
16. Bentson JR, Wilson GH. Cerebral angiography: normal anatomy and variations in adults and children. Semin Roentgenol 1971;6(1):17–33.
17. Numaguchi Y, Hoffman JC, Sones PJ. Femoral percutaneous catheterization in infants and small children for cerebral angiography. Radiology 1975;116(02):451.
18. Cerullo LJ, Rajakulasingam K, Raimondi AJ. Femoral-cerebral angiography in infants and children. Analysis and comparison with direct puncture/retrograde brachial technique. Childs Brain 1980;6(1):1–12.
19. Valk J. Angiography with metrizamide in neuroradiological examinations. Diagn Imag 1979;48(4):199–204.
20. Obenchain TG, Clark R, Hanafee W, et al. Complication rate of selective cerebral angiography in infants and children. A comparison with a similar adult series. Radiology 1970;95(3):669–73.
21. Harrington GJ, Cameron A. An easy technique for cerebral angiography in infants and children. Australas Radiol 1969;13(3):284–6.
22. Newton TH, Gooding CA. Catheter techniques in pediatric cerebral angiography. Am J Roentgenol Radium Ther Nucl Med 1968;104(1):63–5.
23. Takahashi M, Kawanami H. Catheter cerebral angiography in children: analysis of 67 examinations. Clin Radiol 1971;22(3):308–11.
24. Raimondi AJ, Di Rocco C. The physiopathogenetic basis for the angiographic diagnosis of bacterial infections of the brain and its coverings in children. II. Cerebritis and brain abscess. Childs Brain 1979;5(4):398–407.
25. Carrillo R. Cerebral angiography and evaluation of functional status of shunts in hydrocephalic children. Childs Brain 1977;3(4):238–48.
26. Parvey LS, Gerald B. Arteriographic diagnosis of brain death in children. Pediatr Radiol 1976;4(2):79–82.

27. Di Chiro G. Development of spinal cord angiography. Acta Radiol Diagn 1972;13(0):767–70.

28. Perry B. Spinal vascular malformations: an historical perspective. Neurosurg Focus 2006;21(6):E11.

29. Gautam Ayushi, Motaghi Mina, Gailloud Philippe. Safety of diagnostic spinal angiography in children. J Neurointerv Surg 2021;13(4):390–4. Doi:10.1136/neurintsurg-2020-015906.

30. Vogelsang H. Neuroradiological diagnosis of intra-dural spinal angiomas in children. Dev Med Child Neurol 1974;16(1):81–5.

31. Ayushi G, Mina M, Philippe G. Safety of diagnostic spinal angiography in children. J Neurointerventional Surg 2021;13(4):390–4.

32. Lin N, Smith ER, Michael SR, et al. Safety of neuro-angiography and embolization in children: complication analysis of 697 consecutive procedures in 394 patients. J Neurosurg Pediatr 2015;16(4):432–8.

33. Wolfe TJ, Hussain SI, Lynch JR, et al. Pediatric cerebral angiography: analysis of utilization and findings. Pediatr Neurol 2009;40(2):98–101.

34. Keisuke I, Mitsuo I, Kobayashi H, et al. Temporal profile of angiographical stages of moyamoya disease: when does moyamoya disease progress? Neurol Res 2003;25(4):405–10.

35. Ganesan V, Savvy L, Chong WK, et al. Conventional cerebral angiography in children with ischemic stroke. Pediatr Neurol 1999;20(1):38–42.

36. Sabri A, Robbs JV, Maharajh J, et al. Descriptive retrospective analysis of the diagnostic yield and morbidity of four vessel catheter-directed cerebral angiography and multidetector computed tomographic angiography (MDCTA) performed at Inkosi Albert Luthuli Central Hospital (IALCH). Eur J Radiol 2011;80(2):498–501.

37. Alexander C F, Ashley R, Singh V. Primary intraventricular hemorrhage: yield of diagnostic angiography and clinical outcome. Neurocritical Care 2008;8(3):330–6.

38. Zhu XL, Chan MS, Poon WS. Spontaneous intracranial hemorrhage: which patients need diagnostic cerebral angiography? A prospective study of 206 cases and review of the literature. Stroke 1997;28(7):1406–9.

39. Despina E, Tim C, Dawn S, et al. Investigation of childhood central nervous system vasculitis: magnetic resonance angiography versus catheter cerebral angiography. Dev Med Child Neurol 2010;52(9):863–7.

40. Michael F, Heather G, Roth S, et al. Angiographic analysis of ophthalmic artery flow direction in children undergoing chemosurgery for retinoblastoma compared to age-matched controls. Intervent Neuroradiol 2023. https://doi.org/10.1177/15910199231174538. 15910199231174538.

41. Heran Manraj KS, Abruzzo Todd A. Diagnostic cerebral angiography and the Wada test in pediatric patients. Tech Vasc Intervent Radiol 2011;14(1):42–9.

42. Ellis MJ, Kulkarni AV, Drake JM, et al. Intraoperative angiography during microsurgical removal of arteriovenous malformations in children. J Neurosurg Pediatr 2010;6(5):435–43.

43. Chaudhary N, Lucas E, Martinez M, et al. Pediatric diagnostic cerebral angiography: practice recommendations from the SNIS Pediatric Committee. J Neurointerventional Surg 2021;13(8):762–6.

44. Nadine M, Robertson F, Ganesan V. Towards evidence based medicine for paediatricians. Question 2: neurological complications of diagnostic cerebral catheter angiography in children. Arch Dis Child 2014;99(5):483–5.

45. Lee SB, Jin CY, Soo-Hyun K, et al. Transradial cerebral angiography: is it feasible and safe for children? Cardiovasc Intervent Radiol 2022;45(4):504–9.

46. Schneider T, Emily W, Pearl Monica S. Analysis of radiation doses incurred during diagnostic cerebral angiography after the implementation of dose reduction strategies. J Neurointerventional Surg 2017;9(4):384–8.

47. Choi JW, Moon WJ. Gadolinium deposition in the brain: current updates. Korean J Radiol 2019 Jan;20(1):134–47.

48. Lauzier DC, Osbun JW, Chatterjee AR, et al. Safety of pediatric cerebral angiography. J Neurosurg Pediatr 2021 Nov 5;29(2):192–9.

49. Peng Ke, Jian Li, Fu-Hai Ji, et al. Dexmedetomidine compared with propofol for pediatric sedation during cerebral angiography. J Res Med Sci 2014;19(6):549–54.

50. Zuckerman Scott L, Bhatia R, Crystiana T, et al. Prospective series of two hours supine rest after 4fr sheath-based diagnostic cerebral angiography: Outcomes, productivity and cost. Intervent Neuroradiol 2015;21(1):114–9.

51. Philippe G. Spinal vascular malformations: angiographic evaluation and endovascular management. Handb Clin Neurol 2021;176:267–304.

52. Andraska EA, Jackson T, Chen H, et al. Natural history of iatrogenic pediatric femoral artery injury. Ann Vasc Surg 2017 Jul;42:205–13.

53. Alshehri H, Dmytriw AA, Bhatia K, et al. Transradial neuroendovascular procedures in adolescents: initial single-center experience. AJNR Am J Neuroradiol 2021 Aug;42(8):1492–6.

54. Al Saiegh F, Chalouhi N, Sweid A, et al. Intra-arterial chemotherapy for retinoblastoma via the transradial route: technique, feasibility, and case series. Clin Neurol Neurosurg 2020 Jul;194:105824.

55. Srinivasan VM, Hadley Caroline C, Marc P, et al. Feasibility and safety of transradial access for pediatric neurointerventions. J Neurointerventional Surg 2020;12(9):893–6.

56. Shoji S, Hasegawa H, Tomoyoshi O, et al. Safety and feasibility of the distal transradial approach: a novel technique for diagnostic cerebral angiography. Intervent Neuroradiol 2020;26(6):713–8.

57. Burrows PE, Benson LN, Williams WG, et al. Iliofemoral arterial complications of balloon angioplasty for systemic obstructions in infants and children. Circulation 1990;82(5):1697–704.

58. Chen K, Demi D, Orbach DB, et al. Low profile sheaths in pediatric neurointervention: a multicenter experience. J Neurointerventional Surg 2022;14(11):1135–8.

59. Chaudhary N, Elijovich L, Martinez M, et al. alPediatric diagnostic cerebral angiography: practice recommendations from the SNIS Pediatric CommitteeJournal of NeuroInterventional Surgery, 13, 2021. p. 762–6.

60. Kappel Ari D, Orbach DB. Standard umbilical artery catheters used as diagnostic and neurointerventional guide catheters in the treatment of neonatal cerebrovascular malformations. J Neurointerventional Surg 2023;15(4):375–9.

61. Strauss KJ, Racadio JM, Abruzzo TA, et al. Comparison of pediatric radiation dose and vessel visibility on angiographic systems using piglets as a surrogate: antiscatter grid removal vs. lower detector air kerma settings with a grid - a preclinical investigation. J Appl Clin Med Phys 2015 Sep 8;16(5):408–17. PMID: 26699297; PMCID: PMC5690159.

62. Senthilnathan S, Gauvreau K, Marshall AC, et al. Contrast administration in pediatric cardiac catheterization: dose and adverse events. Cathet Cardiovasc Interv 2009 May 1;73(6):814–20. PMID: 19133670; PMCID: PMC7199104.

63. Cruz AS, Khattar NK, Weiner GM, et al. Preventing air microembolism in cerebral angiography: a JNIS fellow's perspective. J Neurointerventional Surg 2024 Mar 14;16(4):331–2. PMID: 38485204.

64. Muthusami P, Shkumat N, Rea V, et al. CT reconstruction and MRI fusion of 3D rotational angiography in the evaluation of pediatric cerebrovascular lesions. Neuroradiology 2017 Jun;59(6):625–33.

65. Shkumat NA, Shroff MM, Muthusami P. Radiation dosimetry of 3D rotational neuroangiography and 2D-DSA in children. AJNR Am J Neuroradiol 2018 Apr;39(4):727–33.

66. Hilal SK, Keim HA. Selective spinal angiography in adolescent scoliosis. Radiology 1972;102(2):349–59.

67. Clark RA, Jacobson Jillian C, Murphy Joseph T. Preoperative spinal angiography decreases risk of spinal ischemia in pediatric posterior thoracic tumor resection. Pediatr Surg Int 2022;38(10):1427–34.

68. Yadav N, Hima P, Baburao KG. Spinal cord infarction: clinical and radiological features. J Stroke Cerebrovasc Dis 2018;27(10):2810–21.

69. Abdel R, Ahmed AK, Hortensia A, et al. Imaging spectrum of CNS vasculitis. Radiographics 2014;34(4):873–94.

70. Philippe G. Diagnostic inefficiency of nonselective spinal angiography (Flush Aortography) in the evaluation of the normal and pathological spinal vasculature. Curr Probl Diagn Radiol 2016;45(3):180–4.

71. Pettersson H, Fitz CR, Harwood-Nash DC, et al. Iatrogenic embolization: complication of pediatric cerebral angiography. AJNR Am J Neuroradiol 1981;2(4):357–61.

72. Heiserman JE, Dean BL, Hodak JA, et al. Neurologic complications of cerebral angiography. AJNR Am J Neuroradiol 1994;15(8):1401–7 [discussion 1408-1411].

73. Robertson RL, Chavali RV, Robson CD, et al. Neurologic complications of cerebral angiography in childhood moyamoya syndrome. Pediatr Radiol 1998;28(11):824–9.

74. Thiex R, Norbash AM, Frerichs KU. The safety of dedicated-team catheter-based diagnostic cerebral angiography in the era of advanced noninvasive imaging. AJNR Am J Neuroradiol 2010;31(2):230–4.

75. Hoffman Caitlin E, Alejandro S, Lauren R, et al. Complications of cerebral angiography in children younger than 3 years of age. J Neurosurg Pediatr 2014;13(4):414–9.

76. Burger Ingrid M, Murphy Kieran J, Jordan Lori C, et al. Safety of cerebral digital subtraction angiography in children: complication rate analysis in 241 consecutive diagnostic angiograms. Stroke 2006;37(10):2535–9.

77. Dawkins AA, Evans AL, Wattam J, et al. Complications of cerebral angiography: a prospective analysis of 2,924 consecutive procedures. Neuroradiology 2007;49(9):753–9.

78. Alghamdi I, Dmytriw AA, Amirabadi A, et al. Clinical and subclinical microemboli following neuroangiography in children. J Neurointerventional Surg 2023. https://doi.org/10.1136/jnis-2023-020686.

79. Bendszus M, Koltzenburg M, Burger R, et al. Silent embolism in diagnostic cerebral angiography and neurointerventional procedures: a prospective study. Lancet 1999;354(9190):1594–7.

80. Bashir Q, Asim I, Anwar BA. Safety of diagnostic cerebral and spinal digital subtraction angiography in a developing country: a single-center experience. Interv Neurol 2018;7(1–2):99–109.

81. da Silva PSL, Kubo EY, Fonseca M, et al. Severe liver and renal injuries following cerebral angiography: late life-threatening complications of nonionic contrast medium administration. Childs Nerv Syst 2016;32(4):733–7.

82. Struelens L, Vanhavere F, Bosmans H, et al. Skin dose measurements on patients for diagnostic and interventional neuroradiology: a multicentre study. Radiat Protect Dosim 2005;114(1–3):143–6.

83. Eric G, LoPresti MA, Kan P, et al. The role of spinal angiography in the evaluation and treatment of pediatric spinal vascular pathology: a case series and systematic review. Childs Nerv Syst 2020;36(2):325–32.

Neurovascular Malformations in the Fetus and Neonate

Ayman M. Qureshi, MBChB, MMed, FRCR[a,b,*],
Adam Rennie, MBBS, BMSc, FRCR[a,b,c],
Fergus Robertson, MD, MA, MRCP, FRCR[a,b,c]

KEYWORDS

- Vein of Galen malformation • Non-Galenic choroidal arteriovenous fistula • Dural sinus malformation
- Pial arteriovenous fistula • Embolization

KEY POINTS

- Vein of Galen malformations (VOGMs) are the most common congenital neurovascular malformation and are a type of arteriovenous fistula involving the midline primitive choroidal venous circulation.
- Complications of VOGM, which may result in cardiopulmonary overload and brain injury, vary according to patient age, severity of arteriovenous shunting, and architecture of the venous outflow tract.
- Dural sinus malformations are characterized by massively dilated intracranial dural venous sinuses that may undergo variable degrees of thrombosis, and can acquire multifocal arteriovenous shunts.
- Pial arteriovenous fistulae are high-flow shunts representing direct arterial to venous communication of pial blood vessels, with no definable nidus. Over half are associated with germline mutations.

INTRODUCTION

Neurovascular malformations developing in-utero children are rare. Notably, the common variety of cerebral (nidal) arteriovenous malformations that were once thought to be congenital are now believed to form postnatally in most cases and are rarely if ever detected prenatally. The congenital neurovascular malformations covered in this study have major clinical significance and are commonly found by prenatal ultrasound in the third trimester, with the majority comprising high-flow arteriovenous shunts. The high-flow nature of this group of lesions can lead to both neurologic and systemic consequences. The susceptibility of affected patients to right heart overload is one of the key clinical factors distinguishing fetal arteriovenous (AV) shunts from those seen in older children and adults. Three clinically significant neurovascular malformations are commonly recognized to develop in utero: vein of Galen malformations (VOGMs), dural sinus malformations (DSMs), and pial arteriovenous fistulas (PAVFs).[1] Non-Galenic choroidal AV fistulas (non-midline lesions), which are frequently misdiagnosed as VOGM (midline lesions), are embryologically and anatomically distinct from VOGM and PAVF but have overlapping clinical presentations. These former lesions, which comprise AV fistulas involving the choroidal veins in the choroid plexus of the lateral ventricles and in the

[a] Lysholm Department of Neuroradiology, National Hospital for Neurology & Neurosurgery, Queen Square, London WC1N 3BG; [b] National Hospital for Neurology & Neurosurgery, UCLH NHS Foundation Trust; [c] Great Ormond Street Hospital for Children NHS Foundation Trust
* Corresponding author. Lysholm Department of Neuroradiology, National Hospital for Neurology and Neurosurgery, 8 - 11 Queen Square, London, WC1N 3BG1.
E-mail address: aymanqm@yahoo.com

Neuroimag Clin N Am 34 (2024) 531–543
https://doi.org/10.1016/j.nic.2024.08.008
1052-5149/24/Crown Copyright © 2024 Published by Elsevier Inc. All rights reserved, including those for text and data mining, AI training, and similar technologies.

adjacent choroid fissure, will not be covered in this study. In this study, the authors discuss the pathology, imaging characteristics, and management of VOGM, DSM, and PAVF.

VEIN OF GALEN MALFORMATIONS

VOGMs are the most common congenital AV shunting lesions.[2] VOGMs are characterized by macrofistulous connections between choroidal, pericallosal, or collicular arteries and the embryonic precursor of the vein of Galen, the median prosencephalic vein of Markowski (MPVM), and/or its midline venous tributaries within the tela choroidea of the third ventricle.[3] The term "VOGM" is therefore a misnomer in the literal sense but has persisted and remains appropriate because the development of the vein of Galen is closely tied to the fate of the MPVM. The range of variant Galenic venous systems that form when normal development is interrupted by arterialization of the MPVM can be considered malformations of the vein of Galen, even though these variants are not the index malformation that initiated the aberrant developmental sequence.

Embryology

As the neural tube grows, the early supplying, peripherally located vascular network (the meninx primitiva), becomes insufficient, prompting invagination of portions of this vasculature (choroid) into the neural canal, allowing both a superficial and deep supply to the developing brain vesicles. The inner lumens of the tube and choroid eventually form the ventricles and choroid plexus, respectively. The metabolically active choroid plexus earns itself a dedicated blood supply. At 5 weeks gestation, the developing internal carotid artery and longitudinal neural system of vessels (the precursor to the vertebrobasilar system) sprout the supplying anterior choroidal, posterior choroidal, and collicular arteries.[4]

The draining venous system of the developing brain forms after the arteries. They can be divided into a superficial and deep system. The MPVM is the earliest vein to drain the deeply located choroid plexi, doing so via the falcine sinus to a developing interhemispheric sinus (future superior sagittal sinus). As the internal cerebral veins (ICVs) develop (draining the deep white matter, later developing basal ganglia, and portions of the diencephalon), they annex the drainage of the choroid plexus from the MPVM. The MPVM subsequently involutes, leaving only its most caudal portion into which the ICVs drain, forming the vein of Galen. This occurs by 11 weeks, typically corresponding to regression of the falcine

sinus, with vein of Galen drainage into the straight sinus.[3,5]

A VOGM results from abnormal AV shunting into the MPVM and/or its midline choroidal venous tributaries. The trigger or cause for this is unknown. Hypotheses include arterialization following venous thrombosis (in a manner similar to that described in the pathogenesis of dural AV fistulae[6]), or regional ischemia.[2] While broadly sporadic, genetic mutations have been described in a few cases and are believed to correspond to heritable vulnerability traits that interact with strategically timed and anatomically targeted injury factors capable of disrupting normal development at a stage of temporal vulnerability. Mutations associated with VOGM have been found in a diversity of genes that regulate normal vascular development including the Ephrin type-B receptor 4 and Ras GTPase-activating protein 1 (RASA1) genes (associated with Capillary Malformation—Arteriovenous Malformation/CM- AVM 1 & 2, respectively), activin A receptor like 1 (ACVRL1), and endoglin (ENG) genes (both described in hereditary hemorrhagic telangiectasia [HHT]).[7,8]

Arterial Supply

Arterial supply to a VOGM is typically through the anterior and posterior choroidal arteries (including subependymal branches) and the limbic arcade (via the anterior and posterior pericallosal arteries). Occasionally, thalamoperforating, middle cerebral artery, basilar circumflex, and dural arterial branches may be recruited.[9]

Three types of lesions are recognized, based on angioarchitecture[1]:

- *Choroidal type*: characterized by a complex network of arterialized choroidal veins in the cistern of the velum interpositum, creating a "nidus" of sorts, that drains into the MPVM. The multifocal choroidal AV shunt zone is located in the midline, distinguishing this malformation from its closely related cousin, the non-Galenic choroidal AV fistula. Choroidal-type VOGMs are reported to have a more aggressive neonatal clinical course presenting with heart failure.
- *Mural type*: consisting of a smaller number of feeding arteries that shunt directly into the wall of the MPVM in a macrofistulous manner.
- *Mixed type*: consisting of both choroidal-type and mural-type AV shunts (**Fig. 1**).

Venous Drainage

AV shunting into the MPVM and/or its choroidal venous tributaries prevents its involution, resulting

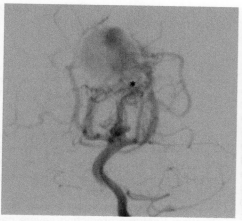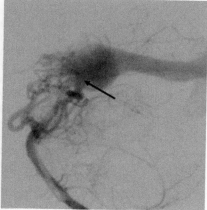

Fig. 1. Catheter-directed angiography in a neonate with antenatally diagnosed vein of Galen malformation (VOGM) presenting with heart failure showing a mixed type VOGM, with choroidal (*asterisk*) and fistulous (*black arrow*) components.

in persistence of the falcine sinus, which drains to the superior sagittal sinus. In most instances, the straight sinus is absent. The fate of the tributaries of the vein of Galen is debated. A previous theory was that there is no communication between the deep venous system of the brain (ICVs) and the VOGM.[1,9] While the basal vein of Rosenthal was never seen to communicate with the aneurysmal pouch in Raybaud's series,[3] the ICVs have been found to drain into the VOGM in up to one-third of patients.[10] The more common configuration is characterized by drainage of the ICVs to the thalamic and subsequently lateral mesencephalic veins to the superior petrosal sinus through the petrosal veins (resulting in the typical "epsilon appearance"). This may be present with or without drainage into the MPVM. It is important, albeit difficult, to look for these venous drainage patterns on cross-sectional imaging, given their clinical and treatment implications. Jugular bulb stenosis (also known as jugular bulb dysplasia) may be acquired in infants with VOGM. High-flow venopathy has been implicated as the underlying mechanism, though developmental processes have been cited as well. A few months after birth, the maturing cavernous sinuses (anterior venous confluences) begin to drain annex the drainage of the sylvian veins. This "cavernous capture" provides an alternate low-pressure route of venous drainage for the developing brain that would otherwise have to compete with the VOGM for venous drainage through the high-pressure posterior venous confluence. Failure of cavernous capture is particularly harmful to the developing brain in patients with jugular bulb stenosis where it often results in rapidly progressive venous congestive encephalopathy.

Clinical Features

The physiologic effects of AV shunting in VOGM predominantly impact the cardiac, pulmonary, and nervous systems, the former tending to manifest earlier.

Cardiac Effects

AV shunting increases right heart preload (volume overload) leading to pulmonary hypertension, which later increases right heart afterload (pressure overload). Right-sided heart failure occurs first and is followed by left heart failure. Large shunts can cause heart failure in utero, with secondary multisystem failure. Evidence of this on antenatal imaging indicates a poor prognosis.[11]

More often, cardiac failure develops and manifests after birth. Following delivery, exclusion of placental circulation rapidly increases blood flow through the VOGM, and the secondary increase in pulmonary blood flow increases the cardiac output manifold.[12–14] An aggressive clinical course can lead to multisystemic effects including renal failure, pulmonary failure, liver failure, and brain damage, and management of postnatal cardiac failure becomes paramount following delivery. Notably, cardiac failure and its complications may be mitigated or prevented altogether when the venous outflow tract of the VOGM is constricted enough to attenuate the pressure of shunted blood returning to the right heart. The important role that the venous outflow tract of the VOGM plays in the development of heart failure underlies the association of fetal and neonatal MRI biomarkers with an aggressive neonatal course.[15]

Neurologic Effects

Intracranial cerebral venous hypertension is the major driver behind neurologic deterioration in VOGM. Elevated venous pressure results from the large AV shunt but is exacerbated by jugular bulb stenosis.[16] A hydrovenous disorder occurs secondary to an impairment of transmedullary cerebrospinal fluid (CSF) absorption leading to interstitial edema and communicating hydrocephalus.[17,18] Age at presentation is influenced by the status of the jugular bulbs, cranial sutures, and availability of alternative cerebral venous drainage pathways including cavernous capture and its timing. For example, macrocrania occurs prior to closure of the cranial sutures, and, hydrocephalus may not develop in the setting of patulous jugular bulbs and cavernous capture.

The combined effects of cerebral venous hypertension, ischemia from steal phenomenon, and cardiac insufficiency cause profound global cerebral hypoperfusion. When mild or moderate, parenchymal calcification and/or white matter lesions may be observed on imaging, but when advanced, there is encephaloclastic parenchymal destruction—the so-called "melting brain syndrome"[1] (Fig. 2).

Seizures can occur although less frequently, and hemorrhage is rare.

Natural History

Untreated, VOGMs have a 6% risk of sudden death, the overwhelming majority (94%) being neonates.[19] In a population-based neonatal cohort, 40% of patients with VOGM did not survive the neonatal period, and half of the survivors had a poor neurocognitive outcome.[20]

Diagnosis and Imaging Features

Prenatal diagnosis of VOGM is increasingly made by screening ultrasound, typically late in the second or third trimester. Imaging features on sonography include a hypoechoic/cystic midline structure within the brain, with flow demonstrated on Doppler interrogation. The diagnosis is confirmed on fetal MRI, where an assessment of the parenchyma and ventricles can be made in greater detail[21] (Fig. 3).

Prenatal echocardiography allows for prognostication. Features predicting severe cardiac failure include an increased cardio–thoracic ratio, right ventricular enlargement, interventricular septum deviation, pulmonary hypertension, bidirectional or right-to-left shunting through the ductus arteriosus, diastolic reversal of flow in the descending thoracic aorta, and aortic and tricuspid regurgitation.[14,22]

Fetal and early neonatal brain MRI findings can also be used to predict outcome. Diffusion-weighted MRI, Fluid Attenuated Inversion Recovery (FLAIR) images, and susceptibility-weighted MRI are key to assessing brain parenchymal health, early ischemic changes, and/or calcification. Time-of-flight magnetic resonance angiogram (MRA) is useful to characterize the feeders to the malformation, while magnetic resonance venogram (MRV) and 3 dimensional contrast enhanced magnetic resonance imaging (CEMRI) are useful to understand venous anatomy including deep veins and

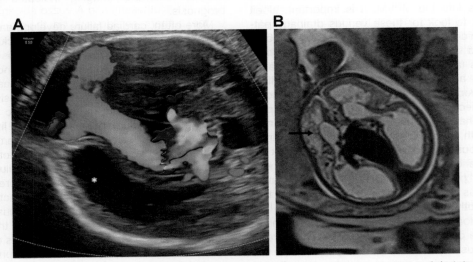

Fig. 2. Melting brain syndrome. Prenatal Doppler ultrasound (*A*) depicting flow in a VOGM and draining falcine sinus. Note the ventriculomegaly (*asterisk*) and thinning of the cerebral mantle. Axial T2 (*B*) confirms hydrocephalus and diffuse parenchymal destruction with cavitation (*arrow*).

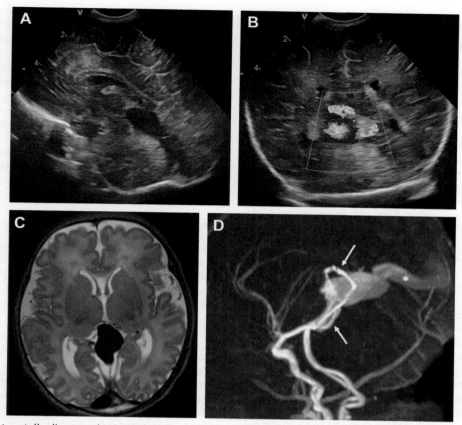

Fig. 3. Antenatally diagnosed VGAM. (*A*) Sagittal ultrasound image though the midline demonstrating a hypo-echoic structure in the velum interpositum. (*B*) Turbulent flow is shown on Doppler interrogation in the coronal plane. (*C*) Axial T2-weighted MR image in the same patient. The hypointense structure in the midline represents the dilated venous pouch. (*D*) Sagittal maximum intensity projection (MIP) image from a time-of-flight MRA showing choroidal branches of the posterior cerebral artery (PCA) (*arrows*) shunting to a venous pouch, which drains via the falcine sinus (*asterisk*).

the dural sinuses. The maximum mediolateral diameter of the narrowest craniocaudal segment of the straight sinus/falcine sinus draining the VOGM serves as a marker of flow resistance between the VOGM and the right heart. The more severe the narrowing the greater the resistance, and the more protection is afforded the right heart against the volume and pressure overload of the VOGM. Wider diameters have been found to predict cardiorespiratory failure after birth—almost 90% of patients with diameters over 8 mm will have an aggressive postnatal course.[15]

MANAGEMENT
Medical

This is directed at cardiac and respiratory failure following delivery, aiming to improve tissue perfusion and oxygenation. Intubation and ventilation and correcting anemia serve to normalize oxygen saturation. Administration of diuretics reduces cardiac preload, while digoxin or β-adrenergic agents such as dopamine, dobutamine, and adrenalin increase cardiac contractility. Sodium nitroprusside, glyceryl trinitrite, and phosphodiesterase inhibitors also play a role in treating cardiac failure.[23]

Interventional

Definitive treatment is directed at occlusion or reduction of the AV shunts. This is achieved through catheter-directed embolization. The timing of embolization is guided by neonatal presentation. The Bicêtre score[1] was developed to prognosticate and triage neonates for treatment. It assesses cardiac, respiratory, neurologic, renal, and hepatic function. Each organ system is scored to a maximum of 5 points, with lower scores indicating poorer function. Scores of less than 8 indicate a grave prognosis and preclude treatment because of futility. Patients with scores of 8 to 12 generally have cardiac failure resistant to medical therapy, and urgent intervention is indicated. Scores above 12 allow a delayed embolization, typically when the child is 4 to 6 months old. Embolization performed during this period is favored because complication rates are considerably lower and clinical outcomes better.

Early endovascular treatment in the neonate is usually performed through a trans-arterial route, via the femoral artery or umbilical artery. Selective microcatherization of the distal feeding arteries permits embolization, ideally as close to the AV junction as possible. A host of agents are available for use, with n-butyl-cyanoacrylate of varying concentrations being historically the most popular choice. Slower polymerizing liquid embolic agents such as Onyx (Medtronic) and Squid (Emboflu) have surged in use, with or without adjunctive coiling. This approach purportedly allows a more controlled embolization, lowering the risk of complications. Transvenous access provides an alternate route for VOGM embolization. Before embarking on such an approach, a careful evaluation of the AV shunt zone and deep venous anatomy should be performed. Internal cerebral venous drainage to the MPVM risks catastrophic venous infarction post-trans-venous embolization.[10,24,25] Other factors deemed to increase the risk of periprocedural complications include the use of larger caliber microcatheters, and embolization of proximal feeding vessels prior to more distal fistulae.[24]

In high-risk fetuses, in-utero VOGM embolization has recently been described. In the first reported case, sonographic guidance was employed for trans-uterine placement of a needle into the falcine sinus allowing delivery of a coiling microcatheter into the VOGM venous varix, subsequently reducing shunting, with a good postnatal outcome.[26] This has set the stage for a clinical trial, which is underway.[27]

Finally, endovascular venoplasty and stenting of the jugular bulb have been attempted in patients with venous hypertension and jugular bulb stenosis.[28,29] Although these case studies produced favorable outcomes, evidence is limited, and continued monitoring is necessary due to the risk of restenosis.

Surgical

Microsurgical approaches to VOGM have historically been shown to result in poor outcomes. In one series and literature review published in 1987, there was 78% mortality in neonates. While mortality figures improved to 31.7% in infants, nearly half had significant neurologic deficits.[30]

The role of CSF diversion for hydrocephalus in VOGM is controversial. A high frequency of complications including intractable seizures, intraventricular hemorrhage, and subdural hygromas/hematomas has been described following ventricular catheter placement.[31] Embolization for AV shunt control is the first-line approach for hydrovenous disorder in VOGM.

Gamma Knife radiosurgery has a role in the treatment of VOGM,[32,33] although most cases have been described to treat residual AV shunting following prior embolization of larger fistulae.

Treatment Outcome

In a meta-analysis on outcome following endovascular treatment of VOGM, 62% of patients had a good outcome, although this was significantly less likely in neonatal presenters and patients with congestive cardiac failure.[34]

DURAL SINUS MALFORMATIONS

Dural AV shunts are rare in children. Although different entities are described (including infantile dural AV shunts and adult-type dural AV shunts), the commonest—and only one that has been diagnosed in utero—is the DSM.[35] Lesions are characterized by massively dilated dural sinuses. Overgrowth of the dural venous sinuses is considered to be the initial phase in the development of these lesions. In some cases, partial or complete venous sinus thrombosis occurs, and this may be symptomatic in utero or in the neonatal period. A fraction of these cases go on to develop dural AV shunting in utero or in the neonatal period. There are 2 discrete subtypes:[1,36]

1. DSM with giant lakes/pouches involving the posterior sinuses (also referred to as torcular DSMs), with or without AV shunting. These are more common and have poorer outcomes.
2. DSM of the jugular bulb and sigmoid sinus. These tend to be associated with a high-flow fistula and have an initial benign course until dural sinus and jugular bulb stenosis set in.

Embryology and Anatomy

The transverse sinuses normally progressively dilate between 4–7 months of gestation. This is a result of the growing cerebrum with its venous dependence on the posterior sinuses, coupled with immature and narrow jugular sinuses. Postnatally, these structures assume a conventional configuration with normalized transverse sinus caliber and patulous jugular bulbs.[37] Some authors have proposed that a DSM develops when arterialization of the dilated dural sinuses occurs in utero causing them to persist.[38,39] This model does not completely account for cases of venous sinus overgrowth without AV shunting seen in some neonates. Since varying degrees of spontaneous thrombosis occur in overgrown venous sinuses and venous sinus thrombosis is a known cause of dural AV fistulae, it is possible that thrombosis plays a role in the development of dural AV shunts in DSM. Although a RASA1 mutation has been described in a patient with torcular DSM and high-flow fistulae,[40] there are no strong genetic associations.

Arterial supply to DSMs is chiefly through the middle meningeal and occipital arteries. However, any dural artery including pial-dural branches can conceivably supply a DSM[41] (Fig. 4).

As noted, thrombosis within the overgrown dilated venous sinuses is a frequent occurrence,[39,42]

the extent of which has implications on presentation and outcome.

Clinical Features

Symptoms in children with DSM are governed by the extent of cerebral venous outflow obstruction, and less so, degree of AV shunting. Lateral DSMs are mild in the majority of cases, due to presence of the contralateral drainage pathway. Torcular DSMs are prone to compromising cerebral venous drainage and have a greater tendency to exhibit an aggressive clinical course. Nearly all the available literature pertains to the management and outcome of this latter entity. While DSMs may manifest in neonates, they typically present after a few months. Macrocrania is the most common symptom, followed by sequalae of cerebral venous hypertension such as seizures, neurodevelopmental delay, hydrocephalus, intracranial hemorrhage, and in severe cases, "melting brain

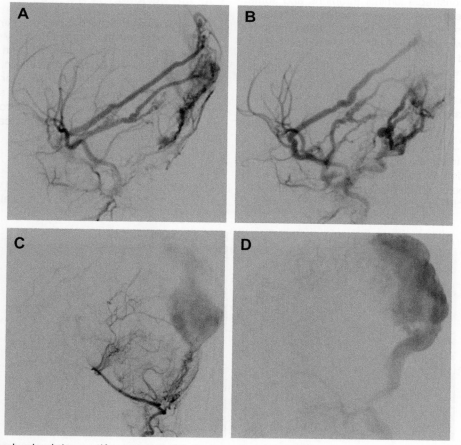

Fig. 4. Torcular dural sinus malformation (DSM). Catheter-directed angiography in bilateral common carotid (A, B) and left vertebral (C) arteries demonstrating dural supply to a large torcular venous lake. Venous phase (D) reveals its true size and extent.

syndrome." This is exacerbated by sinus thrombosis, which in advanced cases can result in consumptive coagulopathy. Unlike VOGM, cardiac failure is infrequent.[35,36]

Diagnosis and Imaging

DSMs may be diagnosed in utero by ultrasound late in the second trimester,[42] characterized by a cystic midline (torcular/superior sagittal sinus DSM) or lateral (jugular DSM) lesion. They are distinguished from VOGM by their dural location[43] (**Fig. 5**) and in torcular DSMs at least, by slower flow on Doppler interrogation.[44] MRI helps to confirm the diagnosis and assess for the presence of sinus arterialization and thrombosis, and for complications such as hydrocephalus, hemorrhage, and parenchymal damage (**Fig. 6**).

Prenatally diagnosed DSM may spontaneously decrease in size, some after a period of initial enlargement. Spontaneous in-utero regression is irreversible and predicts a good neurologic outcome.[41] Many prenatally diagnosed DSM have demonstrable luminal thrombus and some have in-utero AV shunting. In a series of 13 fetuses with DSMs,[45] all showed thrombosis on prenatal imaging, which progressed on follow-up imaging performed in 10 cases. This was accompanied by a progressive reduction in size of the dilated sinus, such that complete regression was demonstrated in 7 cases. A similar course has been shown in a separate series of 16 cases.[46]

Management

Definitive treatment of DSMs is a balance between embolization of arterial feeders and management of thrombosis of the giant dural sinus. Embolization is achieved through use of coils or liquid embolic agents. This is performed in a staged manner to prevent sudden thrombosis of the DSM precipitated by abrupt flow deceleration,[1] which poses a risk of parenchymal injury from worsening cerebral venous hypertension. Adjunctive anticoagulation aids in controlling the rate of thrombosis and has been utilized with positive outcomes.[42,47,48]

Natural History and Outcome

It is increasingly recognized that outcomes from DSMs are not as poor as once thought.[38] Favorable features include non-torcular DSMs, presence of alternate venous drainage pathways (cavernous capture), and absence of arterialization, hydrocephalus, seizures, parenchymal injury, or jugular bulb stenoses. Progressive spontaneous thrombosis of the venous sac is also associated with good outcome and with spontaneous DSM regression in some cases, although close monitoring is advocated.[36,39,46]

PIAL ARTERIOVENOUS FISTULAS

PAVFs represent a distinct subtype of intracranial vascular malformation, characterized by a direct macrofistulous communication between one or more pial arteries and a solitary pial vein, without an intervening nidus. PAVFs account for roughly 4.2% of all central nervous system AV shunt lesions (excluding VOGM) and are disproportionately represented in children.[49] Most cases are considered congenital.

Embryology and Anatomy

At 8 weeks of gestation, both arteries and veins are simply endothelial tubes, which typically cross

A   **B**

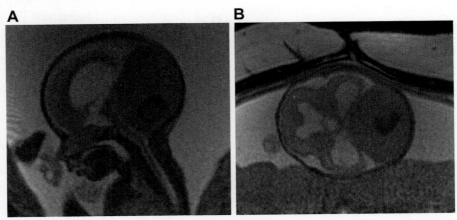

Fig. 5. Fetal MRI in torcular dural sinus malformation (DSM). Sagittal (*A*) and axial (*B*) T2-WI showing the large posterior midline venous lake with brainstem compression and resultant hydrocephalus. Hypointense structure within the torcular venous lake suggests thrombus formation.

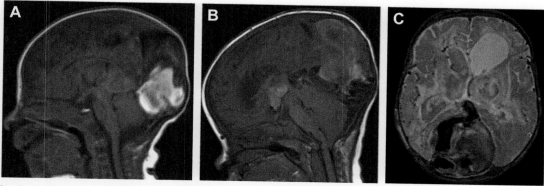

Fig. 6. Dural sinus malformation (DSM) in a 2 week old neonate with heart failure and macrocephaly. (*A*) MRI shows a partially thrombosed torcular DSM. Despite endovascular treatment, the DSM progressively enlarged and thrombosed with worsening mass effect, hydrocephalus, venous hypertension, and intraventricular hemorrhage (*B, C*). This underscores the importance of aggressive post-interventional anticoagulation.

each other perpendicularly or obliquely, increasing their surface area of contact the closer to parallel they course. The chance of AV fistula formation is thought to be greater in this latter arrangement.[50] Another theory is that primitive "capillary nets" exist between developing arteries and veins, allowing shunting of blood between them. When these fail to develop and mature into a normal capillary network, an AV shunt results.[51] Over half of PAVFs are associated with germline mutations in ENG, ACVRL1, or RASA1.[52]

The shunting zone in PAVFs occurs in a subpial location. There may be one or more cortical/pial arterial feeders that converge on a pial vein pouch through single or multiple macrofistulous connections. Due to the high-flow nature of these lesions, marked variceal dilatation of the arterialized venous pouch and extensive ectasia of its draining veins are common[53–55] (see **Fig. 5**). Arterial steal phenomenon can cause feeding artery hypertrophy, while adjacent arteries are smaller until recruited via pial collaterals.

Clinical Features

Presentation of PAVF varies by age. Neonates are more likely to present with heart failure, while infants and children tend to present with symptoms secondary to cerebral venous hypertension including seizures, developmental delay, hydrocephalus, and macrocephaly. Intracranial hemorrhage may occur secondary to rupture of flow-related aneurysms, variceal venous pouches, or venous ectasias. As patients age, the likelihood of hemorrhagic venous infarction due to worsening cerebral venous hypertension and cerebral venous congestion increases.[1,49,56]

Aside from symptoms attributable to the PAVF, manifestations of HHT or CM-AVM syndrome including epistaxis, pulmonary AVM, and mucocutaneous stigmata may be apparent.[52]

Diagnosis and Imaging

PAVFs can be diagnosed antenatally,[57] or more commonly postnatally. Sonographically, they are anechoic structures with high turbulent flow on Doppler. Peripheral, superficially draining lesions are distinguishable from a VOGM; however, deep-seated lesions draining via the vein of Galen are more challenging to differentiate.[58] MRI confirms the diagnosis and aids in assessing the brain parenchyma and ventricular dimensions. As in VOGM, cardiomegaly, tricuspid regurgitation and superior vena cava dilatation may be observed.

Later presentations in infancy or early childhood are best studied by MRI, with MRA and MRV. In some children who present emergently with hemorrhage, computed tomography (CT) with computed tomography angiogram (CTA) might be more reasonable and can provide necessary information needed to plan an urgent intervention.

Given the high likelihood of HHT or CM-AVM syndrome, bubble contrast echocardiography should be performed prior to catheter-directed angiography or endovascular intervention. Catheter-directed angiography is crucial to understanding angio-anatomy and flow-related phenomena including shunting zones, venous congestion, and steal phenomenon.

Management

Fistulous disconnection is often performed endovascularly, by use of coils, vascular plugs, glue or other liquid embolics, and even detachable balloons (**Fig. 7**). Precise occlusion at the fistulous junction can be challenging due to the high flow.

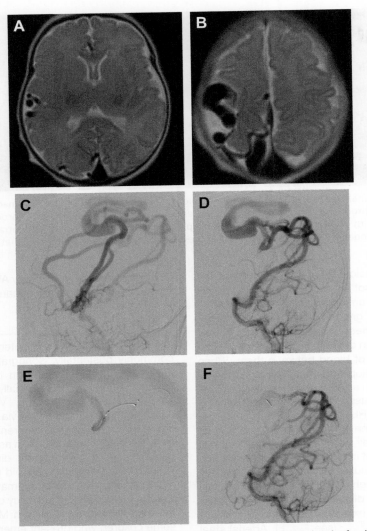

Fig. 7. Right parietal pial arteriovenous fistula (PAVF). (*A, B*) MRI showing dilated right feeding middle cerebral arterial branches (*A*) and ectatic draining cortical vein (*B*). (*C, D*) Catheter-directed angiography showing the enlarged feeders from anterior, middle, and posterior cerebral arteries. (*E, F*) Coil embolization with significantly reduced flow through the fistula.

Surgical disconnection can be considered for lesions with unfavorable angioarchitecture for endovascular treatment (eg, multihole fistulae), with good outcomes.[53,59]

Following treatment, consideration is given to blood pressure management, due to the risk of cerebral edema and reperfusion hemorrhage. Practice varies between hypotension and normotension in countering normal perfusion pressure breakthrough, and occlusive hyperemia, respectively. When possible, staged treatment may aid in adjustment of regional hemodynamics.[60] Abrupt slowing of blood flow in ectatic draining venous can trigger aggressive thrombosis necessitating anticoagulation.

Natural History and Treatment Outcome

Left untreated, PAVFs have a poor prognosis, with a high risk of hemorrhage and mortality.[61] Outcomes following treatment relate to age at presentation (with neonates and infants more likely to do worse), and complexity of lesion angioarchitecture.[56] Clinical series have demonstrated good outcome in 72% to 92% of successfully treated cases.[49,56,62]

SUMMARY

The authors explore the characteristics, embryology, clinical manifestations, diagnostic approaches, and management of fetal neurovascular malformations. Their diverse anatomic features and presentations underscore the importance of a tailored, multidisciplinary approach to diagnosis and treatment. Advances in endovascular treatment have greatly improved outcomes. Individual patient factors require refined therapeutic strategies to improve prognosis and mitigate risks.

ACKNOWLEDGMENTS

The authors thank Dr. Felice D'Arco, Neuroradiologist at the Great Ormond Street Hospital, for his assistance in case selection.

DISCLOSURE

The authors have no conflicts of interest to declare.

REFERENCES

1. Lasjaunias P, ter Brugge KG, Berenstein A. Surgical neuroangiography. Springer Berlin Heidelberg; 2006. https://doi.org/10.1007/978-3-540-68320-9.
2. Klostranec JM, Krings T. Cerebral neurovascular embryology, anatomic variations, and congenital brain arteriovenous lesions. J NeuroIntervent Surg 2022; 14(9):910–9. https://doi.org/10.1136/neurintsurg-2021-018607.
3. Raybaud CA, Strother CM, Hald JK. Aneurysms of the vein of Galen: embryonic considerations and anatomical features relating to the pathogenesis of the malformation. Neuroradiology 1989;31(2): 109–28. https://doi.org/10.1007/BF00698838.
4. Byrne JV. Tutorials in endovascular Neurosurgery and interventional Neuroradiology. Springer International Publishing; 2017. https://doi.org/10.1007/978-3-319-54835-7.
5. Pearl M, Gregg L, Gandhi D. Cerebral venous development in relation to developmental venous anomalies and vein of galen aneurysmal malformations. Seminars Ultrasound, CT MRI 2011;32(3):252–63. https://doi.org/10.1053/j.sult.2011.02.001.
6. Houser OW, Campbell JK, Campbell RJ, et al. Arteriovenous malformation affecting the transverse dural venous sinus–an acquired lesion. Mayo Clin Proc 1979;54(10):651–61.
7. Duran D, Karschnia P, Gaillard JR, et al. Human genetics and molecular mechanisms of vein of Galen malformation. J Neurosurg Pediatr 2018;21(4):367–74. https://doi.org/10.3171/2017.9.PEDS17365.
8. Tas B, Starnoni D, Smajda S, et al. Arteriovenous cerebral high flow shunts in children: from genotype to phenotype. Front Pediatr 2022;10:871565. https://doi.org/10.3389/fped.2022.871565.
9. Alvarez H, Garcia Monaco R, Rodesch G, et al. Vein of galen aneurysmal malformations. Neuroimaging

Clin 2007;17(2):189–206. https://doi.org/10.1016/j.nic.2007.02.005.
10. Kortman H, Navaei E, Raybaud CA, et al. Deep venous communication in vein of Galen malformations: incidence, Imaging, and Implications for treatment. J NeuroIntervent Surg 2021;13(3):290–3. https://doi.org/10.1136/neurintsurg-2020-016224.
11. Deloison B, Chalouhi GE, Sonigo P, et al. Hidden mortality of prenatally diagnosed vein of Galen aneurysmal malformation: retrospective study and review of the literature. Ultrasound Obstet Gynecol 2012;40(6):652–8. https://doi.org/10.1002/uog.11188.
12. Marcelletti C, Picardo S. Dynamics of changes from fetal to postnatal circulation. In: Raimondi AJ, Choux M, Di Rocco C, editors. Cerebrovascular diseases in children. principles of pediatric neurosurgery. New York: Springer; 1992. p. 1–8. https://doi.org/10.1007/978-1-4612-2800-4_1.
13. Hoang S, Choudhri O, Edwards M, et al. Vein of galen malformation. FOC 2009;27(5):E8. https://doi.org/10.3171/2009.8.FOCUS09168.
14. Buratti S, Mallamaci M, Tuo G, et al. Vein of Galen aneurysmal malformation in newborns: a retrospective study to describe a paradigm of treatment and identify risk factors of adverse outcome in a referral center. Front Pediatr 2023;11:1193738. https://doi.org/10.3389/fped.2023.1193738.
15. Arko L, Lambrych M, Montaser A, et al. Fetal and neonatal MRI predictors of aggressive early clinical course in vein of galen malformation. AJNR Am J Neuroradiol 2020;41(6):1105–11. https://doi.org/10.3174/ajnr.A6585.
16. Saliou G, Dirks P, Slater LA, et al. Is jugular bulb stenosis in vein of Galen aneurysmal malformation associated with bony remodeling of the jugular foramina? PED 2016;18(1):92–6. https://doi.org/10.3171/2015.12.PEDS15310.
17. Geibprasert S, Pereira V, Krings T, et al. Hydrocephalus in unruptured brain arteriovenous malformations: pathomechanical considerations, therapeutic implications, and clinical course: clinical article. JNS 2009;110(3):500–7. https://doi.org/10.3171/2008.7.JNS0815.
18. Klostranec JM, Vucevic D, Bhatia KD, et al. Current concepts in intracranial interstitial fluid transport and the glymphatic system: part II—imaging techniques and clinical applications. Radiology 2021;301(3): 516–32. https://doi.org/10.1148/radiol.2021204088.
19. Yan J, Gopaul R, Wen J, et al. The natural progression of VGAMs and the need for urgent medical attention: a systematic review and meta-analysis. J NeuroIntervent Surg 2017;9(6):564–70. https://doi.org/10.1136/neurintsurg-2015-012212.
20. Lecce F, Robertson F, Rennie A, et al. Cross-sectional study of a United Kingdom cohort of neonatal vein of galen malformation. Ann Neurol 2018;84(4):547–55. https://doi.org/10.1002/ana.25316.

21. Bhattacharya JJ. Vein of galen malformations. J Neurol Neurosurg Psychiatr 2003;74(90001):42i–444i. https://doi.org/10.1136/jnnp.74.suppl_1.i42.

22. Gillet De Thorey A, Ozanne A, Melki J, et al. State of the art of antenatal diagnosis and management of vein of Galen aneurysmal malformations. Prenat Diagn 2022;42(9):1073–80. https://doi.org/10.1002/pd.6203.

23. Frawley GP, Dargaville PA, Mitchell PJ, et al. Clinical course and medical management of neonates with severe cardiac failure related to vein of Galen malformation. Arch Dis Child Fetal Neonatal Ed 2002; 87(2):F144. https://doi.org/10.1136/fn.87.2.F144.

24. Bhatia K, Mendes Pereira V, Krings T, et al. Factors contributing to major neurological complications from vein of galen malformation embolization. JAMA Neurol 2020;77(8):992. https://doi.org/10.1001/jamaneurol.2020.0825.

25. Matsoukas S, Shigematsu T, Bazil MJ, et al. Transvenous embolization of vein of galen aneurysmal malformations with coils as a final procedure for cure: a single- institution experience of 18 years. Interv Neuroradiol 2022. https://doi.org/10.1177/15910199221135066. 159101992211350.

26. Orbach DB, Wilkins-Haug LE, Benson CB, et al. Transuterine ultrasound-guided fetal embolization of vein of galen malformation, eliminating postnatal pathophysiology. Stroke 2023;54(6):e231–2. https://doi.org/10.1161/STROKEAHA.123.043421.

27. See AP, Wilkins-Haug LE, Benson CB, et al. Percutaneous transuterine fetal cerebral embolisation to treat vein of Galen malformations at risk of urgent neonatal decompensation: study protocol for a clinical trial of safety and feasibility. BMJ Open 2022;12(5):e058147. https://doi.org/10.1136/bmjopen-2021-058147.

28. Brew S, Taylor W, Reddington A. Stenting of a venous stenosis in vein of galen aneurysmal malformation: a case report. Interv Neuroradiol 2001;7(3):237–40. https://doi.org/10.1177/159101990100700309.

29. Gupta G, Rallo MS, Goldrich DY, et al. Management of jugular bulb stenosis in pediatric vein of galen malformation: a novel management paradigm. Pediatr Neurosurg 2021;56(6):584–90. https://doi.org/10.1159/000517653.

30. Johnston IH, Whittle IR, Besser M, et al. Vein of galen malformation: diagnosis and management. Neurosurgery 1987;20(5):747–58. https://doi.org/10.1227/00006123-198705000-00013.

31. Schneider SJ, Wisoff JS, Epstein FJ. Complications of ventriculoperitoneal shunt procedures or hydrocephalus associated with vein of Galen malformations in childhood. Neurosurgery 1992;30(5):706–8.

32. Triffo WJ, Bourland JD, Couture DE, et al. Definitive treatment of vein of Galen aneurysmal malformation with stereotactic radiosurgery: report of 2 cases. JNS 2014;120(1):120–5. https://doi.org/10.3171/2013.6.JNS121897.

33. Payne BR, Prasad D, Steiner M, et al. Gamma surgery for vein of Galen malformations. J Neurosurg 2000;93(2):229–36. https://doi.org/10.3171/jns.2000.93.2.0229.

34. Brinjikji W, Zhu YQ, Lanzino G, et al. Risk factors for growth of intracranial aneurysms: a systematic review and meta-analysis. Am J Neuroradiol 2016; 37(4):615–20. https://doi.org/10.3174/ajnr.A4575.

35. Lasjaunias P, Magufis G, Goulao A, et al. Anatomoclinical aspects of dural arteriovenous shunts in children: review of 29 cases. Interv Neuroradiol 1996;2(3):179–91. https://doi.org/10.1177/159101999600200303.

36. Barbosa M, Mahadevan J, Weon YC, et al. Dural sinus malformations (DSM) with giant lakes, in neonates and infants: review of 30 consecutive cases. Interv Neuroradiol 2003;9(4):407–24. https://doi.org/10.1177/159101990300900413.

37. Okudera T, Huang YP, Ohta T, et al. Development of posterior fossa dural sinuses, emissary veins, and jugular bulb: morphological and radiologic study. AJNR Am J Neuroradiol 1994;15(10):1871–83.

38. Robertson F. Torcular dural sinus malformation. J NeuroIntervent Surg 2018;10(5):423. https://doi.org/10.1136/neurintsurg-2017-013654.

39. Yang E, Storey A, Olson HE, et al. Imaging features and prognostic factors in fetal and postnatal torcular dural sinus malformations, part II: synthesis of the literature and patient management. J NeuroIntervent Surg 2018;10(5):471–5. https://doi.org/10.1136/neurintsurg-2017-013343.

40. Grillner P, Söderman M, Holmin S, et al. A spectrum of intracranial vascular high-flow arteriovenous shunts in RASA1 mutations. Childs Nerv Syst 2016;32(4):709–15. https://doi.org/10.1007/s00381-015-2940-y.

41. Liby P, Lomachinsky V, Petrak B, et al. Torcular dural sinus malformations: a single- center case series and a review of literature. Childs Nerv Syst 2020; 36(2):333–41. https://doi.org/10.1007/s00381-019-04280-3.

42. Yang E, Storey A, Olson HE, et al. Imaging features and prognostic factors in fetal and postnatal torcular dural sinus malformations, part I: review of experience at Boston Children's Hospital. J NeuroIntervent Surg. 2018;10(5):467–70. https://doi.org/10.1136/neurintsurg-2017-013344.

43. Komiyama M, Ishiguro T, Kitano S, et al. Serial antenatal sonographic observation of cerebral dural sinus malformation. AJNR Am J Neuroradiol 2004; 25(8):1446–8.

44. Tessler F, Dion J, Vinuela F, et al. Cranial arteriovenous malformations in neonates: color Doppler imaging with angiographic correlation. Am J Roentgenol 1989;153(5):1027–30. https://doi.org/10.2214/ajr.153.5.1027.

45. Merzoug V, Flunker S, Drissi C, et al. Dural sinus malformation (DSM) in fetuses. Diagnostic value of

prenatal MRI and follow-up. Eur Radiol 2008;18(4): 692–9. https://doi.org/10.1007/s00330-007-0783-y.

46. Goldman-Yassen AE, Shifrin A, Mirsky DM, et al. Torcular dural sinus malformation: fetal and postnatal imaging findings and their associations with clinical outcomes. Pediatr Neurol 2022;135:28–37. https://doi.org/10.1016/j.pediatrneurol.2022.07.004.

47. Saliou G, Deiva K, Möhlenbruch MA, et al. Anticoagulation helps shrink giant venous lakes and arteriovenous fistulas in dural sinus malformation. J NeuroIntervent Surg 2023. https://doi.org/10.1136/jnis-2022-019923. jnis-2022-019923.

48. Ku JC, Hanak B, Muthusami P, et al. Improving long-term outcomes in pediatric torcular dural sinus malformations with embolization and anticoagulation: a retrospective review of the hospital for sick children experience. J Neurosurg Pediatr 2021;28(4):469–75. https://doi.org/10.3171/2021.3.PEDS20921.

49. Weon YC, Yoshida Y, Sachet M, et al. Supratentorial cerebral arteriovenous fistulas (AVFs) in children: review of 41 cases with 63 non choroidal single-hole AVFs. Acta Neurochir 2005;147(1):17–31. https://doi.org/10.1007/s00701-004-0341-1.

50. Padget DH. The cranial venous system in man in reference to development, adult configuration, and relation to the arteries. Am J Anat 1956;98(3): 307–55. https://doi.org/10.1002/aja.1000980302.

51. Paramasivam S, Toma N, Niimi Y, et al. Development, clinical presentation and endovascular management of congenital intracranial pial arteriovenous fistulas. J NeuroIntervent Surg 2013;5(3):184–90. https://doi.org/10.1136/neurintsurg-2011-010241.

52. Saliou G, Eyries M, Iacobucci M, et al. Clinical and genetic findings in children with central nervous system arteriovenous fistulas. Ann Neurol 2017;82(6): 972–80. https://doi.org/10.1002/ana.25106.

53. Hoh BL, Putman CM, Budzik RF, et al. Surgical and endovascular flow disconnection of intracranial pial single-channel arteriovenous fistulae. Neurosurgery 2001;49(6):1351–64. https://doi.org/10.1097/00006123-200112000-00011.

54. ViñUela F, Drake CG, Fox AJ, et al. Giant intracranial varices secondary to high- flow arteriovenous fistulae. J Neurosurg 1987;66(2):198–203. https://doi.org/10.3171/jns.1987.66.2.0198.

55. Barnwell SL, Ciricillo SF, Halbach VV, et al. Intracerebral arteriovenous fistulas associated with intraparenchymal varix in childhood: case reports. Neurosurgery 1990;26(1):122–5. https://doi.org/10.1097/00006123-199001000-00017.

56. Hetts SW, Keenan K, Fullerton HJ, et al. Pediatric intracranial nongalenic pial arteriovenous fistulas: clinical features, angioarchitecture, and outcomes. AJNR Am J Neuroradiol 2012;33(9):1710–9. https://doi.org/10.3174/ajnr.A3194.

57. Martínez-Payo C, Sancho Saúco J, Miralles M, et al. Nongalenic pial arteriovenous fistula: prenatal diagnosis. J Clin Ultrasound 2017;45(9):621–5. https://doi.org/10.1002/jcu.22478.

58. Garel C, Azarian M, Lasjaunias P, et al. Pial arteriovenous fistulas: dilemmas in prenatal diagnosis, counseling and postnatal treatment. Report of three cases. Ultrasound Obstet Gynecol 2005;26(3): 293–6. https://doi.org/10.1002/uog.1957.

59. Lee JY, Son YJ, Kim JE. Intracranial pial arteriovenous fistulas. Journal of Korean Neurosurgical Society 2008;44(2):101. https://doi.org/10.3340/jkns.2008.44.2.101.

60. Rangel-Castilla L, Spetzler RF, Nakaji P. Normal perfusion pressure breakthrough theory: a reappraisal after 35 years. Neurosurg Rev 2015;38(3):399–405. https://doi.org/10.1007/s10143-014-0600-4.

61. Nelson K, Nimi Y, Lasjaunias P, et al. Endovascular embolization of congenital intracranial pial arteriovenous fistulas. Neuroimaging Clin 1992;2(01):309–17.

62. Yoshida Y, Weon YC, Sachet M, et al. Posterior cranial fossa single-hole arteriovenous fistulae in children: 14 consecutive cases. Neuroradiology 2004; 46(6):474–81. https://doi.org/10.1007/s00234-004-1176-4.

Intracranial Vascular Malformations in Children

Sulaiman Karim, BS[a,b], Samagra Jain, BS[c], Mesha L. Martinez, MD[d,e], Karen Chen, MD[b,e,f],*

KEYWORDS

- Intracranial vascular malformation • Pediatric • Neuroimaging • Diagnostic imaging
- Neurovascular care • Patient safety

KEY POINTS

- Intracranial vascular malformations (IVM) in children present significant diagnostic challenges due to anatomic and pathologic complexity that varies widely across a diverse range of developmental stages.
- Advanced neuroimaging techniques are crucial for accurate diagnostic assessment and treatment planning, with conventional contrast-enhanced MRI, catheter-directed DSA, and advanced MRI techniques such as ASL and TRICKS playing key roles.
- Technological advances have significantly improved the diagnostic and treatment landscape for pediatric patients with IVM, offering less invasive and more accurate neuroimaging evaluation methods.
- Foundational principles of pediatric neuroimaging include the minimization of patient exposure to ionizing radiation.

INTRODUCTION

Vascular malformations are native host blood vessels (nonneoplastic), vascular tissues, or vascular networks with aberrant form, structure, and/or organization but the normal mitotic turnover of endothelial cells and other cellular elements. In contrast, proliferative vascular anomalies or vascular tumors such as hemangiomas feature abnormal proliferation of endothelial cells or other cellular constituents of vascular tissue. Intracranial vascular malformations (IVM) are broadly differentiated into shunting lesions (arteriovenous shunting), and nonshunting lesions, including transitional lesions.

Non-shunting IVM includes venous anomalies (typical and atypical developmental venous anomalies, simple varices, and sinus pericranii), cerebral cavernous malformations (CCM), and telangiectasias or cerebral capillary malformations. More recently, nonshunting "pure arterial malformations" have been described as a unique form of IVM; however, these have not been consistently reported. Shunting IVM includes pial, dural, and choroidal types. Nidal-type pial arteriovenous malformations (AVM) and pial arteriovenous fistulae (AVF) are the most common forms of pial AV shunts. Micro-AVM and cerebral proliferative angiopathy (CPA) may be considered atypical and rare forms of pial AV shunts, with micro-AVM primarily encountered in the hereditary hemorrhagic telangiectasia (HHT) population. It should be noted that while "proliferative" is part of the CPA name, the intended meaning of the term in

[a] Texas Tech University Health Science Center School of Medicine, 3601 4th Street, Lubbock, TX 79430, USA; [b] Edward B. Singleton Department of Radiology, Texas Children's Hospital, 6701 Fannin Street, Suite 470, Houston, TX 77030, USA; [c] Baylor College of Medicine, 1 Baylor Plaza, Houston, TX 77030, USA; [d] Department of Radiology, Texas Children's Hospital, 9835 North Lake Creek Parkway, Suite PA120, Austin, TX 78717, USA; [e] Department of Radiology, Baylor College of Medicine, Houston, TX, USA; [f] Department of Neurosurgery, Baylor College of Medicine, Houston, TX, USA
* Corresponding author. 6701 Fannin Street, Suite 470, Houston, TX 77030.
E-mail address: Kxchen1@texaschildrens.org

Neuroimag Clin N Am 34 (2024) 545–565
https://doi.org/10.1016/j.nic.2024.08.009
1052-5149/24/© 2024 Elsevier Inc. All rights reserved, including those for text and data mining, AI training, and similar technologies.

this context is not to convey something about mitotic activity but to describe the pial and transdural recruitment of arterial supply that is characteristic of this lesion. Choroidal arteriovenous shunts include midline lesions, that is, vein of Galen malformations (VOGM), and non-midline lesions, that is, non-Galenic choroidal arteriovenous fistulae. Dural vascular malformations include dural sinus malformations (DSM), infantile DAVF, and adult-type DAVF. Pial AVF, VOGM, non-Galenic choroidal arteriovenous fistulae, and DSM are primitive lesions that form during early fetal development. These lesions are specifically addressed in the article by Qureshi AM, et al.

Cerebral capilllary malformations (CM), or telangiectasias, can be considered transitional vascular malformations. "Transitional" is meant to indicate that this form of vascular malformation is a precursor to the AVM phenotype. The concept of a transitional AVM state is supported by extensive preclinical and clinical data. In a well-established preclinical model of brain AVM caused by constitutive expression of Notch 4, the brain AVM lesion is initiated by non-sprouting or intussceptive angiogenesis (angioectasia) of embryonic vessels in the "capillary" region of the developing circulation.[1] This intermediate state of progression toward the definitive AVM phenotype is considered a "transitional state" which can be expressed in the setting of HHT or more rarely encountered as a sporadic lesion. Notably, hybrid forms of vascular malformation with intermixed or mosaic compartments of AVM and CM, or AVM and DVA, are not unusual in children.

This article aims to provide a focused overview of the pediatric IVM that are most commonly revealed by clinical neuroimaging studies obtained in a neuropediatric hospital or clinic, specifically nidal type pial arteriovenous malformations (A.K.A. cerebral AVM or brain AVM), cerebral cavernous malformations (CCM), cerebral capillary malformations (CM), and developmental venous anomalies (DVA). This article will strive to highlight the importance of advanced diagnostic imaging in the evaluation of these entities, and how neuroimaging diagnosis can provide a framework for therapeutic strategies in affected patients.

Nidal-type Pial Arteriovenous Malformations

Nidal-type pial arteriovenous malformations (AVM) are characterized by arteriovenous shunting through a complex inter-anastomosing, plexiform network of ectatic and dysplastic (angiomatous) blood vessels, described as a *nidus*, derived from the Latin word for "nest."[2,3] As specific genetic and cellular processes involved in the formation of cerebral AVMs are elucidated in astonishing detail, it has become clear that the pathogenesis of these lesions is a multifactorial process. Though AVM was once believed to arise solely from disordered embryogenesis, recent evidence suggests that the AVM phenotype is the product of a dynamic interaction between environmental factors (tissue injury, inflammation, hypoxemia, and disordered blood flow dynamics) and immature developing vascular tissues with genetically programmed vulnerabilities that are both inherited and acquired through somatic mutations.[4] This model of AVM pathogenesis is also borne out by reports of postnatal de novo AVM cases that develop between 5 and 10 years of age.[5] Several genes have been directly linked to the development of cerebral AVMs including SMAD4, ACVRL1, GDF2, and ENG[6] in Hereditary Hemorrhagic Telangiectasia (HHT), and RASA1, EPHB4, EFNB2 in Capillary Malformation-Arteriovenous Malformation (CM-AVM) syndrome. Interestingly, one of these CM-AVM mutations, EFNB2, has also been implicated in the pathogenesis of VOGM.[7] Somatic activating mutations in the KRAS and BRAF genes have also been identified in the endothelial cells of sporadic cerebral AVM from adults in 55% and 7% of cases, respectively.[8] Although our knowledge of the molecular phenotypes expressed by vascular cells in normal and abnormal blood vessels is rapidly expanding, arteriovenous shunt lesions remain angiographic diagnoses.[9]

Arteriovenous shunts are defined on catheter-directed digital subtraction angiography (DSA) by the finding of draining veins that fill directly from arterial feeders without an associated angiographic blush separating the two phases. An angiographic blush is the defining feature of capillary vessels. It corresponds to the angiographic appearance of vessels that are too small to be distinguished as discrete structures by modern catheter-directed DSA. In angiographic terms, the arteriovenous "shunt zone" is the precise spatial location whereby blood transits directly from artery to vein. While histopathologic descriptions of AVM and AVF exist, the microscopic findings are subjective, ambiguous, nonquantitative, non-specific, and inconsistent. Most notably, the precise identity of blood vessels as arteries, capillaries, or veins cannot be assessed, and the path of blood flow cannot be traced when conventional histopathological methods are applied to explanted clinical specimens that have been distorted by the processes of surgical cautery, excision, and laboratory processing. Given the absence of widely accepted rigorous, objective, and reliable criteria for histopathologic diagnosis, catheter-directed DSA remains the only reliable method for the definitive diagnosis of AVM and AVF within the CNS.

While molecular diagnosis does not yet enable the definitive diagnosis of specific IVM phenotypes, genetic testing plays an essential role in contemporary pediatric neurovascular care and frequently serves as an indication for neuroimaging studies. In children with genetically confirmed HHT or CM-AVM syndrome, screening brain MRI studies are recommended for the early detection of brain AVM/AVF, and follow-up MRI imaging studies are periodically obtained through childhood to detect de novo AVM. Although the incidence of spinal cord AVM is estimated to be upwards of 0.5% in this population, spinal MRI screening guidelines have not been widely adopted, though many have encouraged this[10]

Despite the central role of neuroimaging diagnosis in patients with IVM, further progress in the field of vascular malformation diagnosis and treatment will strongly rely on advances in cell-specific molecular phenotype expression.

The incidence of cerebral AVM within the population ranges from 1.1 to 1.4 cases per 100,000 person-years.[11] About 12% to 21% of cerebral AVMs are present in childhood.[12] Approximately 75% to 80% of pediatric patients are identified after hemorrhagic stroke vs. 36% to 38% of adult patients, with AVM being responsible for approximately 50% of hemorrhagic stroke in children.[11,13] A Randomized Trial of Unruptured Brain AVMs (ARUBA) determined that the annual cumulative risk of bleeding from previously unruptured and untreated cerebral AVM in adults is approximately 2.2%.[14,15] Factors that have been variably associated with an increased risk of cerebral AVM hemorrhage include a history of previous hemorrhage, female sex, an infratentorial or deep brain location, smaller AVM volume, predominantly deep venous drainage, the presence of associated flow-related aneurysms, and a diffuse AVM nidus morphology.[2,16,17] First-time cerebral AVM hemorrhage is associated with a mortality of 12% and a 40% rate of serious permanent neurologic morbidity in survivors. Notably, rebleeding is associated with significant additive morbidity, and the mortality rate for each hemorrhage event can be as high as 25%.[2] Cerebral AVM in children sustain higher rates of re-hemorrhage compared with adults.[18,19] Furthermore, since estimates of annual AVM hemorrhage risk are cumulative, lifetime risks of AVM hemorrhage are much higher in the pediatric population.

The neuropathological effects and clinical complications of cerebral AVM are direct manifestations of the pial hemodynamic derangements caused by arteriovenous shunting. Cerebral arteriovenous shunting (1) markedly elevates vascular wall tension stresses, causing a flow-dependent cumulative mural damage process that leads to the formation of flow-related aneurysms and venous ectasias that exert mass effect and can hemorrhage, (2) steals perfusion from brain tissue and (3) elevates luminal pressure in regional veins causing cerebral venous hypertension and congestion. The combined effects of perfusion steal and venous dysfunction lead to the pathologic depolarization of cortical neurons and seizures, infarction, and hemorrhage. Intracerebral hemorrhage is the most frequent presentation of cerebral AVM in the pediatric population (**Fig. 1**).[13,20] Nonetheless, cerebral AVM may also be found incidentally during the neuroimaging evaluation of children presenting with headache, seizure (**Fig. 2**), or focal neurologic deficit resulting from mass effect or cerebral ischemia.[2,21]

Imaging ruptured cerebral AVMs often begins in the emergency department with noncontrast computed tomography (CT). Noncontrast CT reveals the size and distribution of hemorrhage and associated complications such as mass effect, midline shift and hydrocephalus. In a minority of cases, calcifications may be a clue to the presence of underlying AVM. If noncontrast CT reveals nontraumatic intracranial hemorrhage in a child, CT angiography should be obtained while the patient is still on the table if possible. If the patient is neurologically stable, and immediate cerebral decompressive surgery is not needed, magnetic resonance imaging (MRI) with Gadolinium and time-of-flight MR angiography is favored for a more detailed understanding of the anatomy (parenchymal, cisternal, ventricular, and vascular), underlying hemorrhagic pathology, hemodynamic and parenchymal alterations caused by the AVM and associated hemorrhage. MRI findings can be used to guide the conduct and interpretation of catheter-directed DSA and the formulation of a comprehensive treatment plan. Catheter-directed DSA is critically important to understand the angioanatomy of AVM feeding arteries, their relationship to brain parenchymal supply, AVM venous drainage and its relationship to cerebral venous drainage, as well as the presence and location of high-risk features such as flow-related aneurysms, draining vein stenosis and venous hypertension. Catheter-directed DSA is uniquely able to differentiate AVM nidus from angiomatous artery-to-artery collaterals recruited to supply AVM or to reconstitute occluded arteries. Perhaps most importantly, catheter-directed DSA can be correlated with brain MRI to delineate the precise cause and location of AVM hemorrhage for neuroendovascular and microneurosurgical treatment planning.[22] In recent years, advances in time-resolved MRA

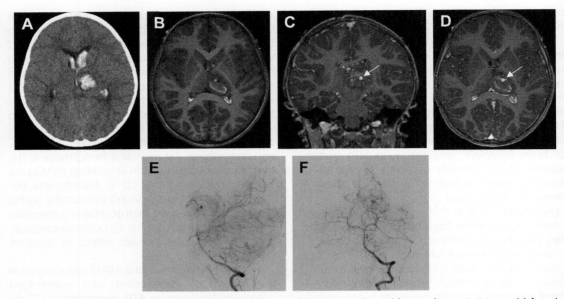

Fig. 1. Arteriovenous malformation (AVM) presenting with intraparenchymal hemorrhage. A 4-year-old female with acute onset right-sided weakness and dysarthria with transient loss of consciousness. (*A*) Noncontrast CT and (*B*) axial T1-weighted MRI images show left thalamic hemorrhage with intraventricular extension. (*C, D*) There is abnormal enhancing vascularity on postcontrast MR images within which a saccular lesion is identified on both coronal and axial images. This nodule corresponds to an intranidal aneurysm arising from thalamoperforating arteries. (*E, F*) Catheter-directed DSA showing a small dysplastic vascular focus with early subependymal venous drainage visualized in the late arterial phase and an associated nidal aneurysm, the presumed rupture point.

has led to its increasing use with reliable results,[23] though the spatial and temporal resolution of catheter-directed DSA is yet to be surpassed.

Several neuroimaging challenges emerge in the preoperative imaging assessment of the child with cerebral AVM hemorrhage, including the potential obfuscation of AVM nidus and arterial feeders by hemorrhage effects (mechanical compression of AVM vasculature and spasm of AVM feeding arteries).[22,24] In these cases, delayed repeat imaging on the order of weeks to months with MRI and catheter-directed DSA is often used for more accurate characterization and definitive treatment planning. Functional brain MRI and tractography play an important role in characterizing anatomically related treatment risks. Pitfalls to consider in the setting of hemorrhagic stroke are that perilesional hemodynamics in patients with brain AVM

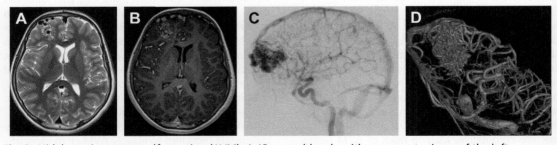

Fig. 2. Nidal arteriovenous malformation (AVM). A 13-year-old male with new onset seizure of the left upper extremity. (*A*) T2 weighted MR images demonstrate abnormal right frontal vascularity with associated enhancing vascular structures on (*B*) postcontrast T1 weighted images. (*C*) Lateral view of right internal carotid catheter-directed digital subtraction angiography demonstrates a compact AVM nidus with early venous drainage to the superior sagittal sinus, Spetzler Martin grade 2. (*D*) Oblique-shaded surface display images reconstructed from rotational angiography demonstrate a characteristic cone-shaped nidus with an apex oriented toward the ventricle.

can mask BOLD contrast, and tractography is highly sensitive to vasogenic edema. Tractography and fMRI are both highly sensitive to magnetic susceptibility caused by hemorrhage or embolic agents containing metals. Further imaging challenges, beyond those discussed here, will be examined in subsequent sections of this article, and in the articles on cross-sectional imaging and catheter-directed DSA by Shroff MM, et al. and Martinez M, et al. respectively.

Multidisciplinary management of children with cerebral AVM involves extensive collaboration between neuropediatric intensivists, pediatric anesthesiologists, pediatric neuroradiologists, neurointerventionists, radiation oncologists, pediatric neurosurgeons, and vascular microneurosurgical specialists. Compared with adults with cerebral AVM, children with cerebral AVM have a higher life-time risk of fatal or disabling hemorrhage, a higher rebleeding rate, a higher long-term risk of recurrence after initial AVM elimination, and a better prognosis for functional recovery due to age-related neuroplasticity. All of these factors favor a more aggressive management approach to the child with cerebral AVM.[2] Treatment strategies vary based on the size and location of the AVM, rupture status, and the presence of high-risk features on catheter-directed DSA. If possible, treatment plans are formulated to achieve complete AVM elimination (cure), though palliative treatment strategies are sometimes preferable considering prohibitive treatment-related risks. Microneurosurgical risks are typically assessed using the Spetzler-Martin Grading (SMG) system with additional considerations of patient age, history of rupture, and distribution of the nidus.[25] Microneurosurgical resection or endovascular embolization with curative intent is generally preferred for smaller AVM (SMG I and II), while stereotactic radiosurgery (SRS) is favored for small AVM that are considered inoperable due to deep or eloquent locations.[3,26]

Larger or more complicated AVMs are best addressed with a multimodal treatment strategy. Endovascular AVM embolization plays an important role in stabilizing high-risk features and as a pre-operative adjunct for the microneurosurgical resection of complicated AVM (SM III). Endovascular stabilization of high-risk features may be leveraged to reduce the short-term risk of rebleeding in patients with ruptured AVMs or to palliate patients with incurable AVM. SRS carries a higher risk of negative cognitive impact in patients less than 10 years of age, and the success rate is limited to some degree by AVM size. This is because as AVM size increases, the probability of cure goes down and the risk of serious treatment-related

morbidity goes up. Consequently, very large AVM (SMG IV and V) have historically been considered untreatable and have been most often managed by palliation alone. Newer techniques of volume-fractionated SRS approaches combined with the pre- or post-radiation embolization of high-flow features and microneurosurgical resection of residual disease are leading to successful cures and satisfactory neurologic outcomes for many patients with SMG IV or V AVM[27]

Cerebral proliferative angiopathy

Cerebral Proliferative Angiopathy is a rare hypervascular shunting intracranial vascular malformation that should be differentiated from nidal AVM. It is believed to be caused by disorganized angiogenesis triggered by an unknown mechanism (ischemia being a possible candidate), and is characterized by a large and diffuse collection of dysplastic and ectatic vessels, with normal brain parenchyma interspersed in between vascular elements. It was described by Lasjaunias and colleagues[28] based on typical clinical and angiographic descriptors. It has usually been described in adolescents and young adults, with a predominance in young females. Patients typically present with seizures, headaches, and recurrent strokes, symptoms secondary to steal phenomena, while hemorrhagic presentation is rare.[29]

Angiographic features include a large and diffuse area of capillary angioectasia and venous dilatations (often lobar, multilobar, or holohemispheric), consisting of multiple arteriovenous transitions fed by enlarged pial and often transdural arteries, with small-sized draining veins relative to lesional size (**Fig. 3**). Normal brain parenchyma in between vascular elements can be appreciated on T2-weighted MR images, and areas of gliosis due to chronic ischemia can be identified in the peri-CPA brain on FLAIR images. With time, increased recruitment of pial and transdural arteries can be seen secondary to exuberant angiogenesis, as well as the stenosis of proximal large arteries. Cerebrovascular reserve (CVR) studies have shown severely impaired perilesional CVR, more so than in nidal AVM, pointing to chronic perilesional hypoperfusion which serves as a driver for angiogenesis[30]

There are no guidelines for the treatment of CPA, with conservative management being chosen most often. Medical therapies for seizures and headaches can be supplemented with targeted embolization or gamma knife treatment, albeit with unsatisfactory and incomplete results. Revascularization surgeries such as multiple burr holes, pial synangiosis, and encephaloduroarteriosynangiosis have also been tried, with mixed

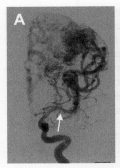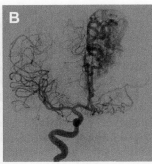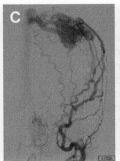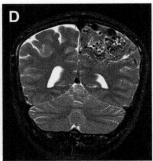

Fig. 3. Cerebral proliferative angiopathy (CPA). 9-year-old girl with intermittent numbness and weakness of the right arm and face. (*A, B*) Catheter-directed cerebral angiography showing classical features of CPA including a large and diffuse area of arteriovenous shunting in the left parietal lobe with transmedullary extension. Hypertrophied cortical and perforating feeding arteries supply the CPA lesion, stealing from the contralateral hemisphere and draining into relatively smaller veins. Note can be made of stenosis of the mid-segment of the left middle cerebral artery (*white arrow* in *A*). (*C*) Left external carotid injection showing large and tortuous meningeal arteries supplying the lesion. (*D*) coronal T2-weighted MRI image showing the lesion in the left parietal lobe with areas of interspersed normal brain parenchyma. Gliosis can be recognized in the form of gyral thinning in the perilesional brain.

results[31] Serial imaging with MRI and MRA is required to assess for evolving ischemia, proximal arterial stenosis, flow-related aneurysms or signs of hemorrhage.

Cerebral Cavernous Malformations

Cerebral cavernous malformations (CCM), also known as cavernomas, are congenital or acquired focal intraparenchymal brain lesions comprising cystic, thin-walled sinusoids partitioned by collagenous stroma, lined by endothelial cells and filled with blood in various stages of thrombus formation and organization, without intervening brain parenchyma or blood vessels.[32] Although some authors have considered these lesions to be tumors rather than vascular malformations, the architecture, and cellular composition are more consistent with a harmatomatous growth of vascular tissue, and therefore most cerebrovascular specialists regard CCM as a type of vascular malformation. Notably, CCM contains slow-flowing or completely stagnant blood under low pressure.[33] Arteriovenous shunting, feeding arteries, and draining veins are conspicuously absent.[34] As a result, the risk of bleeding is relatively low, and the effects of bleeding are relatively mild in comparison to AVM. Gross specimens of excised CCM appear reddish-blue (often compared with mulberries) and are typically associated with hemosiderin deposits due to recurrent intralesional and perilesional microhemorrhages.[32,35]

As with other vascular malformations, an interaction between environmental factors and genetic factors is required to express the CCM phenotype,

and a mixture of sporadic and familial disease patterns is encountered. Pial vascular injury initiated by environmental factors (ie, venous insufficiency or radiation injury) is believed to cause extravascular leakage of blood products which triggers a fibroblastic reaction involving collagen deposition and neovascularization. In genetically susceptible individuals, defective angiogenesis and aberrant tissue remodeling results in the development of the CCM lesion. Heritable loss of function mutations in the KRIT1 (CCM1), Malcavernin (CCM2), and PDCD10 (CCM3) genes are known to cause different familial CCM syndromes. In familial forms of CCM, biallelic loss of function caused by a second hit somatic mutation reveals the CCM phenotype in patients that inherit a germline mutation in one allele. Recent studies suggest that the CCM phenotype is dependent on the unchecked activation of intracellular signaling pathways, such as the Rho/ROCK, MEKK3-KLF2/3, and PI3K/Akt networks.[34,36] Additionally, mutations in the PIK3CA and MAP3K3 genes have been identified in some cases.[37,38] Each of these pathways plays a central role in endothelial cell migration, adhesion, proliferation, and intercellular tight junction maintenance with further effects on vascular permeability, vessel wall assembly, and angiogenesis.[34,35,36] Familial CCM syndromes are notable for a higher lifetime risk of de novo CCM formation, ranging from 0.5 to 3.0 new CCM per year which varies by specific underlying gene mutation[39]

CCM has an incidence of 0.4% to 0.8% in adult populations.[40] The majority of CCMs are sporadic (nonfamilial) and can range in size from punctate to several centimeters.[41] Sporadic CCM can be acquired as a result of pathologic changes induced by ionizing radiation (ie, therapeutic cranial radiation) or venous insufficiency within the drainage territory of a developmental venous anomaly (DVA). While sporadic CCMs are usually solitary, multiple lesions may be clustered within a therapeutic radiation field or within the venous drainage territory of a DVA. While sporadic CCM usually manifests as a single lesion, patients with familial CCM usually express multiple CCM. Consequently, genetic screening is recommended for patients with a family history of CCM or with multiple CCM that are not clustered in the venous drainage territory of a DVA or therapeutic radiation treatment field. Screening brain MRI, beginning at the age of 5 years, is recommended for first-degree relatives of individuals with familial CCM. While 15% of patients with familial CCM also have spinal cord cavernomas, imaging of the spine is generally not recommended as a screening study in the absence of myelopathic symptoms[39] While only 10% of CCM in the pediatric population are familial, 17% of pediatric patients with CCM have multiple lesions.

CCM may present with seizures, headaches, or focal neurologic deficits that are the result of intralesional and/or perilesional bleeding. While evidence of remote and recent CCM bleeding can be revealed by MRI studies, asymptomatic imaging findings in the absence of acute symptoms are not regarded as a hemorrhage event under current Angioma Alliance consensus guidelines.[32,35]

CCM is often found incidentally in routine neuroimaging studies. On noncontrast CT imaging, CCM appears as focal, variably hyperdense intra-axial lesions with indistinct margins, often with a stippled pattern caused by the admixture of calcification and hemorrhage. On MRI, unruptured CCM is typically manifest as a reticulated core of heterogenous T1 and T2 weighted signal hyperintensity with a sharply marginated hemosiderin ring best appreciated on T2-weighted sequences, the so-called "popcorn" appearance (Fig. 4).[35,42] CCM characteristically demonstrates intense blooming artifact on susceptibility-weighted imaging (SWI) sequences. While CCM does not typically enhance with intravenously administered contrast media, contrast is useful to delineate related venous anomalies and tumors in familial cases (CCM3). Acutely ruptured CCM in symptomatic patients will demonstrate blood products outside the hemosiderin ring of the index lesion. Fluid-fluid levels, perilesional vasogenic edema, mass effect, and an increase in lesion size that is more than 20% are additional imaging biomarkers of acute bleeding. Although in acutely ruptured CCM, acute hemorrhage can mask the underlying CCM, an underlying CCM should be suspected when a perilesional T1 hyperintense cloud is present.[43] Atypical MRI neuroimaging patterns that can be displayed by CCM include (1) solitary uniformly T1 hyperintense intraparenchymal lesions with sharply demarcated rounded borders, (2) widely distributed intra-parenchymal foci that are hypointense on T1 and T2 weighted imaging and (3) innumerable diffusely distributed punctate intra-parenchymal lesions exclusively seen as hypointense blooming foci on SWI sequences.[44] Notably, large numbers of small or punctate lesions on SWI images in the absence of one or larger typical lesions are not likely to be CCM, and other causes should be considered (ie, amyloid angiopathy or metastases). CCMs are generally angiographically occult, and prior to the advent of MRI were known as angiographically occult vascular malformations (AOVM). Consequently, catheter-directed angiography is not typically indicated for the evaluation of CCM.

In the general population, the risk of first-time hemorrhage from an incidentally discovered CCM is estimated to be 0.08% per lesion per year.[35] In children, the overall risk of bleeding from a CCM is approximately 0.5% per lesion per year, and adjacent DVA is found in up to 20% of patients.[45] Similar to adults, a significant portion of pediatric CCM are supratentorial in location, with 92% found in lobar structures and 8% found in deep subcortical structures (Fig. 5). Significant risk factors for hemorrhage include prior hemorrhagic presentation, and brainstem location[46] As compared with adults, children with CCM have a higher lifetime probability of bleeding due to the cumulative nature of hemorrhage risk. Punctate lesions that are only present on SWI sequences have a significantly lower risk of bleeding than larger CCM with typical MRI features.

The management of CCM involves 3 principal approaches: conservative treatment with observation alone, microneurosurgical resection, and SRS. The selection of treatment approach is guided by factors such as clinical presentation, lesion size and location, hemorrhage status, as well as the patient's neurologic function and overall health status. Microneurosurgical resection is favored for symptomatic CCM located in accessible brain regions, due to high success rates and possibility for relief from medically refractory epilepsy.[35] For CCMs situated in deep regions, operative risks are weighed against the quality-of-life implications of disease's natural history.

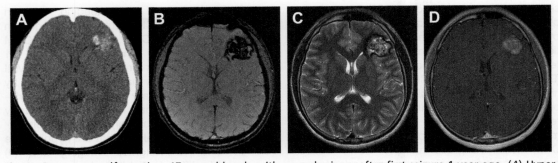

Fig. 4. Cavernous malformation. 17-year-old male with second seizure after first seizure 1 year ago. (*A*) Hyperdensity on non-contrast CT scan corresponds to acute and chronic blood products in the left frontal lobe, also seen on MRI, evidenced by (*B*). susceptibility artifact on SWI. (*C*) Hemosiderin deposition along the periphery of the lesion represents chronic blood products deposited from prior hemorrhage. Mixed T2 hyper- and hypointense signals are pathognomonic for cavernous malformations along with (*D*). intrinsic T1-hyperintensity without enhancement on postcontrast images.

Cerebral Capillary Malformations and Telangiectasias

Cerebral capillary malformations (CM) are focal collections of abnormally dilated microvascular channels within the brain parenchyma. Pathologic descriptions of clinical specimens have identified the abnormally ectatic vessels as capillaries in some reports and postcapillary venules in other reports, though the criteria for taxonomy is not clear and likely unsound because conventional histologic techniques are ill-equipped to differentiate capillaries from postcapillary venules. The findings on catheter-directed DSA, which show progressive

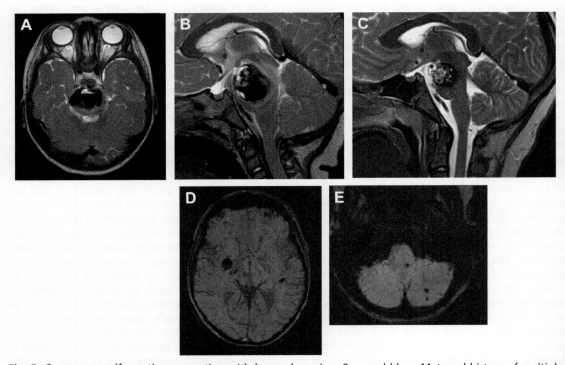

Fig. 5. Cavernous malformation presenting with hemorrhage in a 2-year-old boy. Maternal history of multiple intracranial cavernous malformations in the setting of KRIT-1 mutation. (*A, B*) Axial and sagittal T2-weighted MRI at the time of hemorrhage showed a midbrain-pontine lesion with blood-blood levels and perilesional edema causing mass effect. The lesion remained stable for 9 years and was followed with MRI. MRI at the age of 10 years showing the classical mixed intralesional signals on (*C*). T2-weighted imaging. (*D, E*). Multiple other supratentorial and infratentorial cavernomas are seen on SWI images.

intensification of an indistinct blush, devoid of discrete vessels, seen in the late arterial and capillary phase of angiography followed by the appearance of architecturally normal local draining veins, suggest that the ectatic vessels indeed correspond to capillaries. As noted in the introductory remarks to this article, CM can be considered a type of transitional vascular malformation, or intermediate state along the continuum between normal vascular architecture and the definitive AVM phenotype. Sporadic and hereditary patterns of cerebral CM exist, with the latter being expressed primarily in HHT. As noted previously, hybrid cerebral vascular malformations containing a mosaic arrangement of CM and AVM compartments within the same lesion are sometimes encountered as sporadic lesions in the pediatric population.

Although the term "telangiectasia" is often used interchangeably with CM, it is unclear if both terms describe a single type of vascular malformation or a range of similar vascular malformation phenotypes with overlapping neuroimaging features. Telangiectasia combines the Greek words telos (for terminal), angeion, (for vessel), and ektasis (for expansion). In the neuroimaging and neuropathology literature, telangiectasias are solitary sporadic central nervous system (CNS) vascular malformations that are usually found incidentally on brain MRI or at autopsy, though large and giant forms have been reported to cause symptoms.[47] In the HHT literature, the term telangiectasia is usually reserved for mucocutaneous vascular malformations, while the CM designation describes a specific type of CNS vascular malformation found in the parenchyma of the brain. Given the similarities in clinical behavior, neuroimaging appearances, and histopathological descriptions, the terms telangiectasia and CM will be considered synonymous in this report. The term CM will be used preferentially because it is believed to more properly convey the pathogenetic essence of the index malformation.

Cerebral CM are optimally portrayed on postcontrast T1-weighted images. Isolated sporadic cerebral CM have a predilection for the infratentorial CNS (pons > cerebellum > medulla > spinal cord) though supratentorial cerebral lesions involving the gray-white junction are also reported.[48] In HHT, cerebral CM shows a similar order of preference but as many as 30% are found in the cerebrum.[49] Cerebral CM typically appears as poorly demarcated subcentimeter foci of parenchymal contrast enhancement with faint borders, as if lightly applied by a paintbrush, an appearance which has been described as "brush bristle enhancement" (Fig. 6). There is typically no associated T2-FLAIR signal abnormality or evidence of hemosiderin deposition on susceptibility-weighted imaging to suggest local edema or hemorrhage.[50] As stated previously, catheter-directed DSA shows the progressive intensification of a focal blush in the late arterial phase and capillary phase, without feeding arteries or early draining veins.

In patients with HHT, cerebral CM is the most common intracranial vascular lesion.[51] Screening MRI studies obtained for patients with HHT frequently demonstrate multiple cerebral CM on contrast-enhanced and arterial spin labeling sequences, and differentiation of cerebral CM from micro-AVM by MRI alone can be difficult in this setting.[48,52] Micro-AVM are nidal-type pial AVM with a nidus that is less than or equal to 1 cm. Cerebral micro-AVM are considered rare outside the HHT population. In contrast to cerebral CM, cerebral micro-AVM have a compact nidus comprising macro-angiomatous vessels that are variably differentiated as discrete vascular structures on conventional MRI sequences. Micro-AVM, unlike cerebral CM, is often associated with perilesional parenchymal T2 FLAIR signal hyperintensity corresponding to gliosis, and encephalomalacia. In contradistinction to cerebral CM, micro-AVM is supplied by distinct feeding arteries and directly drained by 1 or 2 veins (Figs. 7 and 8).[51] Catheter-directed DSA will frequently reveal juxta-nidal tapered stenoses of feeding arteries and draining veins which are pathognomonic. While the natural history of the cerebral CM is benign in the HHT population, with no reports of hemorrhage in the published literature,[53,54] hemorrhagic stroke due to microAVM rupture is well reported in the general population.[49] Whether the natural history of micro-AVM in the HHT population differs from that of sporadic micro-AVM is not yet clear. There is broad consensus nonetheless that cerebral CM, whether sporadic or associated with HHT, should be considered "do not touch" lesions.[55] However, follow-up is required to watch for the development of micro-AVM in the setting of HHT.

Because of the syndromic associations with intracranial and/or intraspinal vascular malformations, we will briefly address cutaneous capillary and venous malformations expressed by neurocutaneous disorders. Most cutaneous capillary and venous malformations are solitary and not associated with neuroaxial manifestations. On the other hand, large, segmental, or multifocal cutaneous CM should prompt further imaging of the brain and spine, as they are associated with multisystem syndromic disorders and vascular malformations in deeper tissues.[56]

Another syndromic condition in which cutaneous CM is associated with neuroaxial lesions

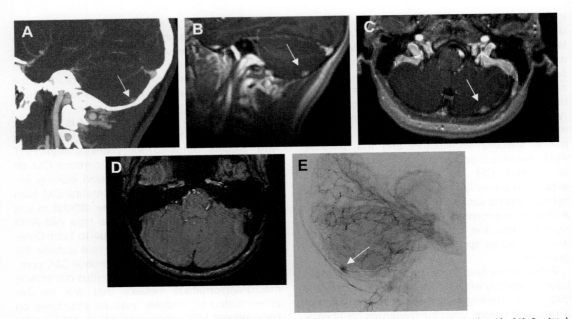

Fig. 6. Capillary malformation. 11-year-old girl with hereditary hemorrhagic telangiectasia (HHT). (*A*) Sagittal CTA image, (*B*) sagittal and (*C*) axial gadolinium-enhanced MRI images show a punctate focus of enhancement along the posterior cerebellar cortex (*arrows*). (*D*) No abnormal susceptibility is seen on SWI images. In the setting of HHT, evolution into a micro-arteriovenous malformation also needs to be considered. (*E*) Catheter-directed DSA showing a typical focal blush (*arrow*) in the capillary phase of a vertebral artery injection in the lateral plane.

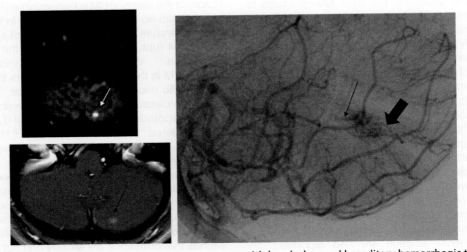

Fig. 7. Micro-arteriovenous malformation. Young woman with headaches and hereditary hemorrhagic telangiectasia due to ACVRL-1 mutation. Arterial spin labeling (ASL) axial imaging shows intense focal flow-related enhancement in the left posterior inferior cerebellum (*thin white arrow*). Gadolinium-enhanced axial T1-weighted image through the posterior fossa demonstrates a focus of parenchymal enhancement without vascular flow voids or discrete enhancing vascular structures (*thin black arrow*). The differential diagnosis includes cerebral capillary malformation (CM) and micro-arteriovenous malformation (AVM). Catheter-directed digital subtraction angiography (DSA), late arterial phase of lateral projection left vertebral artery injection, shows a sub-centimeter nidus supplied by a branch of the left posterior inferior cerebellar artery (*thick arrow*) with a solitary draining vein (*thin arrow*) confirming the diagnosis of micro-AVM.

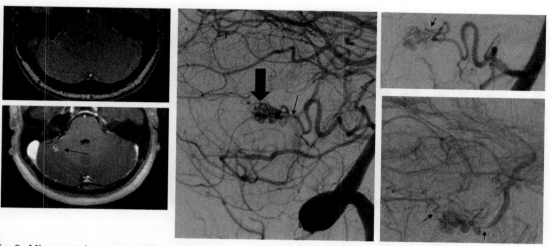

Fig. 8. Micro-arteriovenous malformation. Young woman with hereditary hemorrhagic telangiectasia due to Endoglin mutation and multiple pulmonary arteriovenous malformations (AVMs). Time of flight magnetic resonance angiography axial source image shows a subcentimeter compact cluster of vessels in the right posterior inferior cerebellum (*thin black arrow*). T1 weighted Gadolinium-enhanced axial image through the posterior fossa shows contrast enhancement of discrete vascular structures in the index region (*thin black arrow*). The differential diagnosis includes cerebral capillary malformation (CM) and micro-arteriovenous malformation (AVM). Catheter-directed digital subtraction angiography (DSA), early arterial phase of lateral projection right vertebral artery injection, shows a sub-centimeter angiomatous nidus (*thick arrow*) supplied by a branch of the right posterior inferior cerebellar artery (thin *arrow*) confirming the diagnosis of micro-AVM. Frame acquired earlier in the angiographic series magnified to show tapered stenosis of the AVM feeding artery (thick *arrow*). Frames acquired later in the angiographic series were magnified to show two AVM draining veins with tapered stenoses (*thin arrows*).

is the CM-AVM syndrome (RASA-1 mutation, **Fig. 9**). This condition is characterized by multiple small cutaneous CMs and arteriovenous shunts in the brain, face/head/neck, and viscera.[57,58] In Klippel-Trenaunay Weber syndrome, a form of PIK3CA-related overgrowth syndrome (PROS), there is a characteristic triad of extensive venous malformations, soft tissue, and bone hypertrophy resulting in limb overgrowth, and cutaneous CM.[59] In CLOVES, another type of PROS, cutaneous CM is associated with truncal venous malformations, lymphatic malformations, lipomatous overgrowth, and a diverse range of spinal vascular malformations including low flow lesions (venous and lymphatic), and arteriovenous shunt lesions. When syndromic cutaneous CM is suspected, further workup including comprehensive MR imaging and genetic testing should be pursued. Catheter-directed DSA is indicated if there is suspicion of an arteriovenous shunt within the neuroaxis.[60] The article by Shaibani A, et al. in this book provides an in-depth overview of spinal vascular malformations in childhood.

Segmental cutaneous CM, commonly known as port-wine stains (PWS), are characteristic manifestations of the cerebrofacial venous metameric syndrome known as Sturge-Weber syndrome

(SWS), also called encephalotrigeminal angiomatosis. SWS is a congenital neurocutaneous disorder that results in a metameric failure of normal cerebral venous development and cerebral hypoperfusion with secondary cerebral calcification and atrophy. Affected patients usually develop intractable epilepsy in the first year of life and suffer severe neurologic and ophthalmologic deficits.[61] Ultrasonography with color Doppler is a common first-line imaging modality for cutaneous CMs given its widespread availability and noninvasiveness. A superficial hypoechoic region with increased vascularity is a characteristic ultrasound finding.[62] Late-stage neuroimaging findings of SWS, after the onset of hemi-convulsive seizures, may include venous leptomeningeal angiomatosis with cortical atrophy, gyral enhancement (**Fig. 10**), calcifications of the cerebral cortex and white matter, calvarial thickening and choroid plexus hypertrophy.[62] In asymptomatic infants, abnormalities of cerebral perfusion and metabolism may be the only neuroimaging manifestations.[63] Segmental cutaneous CM is similarly expressed in individuals with cerebrofacial arteriovenous metameric syndrome. For example, the Wyburn Mason syndrome (**Fig. 11**) is characterized by a metameric AVM within the diencephalon, optic tract, optic

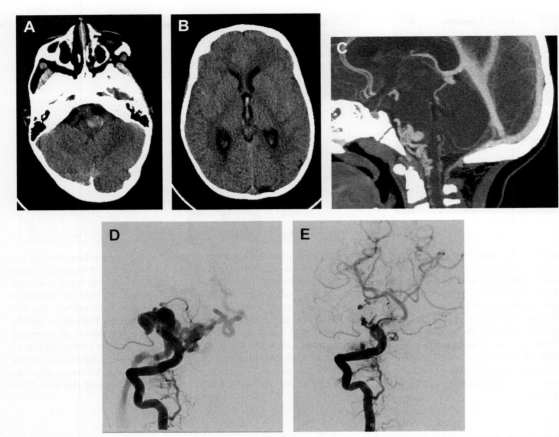

Fig. 9. Capillary malformation-arteriovenous malformation syndrome. A 3-year-old female presented with a sudden headache and loss of consciousness. (*A*) Plain CT showing a hyperdense structure anterolateral to the brainstem with mass effect. (*B*) Intraventricular hemorrhage is seen in the third ventricle. (*C*) CTA shows serpiginous vessels anterior to the brainstem and a large sac indenting the brainstem. (*D*) Catheter-directed DSA, right vertebral artery injection frontal projection showing an arteriovenous fistula arising from a brainstem perforator. The large sac seen on cross-sectional imaging is identified as a venous pouch at the arteriovenous transition (*arrow*). Due to the high-flow nature of the shunt, there is no intracranial flow into the basilar artery from this side, as well as steal from the contralateral vertebral artery (not shown here) (*E*). Right vertebral artery angiography following coil and glue embolization. Positive RASA1 mutation was found on genetic testing.

nerve, and neural retina.[64] A segmental cutaneous CM is variably expressed within the segmental dermatome of the affected metamere.

Developmental venous anomalies

Cerebral developmental venous anomalies (DVA) are among the most common cerebral vascular malformations with an incidence rate of 2.6%.[65] A cerebral DVA is a hypertrophic transcerebral medullary vein (DVA collecting vein) that has expansively remodeled and extended across the deep-superficial medullary venous watershed to annex the territory of neighboring medullary veins on the opposing side of the watershed through subpial or subependymal anastomoses. The annexed medullary veins and the anastomoses which join them to the hypertrophic transcerebral medullary

vein constitute the "caput medusa" formation of the DVA. The venous radicles of the caput medusa radially converge on the afferent pole of the hypertrophic medullary collecting vein in a subpial or subependymal location.

In the normal developmental process, the venous outflow of the brain is balanced between a superficial centrifugally directed (ventriculofugal) system for the cortical and immediate subcortical regions, and a deeper centripetally directed (ventriculopetal) subependymal system for the deep white matter and basal ganglia structures. Anastomoses between the radially oriented ventriculofugal and ventriculopetal medullary veins enable the redistribution of flow when the opposing system is compromised early in development. The process which results in this anatomic variant is

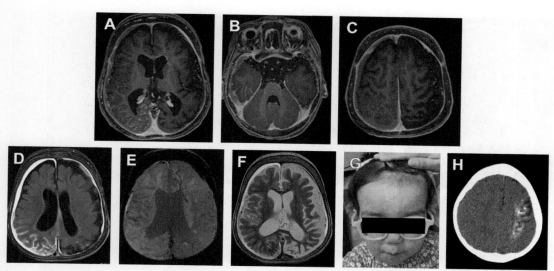

Fig. 10. Sturge Weber syndrome (SWS) in a 4-year-old female. (*A–D*) Post-gadolinium images show diffuse bilateral leptomeningeal enhancement and volume loss, left greater than right, resulting in chronic extra-axial collections and ex vacuo dilatation of the ventricles. (*E*) SWI image showing increased susceptibility from slow-flowing blood in the subependymal venous system. (*F*) On T2 weighted images, serpiginous ectatic vasculature is identified in the CSF space of the left cerebral convexity. (*G*) There is a corresponding bilateral port wine stain of the V1 and V2 dermatomes. (*H*) Plain CT image in another child with SWS showing tram-track calcifications in the left parietal region. The child had a V2-distribution port-wine stain.

believed to be initiated early in fetal development when thrombosis or developmental failure of local draining veins, on the pial or ependymal surface of the brain, forces a redistribution of venous outflow from hemodynamically stranded medullary veins into the nearest medullary vein with a patent drainage pathway on the opposing side of the deep-superficial medullary venous watershed. The DVA is therefore considered an adaptive response to a developmental constraint imposed by pathologic loss of normal venous drainage pathways. While thrombosis or developmental failure of draining veins is the most widely agreed upon trigger for the redistribution of medullary venous drainage that leads to DVA formation, alternative theories have focused on disturbances of fetal brain development that result in asymmetric "hemodynamic demand" across the medullary venous watershed.[66–68] This would explain the occurrence of DVA in conjunction with malformations of cortical development.

DVA vary widely in size and complexity. An isolated simple DVA has a single transcerebral medullary collecting vein that receives the drainage of one caput medusa formation serving a sublobar brain region (**Fig. 12**). Complex DVAs receive the venous drainage of lobar, multi-lobar, or hemispheric brain regions, and can have multiple hypertrophic transcerebral medullary collecting veins.

DVAs are considered anatomic variants with a benign natural history.[69] Isolated simple DVA generally has limited clinical significance when found incidentally. While the vast majority are incidental findings on neuroimaging studies, symptomatic DVA is occasionally encountered. In some cases, an associated vascular or nonvascular lesion within the venous drainage territory of the DVA may be the cause of symptoms rather than the DVA itself. The most common vascular lesion associated with DVA is CCM within the corresponding venous drainage territory. CM and pial AV shunt lesions are similarly associated, but less commonly. Notably, dural arteriovenous shunts, orbital lymphatic malformations, extracranial head and neck venous malformations, sinus pericranii, and AVM of the face/head/neck are also reported associations.[70,71]

DVA is responsible for the venous drainage of the normal brain within a large region that is depleted of its venous reserve.[72] Consequently, pathologic or iatrogenic occlusion of a DVA usually results in extensive hemorrhagic venous infarction. Care must be taken during microneurosurgical and endovascular procedures to avoid compromising DVAs and disrupting cerebral venous drainage. In the majority of patients who are symptomatic from the DVA itself, thrombosis of the DVA collecting vein is the cause, though complex DVAs may also cause symptoms due

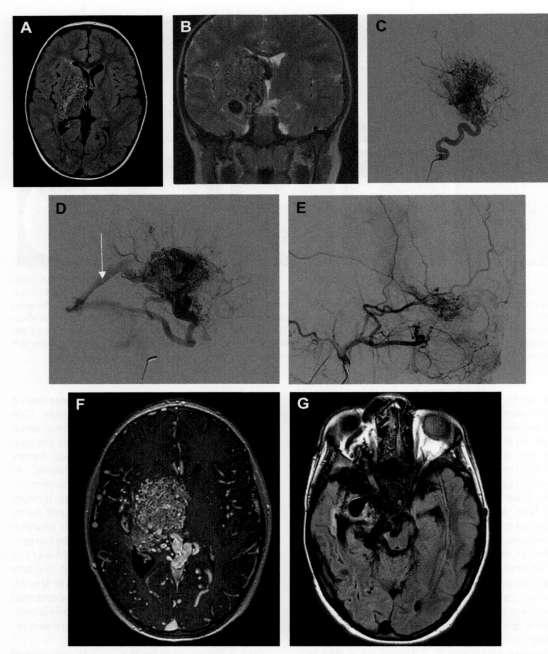

Fig. 11. Wyburn mason syndrome. A 5-year-old boy presented with left-sided facial droop. MRI was performed as part of a code stroke work-up. (*A*) Axial FLAIR and (*B*) Coronal T2-weighted images show a diffuse proliferation of ectatic vessels in the right gangliocapsular and thalamic regions. No hemorrhage was identified. Catheter-directed DSA was performed, which showed a proliferative angiopathy seen in (*C*). early arterial phase of right internal carotid injection, with prominent early veins into superficial and deep venous systems, seen in (*D*) late arterial phase. On right external carotid angiography, (*E*) prominent orbital hypervascularity (*arrow*) was noted via the meningo-ophthalmic system. (*F*) Subsequent MR imaging at age 8 years and (*G*) at age 14 years show increased vascular proliferation in the brain parenchyma with volume loss and in the ipsilateral orbit, with contiguous progression along the chiasma and optic nerve.

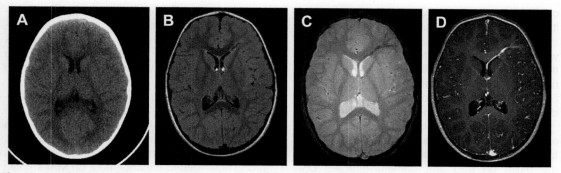

Fig. 12. Developmental venous anomaly. A 3-year-old boy presented with lethargy. (*A*) Plain CT showed no abnormality. MRI was performed including (*B*) FLAIR, (*C*) gradient recalled, and (*D*) post-gadolinium images, which show a caput medusae of left frontal subcortical veins draining centripetally via a transmedullary collector vein into the subependymal system. Some surrounding FLAIR hyperintensity suggests mild congestive changes.

to mass effect.[73] Risk factors for DVA thrombosis include oral contraceptives, dehydration, thrombophilia, and sickle cell crisis. Thrombosis of a DVA can cause intraparenchymal hemorrhage in infants and small children, and the caput-medusa of a thrombosed hypertrophic transcerebral medullary collecting vein can be mistaken for AVM nidus on contrast-enhanced CT imaging. Thin-section, multiphase CECT can reveal the true nature, but adequate CECT is challenging to obtain reliably in this population, often necessitating MRI with contrast and SWI imaging to identify thrombus in the hypertrophic transcerebral medullary collecting vein. Catheter-directed DSA with its inherent risks in this age group can be avoided with knowledge of this phenomenon and appropriate use of cross-sectional imaging. Most complications of DVA tend to present later in life as they are considered a sequela of long-standing shear-induced intimal hyperplasia within the hypertrophic transcerebral medullary collecting vein, resulting in venous hypertension, edema, and chronic ischemia.[74]

DVA is commonly detected as incidental findings on contrast-enhanced (CE) computed tomography (CT) or magnetic resonance imaging (MRI) scans.[75] Noncontrast CT imaging often reveals a subtle linear hyperdensity corresponding to the hypertrophic transcerebral medullary collecting vein of the DVA. Calcifications occasionally found in the drainage territory of the caput medusa may be related to dystrophic calcification or a CCM. DVA medullary collecting veins can be seen as conspicuous transcerebral flow voids on T2 weighted MRI sequences. CECT or CEMRI will reveal the venous radicles of the caput medusa as well as the hypertrophic transcerebral medullary collecting vein. Susceptibility-weighted imaging (SWI) in particular is useful for the thorough

evaluation of a DVA and associated abnormalities due to the presence of deoxygenated blood.[76,77] SWI imaging delineates the different components of the DVA, and highlights associated CCM in the venous drainage territory of the caput medusa. Transcranial ultrasound appearances of DVA have recently been described in neonates: hyperechoic brain parenchyma in the draining territories and venous waveforms are typical findings. Further imaging workup is rarely indicated for isolated asymptomatic DVA detected on CT or noncontrast MRI but when an associated vascular malformation is suspected, or detailed preoperative planning is required for microneurosurgery, contrast-enhanced MRI, MRA and MRV is indicated. Catheter-directed DSA may be further indicated to evaluate symptomatic DVA, atypical DVA, associated AVM/AVF or for planning microneurosurgery in the region of the DVA.[78]

A spectrum of atypical DVA phenotypes, which may be considered to exist along a continuum, is recognized from catheter-directed angiography. Type 1 and type 2 atypical DVA are characterized by a dense, hyperemic capillary blush (A.K.A. tissue stain) in the venous drainage territory of a DVA caput medusa. Type 2 atypical DVA are further differentiated by enlarged arterial feeders supplying the hyperemic capillary blush.[77] Type 3 lesions consist of a nidal type pial AVM or AVF within the venous drainage territory of a DVA caput medusa. While the caput medusa and corresponding hypertrophic medullary collecting vein of the type 1 and type 2 atypical DVA appear early in relation to normal brain parenchymal draining veins on catheter-directed DSA, this must be differentiated from true "arteriovenous shunting".[79]

Since the blood flowing into the atypical DVA caput medusa initially passes through an ectatic capillary network, arteriovenous shunting is definitively absent. The hypertrophic medullary collecting vein appears before normal brain parenchymal veins due to decreased tissue transit time, rather than arteriovenous shunting. A similar phenomenon is observed in the setting of acute brain infarction due to auto-regulatory precapillary arteriolar dilatation (A.K.A. luxury perfusion).

The basis of the dense hyperemic capillary blush or tissue stain in type 1 and 2 atypical DVA is not fully known. Since the neuroimaging features of the blush on MRI and catheter-directed DSA closely resemble that of cerebral CM, a popular model of atypical DVA phenotypes conceptualizes type 1 and type 2 lesions as sequential transitional states along a continuum to the type 3 lesion.[79] In this model, the atypical DVA is a hybrid lesion comprising 2 separate entities: (1) the DVA and (2) an error of vascular network segmentation and differentiation within the venous drainage territory of the DVA caput medusa (Fig. 13). The spectrum of phenotypes that may result from errors of vascular network segmentation and differentiation include CM (in atypical DVA types 1 and 2) and AVM (in atypical DVA type 3). Alternative theories suggest that the hyperemic capillary blush of type 1 and type 2 atypical DVAs is the consequence of autoregulatory precapillary arteriolar dilatation induced by impaired tissue perfusion in the venous drainage territory of the DVA caput medusa. Type 1 and 2 atypical DVAs are known to display flow-related enhancement on ASL imaging.[80]

While type 1 and type 2 atypical DVA are associated with a risk of cerebral hemorrhage, the risks have not been well characterized and the mechanisms have not yet been established. Since type 3 lesions have a pial AVM component, strong flow-related enhancement on MRI studies is typical, and the risk of bleeding should be concordant with what has been reported for pial AVM.

Novel imaging applications for intracranial vascular malformations in children

Advances in MRI-based imaging technologies have facilitated detailed insights into the structural and functional aspects of IVM in children. High-resolution magnetic resonance imaging (MRI) and functional MRI (fMRI) have long been used to evaluate pediatric neurovascular disease and offer powerful detail about morphologic and hemodynamic characteristics. More recent advances such as flow-sensitive arterial spin labeling (ASL),

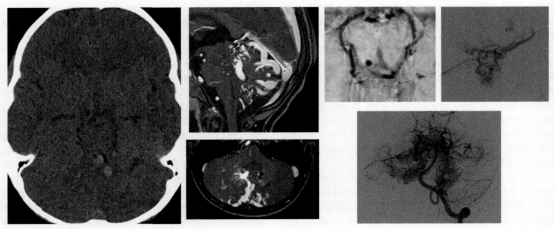

Fig. 13. Hybrid central nervous system vascular malformation involving diffuse cerebellar capillary malformation with mosaic compartments of arteriovenous malformation within the venous drainage territory of complex atypical infratentorial developmental venous anomaly. A 7-year-old girl with headache, nausea, emesis, ataxia, and nystagmus. Axial noncontrast CT image shows acute hemorrhage in the left superior cerebellar peduncle (*think black arrow*) extending into the fourth ventricle (*thick black arrow*). Sagittal and axial T1 weighted Gadolinium-enhanced axial image through the posterior fossa show multiple hypertrophic transcerebral medullary collecting veins of a complex infratentorial developmental venous anomaly involving the cerebellum and brainstem bilaterally. Axial susceptibility-weighted image reveals a small cerebral cavernous malformation in the midbrain tecum (*thin black arrow*). Catheter-directed digital subtraction angiography (DSA), arterial phase of frontal projection left vertebral artery injection, shows a diffuse butterfly-shaped capillary malformation involving the cerebellar hemispheres bilaterally. Microcatheter angiogram (early arterial phase, lateral projection) of a left superior cerebellar artery branch supplying the left superior cerebellar peduncle reveals a compartment of hemorrhagic arteriovenous malformation nidus with a single draining vein (*thin arrow*).

time-resolved contrast-enhanced or spin-labeled magnetic resonance angiography (MRA), and 4D flow MRI have dramatically improved the accuracy of neuroimaging diagnosis and treatment planning for children with neurovascular disease.

ASL magnetically labels protons in arterial blood, replacing the need for exogenous contrast agents, whereby T1 signal decay occurs before normal capillary transit time. Flow-related enhancement on ASL sequences is seen in a variety of high-flow lesions including vascular malformations, vascular tumors and inflammatory disorders. While non-specific, flow-related enhancement on ASL sequences can reveal a high-flow lesion with exquisite sensitivity and conspicuity.[81] ASL sequences are a powerful tool for the detection of small high-flow lesions in the setting of hemorrhagic stroke and in patients with HHT.[82,83]

Time-resolved spin-labeled MRA distinguishes itself through its capacity to dynamically assess blood flow and depict angioarchitecture. Serial imaging across arterial, capillary, and venous phases offers greater diagnostic accuracy for venous drainage depiction in brain AVMs than 3D time-of-flight MRA, which lacks temporal hemodynamic information, and time-resolved contrast-enhanced MRA, which suffers from dense venous opacification over the required acquisition time, obscuring the areas of interest.[84] Another technique that utilizes single vessel-selective time-resolved spin-labeled MRA, allows one to spin-label blood in a specific vessel to interrogate its territorial distribution and individual contribution to the arterial supply of a vascular malformation. Using this approach, one group achieved greater diagnostic accuracy in identifying the feeding vessels of dural arteriovenous fistulae[85] and both feeding vessels and draining veins in brain AVMs.[86] The downside of this technique is that acquisition time for each vessel is approximately 5 minutes so a 4-vessel study would require 20 minutes of scan time, an opportunity cost that would impact many departments' MRI schedules.

Finally, 4D Flow MRI captures data along the time dimension and provides quantitative flow data such as velocity, volume, and wall shear inside specific vessels.[87,88] This technique offers detailed quantitative assessments of blood flow in specific vessels before and after intervention. Limitations include the lack of spatial resolution to capture small vessel hemodynamics (ie, AVM feeding arteries and draining veins) as well as a limited accuracy in capturing a wide range of flow velocities. This technique also suffers from long scan times, ranging from 5 to 20 minutes, along with personnel constraints due to cumbersome postprocessing requirements.[87]

Blood pool agents such as Ferumoxytol and gadofosveset trisodium have been used to provide extended intravascular enhancement and to increase spatial and contrast resolution.[81] Ferumoxytol is an iron oxide nanoparticle with a plasma half-life of 14 to 21 hours.[89] On delayed imaging at 24 hours postadministration, it has been useful in identifying intracranial tumors by virtue of blood-brain barrier disruption.[89] Since the Ferumoxytol nanoparticle is taken up and retained by macrophages, which are abundant in inflammatory tissues, Ferumoxytol enhancement on delayed images has been used to monitor inflammatory changes in brain AVM and aneurysms, which may be a surrogate of silent intralesional hemorrhage.[90] Others have used delayed Ferumoxytol enhancement to detect the recurrence of pediatric cerebral AVM.[91] The persistence of blood pool agents on delayed imaging has been noted to produce artifacts in subsequent MRI studies. This can be confused for pathology if the reading neuroradiologist is not aware of prior administration.[92] Therefore, the utilization of this agent for pediatric IVM must be performed with full view of their imaging needs over time. Gadofosveset trisodium binds to human serum albumin resulting in extended intravascular contrast enhancement[93] that yields crisp MRA imaging with uniform vascular opacification.[81,94] However, comparative studies with gadolinium-based MRA for IVM are lacking, with at least one report demonstrating superior image quality with gadofosveset trisodium, without statistically significant increased accuracy compared with TOF MRA.[95]

SUMMARY

IVM in children represents a diagnostic and therapeutic challenge, necessitating the use of advanced diagnostic neuroimaging approaches, including catheter-directed DSA, and the collaboration of multidisciplinary teams. Advances in neuroimaging have enabled improved outcomes for children with IVM. The emergence of novel imaging applications and techniques such as ASL, time-resolved spin-labeled MRA, 4D flow MRI, and alternative MRI contrast agents promise further improvements. These innovations supplement traditional diagnostic methods such as CT and catheter-directed DSA, providing comprehensive vascular and soft tissue depiction without exposing patients to ionizing radiation. These advanced modalities not only offer detailed views into vascular structure and function, which are critical for treatment planning but also pave the way for more accurate and minimally invasive interventions.

CLINICS CARE POINTS

- Treatment approaches are based on the specific type of vascular malformation, its location, and patient's neurological status which requires a multidisciplinary approach combining neurosurigcal, endovascular, and radiosurgical techniques to optimize outcomes for complex cases.

- Advanced neuroimaging techniques, such as MRI with ASL and TRICKS, and catheter digital subtraction angiography, are needed to accurately diagnose and plan treatment for pediatric patients with intracranial vascular malformations.

- Differentiating shunting and non-shunting lesions is key in assessing risk in choosing between conservative management and more aggressive surgical or endovascular interventions.

REFERENCES

1. Murphy PA, Kim TN, Huang L, et al. Constitutively active Notch4 receptor elicits brain arteriovenous malformations through enlargement of capillary-like vessels. Proc Natl Acad Sci USA 2014;111(50):18007–12.

2. El-Ghanem M, Kass-Hout T, Kass-Hout O, et al. Arteriovenous malformations in the pediatric population: review of the existing literature. Interv Neurol 2016; 5(3–4):218–25.

3. Van Beijnum J, Van Der Worp HB, Buis DR, et al. Treatment of brain arteriovenous malformations: a systematic review and meta-analysis. JAMA 2011; 306(18):2011.

4. Moftakhar P, Hauptman JS, Malkasian D, et al. Cerebral arteriovenous malformations. Part 2: physiology. FOC 2009;26(5):E11.

5. Tasiou A, Tzerefos C, Alleyne CH, et al. Arteriovenous malformations: congenital or acquired lesions? World Neurosurgery 2020;134:e799–807.

6. Shovlin CL, Simeoni I, Downes K, et al. Mutational and phenotypic characterization of hereditary hemorrhagic telangiectasia. Blood 2020;136(17):1907–18.

7. Zeng X, Hunt A, Jin SC, et al. EphrinB2-EphB4-RASA1 Signaling in human cerebrovascular development and disease. Trends Mol Med 2019;25(4): 265–86.

8. Bameri O, Salarzaei M, Parooie F. KRAS/BRAF mutations in brain arteriovenous malformations: A systematic review and meta-analysis. Intervent Neuroradiol 2021;27(4):539–46.

9. Winkler EA, Kim CN, Ross JM, et al. A single-cell atlas of the normal and malformed human brain vasculature. Science 2022;375(6584).

10. Eli I, Gamboa NT, Joyce EJ, et al. Clinical presentation and treatment paradigms in patients with hereditary hemorrhagic telangiectasia and spinal vascular malformations. J Clin Neurosci 2018;50:51–7.

11. Abecassis IJ, Xu DS, Batjer HH, et al. Natural history of brain arteriovenous malformations: a systematic review. Neurosurg Focus 2014;37(3):E7.

12. Lu AY, Winkler EA, Garcia JH, et al. A comparison of incidental and symptomatic unruptured brain arteriovenous malformations in children. J Neurosurg Pediatr 2023;1–6. https://doi.org/10.3171/2023.1. PEDS22541.

13. Di Rocco C, Tamburrini G, Rollo M. Cerebral arteriovenous malformations in children. Acta Neurochir (Wien) 2000;142(2):145–56. discussion 156-158.

14. Mohr JP, Parides MK, Stapf C, et al. Medical management with or without interventional therapy for unruptured brain arteriovenous malformations (ARUBA): a multicentre, non-blinded, randomised trial. Lancet 2014;383(9917):614–21.

15. Dicpinigaitis A, Ogulnick J, Cooper J, et al. Increased incidence of ruptured cerebral arteriovenous malformations and mortality in the United States: unintended consequences of the aruba trial? J Neurointerv Surg 2022;14:A29.

16. Gross BA, Du R. Natural history of cerebral arteriovenous malformations: a meta-analysis: Clinical article. JNS 2013;118(2):437–43.

17. Ding D, Starke RM, Kano H, et al. International multi-center cohort study of pediatric brain arteriovenous malformations. Part 1: Predictors of hemorrhagic presentation. PED 2017;19(2):127–35.

18. Yamada S, Takagi Y, Nozaki K, et al. Risk factors for subsequent hemorrhage in patients with cerebral arteriovenous malformations. JNS 2007;107(5): 965–72.

19. Hernesniemi JA, Dashti R, Juvela S, et al. Natural history of brain arteriovenous malformations: a long-term follow-up study of risk of hemorrhage in 238 patients. Neurosurgery 2008;63(5):823–31.

20. Pepper J, Lamin S, Thomas A, et al. Clinical features and outcome in pediatric arteriovenous malformation: institutional multimodality treatment. Childs Nerv Syst 2023;39(4):975–82.

21. Ozpinar A, Mendez G, Abla AA. Epidemiology, genetics, pathophysiology, and prognostic classifications of cerebral arteriovenous malformations. Handb Clin Neurol 2017;143:5–13.

22. Sporns PB, Psychogios MN, Fullerton HJ, et al. Neuroimaging of pediatric intracerebral hemorrhage. JCM 2020;9(5):1518.

23. Cheng YC, Chen HC, Wu CH, et al. Magnetic resonance angiography in the diagnosis of cerebral arteriovenous malformation and dural arteriovenous fistulas: comparison of time-resolved magnetic resonance angiography and three dimensional time-of-

flight magnetic resonance angiography. Iran J Radiol 2016;13(2):e19814.

24. Karhunen PJ, Penttilä A, Erkinjuntti T. Arteriovenous malformation of the brain: Imaging by postmortem angiography. Forensic Sci Int 1990;48(1):9–19.

25. Davies JM, Kim H, Young WL, et al. Classification schemes for arteriovenous malformations. Neurosurg Clin 2012;23(1):43–53.

26. Spetzler RF, Ponce FA. A 3-tier classification of cerebral arteriovenous malformations: Clinical article. JNS 2011;114(3):842–9.

27. Seymour ZA, Sneed PK, Gupta N, et al. Volume-staged radiosurgery for large arteriovenous malformations: an evolving paradigm. J Neurosurg 2016; 124(1):163–74.

28. Lasjaunias PL, Landrieu P, Rodesch G, et al. Cerebral proliferative angiopathy: clinical and angiographic description of an entity different from cerebral AVMs. Stroke 2008;39:878–85.

29. Brown NJ, Lien BV, Ehresman J, et al. Proliferative angiopathy: a systematic review. Stroke Vasc Interv Neurol 2024;4(3):e001186.

30. Fierstra J, Spieth S, Tran L, et al. Severely impaired cerebrovascular reserve in patients with cerebral proliferative angiopathy. J Neurosurg Pediatr 2011;8:310–5.

31. Kono K, Terada T. Encephaloduroarteriosynangiosis for cerebral proliferative angiopathy with cerebral ischemia. J Neurosurg 2014;121:1411–5.

32. Ene C, Kaul A, Kim L. Natural history of cerebral cavernous malformations. Handb Clin Neurol 2017; 143:227–32. Elsevier.

33. Berg MJ, Vay T. Clinical features and medical management of cavernous malformations. In: Rigamonti D, editor. Cavernous malformations of the nervous system. 1st edition. Cambridge, UK: Cambridge University Press; 2011. p. 65–78.

34. Meyers PM, Halbach VD, Barkovich AJ. Anomalies of cerebral vasculature: diagnostic and endovascular considerations. In: Barkovich AJ, editor. Pediatric neuroimaging. 4th edition. Philadelphia, PA: Lippincott Williams & Wilkins; 2005. p. 869–918.

35. Akers A, Al-Shahi Salman R, A Awad I, et al. Synopsis of guidelines for the clinical management of cerebral cavernous malformations: consensus recommendations based on systematic literature review by the angioma alliance scientific advisory board clinical experts panel. Neurosurgery 2017; 80(5):665–80.

36. Denier C, Labauge P, Bergametti F, et al. Genotype–phenotype correlations in cerebral cavernous malformations patients. Ann Neurol 2006;60(5):550–6.

37. Peyre M, Miyagishima D, Bielle F, et al. Somatic PIK3CA mutations in sporadic cerebral cavernous malformations. N Engl J Med 2021;385(11):996–1004.

38. Weng J, Yang Y, Song D, et al. Somatic MAP3K3 mutation defines a subclass of cerebral cavernous malformation. Am J Hum Genet 2021;108(5):942–50.

39. Mabray MC, Starcevich J, Hallstrom J, et al. High prevalence of spinal cord cavernous malformations in the familial cerebral cavernous malformations type 1 cohort. AJNR Am J Neuroradiol 2020;41(6): 1126–30.

40. Mouchtouris N, Chalouhi N, Chitale A, et al. Management of Cerebral Cavernous Malformations: From Diagnosis to Treatment. Sci World J 2015;2015:1–8.

41. Stapleton CJ, Barker FG. Cranial cavernous malformations: natural history and treatment. Stroke 2018;49(4):1029–35.

42. Al-Shahi SR, Berg MJ, Morrison L, et al. Hemorrhage from cavernous malformations of the brain: definition and reporting standards. Stroke 2008;39(12):3222–30.

43. Yun TJ, Na DG, Kwon BJ, et al. A T1 hyperintense perilesional signal aids in the differentiation of a cavernous angioma from other hemorrhagic masses. AJNR Am J Neuroradiol 2008;29(3):494–500.

44. Zabramski JM, Wascher TM, Spetzler RF, et al. The natural history of familial cavernous malformations: results of an ongoing study. J Neurosurg 1994; 80(3):422–32.

45. Michael GZG, Srinivasan V, Mohan A, et al. Pediatric cerebral cavernous malformations: Genetics, pathogenesis, and management. Surg Neurol Int 2016; 7(45):1127.

46. Gross BA, Moon K, Mcdougall CG. Endovascular management of arteriovenous malformations. Handb Clin Neurol 2017;143:59–68. Elsevier.

47. Sayama CM, Osborn AG, Chin SS, et al. Capillary telangiectasias: clinical, radiographic, and histopathological features: Clinical article. JNS 2010; 113(4):709–14.

48. Hetts SW, Shieh JT, Ohliger MA, et al. Hereditary hemorrhagic telangiectasia: the convergence of genotype, phenotype, and imaging in modern diagnosis and management of a multisystem disease. Radiology 2021;300(1):17–30.

49. Brinjikji W, Iyer VN, Yamaki V, et al. Neurovascular manifestations of hereditary hemorrhagic telangiectasia: a consecutive series of 376 patients during 15 years. AJNR Am J Neuroradiol 2016;37(8): 1479–86.

50. Castillo M, Morrison T, Shaw JA, et al. MR imaging and histologic features of capillary telangiectasia of the basal ganglia. AJNR Am J Neuroradiol 2001; 22(8):1553–5.

51. Krings T, Kim H, Power S, et al. Neurovascular manifestations in hereditary hemorrhagic telangiectasia: imaging features and genotype-phenotype correlations. AJNR Am J Neuroradiol 2015;36(5):863–70.

52. Faughnan ME, Mager JJ, Hetts SW, et al. Second International guidelines for the diagnosis and management of hereditary hemorrhagic telangiectasia. Ann Intern Med 2020;173(12):989–1001.

53. Brinjikji W, Iyer VN, Lanzino G, et al. Natural history of brain capillary vascular malformations in hereditary

hemorrhagic telangiectasia patients. J NeuroIntervent Surg 2017;9(1):26–8.

54. Matsubara S, Mandzia JL, ter Brugge K, et al. Angiographic and clinical characteristics of patients with cerebral arteriovenous malformations associated with hereditary hemorrhagic telangiectasia. AJNR Am J Neuroradiol 2000;21(6):1016–20.

55. Krings T, Ozanne A, Chng SM, et al. Neurovascular phenotypes in hereditary haemorrhagic telangiectasia patients according to age: Review of 50 consecutive patients aged 1 day–60 years. Neuroradiology 2005;47(10):711–20.

56. Maguiness SM, Liang MG. Management of capillary malformations. Clin Plast Surg 2011;38(1):65–73.

57. Bayrak-Toydemir P, Stevenson DA. Capillary malformation-arteriovenous malformation syndrome. In: Adam MP, Feldman J, Mirzaa GM, et al, editors. GeneReviews®. University of Washington, Seattle; 1993. Available at: http://www.ncbi.nlm.nih.gov/books/NBK52764/. [Accessed 25 March 2024].

58. Valdivielso-Ramos M, Martin-Santiago A, Azaña JM, et al. Capillary malformation—arteriovenous malformation syndrome: a multicentre study. Clin Exp Dermatol 2021;46(2):300–5.

59. Glovkzki P, Driscoll DJ. Klippel–Trenaunay syndrome: current management. Phlebology 2007; 22(6):291–8.

60. Gangopadhyay AN, Tiwari P. Capillary malformation. In: Khanna AK, Tiwary SK, editors. Vascular malformations. Singapore: Springer; 2021. p. 73–82.

61. Yan H, Hu M, Cui Y, et al. Clinical characteristics of infants with port-wine stain and glaucoma secondary to Sturge–Weber Syndrome. BMC Ophthalmol 2022;22(1):260.

62. Hussein A, Malguria N. Imaging of vascular malformations. Radiol Clin 2020;58(4):815–30.

63. Clifford SM, Ghosh A, Zandifar A, et al. Arterial spin-labeled (ASL) perfusion in children with Sturge-Weber syndrome: a retrospective cross-sectional study. Neuroradiology 2023;65(12):1825–34.

64. O'Loughlin L, Groves ML, Miller NR, et al. Cerebrofacial arteriovenous metameric syndrome (CAMS): a spectrum disorder of craniofacial vascular malformations. Childs Nerv Syst 2017;33(3):513–6.

65. San Millán Ruíz D, Yilmaz H, Gailloud P. Cerebral developmental venous anomalies: current concepts. Ann Neurol 2009;66(3):271–83.

66. Mooney MA, Zabramski JM. Developmental venous anomalies. Handb Clin Neurol 2017;143:279–82. Elsevier.

67. Lasjaunias P, Burrows P, Planet C. Developmental venous anomalies (DVA): The so-called venous angioma. Neurosurg Rev 1986;9(3):233–42.

68. Saito Y, Kobayashi N. Cerebral venous angiomas: clinical evaluation and possible etiology. Radiology 1981;139(1):87–94.

69. Hon JM, Bhattacharya JJ, Counsell CE, et al. The presentation and clinical course of intracranial developmental venous anomalies in adults: a systematic review and prospective, population-based study. Stroke 2009;40(6):1980–5.

70. Huber G, Henkes H, Hermes M, et al. Regional association of developmental venous anomalies with angiographically occult vascular malformations. Eur Radiol 1996;6(1):30–7.

71. Boukobza M, Enjolras O, Guichard JP, et al. Cerebral developmental venous anomalies associated with head and neck venous malformations. Am J Neuroradiol 1996;17(5):987.

72. San Millán Ruíz D, Gailloud P. Cerebral developmental venous anomalies. Childs Nerv Syst 2010; 26(10):1395–406.

73. Pereira VM, Geibprasert S, Krings T, et al. Pathomechanisms of symptomatic developmental venous anomalies. Stroke 2008;39(12):3201–15.

74. Santucci GM, Leach JL, Ying J, et al. Brain parenchymal signal abnormalities associated with developmental venous anomalies: detailed MR imaging assessment. AJNR Am J Neuroradiol 2008;29(7): 1317–23.

75. Rigamonti D, Spetzler RF, Drayer BP, et al. Appearance of venous malformations on magnetic resonance imaging. J Neurosurg 1988;69(4):535–9.

76. Takasugi M, Fujii S, Shinohara Y, et al. Parenchymal hypointense foci associated with developmental venous anomalies: evaluation by phase-sensitive MR imaging at 3T. AJNR Am J Neuroradiol 2013; 34(10):1940–4.

77. Horsch S, Govaert P, Cowan FM, et al. Developmental venous anomaly in the newborn brain. Neuroradiology 2014;56(7):579–88.

78. Hanson EH, Roach CJ, Ringdahl EN, et al. Developmental venous anomalies: appearance on whole-brain CT digital subtraction angiography and CT perfusion. Neuroradiology 2011;53(5):331–41.

79. Abruzzo T, Muthusami P, Hui F. Arterial spin-labeling imaging features of atypical cerebral developmental venous anomaly phenotypes. AJNR Am J Neuroradiol 2024;45(7):E24.

80. Yoo DH, Sohn CH, Kang HS, et al. Arterial spin-labeling MR imaging for the differential diagnosis of venous-predominant AVMs and developmental venous anomalies. AJNR Am J Neuroradiol 2023; 44(8):916–21.

81. Tranvinh E, Heit JJ, Hacein-Bey L, et al. Contemporary imaging of cerebral arteriovenous malformations. Am J Roentgenol 2017;208(6):1320–30.

82. Le TT, Fischbein NJ, André JB, et al. Identification of venous signal on arterial spin labeling improves diagnosis of dural arteriovenous fistulas and small arteriovenous malformations. AJNR Am J Neuroradiol 2012;33(1):61–8.

83. Sunwoo L, Sohn CH, Lee JY, et al. Evaluation of the degree of arteriovenous shunting in intracranial arteriovenous malformations using pseudo-continuous arterial spin labeling magnetic resonance imaging. Neuroradiology 2015;57(8):775–82.

84. Raoult H, Bannier E, Robert B, et al. Time-resolved spin-labeled MR angiography for the depiction of cerebral arteriovenous malformations: a comparison of techniques. Radiology 2014;271(2):524–33.

85. Togao O, Obara M, Kikuchi K, et al. Vessel-selective 4D-MRA using superselective pseudocontinuous arterial spin-labeling with keyhole and view-sharing for visualizing intracranial dural AVFs. AJNR Am J Neuroradiol 2022;43(3):368–75.

86. Togao O, Obara M, Helle M, et al. Vessel-selective 4D-MR angiography using super-selective pseudo-continuous arterial spin labeling may be a useful tool for assessing brain AVM hemodynamics. Eur Radiol 2020;30(12):6452–63.

87. Schnell S, Wu C, Ansari SA. Four-dimensional MRI flow examinations in cerebral and extracerebral vessels - ready for clinical routine? Curr Opin Neurol 2016;29(4):419–28.

88. Turski P, Scarano A, Hartman E, et al. Neurovascular 4DFlow MRI (Phase Contrast MRA): emerging clinical applications. Neurovasc Imaging 2016;2(1):8.

89. Toth GB, Varallyay CG, Horvath A, et al. Current and potential imaging applications of ferumoxytol for magnetic resonance imaging. Kidney Int 2017; 92(1):47–66.

90. Hasan DM, Amans M, Tihan T, et al. Ferumoxytol-enhanced MRI to image inflammation within human brain arteriovenous malformations: a pilot investigation. Transl Stroke Res 2012;3(S1):166–73.

91. Huang Y, Singer TG, Iv M, et al. Ferumoxytol-enhanced MRI for surveillance of pediatric cerebral arteriovenous malformations. J Neurosurg Pediatr 2019;24(4):407–14.

92. Hanreck JC, Gerasymchuk M, Nayate AP. Head and neck vessel magnetic resonance angiography appearance and artifacts after therapeutic intravenous ferumoxytol infusion. BJR Case Rep 2023; 9(3):20230014.

93. Goyen M. Gadofosveset-enhanced magnetic resonance angiography. Vasc Health Risk Manag 2008; 4(1):1–9.

94. Kramer LA, Cohen AM, Hasan KM, et al. Contrast enhanced MR venography with gadofosveset trisodium: evaluation of the intracranial and extracranial venous system: Contrast Enhanced MR. J Magn Reson Imaging 2014;40(3):630–40.

95. Kau T, Gasser J, Celedin S, et al. MR angiographic follow-up of intracranial aneurysms treated with detachable coils: evaluation of a blood-pool contrast medium. AJNR Am J Neuroradiol 2009;30(8): 1524–30.

Intracranial Arterial Aneurysms in Childhood

Kartik D. Bhatia, MBBS, PhD, FRANZCR[a],*, Carmen Parra-Farinas, MD[b]

KEYWORDS

• Aneurysm • Mycotic • Dissection • Vessel sacrifice • Pediatric

KEY POINTS

- Intracranial arterial aneurysms in children are rare.
- Pediatric aneurysms differ from adult aneurysms in etiology, natural history, and management.
- Fusiform, dissecting, and mycotic aneurysms form a greater proportion of aneurysms in children compared with adults.
- Endovascular treatment is the primary interventional approach in children.

INTRODUCTION

Intracranial arterial aneurysms in children differ from adult aneurysms in their etiology, natural history, co-morbidities, and management approaches. Whilst rare, most large pediatric hospitals would encounter several aneurysm cases each year. Historically, most aneurysms presented with subarachnoid hemorrhage (54%–89%).[1–4] However, with advances in non-invasive imaging and increased screening of high-risk populations, unruptured aneurysms will be increasingly detected in children.[5]

In this article, the authors describe the epidemiology, clinical presentation, etiology, natural history, and management of intracranial arterial aneurysms in children.

EPIDEMIOLOGY

Pediatric intracranial arterial aneurysms are rare. They account for approximately 1% of all intracranial aneurysms.[6–8] Population-level incidence data for children are lacking in the literature and this represents an important topic for future research.

The key demographics and risk factors associated with pediatric aneurysms include as follows:

- *Sex:* Pre-pubertal children—M > F (approximately 3:2).[2,7] Post-pubertal—F > M (similar to adult pattern).[1,9]
- *Age:* Most cohorts reported a mean age of 10 to 14 years, with a range extending from neonates to late adolescence.[1,3,9–11]
- *Mortality:* In historic cohorts, the mortality rate ranged from 1.3% to 10.4%.[2–4,9]
- *Etiology:* Dissecting aneurysms are the most common aneurysm type in children <10 years age and saccular aneurysms are the most common in adolescents.[1,2,9] Fusiform, giant, and dissecting aneurysms form a greater proportion of childhood aneurysms relative to adult populations.[1]
- *Prevalence amongst imaged patients:* A retrospective study of 1458 pediatric magnetic resonance angiography (MRA) studies identified underlying aneurysms in 3.3% (n = 49).[5] However, these data are skewed by the higher risk population being imaged.

a Department of Medical Imaging, Sydney Children's Hospital Network, Children's Hospital at Westmead Clinical School, University of Sydney, Corner Hainsworth Street and Hawksebury Road, Westmead, New South Wales 2145, Australia; b Division of Pediatric Interventional Neuroradiology, Hospital for Sick Children, 170 Elizabeth Street, Toronto, ON, M5G1E8, Canada
* Corresponding author. Department of Medical Imaging, Level 2, Children's Hospital at Westmead, Cnr Hainsworth Street and Hawkesbury Road, Westmead, NSW< 2145, Australia
E-mail address: Kartik.Bhatia@health.nsw.gov.au

Neuroimag Clin N Am 34 (2024) 567–578
https://doi.org/10.1016/j.nic.2024.08.011
1052-5149/24/Crown Copyright © 2024 Published by Elsevier Inc. All rights reserved, including those for text and data mining, AI training, and similar technologies.

- *Risk factors for ruptured presentation:* Age <5 years and distal arterial location.[12]
- *Aneurysm features associated with unruptured presentation:* Wide-necked, giant, and internal carotid artery (ICA) aneurysms are predictors of an unruptured presentation.[12]
- *Anatomic distribution—anterior vs posterior circulation:* Approximately 75% in the anterior circulation and 25% in the posterior circulation.[1–3,9]
- *Anatomic distribution—most common:* In children, the most common aneurysm locations are the ICA and vertebrobasilar arteries.[1,2,9] The proportion of middle cerebral artery aneurysms appears similar between children and adults.[1] Anterior cerebral artery (or anterior communicating artery) aneurysms represent only 5% to 10% of cases in children,[1,2] whilst representing approximately one-third of adult aneurysms.

Underlying Systemic Conditions

An underlying systemic or genetic disorder is present in many pediatric patients with intracranial aneurysms. These include as follows:

- Hematological disorders,
- Systemic infection or immunosuppression,
- Phacomatoses, and
- Collagenopathies, elastinopathies, and other connective tissue disorders.

Sickle-cell disease is associated with the development of intracranial aneurysms (often multiple) with aneurysms identified in 1.2% of imaged children.[13]

Intracranial mycotic aneurysms can occur in children with systemic sepsis, endocarditis, or immunosuppression.[2] Aneurysms have been described in children with human immunodeficiency virus[2] and with primary immunodeficiency such as hyper-IgE syndrome.[14]

Phacomatoses including posterior fossa anomalies, hemangioma, arterial anomalies, cardiac anomalies, and eye anomalies (PHACE) syndrome (1 in 7 children affected[15]), tuberous sclerosis (predominantly fusiform ICA aneurysms[16]), and Type 1 neurofibromatosis (approximately 5% affected[17]) carry an increased risk of intracranial aneurysm formation, including in young children. The dilative arteriopathy phenotype of Alagille syndrome, which often featuresdolichoectasia, is commonly associated with childhood intracranial aneurysms.[18] This may warrant screening MR angiography in these populations. Autosomal dominant polycystic kidney disease is associated with saccular aneurysms in adults, but aneurysms have also been demonstrated in children.[19]

Collagenopathies, elastinopathies, and other connective tissue disorders frequently express systemic dissecting arteriopathies and therefore carry an increased risk of developing fusiform, giant, and dissecting aneurysms[1]—see **Fig. 1.** These unusual aneurysm phenotypes are a red flag for an underlying dissecting arteriopathy and clinical genetics consultation should be sought. Intracranial aneurysms have been described in patients with following conditions:

- *Marfan's syndrome:* 7% affected,[20]
- *Ehlers-Danlos syndrome type IV,*[21]
- *Loeys-Dietz syndrome:* 30% affected,[22]
- *COL4A1 mutation,*[23] and
- *Fibromuscular dysplasia:* 5% affected.[24]

Flow-Related Aneurysms

Flow-related aneurysms occur in patients with arterio-venous malformations (AVMs) or other arterio-venous (AV) shunting lesions. Management is centered upon treatment of the AVM to reduce flow. There are case reports of aneurysmal growth after successful treatment of the AVM,[25] suggesting the natural history is not entirely predictable. A retrospective analysis of AVM patients with and without flow-related aneurysms reported no significant difference in the annual hemorrhage rate (1.05% vs 1.35%).[26] Given the alternative etiology and management of flow-related aneurysms, they are not discussed further in this article.

What Proportion of Pediatric Hemorrhagic Stroke Patients Have an Aneurysm?

Intracranial aneurysms were identified in 13% of pediatric patients with hemorrhagic stroke in a population-level study of Northern California.[27] The annual incidence of aneurysmal hemorrhage was 0.18 per 100,000 person-years, highest in 15to 19 years old patients (0.52) and lowest in 5 to 9 years old patients (0.05).[27]

Predictors of an underlying aneurysm in this population of non-traumatic pediatric intracranial hemorrhage included as follows:

- Late adolescent age (15–19 years),
- Syncope or headache as a clinical presentation, and
- Bleeding pattern of pure subarachnoid hemorrhage.[27]

CLINICAL PRESENTATION

In historic cohorts, the most frequents modes of clinical presentation were as follows:

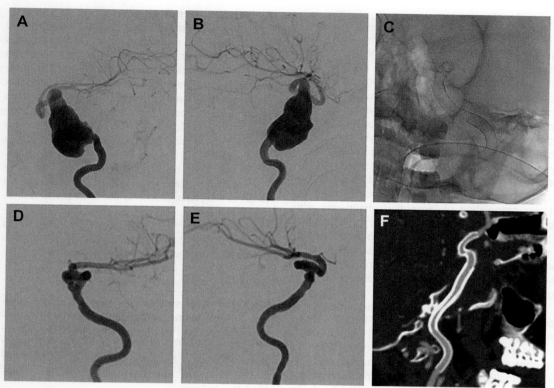

Fig. 1. Fusiform aneurysm: An 8-year-old girl with connective tissue disease presented with complete ptosis, ophthalmoplegia, and progressive visual loss. MR imaging demonstrated multiple fusiform aneurysms at the skull base. (*A, B*) Left interal carotid artery (ICA) digital subtraction angiogram (frontal and lateral) demonstrated a giant fusiform left petro-cavernous ICA aneurysm. There was relative isolation of the left middle cerebral artery (MCA) due to hypoplastic communicating arteries, excluding vessel sacrifice as an option. (*C*) Frontal oblique image following placement of 3 partially overlapping flow-diverter stents (Pipeline Vantage, Medtronic Inc) across the aneurysm. (*D, E*) Follow-up angiogram 5 months later confirmed marked reduction of flow into the aneurysm. (*F*) Reformatted computed tomography (CT) angiogram maximum intensity projection (MIP) of the left ICA 2 days following stent placement demonstrated the patent flow-diverter construct and marked reduction in intra-aneurysmal flow. There was progressive improvement in the patient's left eye opening, movement, and vision over the next 12 months.

- Hemorrhage (32%–78%[2,4,9]),
- Headache (33%–46%[2,9,10]), and
- Non-hemorrhagic neurologic deficit or seizures (36%–39%[2,9]).

Unruptured pediatric intracranial aneurysms are increasingly identified during screening MR angiography performed in high-risk populations.[5]

Dissecting aneurysms most commonly present with hemorrhage in children <5 years old, with headache and neck pain more common in older children.[2] Chronic fusiform aneurysms more often present with mass effect or non-hemorrhagic deficit.[9] Mycotic aneurysms frequently present with rupture.[28] Giant cavernous ICA aneurysms may cause progressive ophthalmoplegia and visual loss–see **Fig. 1**.

Children presenting with ruptured aneurysms tend to have better clinical grades at presentation than adults.[1,2,10] They also appear less likely to suffer clinically significant cerebral vasospasm after aneurysm rupture.[2,9,29]

ANEURYSM MORPHOLOGY

The major aneurysm etiologies in the pediatric population are as follows:

- Dissecting/fusiform aneurysms (19%–45%[2,9,10]), and
- Saccular aneurysms (32%–46%[2,9,10]).

ANEURYSM ETIOLOGY

- Idiopathic aneurysms,[9,30]
- Aneurysms associated with syndromic arteriopathies (10%–20%[9,30]),
- Mycotic (infectious) aneurysms (12%–20%[2,9,10]), and
- Traumatic aneurysms (3%–15%[2,9,10]).

Dissecting/Fusiform Aneurysms

Dissecting/fusiform aneurysms have fusiform or fusi-saccular morphology and typically demonstrate irregularity or stenosis in the pre-aneurysmal or post-aneurysmal segments of the parent vessel.[1,2] They are strongly associated with underlying connective tissue diseases or systemic arteriopathies (eg, Ehlers-Danlos Type IV, Marfan's, Loeys-Dietz, Menkes, osteogenesis imperfecta, fibromuscular dysplasia). Even in dissecting aneurysm cases where a currently characterized arteriopathy cannot be confirmed, a focal or mosaically expressed arteriopathy is likely present, given the strong association of dissecting aneurysms with regional or diffuse arterial tortuosity.[31] Whilst these fusiform aneurysms are presumed to be of dissecting etiology, a distinct preceding traumatic event is not identified in most cases, emphasizing the importance of underlying arteriopathy in affected patients.

Damage to the vessel wall intima ± media followed by intermittent episodes of intramural hematoma, thrombosis, remodeling, and reinjury progressively weakens the vessel wall.[32,33] This pathophysiology subsequently results in the typical fusiform or giant aneurysm morphology. They may present acutely, sub-acutely 2 to 6 weeks after a recent dissection, or as a chronic pathology. In children, the posterior circulation is involved more often than the anterior circulation.[2] These aneurysms are the most common morphologic type encountered in children less than 10 years old, after which saccular aneurysms predominate.[1,2,9]

Presentation is more often non-hemorrhagic (61%),[2] but young children (age <5 years) most often present with rupture.[2] The clinical presentation is determined by the evolution of the presumed dissecting event. If the intimal tear extends across the adventitia, subarachnoid hemorrhage (or carotid-cavernous fistula) will occur. Alternatively, if it does not extend to the adventitia, an intramural hematoma will develop.[32] Re-entry to the vessel lumen more distally or adjacent intraluminal stasis with thrombosis will predispose to embolic strokes. Enlarging fusiform aneurysms may cause mass effect upon adjacent structures (eg, cavernous sinus syndrome)—see Fig. 1.

Mycotic (Infectious) Aneurysms

Mycotic aneurysms comprise approximately 15% of pediatric intracranial aneurysms, can occur at any age, and most often present with hemorrhage.[2,28] Staphylococcus aureus is the most common organism involved,[34] followed by Streptococcus viridans, with gram-negative and fungal infections being less common.[28,32] Underlying bacterial endocarditis, immunodeficiency (including HIV), systemic sepsis, invasive sinus infection, penetrating head injury, or meningitis are all predisposing factors.

Systemic bacterial infection (including endocarditis) typically manifests with multiple aneurysms in the distal arterial circulation due to embolic deposition of organisms in smaller arteries followed by extension of infection outwards through the vessel wall[28,32]—see Fig. 2.

On the other hand, invasive sinus infection or bacterial/fungal meningitis can cause proximal larger aneurysms, closer to the skull base, due to spread of infection from the adventitia inwards toward the lumen[28,32,34]—see Fig. 3. This latter group of patients often has underlying immunosuppression which predisposes to poor outcomes.

Saccular Aneurysms

Saccular aneurysms are the most common aneurysm morphology in adolescents and are uncommon in children less than 8 years old.[1,2] They may be associated with a predisposing systemic condition (such as sickle cell disease)[2,13,19,32] or from hemodynamic stresses due to anatomic variations—see Fig. 4.

Historically, hemorrhage was the most common clinical presentation in children (80%).[2] Into the future, unruptured saccular aneurysms will be increasingly prevalent as non-invasive imaging and screening programs improve.[9,35] Most unruptured saccular aneurysms in children are <7 mm diameter ($\mu = 5$ mm).[35] The most common locations are ICA > middle cerebral artery (MCA) > anterior cerebral artery (ACA) and vertebrobasilar.[2]

Traumatic Aneurysms

Traumatic aneurysms have a distinct preceding traumatic event resulting in focal vessel wall injury. Typically, the child presents with intracranial hemorrhage 2 to 4 weeks following a blunt or less commonly penetrating head injury.[32] If the arterial wall is completely breached, pseudoaneurysm may form, around which a fibrotic capsule/wall may develop. When a pseudoaneurysm is present, post-traumatic dilatations of intradural arteries will be associated with subarachnoid hemorrhage and post-traumatic dilatations of the cavernous ICA will be associated with evidence of direct carotid-cavernous sinus fistula such as asymmetric cavernous sinus enlargement, cortical venous engorgement, ophthalmic venous engorgement, proptosis or abnormal flow-related enhancement of the cavernous sinus on arterial

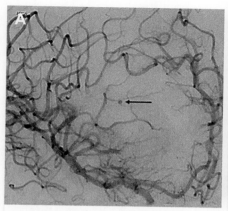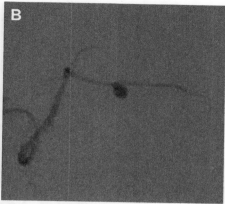

Fig. 2. Mycotic aneurysm (*black arrow*): A 7-year-old girl with a metallic heart valve and bacterial endocarditis, anticoagulated on warfarin, suffered a sudden onset severe headache. CT demonstrated hemorrhage adjacent to the right middle frontal gyrus. (*A*) Catheter-directed angiogram demonstrated a small mycotic aneurysm arising from a distal frontal branch of the right middle cerebral artery. (*B*) Subtracted roadmap demonstrated successful vessel sacrifice and occlusion of the aneurysm using Onyx-18 (Medtronic Inc.).

spin labeling, or time-of-flight MR sequences. The most common locations are the distal anterior cerebral artery (adjacent to the falx cerebri),[36] postcommunicating segment (P2)/quadrigeminal segment (P3) segments of the posterior cerebral artery (adjacent to the tentorial free edge),[37] the skull base,[38] and distal cortical branch arteries[32,39]—see **Fig. 5**.

Unruptured traumatic aneurysms are highly prone to rupture, and pseudoaneurysms are particularly unstable. Ruptured lesions should be secured acutely. Due to the absence of a true vessel wall around the pseudoaneurysm sac and the typical distal arterial location, it can be difficult or impossible to achieve selective occlusion of the lesion while maintaining patency of the parent vessel and vessel sacrifice is favored.[32,36]

NATURAL HISTORY
Unruptured Aneurysms

Unruptured pediatric aneurysms have a favorable natural history in most cases.

- *Size:* Approximately 80% present with a size of <7 mm.[35]
- *Growth:* A study of 60 unruptured aneurysms identified interval growth over time in 13% and a decreased diameter in 10%; the remainder was unchanged.[35] In a separate cohort of 114 aneurysms in 83 patients, 8.4% demonstrated enlargement or a new (de novo) aneurysm on follow-up imaging.[6]
- *Rupture rate:* No aneurysms ruptured during a mean follow-up period of 4 years.[6,35]
- *Management:* These results suggest the majority of unruptured pediatric aneurysms can

be managed conservatively but serial follow-up imaging is essential.

Mycotic aneurysms are an exception to this favorable natural history.

- The risk of rupture is thought to be high in the absence of treatment.
- *Natural history:* Unruptured mycotic aneurysms treated with intravenous antibiotics have a variable natural history including an increase in size in 17% to 22%, no change in 15% to 33%, decreased size in 17% to 18.5%, and resolution in 29% to 33%.[40–42] In summary, only one-half will respond to medical management and one-third will resolve on antibiotic therapy.
- *Intervention:* Unruptured mycotic aneurysms warrant frequent imaging monitoring and a low threshold to intervene where safe to do so.

Similarly, acute dissecting intracranial aneurysms have a poor natural history due to the high risk of stroke or bleeding/re-bleeding[43].

- *Acute presentations:* When the clinical history and imaging are suggestive of a recent acute dissecting event, endovascular treatment should be strongly considered when safe to do so.
- *Chronic presentations:* In chronic cases or where or there is significant uncertainty regarding timing of onset, it would be reasonable to monitor with serial imaging since long-term stability of healed chronic dissections and dissecting aneurysms is not uncommon.
- *Natural history:* Approximately one-quarter of dissecting aneurysms can spontaneously

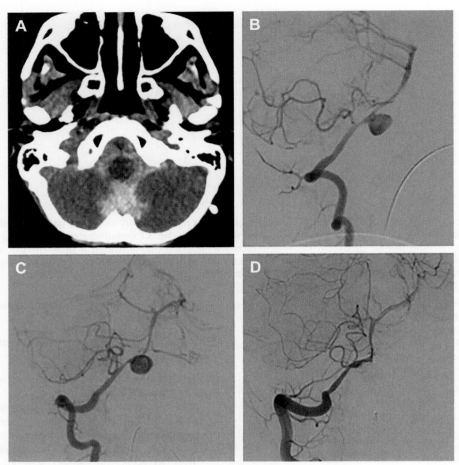

Fig. 3. Mycotic aneurysm: An 8-year-old girl under treatment for relapsed T-cell lymphoma with leptomeningeal seeding developed progressive *Fusarium* fungal meningitis. MR imagingdemonstrated extensive leptomeningeal enhancement in the prepontine cistern and anti-fungal therapy was commenced. She then developed headache and reduced consciousness. (*A*) Non-contrast CT brain demonstrated extensive subarachnoid hemorrhage in the posterior fossa. (*B, C*) Catheter-directed angiogram of the right vertebral artery (frontal and lateral) demonstrated a wide-necked mycotic aneurysm arising from the most distal aspect of the right V4 segment with the dome directed anteriorly. This was immediately adjacent to the leptomeningeal enhancement seen on MR imaging, but no aneurysm was present on prior imaging. Marked spasm of the intradural right vertebral artery and proximal basilar artery is also present. (*D*) Balloon-assisted coiling resulted in control of the aneurysm with minor residual flow in the aneurysm neck. She made an excellent recovery initially, but after several weeks began suffering progressive neurologic deterioration due to worsening fungal meningitis resulting in her death.

heal over time[44] with vascular remodeling or thrombosis.[2]

- *Intervention:* Intervention should thus be focused on ruptured, acutely presenting, or progressively enlarging chronic dissecting aneurysms.

Ruptured Aneurysms

Ruptured intracranial aneurysms in children, just as in adults, should be treated acutely to reduce the risk of rebleeding[2,11].

- *Rebleeding rate:* The rebleeding rate appears higher than in adults (perhaps due to delayed presentations) and may approach 60%.[45,46]
- *Intervention:* In the acute management phase, endovascular treatment is favored in children where possible.[1,10]
- *Outcomes:* Two-thirds (64%–68%) of pediatric patients with aneurysmal subarachnoid hemorrhage who undergo treatment have favorable long-term outcomes (equivalent to mRS 0–2).[45,47]

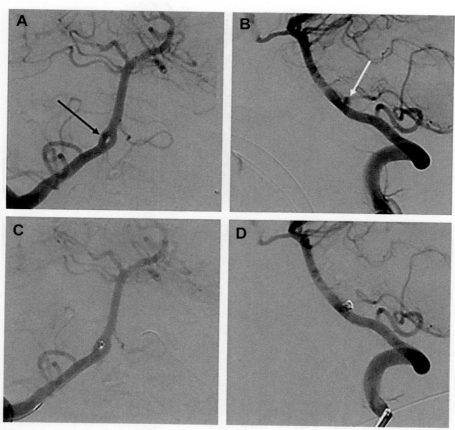

Fig. 4. Saccular aneurysm: A 12-year-old previously healthy boy suffered sudden-onset headache followed by collapse. The Glasgow Coma Score was 3/15. Non-contrast CT demonstrated posterior fossa subarachnoid hemorrhage and hydrocephalus. After ventriculostomy, he underwent catheter-directed angiography. (*A, B*) Right vertebral artery injections (frontal and lateral) demonstrated a congenital fenestration of the proximal basilar artery and a small 2.5 mm posteriorly directed saccular aneurysm arising from the inner right channel of the fenestration. (*C, D*) The aneurysm was successfully treated with endovascular coil embolization. The patient made a complete neurologic recovery and returned to school 6 weeks later. *White and black arrows* indicate the basilar artery fenestration aneurysm.

- *Mortality:* Pediatric patients with ruptured aneurysms who received treatment had mortality in the first year of 13% in a large study of Finnish patients with long-term follow-up.[11] A further 10% of patients died from recurrent subarachnoid hemorrhage over the long term (median 11.0 years) due to de novo aneurysm formation or incomplete occlusion of the initial aneurysm.[11]
- *Long-term mortality:* Amongst patients who survived the first 12 months, there was an excess long-term mortality compared to the whole population of 10% (worse in males).[11]

Cerebral vasospasm following aneurysmal subarachnoid hemorrhage in children appears to cause less morbidity than in adults. In a study comprising 37 children with aneurysmal subarachnoid hemorrhage, 46% had cerebral vasospasm

on angiography (mild 21%, moderate 50%, and severe 29%).[47] However, only 3 patients (8%) had symptomatic vasospasm, which was thought to be associated with poor cerebral collaterals.[47] Low rates of symptomatic vasospasm in children following subarachnoid hemorrhage have also been noted in several other studies.[2,4,48]

MANAGEMENT

The 3 treatment modalities for intracranial aneurysms in children, like in adults, are as follows:

1. Conservative
2. Endovascular, and
3. Micro-neurosurgical.

Treatment decisions should be made by a multi-disciplinary team (MDT) composed of

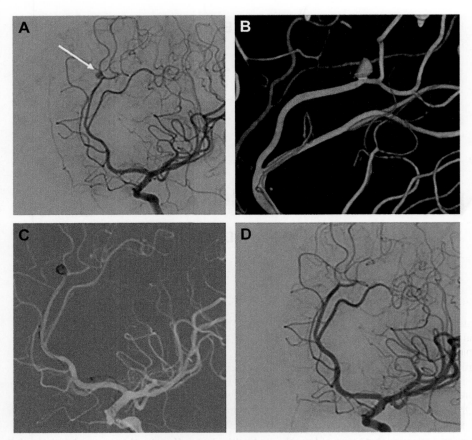

Fig. 5. Traumatic aneurysm: A 11-year-old boy suffered a penetrating traumatic brain injury extending across the left frontal lobe and into the anterior interhemispheric fissure. He subsequently developed a cerebral abscess in the frontal lobe requiring evacuation. MR angiogram 4 weeks after the injury demonstrated a new aneurysm arising from the callosomarginal branch of the left anterior cerebral artery. Both traumatic and mycotic etiologies were considered in the differential diagnosis. (*A, B*) Left ICA injection (transorbital oblique) and 3D rotational angiogram demonstrated a 3-mm probable traumatic aneurysm of the left callosomarginal artery. (*C*) Vessel sacrifice was considered, but fortunately the aneurysm was successfully treated by coil embolization due to its narrow neck. (*D*) Follow-up catheter-directed angiogram 4 months later demonstrated complete cure of the aneurysm with no recurrence. *White arrow* indicates the aneurysm

pediatric or cerebrovascular neurosurgeons, pediatric neurologists, and pediatric neuroendovascular surgeons (interventional neuroradiologists). Recommendations should be informed by the factors outlined below.

Factors to be considered for a treatment recommendation include as follows:

- Rupture status,
- Aneurysm location, morphology, and size,
- Patient age and vessel size,
- Etiology,
- Current clinical status and disability,
- Strength of adjacent collateral vessels,
- Views of the patient's family and carers,
- Likelihood of compliance with a follow-up or anti-platelet regimen,

- Presumed natural history (based on etiology and mechanism of pathogenesis), and
- Estimated risks related to endovascular or micro-neurosurgical treatment.

Conservative Management

Conservative management entails serial monitoring both clinically and radiologically to assess for morphologic change in the aneurysm over time. As discussed earlier, the majority of unruptured pediatric intracranial aneurysms are stable over time.

- Approximately 8% to 13% of patients show interval aneurysm growth or a de novo aneurysm on serial follow-up imaging.[6,35]

- For this reason, conservative management requires serial clinical follow-up and imaging on at least an annual basis initially, with increasingly longer follow-up intervals over time. Children with non-traumatic and non-infectious intracranial arterial aneurysms and those with predisposition syndromes are presumed to have an aneurysmal arteriopathy and require lifelong follow-up to monitor for de novo aneurysm formation. In contrast, children with traumatic and infectious aneurysms which have been treated and cured should not require lifelong imaging surveillance for de novo aneurysm formation over time.
- To minimize ionizing radiation, MR angiography is preferable to computed tomography angiography (CTA) for follow-up imaging.
- Interval aneurysm growth or new symptoms warrant repeat MDT discussion for reconsideration of treatment options.

Conservative management is most appropriately applied to conditions as follows:

- *Unruptured saccular aneurysms*—particularly small aneurysms. Unruptured mycotic aneurysms should be more strongly considered for treatment based on the factors outlined earlier.
- *Unruptured chronic dissecting/fusiform aneurysms:* Acutely presenting unruptured dissecting aneurysms should be strongly considered for definitive treatment based on the factors outlined earlier.

On the other hand, interventional management is most appropriately applied to conditions as follows:

- *Ruptured aneurysms*—these have up to a 60% re-rupture rate.[45,46]
- *Unruptured mycotic or acutely presenting dissecting aneurysms*.

Unruptured acute dissecting aneurysms or mycotic aneurysms with a high risk of treatment-related morbidity may be considered for conservative management on a case-by-case basis as approximately one-quarter will resolve over 4 to 6 weeks with medical management alone (*see Natural History*). A moderate proportion will also stay the same size or shrink. Medical management typically consists of anti-platelet agents for prevention of ischemic stroke in dissecting aneurysms and intravenous antibiotics for mycotic aneurysms. These lesions should be monitored very closely using serial non-invasive angiographic imaging every 1 to 2 weeks, with growth warranting reconsideration of the treatment strategy.

Endovascular Treatment

When definitive intracranial aneurysm treatment is warranted, endovascular treatment is increasingly performed in pediatric settings.[1,9,10,49] The endovascular approach chosen should be based on the etiology, location, and morphology of the aneurysm.

Dissecting/fusiform aneurysms

- Parent vessel sacrifice or trapping (by endovascular or micro-neurosurgical approach) has traditionally been utilized for intracranial ICA fusiform aneurysms,[9,32,50] relying on the circle of Willis and pial collaterals to prevent ischemia. See **Fig. 1**.
- Balloon-test occlusion can be undertaken prior to ICA sacrifice, using venous phase timing on contralateral angiography or electroencephalogram ± single-photon emission computed tomography tracer injection to assess the adequacy of collateral cerebral perfusion for young children requiring general anesthesia.
- MCA, ACA, and posterior cerebral artery (PCA) fusiform aneurysms may require combined parent vessel sacrifice with surgical bypass.[50]
- Reconstructive approaches using flow-diverters are an increasingly popular approach in recent years,[51,52] despite the paucity of trial data for these devices in children. Flow-diverters can also be effectively utilized for giant aneurysms.
- The optimal second anti-platelet agent for use with flow-diverters in children is uncertain, but most cases have utilized clopidogrel.[51,52] Whilst pediatric clopidogrel resistance has been demonstrated in the Chinese population (affecting 31% of patients),[53] clopidogrel has a long established role in pediatric stroke management.[54] Prasugrel has been trialled in children with sickle cell disease.[55]
- Flow reversal (eg, via vertebral artery coil occlusion below the posterior inferior cerebellar artery [PICA] origins) can be considered for progressive fusiform basilar aneurysms.

Distal arterial aneurysms (eg, traumatic and mycotic aneurysms)

- Parent artery sacrifice using coils or liquid embolic agents is favored due to the difficulty of achieving selective occlusion of the target lesion while maintaining parent artery patency in these locations see **Figs. 2** and **5**.[28,32]

- Strong adjacent leptomeningeal collaterals, particularly in young children, will provide a degree of protection against development of a large infarct.[32]
- In older children and those with less robust collaterals, surgical bypass with vessel sacrifice can be considered.[50]

Saccular aneurysms

- May be effectively treated by simple coil embolization of the aneurysm sac, with balloon or stent protection of the parent vessel lumen as appropriate.[32] See **Fig. 4**.
- Some wide-necked aneurysms are suitable for surgical clipping.
- Endovascular reconstruction with flow-diverting stents may also be considered.

MR angiography is typically the optimal imaging modality for follow-up after endovascular treatment, but spatial resolution limits its utility for small distal aneurysms. Similarly, assessment of in-stent stenosis following flow-diversion is limited by susceptibility artifact. For these situations, CT angiography ± formal catheter angiography may be needed.

Surgical Treatment

Whilst endovascular treatment is now the most common interventional approach for pediatric intracranial aneurysms,[49] micro-neurosurgery still plays an essential role in management. In some cases, a combination of endovascular and micro-neurosurgical approaches may be needed. Close collaboration with an experienced cerebrovascular neurosurgeon is essential.

Micro-neurosurgical treatment is of particular use in the following scenarios.

- *Dissecting/fusiform aneurysms* of the ACA, MCA, or PCA that are not suitable for flow diverter placement and which may require aneurysm trapping combined with revascularization (eg, superficial temporal artery [STA]-MCA or occipital-PCA bypass, interposition graft, contralateral ACA side-to-side anastomosis).[50]
- *Saccular aneurysms* that are wide-necked, have unfavorable morphology for coil embolization, or are recurrent after endovascular treatment can be successfully treated with microsurgical clipping.[9]
- *Mycotic aneurysms*, particularly the large base of skull variety,[34] in which placement of a flow diverter may not be suitable due to theoretic risk of infectious seeding causing in-stent thrombosis or septic emboli and cerebral abscesses. This is particularly relevant when vessel sacrifice is not an option. In such cases, trapping and surgical bypass may be required.

SUMMARY

Pediatric intracranial aneurysms differ from adult aneurysms in their etiology, natural history, and management. Unruptured aneurysms can frequently be managed conservatively with serial imaging follow-up. When definitive treatment is indicated, endovascular techniques are increasingly favored.

CLINICS CARE POINTS

- Treatment decision for pediatric intracranial aneurysms are based on the aneurysm type and the associated natural history.
- Many unruptured pediatric intracranial aneurysms can be managed conservatively.
- Acute dissecting, mycotic, and traumatic aneurysms have a higher rupture risk and should be considered for treatment if safe to do so.

REFERENCES

1. Gemmete JJ, Toma AK, Davagnanam I, et al. Pediatric cerebral aneurysms. Neuroimaging Clin N Am 2013;23:771–9.
2. Lasjaunias P, Wuppalapati S, Alvarez H, et al. Intracranial aneurysms in children aged under 15 years: review of 59 consecutive children with 75 aneurysms. Childs Nerv Syst 2005;21:437–50.
3. Mehrotra A, Nair AP, Das KK, et al. Clinical and radiological profiles and outcomes in pediatric patients with intracranial aneurysms. J Neurosurg Pediatr 2012;10:340–6.
4. Koroknay-Pál P, Lehto H, Niemelä M, et al. Long-term outcome of 114 children with cerebral aneurysms. J Neurosurg Pediatr 2012;9:636–45.
5. Khatri D, Zampolin R, Behbahani M, et al. Pediatric brain aneurysms: a review of 1458 brain MR angiograms. Childs Nerv Syst 2023;39:3249–54.
6. Hetts SW, English JD, Dowd CF, et al. Pediatric intracranial aneurysms: new and enlarging aneurysms after index aneurysm treatment or observation. AJNR Am J Neuroradiol 2011;32:2017–22.
7. Gerosa M, Licata C, Fiore DL, et al. Intracranial aneurysms of childhood. Childs Brain 1980;6:295–302.
8. Locksley HB, Sahs AL, Knowler L. Report on the cooperative study of intracranial aneurysms and subarachnoid hemorrhage. Section ii. General

survey of cases in the central registry and characteristics of the sample population. J Neurosurg 1966; 24:922–32.

9. Hetts SW, Narvid J, Sanai N, et al. Intracranial aneurysms in childhood: 27-year single-institution experience. AJNR Am J Neuroradiol 2009;30: 1315–24.

10. Agid R, Souza MP, Reintamm G, et al. The role of endovascular treatment for pediatric aneurysms. Childs Nerv Syst 2005;21:1030–6.

11. Koroknay-Pál P, Laakso A, Lehto H, et al. Long-term excess mortality in pediatric patients with cerebral aneurysms. Stroke 2012;43:2091–6.

12. Chen R, Zhang S, Xiao A, et al. Risk factors for intracranial aneurysm rupture in pediatric patients. Acta Neurochir (Wien) 2022;164:1145–52.

13. Nabavizadeh SA, Vossough A, Ichord RN, et al. Intracranial aneurysms in sickle cell anemia: clinical and imaging findings. J Neurointerventional Surg 2016;8:434–40.

14. Kim Y, Nard JA, Saad A, et al. Cerebral aneurysm in a 12-year-old boy with a $STAT_3$ mutation (hyper-IgE syndrome). Ann Allergy Asthma Immunol 2015; 114:430–1.

15. Hess CP, Fullerton HJ, Metry DW, et al. Cervical and intracranial arterial anomalies in 70 patients with phace syndrome. AJNR Am J Neuroradiol 2010;31: 1980–6.

16. Chihi M, Gembruch O, Darkwah Oppong M, et al. Intracranial aneurysms in patients with tuberous sclerosis complex: a systematic review. J Neurosurg Pediatr 2019;24:174–83.

17. Schievink WI, Riedinger M, Maya MM. Frequency of incidental intracranial aneurysms in neurofibromatosis type 1. Am J Med Genet A 2005;134a:45–8.

18. Carpenter CD, Linscott LL, Leach JL, et al. Spectrum of cerebral arterial and venous abnormalities in alagille syndrome. Pediatr Radiol 2018;48:602–8.

19. Kubo S, Nakajima M, Fukuda K, et al. A 4-year-old girl with autosomal dominant polycystic kidney disease complicated by a ruptured intracranial aneurysm. Eur J Pediatr 2004;163:675–7.

20. Laczynski DJ, Dong S, Kalahasti V, et al. Prevalence of intracranial aneurysms in Marfan syndrome. J Vasc Surg 2023;78:633–7.

21. North KN, Whiteman DA, Pepin MG, et al. Cerebrovascular complications in Ehlers-Danlos syndrome type IV. Ann Neurol 1995;38:960–4.

22. Perez-Vega C, Domingo RA, Tripathi S, et al. Intracranial aneurysms in Loeys-Dietz syndrome: a multicenter propensity-matched analysis. Neurosurgery 2022;91:541–6.

23. Plaisier E, Ronco P. Col4a1-related disorders. In: Adam MP, Feldman J, Mirzaa GM, et al, editors. Genereviews(®). Seattle (WA): University of Washington; 1993. Seattle Copyright © 1993-2024, University of Washington, Seattle. GeneReviews is a registered trademark of the University of Washington, Seattle. All rights reserved.

24. Kadian-Dodov D, Gornik HL, Gu X, et al. Dissection and aneurysm in patients with fibromuscular dysplasia: findings from the U.S. Registry for FMD. J Am Coll Cardiol 2016;68:176–85.

25. Swiątnicki W, Bocher-Schwarz HG, Standhardt H. Growth of flow-related aneurysms following occlusion of cerebral arteriovenous malformation. J Neurol Surg Cent Eur Neurosurg 2023;85(5):534–7.

26. Hung AL, Yang W, Jiang B, et al. The effect of flow-related aneurysms on hemorrhagic risk of intracranial arteriovenous malformations. Neurosurgery 2019;85:466–75.

27. Jordan LC, Johnston SC, Wu YW, et al. The importance of cerebral aneurysms in childhood hemorrhagic stroke: a population-based study. Stroke 2009;40: 400–5.

28. Flores BC, Patel AR, Braga BP, et al. Management of infectious intracranial aneurysms in the pediatric population. Childs Nerv Syst 2016;32:1205–17.

29. Huang J, McGirt MJ, Gailloud P, et al. Intracranial aneurysms in the pediatric population: case series and literature review. Surg Neurol 2005;63:424–32 [discussion 432-423].

30. Aeron G, Abruzzo TA, Jones BV. Clinical and imaging features of intracranial arterial aneurysms in the pediatric population. Radiographics 2012;32:667–81.

31. Chen AM, Karani KB, Taylor JM, et al. Cervicocerebral quantitative arterial tortuosity: a biomarker of arteriopathy in children with intracranial aneurysms. J Neurosurg Pediatr 2019;24:389–96.

32. Krings T, Geibprasert S, terBrugge KG. Pathomechanisms and treatment of pediatric aneurysms. Childs Nerv Syst 2010;26:1309–18.

33. Day AL, Gaposchkin CG, Yu CJ, et al. Spontaneous fusiform middle cerebral artery aneurysms: characteristics and a proposed mechanism of formation. J Neurosurg 2003;99:228–40.

34. Chun JY, Smith W, Halbach VV, et al. Current multimodality management of infectious intracranial aneurysms. Neurosurgery 2001;48:1203–13 [discussion 1213-1204].

35. Bisson DA, Dirks P, Amirabadi A, et al. Unruptured intracranial aneurysms in children: 18 years' experience in a tertiary care pediatric institution. J Neurosurg Pediatr 2019;24:184–9.

36. Nakstad P, Nornes H, Hauge HN. Traumatic aneurysms of the pericallosal arteries. Neuroradiology 1986;28:335–8.

37. Essibayi MA, Kerezoudis P, Keser Z, et al. Traumatic posterior cerebral artery dissection and dissecting aneurysms: a systematic review with an illustrative case report. Intervent Neuroradiol 2023;15910199231162487.

38. Hahn YS, Welling B, Reichman OH, et al. Traumatic intracavernous aneurysm in children: massive

epistaxis without ophthalmic signs. Childs Nerv Syst 1990;6:360–4.

39. Pasqualin A, Mazza C, Cavazzani P, et al. Intracranial aneurysms and subarachnoid hemorrhage in children and adolescents. Childs Nerv Syst 1986;2: 185–90.

40. Zanaty M, Chalouhi N, Starke RM, et al. Endovascular treatment of cerebral mycotic aneurysm: a review of the literature and single center experience. BioMed Res Int 2013;2013:151643.

41. Bartakke S, Kabde U, Muranjan MN, et al. Mycotic aneurysm: an uncommon cause for intra-cranial hemorrhage. Indian J Pediatr 2002;69:905–7.

42. Kannoth S, Thomas SV. Intracranial microbial aneurysm (infectious aneurysm): current options for diagnosis and management. Neurocritical Care 2009;11: 120–9.

43. Fleischer AS, Patton JM, Tindall GT. Cerebral aneurysms of traumatic origin. Surg Neurol 1975;4:233–9.

44. Su TM, Cheng CH, Chen WF, et al. Spontaneous healing and complete disappearance of a ruptured posterior inferior cerebellar artery dissecting aneurysm. J Neurosurg Pediatr 2014;13:503–6.

45. Proust F, Toussaint P, Garniéri J, et al. Pediatric cerebral aneurysms. J Neurosurg 2001;94:733–9.

46. Dagra A, Williams E, Aghili-Mehrizi S, et al. Pediatric subarachnoid hemorrhage: rare events with important implications. Brain Neurol Disord 2022;5.

47. Moftakhar P, Cooke DL, Fullerton HJ, et al. Extent of collateralization predicting symptomatic cerebral vasospasm among pediatric patients: correlations among angiography, transcranial Doppler ultrasonography, and clinical findings. J Neurosurg Pediatr 2015;15: 282–90.

48. Skoch J, Tahir R, Abruzzo T, et al. Predicting symptomatic cerebral vasospasm after aneurysmal subarachnoid hemorrhage with an artificial neural network in a pediatric population. Childs Nerv Syst 2017;33:2153–7.

49. Alawi A, Edgell RC, Elbabaa SK, et al. Treatment of cerebral aneurysms in children: analysis of the kids' inpatient database. J Neurosurg Pediatr 2014;14: 23–30.

50. Kalani MY, Elhadi AM, Ramey W, et al. Revascularization and pediatric aneurysm surgery. J Neurosurg Pediatr 2014;13:641–6.

51. Barburoglu M, Arat A. Flow diverters in the treatment of pediatric cerebrovascular diseases. AJNR Am J Neuroradiol 2017;38:113–8.

52. Santos-Franco JA, Cruz-Argüelles CA, Agustin-Aguilar F, et al. Intracranial aneurysms in pediatric population treated with flow diverters: a single-center experience. Surg Neurol Int 2022;13:522.

53. Zhang M, Meng L, Chen Y, et al. Cyp2c19 polymorphisms and lipoproteins associated with clopidogrel resistance in children with Kawasaki disease in china: a prospective study. Front Cardiovasc Med 2022;9:925518.

54. Soman T, Rafay MF, Hune S, et al. The risks and safety of clopidogrel in pediatric arterial ischemic stroke. Stroke 2006;37:1120–2.

55. Heeney MM, Hoppe CC, Abboud MR, et al. A multinational trial of prasugrel for sickle cell vaso-occlusive events. N Engl J Med 2016;374: 625–35.

Arterial Ischemic Stroke in Children

Nevena Fileva, MD, PhD[a,b], Marta Bertamino, MD, PhD[c], Domenico Tortora, MD, PhD[a], Mariasavina Severino, MD[a],*

KEYWORDS

- Arterial ischemic stroke • Children • Neonates • Imaging • Focal cerebral arteriopathy
- Arterial dissection • Congenital heart disease • Moyamoya

KEY POINTS

- Neuroimaging has an important role in the diagnosis, treatment, and follow-up of children with arterial ischemic stroke (AIS).
- The recommended imaging modality is MRI, with a role for rapid MRI protocols in the revascularization time window.
- CT and CT angiography may be used in children with AIS if MRI is not available and in specific clinical scenarios.
- Arteriopathy is the predominant underlying mechanism in pediatric AIS and the greatest predictor of recurrence and poor outcome.
- Newborns have the highest stroke risk ratio, with high lifelong morbidity, accounting for most cases of hemiparetic cerebral palsy.

INTRODUCTION

The incidence of pediatric arterial ischemic stroke (AIS) ranges between 3 and 25 per 100,000 children/year,[1] with a mortality rate of 4% to 20%.[2] Depending on the patient's age at the initial event, it can be divided into perinatal stroke (between 20 gestational weeks and 1 month of age) and childhood stroke (between the second month of life and 18 years). Differences between the biological sexes and ethnicities are observed, with a higher prevalence among boys and African, Asian, and Hispanic children.[1] The majority of the survivors suffer from life-long disability with motor and cognitive deficits or epilepsy.[1] The unusual nature of pediatric AIS and consequent under-recognition, frequent nonspecific symptoms, and the wide range of differential diagnoses lead to diagnostic delays and misdiagnoses.[3,4] The median time for diagnostic confirmation ranges from 6 to 22 hours, leading to limited possibility of access to modern treatment options.[2,4]

Clinical presentation varies according to age, setting (inpatient vs outpatient), and stroke subtype. As for adults, the most common onset symptoms in pediatric stroke include hemiparesis (67%-90%), speech disturbance (20%-50%), vision disturbance (10%–15%), and ataxia (8%-10%).[1] However, children may also present with non-localizing and/or intermittent symptoms, such as headache (20% to 50%), altered mental status (17% to 38%), and seizures (15%-25%).[1] As a consequence, stroke recognition instruments used in the adult population, such as the FAST (Face Arm Speech Test) and ROSIER (Recognition of Stroke in the Emergency Room), have a reduced sensitivity to depict a pediatric AIS and are insufficient to discriminate between stroke and stroke mimics in the pediatric age group.[5] Therefore, neuroimaging plays a central role in the diagnosis

a Neuroradiology Unit, IRCCS Istituto Giannina Gaslini, Via Gaslini 5, Genova 16147, Italy; b Diagnostic Imaging Department, UMHAT Aleksandrovska, Bul G.Sofiiski 1, Sofia 1431, Bulgaria; c Physical Medicine and Rehabilitation Unit, IRCCS Instituto Giannina Gaslini, Via Gaslini 5, Genoa, Italy
* Corresponding author.
E-mail address: mariasavinaseverino@gaslini.org

Neuroimag Clin N Am 34 (2024) 579–599
https://doi.org/10.1016/j.nic.2024.08.010
1052-5149/24/© 2024 Elsevier Inc. All rights reserved, including those for text and data mining, AI training, and similar technologies.

of this condition in children. Of note, the presence of predisposing conditions, such as sickle cell disease, previous stroke, congenital heart disease, recent trauma, hypercoagulability, history of cerebral radiotherapy, asparaginase therapy, Down syndrome, Moyamoya arteriopathy, and recent infection, should raise the suspicion of stroke even in the absence of focal neurologic symptoms.[2] Finally, to quantify the stroke severity, a child-specific version of the National Institutes of Health Stroke Score (NIHSS) has been developed, that is, the pedNIHSS, that correlates with the initial infarct volume and functional outcome.[6,7] Considering the wide range of pediatric AIS etiology, children with this diagnosis usually undergo in-depth cardiac, hematologic, rheumatologic, and genetic investigations.[1]

Perinatal stroke is a likely underestimated condition with the reported incidence ranging from 1:1600 to 1:3000 live births.[1] Approximately 80% of perinatal strokes are ischemic*Fetal AIS* (20th gestational week–delivery) may be detected on prenatal imaging or in neuropathologic examination in case of stillbirth. *Neonatal AIS* is diagnosed between birth and 28 days of life, usually as a result of acute encephalopathy and seizures.[8] *Presumed perinatal ischemic stroke* is diagnosed in older infants presenting with delayed motor milestones, epilepsy, cerebral palsy, or early handedness. In these cases, it is presumed that the ischemic event occurred within the perinatal period, with clinically cryptic presentation and/or without neuroimaging for definite diagnosis.[1] The main risk factors can be divided into maternal (first pregnancy, twins, preeclampsia, maternal smoking, fever), fetal/intrapartum (male sex, congenital heart disease, hypoglycemia, perinatal hypoxia, Apgar <7 on 5th minute, need for resuscitation) and placental (fetal vascular malperfusion, amniotic fluid inflammation, chorionic villitis).[9] While mortality is low, most neonates with AIS experience persistent neurologic deficits including hemiparesis, and cognitive and speech impairment. The risk of epilepsy is high with rates ranging from 9% to 27.2%.[8] Notably, the risk for epilepsy and poor outcomes can be predicted on imaging and managed with timely referral to rehabilitation services.

In this article, we discuss the neuroimaging techniques and protocols, describe the main underlying causes, and review the current treatment options for pediatric and perinatal AIS.

IMAGING PROTOCOLS

The imaging aims in pediatric AIS are manyfold, including the confirmation of the diagnosis, definition of the type and mechanisms, estimation of

neurologic prognosis, detection of complications, surveillance of arteriopathies, and planning of medical and interventional treatments.[10,11]

Brain MRI

Brain MRI has the greatest diagnostic sensitivity to AIS in the hyperacute and acute phases (up to 24 hours from the onset).[12] Furthermore, brain MRI facilitates the exclusion of other neurologic conditions with stroke-like presentations, that have a high incidence (20%–50%) in the pediatric population.[13,14]

Abbreviated MRI protocols (AKA "quick MRI" or "fast MRI") may be useful to avoid late diagnosis and to select candidates for mechanical thrombectomy in the acute phase. These imaging studies usually last from 5 to 10 minutes (**Table 1**).[15] In this phase of patient care, MR Perfusion imaging may be useful to distinguish the stroke core (ie, the irreversibly infarcted tissue) from the penumbra (ie, the critically hypoperfused tissue doomed to infarct if not reperfused). In the absence of pediatric data, the penumbra is currently defined as noninfarcted tissue (without diffusion restriction) which has a Tmax >6s on Dynamic susceptibility contrast-enhanced (DSC) T2* sequences with bolus-tracking, as it is in adults.[16] However, further studies are needed to define the Tmax that best characterizes the penumbra at different ages in the pediatric population. Moreover, evidence is required to validate arterial spin labeling (ASL) MR perfusion, as a noncontrast technique for this specific purpose. More commonly, clinical-DWI mismatch as described by the DAWN trial is used to determine the role of reperfusion therapies, albeit no pediatric thresholds have been established.

When the etiology of LVO is not evident, it is indicated to complete the fast MRI study, possibly in the same session, with other MRI sequences tailored for the situation. These include any or all of A **full protocol brain MRI** study for pediatric AIS is usually used outside the emergency setting (**Table 2**).[17] Regarding vessel wall imaging (VWI), adequate interpretation of the results requires the knowledge of artifacts (such as those related to slow blood flow) and false-positive cases due to dissection, peri-arterial venous plexi (ie, venous plexus of Rektorzik and peri-arterial venous plexus surrounding cervical vertebral artery), anatomic locations of extracranial and intracranial vasa vasorum and recent endovascular procedures.

In **perinatal AIS**, MRI protocols include both anatomic and vascular sequences that can be extended to the neck (**Table 3**). Notably,

Table 1
Recommended Fast MR imaging protocol for pediatric AIS

Sequence	Plane	Key Role
DWI	Axial	Detection of cytotoxic edema with distribution in vascular territories and definition of the stroke core (tissue with ADC values < 620×10^{-6} mm^2/s)
2D T2-WI (HASTE/SSh TSE) or 2D/3D FLAIR (>2 y)	Axial	Evaluation of signal abnormalities
2D T2* GE or SWI	Axial	Identification of microhemorrhages within the infarction and of asymmetric prominence of the cortical veins in the penumbra area
Intracranial 3D TOF Arterial MRA	Axial	Depiction of large vessel occlusion
MR perfusion (DSC T2* or ASL)	Axial	Qualitative and quantitative information on the brain perfusion; definition of the penumbra as the tissue with a Tmax>6s on DSC T2*

Abbreviations: ADC, apparent diffusion coefficient; ASL, arterial spin labeling; DSC, dynamic susceptibility contrast; DWI, diffusion-weighted imaging, GE, gradient echo; HASTE, Half-Fourier Acquisition Single-shot TSE; MRA, magnetic resonance angiography; s, seconds; SWI, susceptibility-weighted imaging; T2*, T2 star; TOF, time of flight; TSE, turbo spin echo; WI, weighted imaging.

cervicocerebral arterial injuries due to birth trauma, an important cause of neonatal AIS, may be overlooked if the vascular imaging of the neck is not obtained. Contrast injection is usually not needed.[18]

Computed Tomography (CT) Imaging

In the emergency setting, head CT and CT angiography should be performed to evaluate suspected **pediatric AIS** in the case of MR contraindications

Table 2
Recommended full MR imaging protocol for pediatric AIS

Sequence	Plane	Key Role
DWI	Axial	Detection of cytotoxic edema with distribution in vascular territories
2D T2-WI (TSE)	Axial and coronal	Evaluation of signal abnormalities
2D or 3D FLAIR	Axial or sagittal	Evaluation of signal abnormalities (>2 y)
2D or 3D T1-WI (TFE)	Axial or sagittal	(High-resolution) anatomic information
2D T2* GE or SWI	Axial	Identification of microhemorrhages in the infarct and surrounding brain tissue
Intracranial 3D TOF Arterial MRA	Axial	Depiction of intracranial large vessel occlusion, stenosis, aneurysm, leptomeningeal collaterals
Cervical CE MRA (3D spoiled GE)	Coronal	Detection of aortic arch and/or cervical artery anomalies (occlusion, stenosis, pseudoaneurysm, relevant variant)
Pre- and post-contrast BBVWI	Sagittal	Identification of intramural hematomas (dissection) and pattern of vessel wall contrast enhancement
MR perfusion (DSC T2* or ASL)	Axial	Qualitative and quantitative information on brain perfusion in the case of cerebral arteriopathies

Abbreviations: ADC, apparent diffusion coefficient; ASL, arterial spin labeling; BBVWI, black-blood vessel wall imaging; CE, contrast-enhanced; DSC, dynamic susceptibility contrast; DWI, diffusion-weighted imaging; GE, gradient echo; HASTE, Half-Fourier Acquisition Single-shot TSE; MRA: magnetic resonance angiography; s, seconds; SWI, susceptibility-weighted imaging; TFE, turbo field echo; TOF, time of flight; TSE, turbo spin echo; WI, weighted imaging.

Table 3
Recommended Full MR imaging protocol for neonatal AIS

Sequence	Plane	Key Role
DWI	Axial	Detection of cytotoxic edema with distribution in vascular territories
2D T2-WI (TSE)[a]	Axial and coronal	Evaluation of signal abnormalities
2D or 3D T1-WI (TSE or TFE)[a]	Axial and/or sagittal	(High-resolution) anatomic information
2D T2[a] GE or SWI	Axial	Identification of microhemorrhages within the infarction and of asymmetric prominence of the cortical veins in the penumbra area
Intracranial and cervical 3D TOF Arterial MRA	Axial	Depiction of large vessel occlusion, stenosis or irregularities both at the intracranial and cervical level
MR perfusion (ASL)[b]	Axial	Qualitative and quantitative information on the brain perfusion

Abbreviations: ADC, apparent diffusion coefficient; ASL, arterial spin labeling; DWI, diffusion-weighted imaging, GE, gradient echo; MRA, magnetic resonance angiography; s, seconds; SWI, susceptibility-weighted imaging, TOF, time of flight; TSE, turbo spin echo; WI, weighted imaging.
[a] Adjust the sequence parameters for unmyelinated brain.
[b] Optional sequence.

(eg, noncompatible medical devices or dental braces degrading the image quality), organizational delay, lack of MRI access, clinical instability, trauma, or high-risk populations in whom the pretest probability of AIS with intracranial large vessel occlusion (LVO) is high.[18,19] Noncontrast head CT has high sensitivity in detecting hemorrhagic stroke but fails to detect AIS in 34% to 40% of cases, especially in the hyperacute phase and with reduced radiation dose CT protocols that are used in small children.

In children, exposure to the radiation and administration of iodinated contrast via mechanical injectors are considered disadvantages. While in adults with suspect AIS CT angiography is strongly indicated after a negative brain CT, in the pediatric setting the diagnostic approach is more complex. Indeed, neurologic conditions with a possible stroke-like presentation and negative CT examination are highly frequent, especially in early childhood. Therefore, CT angiography of the head and neck after a negative noncontrast head CT may be of low yield and thus obtained more selectively. In most such instances, brain MRI is the next step in diagnostic evaluation. CT angiography of the head and neck should be obtained if time-sensitive revascularization therapies are potentially indicated, particularly in high-risk populations, such as children with cardiac disease or children with prothrombotic conditions.[20–22] CT perfusion is rarely useful in children because of the requisite radiation exposure and lack of meaningful data from pediatric penumbral imaging studies to guide clinical decision-making.[23]

In the case of **perinatal AIS**, nonenhanced head CT should be performed only if MRI is not available or in the presence of non-MRI-compatible medical devices.[24]

Catheter-Directed Digital Subtraction Angiography

Despite being an invasive procedure with ionizing radiation exposure, catheter-directed DSA is still considered a gold standard in the diagnosis of many cerebrovascular pathologies due to higher spatial resolution compared with CTA and MRA, and unparalleled temporal resolution which facilitates the detailed characterization of discrete arterial, capillary and venous circulatory phases/compartments.[25,26] Catheter-directed DSA may be indicated when clinical-laboratory (echocardiography), CT, and/or MRI examinations have not adequately delineated the underlying cause of AIS in a child. Moreover, catheter-directed DSA is useful in cases of posterior circulation stroke, particularly if they are recurrent, since it may reveal subtle dissections of the atlanto-axial (AA) or atlanto-occipital (AO) vertebral artery that are occult on CTA and MRI/MRA. In children with non-traumatic AA or AO vertebral artery dissections, catheter-directed DSA with rotational head maneuvers has an important role in the diagnosis of bow-hunter syndrome.[26,27] Catheter-directed DSA also has a central role in the diagnosis of primary nervous system (CNS) angiitis because of the better delineation of stenotic and ectatic changes in the cortical branch arteries of the brain.[28] Finally, in moyamoya arteriopathy, catheter-directed DSA is indicated for definitive diagnosis, staging, and surgical treatment planning.[29] Catheter-directed DSA is usually not indicated for the diagnosis or management of perinatal AIS.

IMAGING FINDINGS
Perinatal Arterial Ischemic Stroke

Neuroimaging in perinatal AIS has similar aims as in the pediatric age group, confirming the diagnosis, identifying a potential etiology, suggesting the timing of insult, excluding stroke mimics, assisting in treatment decisions, and providing prognostic information. In particular, early diffusion findings correlate with clinical outcomes, especially cerebral palsy.[30,31] The majority of perinatal AIS affects the MCA territory, more often on the left side due to preferential flow direction in fetal and neonatal circulation.[24] Placental thrombi embolizing in the fetal circulation is considered the most probable etiology. Multiple arterial territories may be involved in neonates with meningitis, thrombophilia, and fetal vascular malperfusion.[32,33] Perforator strokes in lenticulostriate and posterior circulation territories are more frequent in preterm neonates.[34]

In the neonatal period, intracranial MRA is positive in 22% to 62% of cases.[35] MRA of the neck vessels may be useful to detect cervical vessel dissection resulting from birth trauma.[36] In newborn infants who undergo acute brain MRI because of clinically suspected AIS (seizures, apnea, or encephalopathy), geographic areas of restricted diffusion correspond to core infarction, and surrounding penumbral regions often fail to show signal hypointensity on ASL sequences. Paradoxically, ASL signal within the core infarction is increased, in such cases. While these changes may be related to tissue reperfusion and/or changes in cerebral blood flow linked to seizure activity, stasis within parenchymal vessels cannot be excluded as the cause.[37]

Congenital heart disease or twin-twin transfusion syndrome may manifest in utero with acute fetal AIS (**Fig. 1**) or in the chronic phase as porencephaly, cerebral volume loss, and malformations of cortical development.[38]

In contradistinction to the broader pediatric population, the risk of recurrence in perinatal AIS is low (around 1%).[39] Long-term MRI follow-up is thus not needed in the absence of specific risk factors and/or extremely rare congenital arteriopathies.[40]

Pediatric Arterial Ischemic Stroke

International Pediatric Stroke Study Investigators (IPSS) developed The Childhood Arterial Ischemic Stroke Standardized Classification and Diagnostic Evaluation (CASCADE) system to categorize childhood strokes according to the underlying cause. It divides AIS into seven subtypes: (1) small vessel arteriopathy, (2) unilateral focal cerebral arteriopathy (FCA), (3) bilateral cerebral arteriopathy, (4) aortic/cervical arteriopathy, (5) cardioembolic, (6) other, and (7) multifactorial.[41] The CASCADE classification at stroke onset may help in predicting the risk of recurrent stroke, progression of arteriopathy, and treatment selection.[42] Stroke recurrence is higher in children with arteriopathies[43] and in the presence of predisposing conditions such as cardiac anomalies, thrombophilia, and sickle cell disease.

Arterial dissection

Intra- and extracranial arterial dissections are among the most common arteriopathies causing AIS in childhood. Children account for 55% to 75% of all intra- and extracranial arterial dissections[26] (**Fig. 2**). Such dissections are often secondary manifestations of an underlying arteriopathy that alters the structural integrity of the arterial wall. In some cases, the underlying arteriopathy is a recognizable multisystem disorder with a verifiable genetic basis as in Marfan's disease and Osteogenesis imperfecta, but in other cases, the underlying arteriopathy may be uncharacterized with arterial tortuosity being the only clue to its presence.[44] In other cases, arterial dissections are complications of musculoskeletal anomalies that exert aberrant dynamic forces on the vertebral artery.[45]

Frequent locations for arterial dissections in children are the atlanto-axial and atlanto-occipital segments of the vertebral artery and the cervical internal carotid artery (ICA). Brain MRI with fat-saturated T1-weighted sequences may depict intramural hematoma. Vascular imaging (CTA, MRA, or catheter-directed DSA) may reveal a double lumen, intimal flap, pseudoaneurysm, and segmental arterial stenosis or occlusion.[20] Catheter-directed DSA is still considered a gold standard in the diagnosis of arterial dissection due to its exquisite sensitivity to subtle luminal distortions. Nevertheless, especially in the pediatric population, brain MRI with cranio-cervical MRA is the preferred modality due to the non-invasiveness and ability to image both the affected vessels and brain parenchyma in one study.[46] In children, particularly males, presenting with posterior circulation AIS, an atlanto-axial (Power's V2) or atlanto-occipital (Power's V3) segment vertebral artery dissection should be further investigated by catheter-directed DSA with provocative head maneuvers once the arterial dissection has healed.

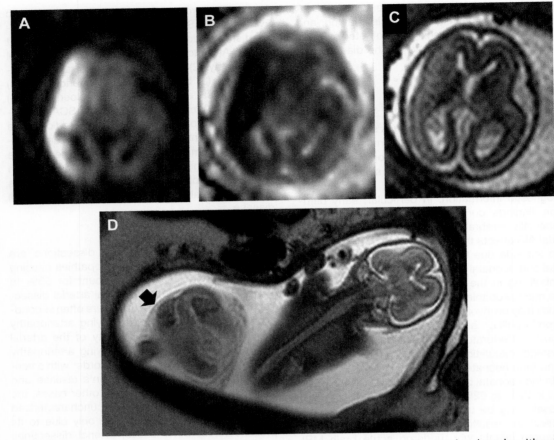

Fig. 1. Twin-to-twin transfusion syndrome complicated by fetal AIS. Fetal MRI at 20 gestational weeks with axial DWI (*A*), corresponding ADC map (*B*), and axial (*C*) and coronal (*D*) T2-weighted image reveals an AIS in the left MCA territory. Note the deceased twin fetus (thick *arrow*).

Dynamic and reversible vertebral artery occlusion, that colocalizes to the site of vertebral artery dissection, upon contralateral head rotation, confirms the diagnosis of bow-hunter syndrome.[20,27]

Cardiac disorders

This group includes embolic AIS caused by congenital heart disease, procedure-related events (extracorporeal membrane oxygenation, catheterization, or surgery), or acquired heart disease.[47] According to the IPSS study, 30% of pediatric strokes can be related to cardiac disorders, with half of cases due to congenital heart disease. Patients tend to have higher mortality, poorer prognosis, and higher recurrence rate compared with other etiologies.[47,48]

Persistent foramen ovale is the most common congenital right-to-left shunt anomaly that may lead to paradoxic embolism. The stroke risk increases corresponding to the size of the communication between the ventricles or in combination with genetic or acquired prothrombotic

abnormality. In selected cases, closure procedures and preventive therapy have proven to decrease the AIS recurrence rates.[48,49]

A cardioembolic source should be suspected when there are signs of asynchronous AIS or multiple vascular territories are affected (particularly bilateral ICA territories or combined involvement of vertebrobasilar and ICA territories) (**Fig. 3**). On vascular imaging, abrupt arterial occlusion without surrounding vessel changes or stenosis is highly suspicious. A meniscus sign, in which contrast media or flow-related signal marginates the convex border of the luminal filling defect, strongly favors embolic vascular occlusion. Simultaneous cortico-subcortical and basal ganglia infarction is a worse prognostic sign. Children with AIS typically undergo cardiac evaluation via transthoracic echocardiography with intravenous with bubble contrast, as well as electrocardiographic monitoring to assess for an arrhythmia.[1] Where acute cardiac assessment is not available, transcranial Doppler can provide a first clue to the existence

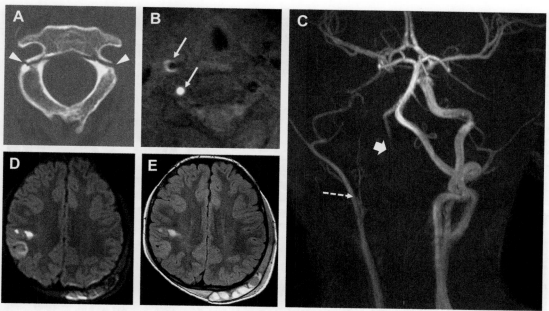

Fig. 2. Post-traumatic arterial dissections in a 7-year-old boy. (*A*) Axial CT scan reveals bilateral hangman fractures of C2 (*arrowheads*). (*B*) Axial fat-suppressed T1-weighted image of the cervical region demonstrates the hematomas in the right ICA and vertebral artery walls (thin *arrows*). (*C*) 3D-TOF MRA shows ICA (dashed *arrow*) and vertebral artery (thick *arrow*) occlusion. (*D*) Axial DWI and (*E*) FLAIR images depict small cortical-subcortical AIS in the right posterior frontal and parietal lobes. Note a subcutaneous hematoma in the left parietooccipital region.

of a right-to-left shunt by detecting microbubbles in the middle cerebral artery (MCA) after intravenous agitated saline injection.[11]

Focal cerebral arteriopathy

The updated definition of focal cerebral arteriopathy (FCA) includes unifocal and unilateral stenosis/irregularity of the intradural ICA, proximal MCA, and/or proximal anterior cerebral artery.[50] It can be divided into 2 main groups: (1) inflammatory subtype (FCA-i) that can occur in cases of active and postinfectious disorders, including postvaricella cerebral arteriopathy; and (2) dissection subtype (FCA-d) affecting the intracerebral vessels.

FCA-i should be suspected in cases of subcortical lateral lenticulostriate territory infarction and/or irregular stenosis involving the intradural ICA and/or its first-order branches. The characteristic stenosis demonstrates luminal beading on vascular imaging studies and vessel wall thickening with concentric mural contrast enhancement on black blood MR vessel wall imaging (Fig. 4). In many affected patients, there is a clinical history of previous or ongoing infection with a range of agents that include varicella-zoster virus and SARS-COVID19.[48,51,52] FCA is covered in more detail in the article on arteriopathies in this book.

The 1-year stroke recurrence rate after FCA reportedly ranges from 19% to 25% and regular follow-up is recommended.[53] Brain MRI with MRA studies at 1.5 to 3, 6, and 12 months are fundamental to distinguish transient from persistent or progressive FCA and to exclude evolution into a moyamoya arteriopathy.[54]

Although FCA-d is often associated with minor trauma, a history of trauma is absent in several cases. Since the intradural ICA and its first-order branches are characteristically involved, there is a mixed subcortical/cortical cerebral infarction. In contrast to the relatively regular beaded stenosis of FCA-i, the vascular lesion of FCA-d is much more irregular, and complete occlusions are common. Other features of dissection may also be apparent such as intimal flap, aneurysmal dilatation, pseudoaneurysm, segmental ectasia, corkscrew tortuosity, and double lumen sign or false lumen. Black blood VWI may demonstrate intramural hematoma, with or without eccentric mural contrast enhancement. Vascular imaging follow-up is required to exclude complications such as pseudoaneurysms.[54]

Cerebral vasculitis

Cerebral vasculitis is classified as (i) primary CNS vasculitis, (ii) idiopathic with isolated CNS

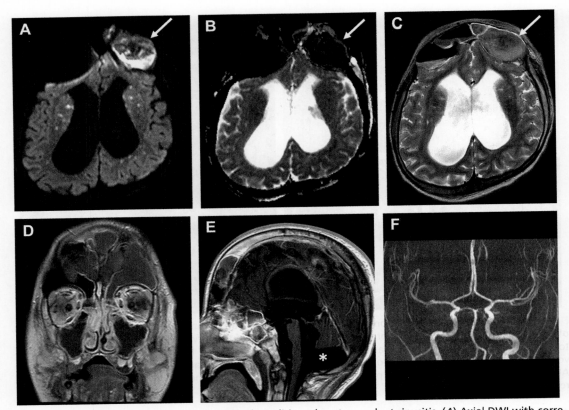

Fig. 3. Embolic AIS in a 13-year-old boy with endocarditis and acute purulent sinusitis. (*A*) Axial DWI with corresponding ADC maps (*B*) and T2-weighted images (*C*) show multiple bilateral small AIS in the basal ganglia and cerebral white matter. Note the mucosal thickening and fluid accumulation in the frontal sinuses with markedly reduced diffusion (thin *arrows*) in keeping with a purulent content. Coronal (*D*) and sagittal (*E*) postcontrast T1-weighted images reveal inflammatory mucosal enhancement in the paranasal sinuses. There is also a persistent Blake pouch cyst (*asterisk*) causing tetraventricular hydrocephalus. (*F*) 3D TOF MRA shows normal intracranial vessels.

involvement, and (iii) secondary CNS vasculitis in the context of systemic diseases due to rheumatological, infective, drug or treatment-related causes (Fig. 5).

Childhood primary angiitis of the central nervous system (cPACNS) is an extremely rare condition with an estimated incidence of around 2.4 cases/1000000/y[55] Two broad subtypes are recognized: (1) angiitis involving large- and medium-sized vessels (angiography-positive cPACNS) and (2) angiitis involving small vessels (angiography-negative cPACNS). CSF inflammatory biomarkers are more frequently found in secondary CNS vasculitis and angiography-negative cPACNS.[55]

Brain MRI may show multiple/bilateral cerebral infarcts, cerebral microhemorrhages, and rarely subarachnoid hemorrhage, variably associated with leptomeningeal and/or parenchymal contrast enhancement. Multifocal intracranial arterial narrowing and/or irregular beading of both large and medium-sized blood vessels may be detected on

MR angiography.[28] MRI black blood VWI with contrast may depict arterial wall thickening and mural enhancement (see **Fig. 5**). Catheter-directed DSA may reveal multifocal segmental narrowing and/or irregular beading involving both medium-sized blood vessels. A negative DSA does not exclude a cPACNS and a neurosurgical biopsy might be needed.[56]

Moyamoya arteriopathy

Moyamoya arteriopathy is a chronic, progressive, noninflammatory intracranial arteriopathy characterized by progressive steno-occlusive disease affecting the internal carotid termination and its branches, along with specific patterns of compensatory arterial collateral formation.[41,57] Moyamoya arteriopathy is bilateral in the vast majority of cases, though unilateral disease has been reported. Signature collateral patterns include moyamoya collaterals (hypertrophic lateral lenticulostriates vascularizing striatocapsular structures),

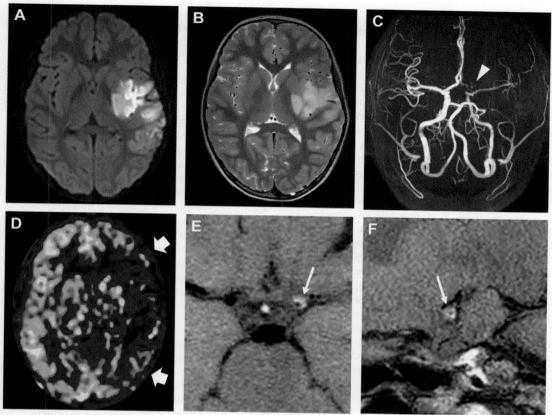

Fig. 4. Inflammatory FCA in a 12-year-old girl. Axial DWI (*A*) and T2-weighted (*B*) images demonstrate an AIS in the left fronto-insulo-temporal and nucleo-capsular region. (*C*) 3D-TOF MRA reveals a focal stenosis involving the left supraclinoid ICA, M1, and A1 segments (*arrowhead*) with the reduced flow in the MCA distal branches. (*D*) ASL flow-sensitive sequences reveal decreased blood flow in the MCA territory (*thick arrows*). (*E, F*) Axial and sagittal VWI demonstrates focal concentric contrast enhancement in the left ICA and M1 vessel wall (*thin arrows*).

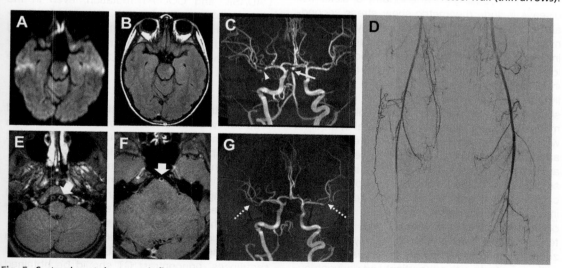

Fig. 5. Systemic autoimmune inflammatory vasculitis with CNS involvement in a 10.5-year-old girl. (*A*) Axial DWI and (*B*) FLAIR images show a left mesencephalic AIS. (*C*) 3D-TOF MRA demonstrates focal stenosis of the basilar artery (*thin arrow*) and right M2 segment (*arrowhead*). (*D*) Catheter-directed DSA reveals lower extremity vasculitis, more severe on the right side. (*E, F*) Black-blood vessel wall imaging reveals basilar and vertebral artery wall thickening with associated concentric mural enhancement (*thick arrows*). (*G*) Follow-up 3D-TOF MRA after 10 years shows the progression of the intracranial stenoses, including at the MCA level (*dashed arrows*).

leptomeningeal collaterals, transdural collaterals, and choroidal collaterals.

Moyamoya causes 6% to 10% of all childhood strokes and TIA in children.[1] This condition is described in further detail in the article on childhood arteriopathies. The natural history includes the occurrence of transient ischemic attacks, ischemic infarcts, or intracerebral hemorrhage. Since medical treatment is not effective in preventing clinical events, patients with advanced cerebral hemodynamic failure and/or neurologic symptoms benefit from surgical revascularization.[58] On imaging, as intracranial ICA stenoses become increasingly worse, there is a progressive increase in hypertrophic lateral lenticulostriate collaterals (Suzuki stages 1 through 3) followed by exhaustion (Suzuki stages 4 through 6). These collaterals have a "puff of smoke" appearance on vascular imaging ("Moyamoya" in Japanese) (Fig. 6). Brain MR perfusion studies with DSC T2* or ASL techniques are useful to depict regions of decreased cerebral perfusion. In combination with acetazolamide injection or induced hypercarbia, these studies can be used to quantify the cerebrovascular reserve and to reveal postrevascularization perfusion improvements.[59–61]

Sickle cell disease

Sickle cell disease is the most common hemoglobinopathy worldwide. It is associated with chronic anemia and vasculopathy with multisystem involvement. The drivers of endothelial injury and dysfunction causing the arteriopathy of sickle cell disease include rheometric shear stress secondary to the sickling of erythrocytes, hypertension, hyperdynamic circulatory changes, and vascular inflammation fueled by hemolysis and iron overload. The main patterns of cerebral arteriopathy in sickle cell disease are progressive large artery intracranial occlusive disease and progressive small vessel cerebral arteriopathy which typically manifests "silent" subcortical cerebral infarctions with cognitive impairment.[51,62] Progressive large artery intracranial occlusive disease demonstrates anatomic heterogeneity and may involve any segment of the anterior circulation or posterior circulation. A moyamoya arteriopathy pattern is not infrequent. Progressive large artery intracranial occlusive disease may present with geographic territorial infarctions or less commonly watershed zone infarctions. In contrast, small vessel arteriopathy manifests with subcortical and periventricular white matter infarctions.[63] This risk of stroke in the setting of progressive large artery intracranial occlusive disease drastically changed after the introduction of preventive chronic blood transfusions.[64] Stem cell transplantation and gene therapy promise to further reduce cerebrovascular morbidity in individuals affected with sickle cell disease.[65]

Infection

Systemic or cerebral infection can be associated with AIS through a variety of mechanisms with patterns that are distinct from those seen in FCA-i. According to the IPSS study, 24% of children presenting with AIS were found to have an active infection at the time of their stroke, most commonly bacterial meningitis (including tuberculous) or viral encephalitis caused by varicella, HIV, Zika, Dengue, herpes, Epstein Barr Virus, CMV, or COVID-19. The stroke mechanisms include the activation of the coagulation cascade and septic emboli.[48] Common neuroradiological findings are multifocal asynchronous AIS, striatocapsular infarction, leptomeningeal contrast enhancement, and stenoses of large and medium-sized intracranial arteries.[47]

Genetic

Pediatric and perinatal stroke can be the manifestation of a genetic condition with simple Mendelian inheritance (Table 4, Fig. 7A–D).[66] In the last decade, next-generation sequencing techniques have revolutionized the diagnostic approach to monogenic stroke, improving overall patient management.[67] Specific clinical-neuroradiological phenotypes have been described that may raise the suspicion of genetic variants in genes associated with hereditary monogenic AIS forms such as CADASIL and COL4A1 mutation, even in the absence of a positive family history.[68,69] Additionally, there are other non-hereditary syndromes associated with congenital arteriopathies and/or AIS, such as the PHACES syndrome (see Fig. 7E-H).[70]

Mineralizing angiopathy

Isolated striatocapsular infarctions in infants and toddlers, without evidence of medium or large vessel abnormalities on vascular imaging should raise suspicion of mineralizing angiopathy.[71] Although initially believed to be a cause of nonperinatal AIS in children less than 18 months of age, mineralizing angiopathy has now been reported as a cause of AIS in children as old as 6 years of age. If pathognomonic findings of multifocal, bilateral basal gangilia calcifications are not revealed by T1-weighted or susceptibility-weighted MRI sequences, noncontrast CT should be obtained for further evaluation. Frontal and parietal lobar calcifications in the corticomedullary junction regions, thalamic calcifications, and calcifications of the dentate nuclei may also be present though these may not be conspicuous on MRI. The

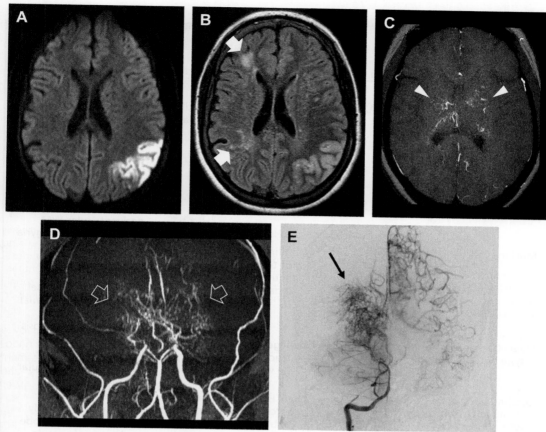

Fig. 6. Moyamoya arteriopathy in a 14-year-old girl. (*A-C*) Brain MRI and MRA at clinical onset. Axial DWI (*A*) and FLAIR (*B*) images show an acute cortical AIS in the left parietal MCA-PCA posterior watershed region. White matter signal changes are noted in the right fronto-parietal MCA-ACA and MCA-PCA watershed regions associated with cortical atrophy (thick *arrows*). (*C, D*) 3D-TOF MRA demonstrates moyamoya collaterals in the basal ganglia (*arrowheads*) and markedly reduced blood flow in bilateral MCAs, ACAs, and PCAs (empty *arrows*). (*E*) Catheter-directed DSA, right vertebral artery injection in the capillary phase, shows delayed retrograde angiographic filling of left MCA cortical branches through leptomeningeal anastomoses supplied by the left PCA, and delayed angiographic filling of moyamoya collateral networks ("puff of smoke") in the right cerebral hemisphere by the stenotic/occluded right PCA (*thin arrow*).

pathophysiology of this entity is poorly understood. In the majority of cases, AIS is associated with minor head trauma (ie, fall from bed) and isolated cases have been associated with thrombophilia. Large case series indicate that minor trauma precedes the onset of stroke symptoms by an average of 60 minutes, suggesting that the trauma precipitates a cascade of events within previously diseased, calcified lenticulostriate arteries which culminates in symptomatic AIS.[72] The literature suggests a favorable neurologic prognosis with adequate rehabilitation. Although recurrent strokes have been reported, sometimes after a period of several years, stroke recurrence is not typical.

Complications of arterial ischemic stroke in children

Regular imaging follow-up is recommended in AIS, especially in the early phases. This is useful to evaluate therapy response and to exclude recurrent subclinical events or complications. In cases of large MCA or cerebellar infarction, secondary malignant edema may occur, and decompressive craniectomy may be indicated. Hemorrhagic transformation is another event that can lead to a change in the therapeutic strategy.[11]

DIFFERENTIAL DIAGNOSIS/STROKE MIMICS IN CHILDREN

Migraine is the most common stroke mimic in children,[73] with an overall prevalence of 10.6%. Migraine headaches may be associated with vomiting and/or auras including visual or sensory disturbances.[13] MRI findings range from normal to multiple focal white matter signal changes or cortical swelling with venous dilatation and gyriform

Table 4
Monogenic conditions associated with stroke and arteriopathies

Disease Name	Gene Symbol	Protein name and Function	Neuroimaging Features
Autosomal Dominant			
ACTA2-related vasculopathy	ACTA2[a]	Actin Alpha 2: contractile protein of the vascular smooth muscle cells	Ischemic AIS, fusiform dilatation of ICA cavernous/clinoid segments, stenosis of terminal ICA segment, initial M1 and A1 segments, absence of "moyamoya" basal collaterals, periventricular WM signal changes, dysgyria
Marfan syndrome	FBN1	Fibrillin 1: structural role for tissue integrity and regulator of cellular signaling events	Ischemic and/or hemorrhagic stroke; dissecting aortic aneurysm; neck vessel dissections; intracranial aneurysms; dural ectasias; kyphoscoliosis
Ehlers-Danlos Syndrome type IV (EDS-IV)	COL3A1	Collagen type III: a major structural component of the vessel wall	Ischemic and/or hemorrhagic stroke; aneurysms and vascular ectasias; dissections
Cerebral autosomal dominant arteriopathy with subcortical infarcts and leukoencephalopathy (CADASIL)	NOTCH3	NOTCH3 (Neurogenic locus notch homolog protein 3): transmembrane receptor protein, role in the survival of vascular smooth muscle cells	Confluent WM signal alterations with early anterior temporal lobe and external capsule involvement and sparing of occipital regions; focal lesions in the BG, thalamus, and pons; frequent cerebral microhemorrhages; late cerebral atrophy
Cathepsin A-related arteriopathy with strokes and leukoencephalopathy (CARASAL)	CTSA[b]	Cathepsin A: stabilizes the protein complex formed by β-galactosidase and neuromidase-1 thus protecting from lysosomal degradation	Confluent WM signal alterations; focal lesions in the BG and thalamus; high T2 signal connecting the middle cerebellar peduncles across the pons (arc sign); rare cerebral microhemorrhages
Autosomal dominant familial porencephaly	COL4A1 COL4A2	Collagen type IV: main component of the basement membranes	Antenatal/perinatal hemorrhagic stroke; microhemorrhages; WM signal alterations; periventricular leukomalacia-like pattern; porencephaly; brain calcifications; schizencephaly; focal cortical dysplasia

(continued on next page)

Table 4
(continued)

Disease Name	Gene Symbol	Protein name and Function	Neuroimaging Features
Pontine autosomal dominant microangiopathy and leukoencephalopathy (PADMAL)	COL4A1[c]	Collagen type IV: main component of the basement membranes	lacunar infarcts predominantly affecting the pons; subcortical and periventricular WM lesions; rare spinal cord involvement; uncommon micro- and macro-hemorrhages; late brainstem atrophy
Neurofibromatosis Type 1 (NF-1)	NF1	Neurofibromin 1: protein regulating Ras signaling pathway, tumor-suppressing function	Ischemic stroke, moyamoya vasculopathy, distal arterial stenoses, aneurysms, focal areas of signal intensity (FASI) typically in the cerebellar WM, brainstem, and BG; optic end extra-optic pathway gliomas, sphenoid wing dysplasia; dural calcifications; scoliosis; neurofibromas; dural ectasia; kyphoscoliosis
Neurofibromatosis type 2 (NF-2)	NF2	Neurofibromin 2: tumor suppressor gene	Ischemic stroke, cerebral arteriopathy, meningiomas, schwannomas (usually from the inferior vestibular division of the vestibulocochlear nerve); spinal ependymoma
Acardi-Goutieres Syndrome 1, dominant (AGS)	TREX1	TREX1 (Three Prime Repair Exonuclease 1): DNA-degrading enzyme	Ischemic stroke; aneurysms; WM signal alterations with frontotemporal predominance or diffuse involvement; deep WM cysts in frontal and temporal regions; cerebral calcifications (may be absent in late onset); cerebral atrophy
Hutchinson-Gilford Progeria Syndrome	LMNA	Progerin, truncated form of the lamin A precursor prelamin A: maintenance of nuclear architecture and stability, as well as genome organization and function	Ischemic stroke; progressive arterial stenoses; craniofacial disproportion with maxillary and mandibular hypoplasia
Alagille syndrome	JAG1, NOTCH2	Jagged1: Transmembrane receptor for the Notch signaling pathway; NOTCH2: Jagged 1 ligand; vascular development, and response in cases of vascular injury	Ischemic and hemorrhagic stroke; aneurysms, dolichoectasia, Moyamoya syndrome, venous anomalies; Chiari 1 anomaly, craniosynostosis, intracranial hypertension, vertebral malformations, midline malformations

(continued on next page)

Table 4
(continued)

Disease Name	Gene Symbol	Protein name and Function	Neuroimaging Features
Williams-Beuren syndrome	*ELN*	Elastin: architectural and mechanical role in blood vessels	Rare moyamoya arteriopathy
Von Hippel–Lindau disease	*VHL*	VHL (Von Hippel–Lindau): tumor suppressor role	Hemorrhagic stroke; craniospinal hemangioblastomas; endolymphatic sac tumor
Autosomal Recessive			
Sickle cell disease (SCD)	HBB (β^S allele)	B Hemoglobin	Ischemic and hemorrhagic strokes; WM signal alterations; cerebral atrophy; moyamoya arteriopathy; vertebral bone infarction, osteomyelitis, and altered marrow signal
Deficiency of adenosine deaminase 2 (DADA-2)	CECR1	Adenosine deaminase 2: growth and development of macrophages, important for the proper immune response and endothelial integrity	Lacunar ischemic infarcts in the nucleo-capsular, midbrain, and thalamic regions; hemorrhagic stroke, microhemorrhages, arterial stenoses with perivascular enhancing tissue in the posterior circulation, small-sized intracranial aneurysms, brain atrophy
Pseudoxanthoma elasticum (PXE)	ABCC6	ABCC6 (ATP-binding cassette sub-family C member 6): transport and deposition of elastic fibers in the vessel wall	Ischemic stroke, intra- and extra-cranial aneurysms, arterial stenosis, tortuosity, and occlusion; segmental hypoplasia/aplasia of the petrous and/or cavernous segments of the ICA often associated with compensating arterial network supplied by external carotid artery branches (carotid rete mirabile)
Cerebral autosomal recessive arteriopathy with subcortical infarcts and leukoencephalopathy (CARASIL)	HTRA1	HTRA1 (High-Temperature Requirement A Serine Peptidase 1): protein quality control under various stress conditions	Diffuse WM changes and multiple lacunar infarctions in the BG and thalamus; microhemorrhages
Ehlers-Danlos syndrome type VIA (EDS-Via)	PLOD1	PLOD1 (Procollagen-Lysine,2-Oxoglutarate 5-Dioxygenase 1): catalyzes the hydroxylation of lysyl residues in collagen-like peptides	Perinatal stroke; hemorrhagic stroke; kyphoscoliosis

(continued on next page)

Table 4
(continued)

Disease Name	Gene Symbol	Protein name and Function	Neuroimaging Features
Grange syndrome	YY1AP1	Yin yang 1–associated protein 1, DNA repair pathway in vascular smooth muscle cells	Hemorrhagic and ischemic stroke; subarachnoid stroke; arterial stenoses and occlusion;
ADAMTS13 thrombotic microangiopathy	ADAMTS13	Extracellular matrix components, part of the coagulation cascade	Ischemic stroke (often multiple)
Acardi-Goutieres Syndromes	RNASEH2A RNASEH2B RNASEH2C SAMHD1 TREX1	Ribonuclease H2 subunit A, B, and C; SAMHD1 (SAM And HD Domain Containing Deoxynucleoside Triphosphate Triphosphohydrolase 1); TREX1: regulation of the innate immune response	Ischemic stroke; aneurysms; arterial stenoses; WM signal alterations with frontotemporal predominance or diffuse involvement; delayed myelination; deep WM cysts in frontal and temporal regions; periventricular leukomalacia-like pattern; cerebral calcifications; cerebral atrophy
Fabry disease	GLA	α-galactosidase, part of the transportation of globotriaosylceramide	Ischemic strokes (mostly posterior circulation); lacunar infarcts; WM signal changes; basilar artery dolichoectasia; subarachnoid hemorrhage
Microcephalic osteodysplastic primordial dwarfism type II (MOPD II)	PCNT	Pericentrin, protein involved in centrosomes function (cell cycle progression)	Ischemic and hemorrhagic strokes, Moyamoya vasculopathy, aneurysms; microcephaly, rare malformations of cortical development
Arterial tortuosity syndrome	SLC2A10	Glucose Transporter 10 (GLUT10): Facilitative glucose transporter	Elongated and tortuous large and medium-sized arteries; aneurysms; rare dissection

Abbreviations: ACA, anterior cerebral artery; BG, basal ganglia; ICA, internal carotid artery; MCA, middle cerebral artery; WM, white matter.
[a] with multiple variants at R179 position.
[b] Single variant at R325 C position.
[c] Variants located at 3'-UTR.

enhancement in the hemiplegic form. No diffusion restriction of the affected areas is detected. Distinct phases of parenchymal hypoperfusion, lasting for several hours, and rebound hyperfusion are often found in migraine with aura (A.K.A. complicated migraine or hemiplegic migraine) and are particularly conspicuous in ASL sequences (**Fig. 8**).[74] In such cases, there is often diffuse pruning of cortical branch arteries on time of flight MRA and dephasing effects on susceptibility-weighted MRI sequences.

Todd's paralysis after seizures is another AIS mimic in children. This post-ictal phenomenon can occur in 13% of seizure cases, including partial or complete hemiparesis lasting between 30 min and 36 hours. Decreased cerebral perfusion owing to cortical spreading depolarizations may be observed without restricted diffusion in the affected brain parenchyma.[11,75]

As a mimic of pediatric stroke, symptomatic facial nerve dysfunction is common. Clinical

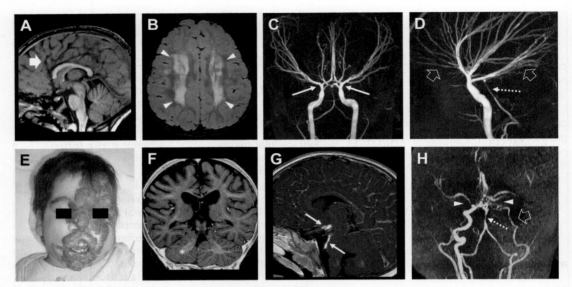

Fig. 7. Genetic and syndromic conditions related to pediatric AIS. (*A-D*) ACTA2-related arteriopathy in a 2-year-old girl. (*A*) Sagittal T1-weighted image reveals a corpus callosum dysmorphism associated with fronto-mesial dysgyria (thick *arrow*). (*B*) Axial FLAIR image reveals confluent white matter signal changes in the cerebral hemispheres (*arrowheads*). (*C, D*) 3D-TOF images show fusiform dilatation and straightening of ICA cavernous/clinoid segments associated with mild stenosis of terminal ICA (thin *arrows*), straightening and narrowing of MCA and ACA branches (empty *arrows*), and absence of moyamoya collaterals. There is severe stenosis and straightening of the basilar artery (dashed *arrow*). (*E–H*) PHACES (posterior fossa malformations, hemangioma, arterial anomalies, coarctation of the aorta/cardiac defects, eye abnormalities, and sternal cleft anomalies) syndrome in an 11-month-old girl. (*E*) Picture showing extended segmental facial hemangioma. (*F*) Coronal inversion recovery T1-weighted image demonstrates right cerebellar hypoplasia with foliar abnormalities (*asterisk*). (*G*) Post-contrast T1-weighted image reveals an intracranial hemangioma located at the brainstem level (thin *arrows*). (*H*) 3D-TOF MRA depicts hypoplasia of the left ICA (empty *arrow*) associated with bilateral terminal ICA stenoses (*arrowheads*) and reduced flow signal in the MCA distributions (moyamoya arteriopathy). There is also a focal narrowing of the basilar artery (dashed *arrow*). Contrast enhancement outlining the cortical and callosal sulci (*G*) corresponds to leptomeningeal collaterals.

neurologic deficits resulting from peripheral facial nerve dysfunction can usually be clinically differentiated from AIS, as central facial nerve palsy resulting from AIS selectively impairs the lower facial muscles and spares the upper facial muscles. In contrast, peripheral facial nerve dysfunction affects the upper and lower facial muscles. Peripheral facial nerve dysfunction is mostly the result of Bell's palsy, infection, or trauma and is frequently associated with abnormal ipsilateral contrast enhancement of the canalicular or tympanic segments of the facial nerve in the absence of brain parenchymal changes on MRI.[76]

Demyelinating diseases, which include multiple sclerosis and acute disseminated encephalomyelitis, can present primarily with acute ataxia and should be included in the differential diagnosis of pediatric AIS, as should tumors. In such cases, brain MRI findings will definitively differentiate AIS from these conditions.[76] In addition, several instances of pediatric stroke are not associated with thromboembolic large vessel occlusion, including arteriopathies, mitochondrial diseases and moyamoya arteriopathies.

TREATMENT
Medical Treatment in Perinatal Arterial Ischemic Stroke

Reperfusion therapies (fibrinolytic agents and MT) and antithrombotic treatment is generally not indicated in neonatal AIS. Secondary stroke prophylaxis with antithrombotoics may occasionally be used in selected cases (ie, severe thrombophilia or cerebral embolism resulting from cardiac disease).[1]

The management of neonatal AIS is currently based on supportive care measures, including the control of seizures, the optimization of oxygenation, and the correction of dehydration and anemia. Early initiation of targeted rehabilitation

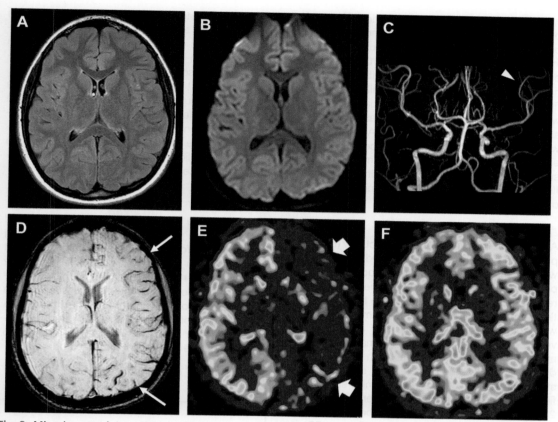

Fig. 8. Migraine attack in a 13-year-old girl presenting with headache, speech disorder and right-sided hypoesthesia, and hypotonia. Axial FLAIR (*A*) and DWI (*B*) images at clinical onset show normal findings. (*C*) 3D-TOF reveals a very mild reduction of flow signal in the left distal MCA branches (*arrowhead*). (*D*) Axial SWI demonstrates increased signal in the left hemispheric cortical veins (thin *arrows*). (*E*) Axial ASL shows reduced cerebral blood flow in the left hemisphere (thick *arrows*). (*F*) Follow-up ASL study performed 3 days later reveals resolution of flow-related signal changes.

therapy has been shown to improve functional outcomes in affected patients.[8]

Reperfusion Therapies for Non-perinatal Pediatric Arterial Ischemic Stroke

Intravenous thrombolytic therapy

Despite the absence of randomized controlled data, intravenous fibrinolytic therapy with alteplase is used to treat nonperinatal AIS, with recent studies showing a more than two-fold increase in utilization across U.S. centers between 2005 and 2019.[77] At least 2 well-designed multi-center study established the safety of intravenous alteplase administered at the standard adult dose and infusion rate within 4.5 hours of AIS onset to eligible children who are 2 to 17 years of age[77,78]. Reluctance to treat children younger than 2 years of age persists since many neuropediatricians do not believe that clinical stroke severity or timing

of stroke onset can be reliably determined in this age group. Tenecteplase is a genetically modified form of tissue plasminogen activator with a prolonged half-life that enables single bolus dosing, and which is engineered to bind to the fibrin component of thrombus such that it selectively converts thrombus-bound plasminogen to plasmin. While tenecteplase is increasingly replacing alteplase for hyperacute reperfusion therapy in adult stroke centers, providers are cautioned about its use in the pediatric population given the absence of pharmacokinetic and safety data in children with AIS.[79] Rapid hyperacute neuroimaging plays a critical role in the selection of patients for intravenous fibrinolytic therapy. Such imaging studies must reliably exclude intracranial hemorrhage and cannot delay the administration of reperfusion therapies. Notably, current American Heart Association guidelines for the early management of AIS in adults do not recommend withholding intravenous fibrinolytic therapy in otherwise eligible patients who demonstrate cerebral microbleeds on brain MRI.[80] Moreover, delaying the administration of fibrinolytic therapy in patients who are considered eligible based on noncontrast CT is discouraged. While intravenous fibrinolytic therapy may be beneficial for patients with adult AIS with Sickle Cell Disease, the hyperacute and acute management of AIS in children with Sickle Cell Disease should be focused on emergent transfusion therapy, administration of supplemental oxygen, hydration with intravenous fluids, maintenance of normothermia and antibiotics if infection is suspected.[80,81]

Endovascular thrombectomy

As in adults, endovascular thrombectomy (EVT) improves neurologic outcomes in pediatric patients with AIS due to acute large vessel occlusion when performed in properly selected patients.[82–84] As a result of diagnostic delays owing to the disproportionately high frequency of stroke mimics in children with acute neurologic deficits and pediatric provider inexperience with stroke, the majority of pediatric stroke patients present with considerable delays. Recently, the Save ChildS study demonstrated that EVT in children has a similar safety profile compared with adults when performed up to 24 hours from the onset of symptoms, especially in patients 7 to 18 years of age. (Sporns PB),[85] The widening of therapeutic windows has thus encouraged the creation of pediatric stroke alert protocols in pediatric referral centers, with the definition of resource-based diagnostic algorithms based on the availability of anesthesiology support, emergency MRI, and neurointerventional expertise. to have retrospect[86]

Most recently, the results of the Save Childs Pro registry, revealed at the 2024 Annual Congress of the International Pediatric Stroke Organization (Sporns PB et al), showed that EVT achieves superior neurologic outcomes relative to the best medical therapy in properly selected children with AIS due to acute intracranial medium or large vessel occlusion. Despite this, the safety and efficacy of MT in children with FCA remains uncertain with several anecdotal cases of poor response to EVT. Moreover, the risk of attempted EVT in the broader population of children with cerebral arteriopathy is considered to be substantial, particularly in patients with moyamoya arteriopathies, collagenopathies, elastinopathies, and other arteriopathies with increased fragility of the arterial wall. This underscores the importance of etiologic determination at the time of initial imaging, and the need for multidisciplinary team discussions on a case-by-case basis.

Nonetheless, there is a strong general consensus that EVT is safe and effective for children with intracranial medium or large vessel occlusions due to embolus, which is either cardiogenic or from a cervical artery dissection. Although penumbral imaging continues to play an important role in the selection of adult patients for EVT, the perfusion metrics that differentiate core infarction, from penumbra, from benign oligemia have not been established for the pediatric population and no meaningful application of penumbral imaging to pediatric patient selection for EVT is possible.[83]

SUMMARY

Confirming the diagnosis of pediatric AIS and determining its etiology is crucial for optimizing treatment and for prognosis. Pediatric AIS should be managed in the context of a multidisciplinary team with expertise in the management of pediatric stroke. Radiologists should be familiar with the pros and cons of each imaging modality and specific findings of different stroke-related pathologies and their most common mimics, more so in the modern era of mechanical thrombectomy.

CLINICS CARE POINTS

- Neuroimaging protocols for AIS in children should be tailored based on the age and timing of presentation.
- Fast MRI protocols with arterial MR angiography and perfusion studies are useful to distinguish between AIS and other causes of acute neurologic presentation in children.
- Full MRI protocols should include additional sequences, such as black blood vessel wall imaging, that may help in the differential diagnosis of pediatric AIS.
- Repeated imaging and follow-up timing will change according to the cause of pediatric or neonatal AIS.

DISCLOSURE

The authors have nothing to disclose.

FUNDING

This work was supported by The Italian Ministry of Health, 5x1000 project n. 5M-2019-23680415.

REFERENCES

1. Ferriero DM, Fullerton HJ, Bernard TJ, et al. Management of stroke in neonates and children: a

scientific statement from the American heart association/American stroke association. Stroke 2019; 50(3):e51–96.

2. Gao L, Lim M, Nguyen D, et al. The incidence of pediatric ischemic stroke: a systematic review and meta-analysis. Int J Stroke 2023;18(7):765–72.

3. DeLaroche AM, Sivaswamy L, Farooqi A, et al. Pediatric stroke and its mimics: limitations of a pediatric stroke clinical pathway. Pediatr Neurol 2018;80: 35–41.

4. Rafay MF, Pontigon AM, Chiang J, et al. Delay to diagnosis in acute pediatric arterial ischemic stroke. Stroke 2009;40(1):58–64.

5. Neville K, Lo W. Sensitivity and specificity of an adult stroke screening tool in childhood ischemic stroke. Pediatr Neurol 2016;58:53–6.

6. Ichord RN, Bastian R, Abraham L, et al. Interrater reliability of the pediatric national Institutes of Health stroke scale (PedNIHSS) in a multicenter study. Stroke 2011;42(3):613–7.

7. Tam D. Calculated decisions: pediatric NIHSS stroke scale (pedNIHSS). Pediatr Emerg Med Pract 2023; 20(5 Suppl):CD1–2.

8. Kirton A, Armstrong-Wells J, Chang T, et al. Symptomatic neonatal arterial ischemic stroke: the international pediatric stroke study. Pediatrics 2011; 128(6):e1402–10.

9. Roy B, Webb A, Walker K, et al. Risk factors for perinatal stroke in term infants: a case-control study in Australia. J Paediatr Child Health 2023;59(4):673–9.

10. Negrotto M, Muthusami P, Wasserman BA, et al. Initial diagnostic evaluation of the child with suspected arterial ischemic stroke. Top Magn Reson Imag 2021;30(5):211–23.

11. Sporns PB, Fullerton HJ, Lee S, et al. Childhood stroke. Nat Rev Dis Prim 2022;8(1):12.

12. Khalaf A, Iv M, Fullerton H, et al. Pediatric stroke imaging. Pediatr Neurol 2018;86:5–18.

13. Mackay MT, Lee M, Yock-Corrales A, et al. Differentiating arterial ischaemic stroke from migraine in the paediatric emergency department. Dev Med Child Neurol 2018;60(11):1117–22.

14. Expert Panel on Pediatric Imaging, Robertson RL, Palasis S, et al. ACR appropriateness criteria(R) cerebrovascular disease-child. J Am Coll Radiol 2020; 17(5S):S36–54.

15. Christy A, Murchison C, Wilson JL. Quick brain magnetic resonance imaging with diffusion-weighted imaging as a first imaging modality in pediatric stroke. Pediatr Neurol 2018;78:55–60.

16. Lee S, Mlynash M, Christensen S, et al. Hyperacute perfusion imaging before pediatric thrombectomy: analysis of the Save ChildS study. Neurology 2023; 100(11):e1148–58.

17. Saunders DE, Thompson C, Gunny R, et al. Magnetic resonance imaging protocols for paediatric neuroradiology. Pediatr Radiol 2007;37(8):789–97.

18. Lee S, Mirsky DM, Beslow LA, et al. Pathways for neuroimaging of neonatal stroke. Pediatr Neurol 2017;69:37–48.

19. Jiang B, Mackay MT, Stence N, et al. Neuroimaging in pediatric stroke. Semin Pediatr Neurol 2022;43: 100989.

20. Little SB, Sarma A, Bajaj M, et al. Imaging of vertebral artery dissection in children: an underrecognized condition with high risk of recurrent stroke. Radiographics 2023;43(12):e230107.

21. Lee S, Ryan KR, Murray J, et al. Multidisciplinary stroke pathway for children supported with ventricular assist devices. ASAIO J 2023;69(4):402–10.

22. Briest RC, Cheung AK, Kandula T, et al. Urgent computed tomography angiography in paediatric stroke. Dev Med Child Neurol 2023;65(1):126–35.

23. Lee S, Jiang B, Heit JJ, et al. Cerebral perfusion in pediatric stroke: children are not little adults. Top Magn Reson Imag 2021;30(5):245–52.

24. Goldman-Yassen AE, Dehkharghani S. Neuroimaging in perinatal stroke and cerebrovascular disease. In: Dehkharghani S, editor. Stroke. Brisbane (AU): Exon Publications; 2021. p. 1–24.

25. Husson B, Lasjaunias P. Radiological approach to disorders of arterial brain vessels associated with childhood arterial stroke-a comparison between MRA and contrast angiography. Pediatr Radiol 2004;34(1):10–5.

26. Nash M, Rafay MF. Craniocervical arterial dissection in children: pathophysiology and management. Pediatr Neurol 2019;95:9–18.

27. Rollins N, Braga B, Hogge A, et al. Dynamic arterial compression in pediatric vertebral arterial dissection. Stroke 2017;48(4):1070–3.

28. Gupta N, Hiremath SB, Aviv RI, et al. Childhood cerebral vasculitis : a multidisciplinary approach. Clin Neuroradiol 2023;33(1):5–20.

29. Storey A, Michael Scott R, Robertson R, et al. Preoperative transdural collateral vessels in moyamoya as radiographic biomarkers of disease. J Neurosurg Pediatr 2017;19(3):289–95.

30. Husson B, Hertz-Pannier L, Renaud C, et al. Motor outcomes after neonatal arterial ischemic stroke related to early MRI data in a prospective study. Pediatrics 2010;126(4):912–8.

31. Mackay MT, Slavova N, Pastore-Wapp M, et al. Pediatric ASPECTS predicts outcomes following acute symptomatic neonatal arterial stroke. Neurology 2020;94(12):e1259–70.

32. Geraldo AF, Parodi A, Bertamino M, et al. Perinatal arterial ischemic stroke in fetal vascular malperfusion: a case series and literature review. AJNR Am J Neuroradiol 2020;41(12):2377–83.

33. Biswas A, Mankad K, Shroff M, et al. Neuroimaging perspectives of perinatal arterial ischemic stroke. Pediatr Neurol 2020;113:56–65.

34. Steggerda SJ, de Vries LS. Neonatal stroke in premature neonates. Semin Perinatol 2021;45(7):151471.

35. Husson B, Hertz-Pannier L, Adamsbaum C, et al. MR angiography findings in infants with neonatal arterial ischemic stroke in the middle cerebral artery territory: a prospective study using circle of Willis MR angiography. Eur J Radiol 2016;85(7):1329–35.

36. Baggio L, Nosadini M, Pelizza MF, et al. Neonatal arterial ischemic stroke secondary to carotid artery dissection: a case report and systematic literature review. Pediatr Neurol 2023;139:13–21.

37. Watson CG, Dehaes M, Gagoski BA, et al. Arterial spin labeling perfusion magnetic resonance imaging performed in acute perinatal stroke reveals hyperperfusion associated with ischemic injury. Stroke 2016;47(6):1514–9.

38. Kirkham FJ, Zafeiriou D, Howe D, et al. Fetal stroke and cerebrovascular disease: advances in understanding from lenticulostriate and venous imaging, alloimmune thrombocytopaenia and monochorionic twins. Eur J Paediatr Neurol 2018;22(6):989–1005.

39. Kurnik K, Kosch A, Strater R, et al. Recurrent thromboembolism in infants and children suffering from symptomatic neonatal arterial stroke: a prospective follow-up study. Stroke 2003;34(12):2887–92.

40. Lehman LL, Beaute J, Kapur K, Danehy AR, Bernson-Leung ME, Malkin H, Rivkin MJ, Trenor CC 3rd. Workup for Perinatal Stroke Does Not Predict Recurrence. Stroke. 2017 Aug;48(8):2078-2083. doi: 10.1161/STROKEAHA.117.017356. Epub 2017 Jul 13. PMID: 28706112

41. Bernard TJ, Manco-Johnson MJ, Lo W, et al. Towards a consensus-based classification of childhood arterial ischemic stroke. Stroke 2012;43(2):371–7.

42. Bohmer M, Niederstadt T, Heindel W, et al. Impact of childhood arterial ischemic stroke standardized classification and diagnostic evaluation classification on further course of arteriopathy and recurrence of childhood stroke. Stroke 2019;50(1):83–7.

43. Fullerton HJ, Wintermark M, Hills NK, et al. Risk of recurrent arterial ischemic stroke in childhood: a prospective international study. Stroke 2016;47(1):53–9.

44. DeVela G, Taylor JM, Zhang B, Linscott LL, Chen AM, Karani KB, Furthmiller A, Leach JL, Vadivelu S, Abruzzo T. Quantitative Arterial Tortuosity Suggests Arteriopathy in Children With Cryptogenic Stroke. Stroke. 2018 Apr;49(4):1011-1014. doi: 10.1161/STROKEAHA.117.020321. Epub 2018 Mar 14. PMID: 29540605.).

45. Baranoski JF, White AC, Chung CY, et al. Mechanical disorders of the cervicocerebral circulation in children and young adults. J Neurointerventional Surg 2023;16(9):939–46.

46. Hedjoudje A, Darcourt J, Bonneville F, et al. The use of intracranial vessel wall imaging in clinical practice. Radiol Clin North Am 2023;61(3):521–33.

47. Yeh HR, Kim EH, Yu JJ, et al. Arterial ischemic stroke in children with congenital heart diseases. Pediatr Int 2022;64(1):e15200.

48. Sun LR, Lynch JK. Advances in the diagnosis and treatment of pediatric arterial ischemic stroke. Neurotherapeutics 2023;20(3):633–54.

49. Elgendy AY, Saver JL, Amin Z, et al. Proposal for updated nomenclature and classification of potential causative mechanism in patent foramen ovale-associated stroke. JAMA Neurol 2020;77(7):878–86.

50. Wintermark M, Hills NK, DeVeber GA, et al. Clinical and imaging characteristics of arteriopathy subtypes in children with arterial ischemic stroke: results of the VIPS study. AJNR Am J Neuroradiol 2017;38(11):2172–9.

51. Perez FA, Oesch G, Amlie-Lefond CM. MRI vessel wall enhancement and other imaging biomarkers in pediatric focal cerebral arteriopathy-inflammatory subtype. Stroke 2020;51(3):853–9.

52. Bertamino M, Signa S, Veneruso M, et al. Expanding the clinical and neuroimaging features of post-varicella arteriopathy of childhood. J Neurol 2021;268(12):4846–65.

53. Fullerton HJ, Stence N, Hills NK, et al. Focal cerebral arteriopathy of childhood: novel severity Score and natural history. Stroke 2018;49(11):2590–6.

54. Fearn ND, Mackay MT. Focal cerebral arteriopathy and childhood stroke. Curr Opin Neurol 2020;33(1):37–46.

55. Smitka M, Bruck N, Engellandt K, et al. Clinical perspective on primary angiitis of the central nervous system in childhood (cPACNS). Frontiers in Pediatrics 2020;8:281.

56. Elbers J, Armstrong D, Yau I, et al. Vascular imaging outcomes of childhood primary angiitis of the central nervous system. Pediatr Neurol 2016;63:53–9.

57. Scott RM, Smith ER. Moyamoya disease and moyamoya syndrome. N Engl J Med 2009;360(12):1226–37.

58. Morello A, Scala M, Schiavetti I, et al. Surgical revascularization as a procedure to prevent neurological complications in children with moyamoya syndrome associated with neurofibromatosis I: a single institution case series. Child's Nerv Syst 2024;40(6):1731–41.

59. Tortora D, Scavetta C, Rebella G, et al. Spatial coefficient of variation applied to arterial spin labeling MRI may contribute to predict surgical revascularization outcomes in pediatric moyamoya vasculopathy. Neuroradiology 2020;62(8):1003–15.

60. Tortora D, Severino M, Pacetti M, et al. Noninvasive assessment of hemodynamic stress distribution after indirect revascularization for pediatric moyamoya vasculopathy. AJNR Am J Neuroradiol 2018;39(6):1157–63.

61. Dlamini N, Shah-Basak P, Leung J, et al. Breath-hold blood oxygen level-dependent MRI: a tool for the

assessment of cerebrovascular reserve in children with moyamoya disease. AJNR Am J Neuroradiol 2018;39(9):1717–23.

62. Alshehri E, Dmytriw AA, Chavhan GB, et al. The role of MRA in pediatric sickle cell disease with normal transcranial Doppler imaging velocities. J Stroke Cerebrovasc Dis 2020;29(7):104864.

63. Mallon D, Doig D, Dixon L, et al. Neuroimaging in sickle cell disease: a review. J Neuroimaging 2020; 30(6):725–35.

64. Rawanduzy CA, Earl E, Mayer G, et al. Pediatric stroke: a review of common etiologies and management strategies. Biomedicines 2022;11(1):2.

65. Booth N, Ngwube A, Appavu B, et al. Reversal of cerebral arteriopathy post-hematopoietic Stem cell transplant for sickle cell disease. Pediatrics 2024; 153(2). e2023062643.

66. Jankovic M, Petrovic B, Novakovic I, et al. The genetic basis of strokes in pediatric populations and insight into new therapeutic options. Int J Mol Sci 2022;23(3):1601.

67. Grossi A, Severino M, Rusmini M, et al. Targeted resequencing in pediatric and perinatal stroke. Eur J Med Genet 2020;63(11):104030.

68. Geraldo AF, Caorsi R, Tortora D, et al. Widening the neuroimaging features of adenosine deaminase 2 deficiency. AJNR Am J Neuroradiol 2021;42(5): 975–9.

69. Gupta N, Miller E, Bhatia A, et al. Imaging review of pediatric monogenic CNS vasculopathy with genetic correlation. Radiographics 2024;44(5):e230087.

70. Tortora D, Severino M, Accogli A, et al. Moyamoya vasculopathy in PHACE syndrome: six new cases and review of the literature. World Neurosurgery 2017;108:291–302.

71. Gorodetsky C, Pulcine E, Krishnan P, et al. Childhood arterial ischemic stroke due to mineralizing angiopathy: an 18-year single-center experience. Dev Med Child Neurol 2021;63(9):1123–6.

72. Bahri R, Sharma RS, Jain V. Mineralizing angiopathy with basal ganglia stroke after minor head trauma; a clinical profile and follow up study of a large series of paediatric patients from North India. Eur J Paediatr Neurol 2021;33:61–7.

73. Mackay MT, Chua ZK, Lee M, et al. Stroke and non-stroke brain attacks in children. Neurology 2014; 82(16):1434–40.

74. Sinha R, Ramji S. Neurovascular disorders in children: an updated practical guide. Transl Pediatr 2021;10(4):1100–16.

75. Brosinski CM. Implementing diagnostic reasoning to differentiate Todd's paralysis from acute ischemic stroke. Adv Emerg Nurs J 2014;36(1):78–86.

76. Caffarelli M, Kimia AA, Torres AR. Acute ataxia in children: a review of the differential diagnosis and evaluation in the emergency department. Pediatr Neurol 2016;65:14–30.

77. Kaur N, Patel S, Ayanbadejo MO, et al. Age-specific trends in intravenous thrombolysis and mechanical thrombectomy utilization in acute ischemic stroke in children under age 18. Int J Stroke 2023;18(4): 469–76.

78. Kossorotoff M, Kerleroux B, Boulouis G, Husson B, Tran Dong K, Eugene F, Damaj L, Ozanne A, Bellesme C, Rolland A, Bourcier R, Triquenot-Bagan A, Marnat G, Neau JP, Joriot S, Perez A, Guillen M, Perivier M, Audic F, Hak JF, Denier C, Naggara O; KidClot Group. Recanalization Treatments for Pediatric Acute Ischemic Stroke in France. JAMA Netw Open. 2022 Sep 1;5(9):e2231343. doi: 10.1001/jamanetworkopen.2022.31343. PMID: 36107427; PMCID: PMC9478769

79. Sun LR, Wilson JL, Waak M, et al. Tenecteplase in acute stroke: what about the children? Stroke 2023;54(7):1950–3.

80. Powers WJ, Rabinstein AA, Ackerson T, et al. Guidelines for the early management of patients with acute ischemic stroke: 2019 update to the 2018 guidelines for the early management of acute ischemic stroke: a guideline for healthcare professionals from the American heart association/American stroke association. Stroke 2019;50(12):e344–418. Epub 2019 Oct 30. Erratum in: Stroke. 2019 Dec;50(12):e440-e441. doi: 10.1161/STR.0000000000000215. PMID: 31662037).

81. Kassim AA, Galadanci NA, Pruthi S, et al. How I treat and manage strokes in sickle cell disease. Blood 2015;125(22):3401–10.

82. Sporns PB, Psychogios MN, Straeter R, et al. Clinical diffusion mismatch to select pediatric patients for embolectomy 6 to 24 hours after stroke: an analysis of the Save ChildS study. Neurology 2021;96(3): e343–51.

83. Bhatia KD, Chowdhury S, Andrews I, et al. Association between thrombectomy and functional outcomes in pediatric patients with acute ischemic stroke from large vessel occlusion. JAMA Neurol 2023;80(9):910–8.

84. Dicpinigaitis AJ, Gandhi CD, Pisapia J, et al. Endovascular thrombectomy for pediatric acute ischemic stroke. Stroke 2022;53(5):1530–9.

85. Kunz WG, Sporns PB, Psychogios MN, et al. Cost-effectiveness of endovascular thrombectomy in childhood stroke: an analysis of the Save ChildS study. J Stroke 2022;24(1):138–47.

86. Shack M, Andrade A, Shah-Basak PP, et al. A pediatric institutional acute stroke protocol improves timely access to stroke treatment. Dev Med Child Neurol 2017;59(1):31–7.

Steno-occlusive Intracranial Large Vessel Arteriopathies in Childhood
A Pattern Oriented Approach to Neuroimaging Diagnosis

Katherine S. Kelson[a], Timothy J. Bernard, MD[a,b], Nicholas V. Stence, MD[a,c],*

KEYWORDS

- Focal cerebral arteriopathy • Intracranial arteriopathy • Intracranial dissection • Moyamoya

KEY POINTS

- Steno-occlusive intracranial large vessel arteriopathies are a common cause of arterial ischemic stroke (AIS) in children, particularly within the anterior cerebral circulation. The wide range of disorders that belongs to this category expresses a limited number of discrete phenotypes whose recognition facilitates diagnosis and treatment.
- Focal cerebral arteriopathy (FCA) is most common of these disorders expressed in childhood with characteristic acute clinical presentation and imaging features involving the intradural internal carotid artery (ICA) distribution unilaterally. It is notable for a significant risk of transient arteriopathy progression complicated by recurrent stroke.
- The moyamoya arteriopathies are a group of disorders characterized by chronic progressive occlusion of the intradural ICA terminus accompanied by specific unique types of collateral vessel formation. It is bilateral in most cases, is a common cause of AIS in children and often requires microneurosurgical revascularization for definitive therapy.
- Multi-focal arteriopathy (MFA) is the least common pattern of steno-occlusive intracranial large vessel disease in children. It is characterized by involvement of the anterior circulation bilaterally, and/or the posterior circulation and is often accompanied by involvement of small to medium size intracranial arteries.
- Intracranial arterial dissection is a specific mural injury process that may occur as a result of major mechanical damage to otherwise normal arteries or may be a manifestation of minor hemodynamic trauma (spontaneous) in the setting of underlying arteriopathy that compromises mural integrity. It may involve the intracranial posterior circulation in children and can frequently result in recurrent stroke.

INTRODUCTION

Steno-occlusive intracranial large vessel arteriopathy is an important cause of arterial ischemic stroke (AIS) in pediatric patients, representing up to 50% of cases.[1] Among the different phenotypic patterns encountered, the focal cerebral arteriopathy (FCA) pattern is most common. The

[a] University of Colorado Anschutz School of Medicine, Aurora, CO, USA; [b] Department of Pediatrics, Section of Child Neurology, University of Colorado Anschutz School of Medicine, Aurora, CO, USA; [c] Department of Radiology, Section of Pediatric Radiology, University of Colorado Anschutz School of Medicine, Aurora, CO, USA
* Corresponding author. 13123 East 16th Avenue, Aurora, CO 80045.
E-mail address: nicholas.stence@cuanschutz.edu

Neuroimag Clin N Am 34 (2024) 601–613
https://doi.org/10.1016/j.nic.2024.08.022
1052-5149/24/© 2024 Elsevier Inc. All rights are reserved, including those for text and data mining, AI training, and similar technologies.

moyamoya arteriopathy phenotype accounts for most remaining cases of childhood AIS due to steno-occlusive intracranial large vessel arteriopathy, with MFA phenotypes being relatively uncommon.[2] Moyamoya arteriopathies (MMA) result from the interaction of vascular injury factors (radiation, mycobacterial infection, and rheometric shear stress caused by sickled erythrocytes) with genetically-programmed segmental vulnerability traits in arteries. Consequently, the moyamoya phenotype can be expressed in many different clinical settings and is variably associated with a variety of syndromic conditions. The congenital cerebrovascular dysplasias expressed in the PHACE syndrome are worth noting here. These may be symptomatic with AIS, are usually monofocal and usually involve the internal carotid artery (ICA). Although any ICA segment may be involved, a moyamoya phenotype is sometimes encountered. These cases are typically recognized by clinical and imaging stigmata of the well-described neurocristopathy. MFA patterns are expressed by a variety of genetic arteriopathies, infectious and autoimmune forms of vasculitis, and in the reversible cerebral vasoconstriction syndrome (RCVS).

Given the high rate of recurrent stroke and varied options for stroke prevention, which may depend on the specific type of arteriopathy diagnosis, early and accurate diagnosis of steno-occlusive intracranial large vessel arteriopathy subtypes is important. We will discuss the subtypes of childhood steno-occlusive intracranial large vessel arteriopathies and important imaging findings to help guide clinical diagnosis.

1. FCA
   a. Definition and Epidemiology

      FCA is an acutely presenting, acquired, monophasic, unilateral monofocal steno-occlusion of the large intracranial arteries of the anterior cerebral circulation, most commonly involving the intradural ICA and its terminal branches.[2] The acute presentation initially expresses signs and symptoms of striatocapsular ischemia, followed by signs and symptoms of cortical ischemia as the primary vascular lesion progresses and collateral failure ensues. The brain imaging findings closely reflect the characteristic clinical course with striatocapsular infarction being the earliest and most consistent brain imaging manifestation. FCA has previously been referred to as transient cerebral arteriopathy, as it often stabilizes or improves months to years after onset.[2] FCA has been further differentiated by subtype based on the dominant underlying mechanism of vessel wall injury (arterial dissection vs mural inflammation). The most widely recognized primary subtypes recently defined by the vascular effects of infection in pediatric stroke (VIPS) trial include FCA-inflammatory (FCA-i), FCA-dissection (FCA-d), and FCA-undetermined.[2] A classification system described by Bernard and colleagues applies the CASCADE criteria to aid in the diagnosis of FCA based on the presence of characteristic lenticulostriate collateral vessels, which are distinct from those encountered in the MMA.[3] Specifically, the lenticulostriate collateral vessels encountered in FCA are bridging collaterals, which do not vascularize the striatum and internal capsule but instead form horizontally-oriented anastomotic bridges with each other in the subarachnoid space to reconstitute distal flow across a severe stenosis within the circle of Willis. In contrast, true moyamoya collaterals are hypertrophied lenticulostriate arteries, which directly vascularize the striatum and internal capsule in an attempt to reach the cortical territory. Notably, the CASCADE criteria recognize a posterior circulation form of FCA, which may be caused by dissection of the intradural vertebral arteries, basilar artery, and/or posterior cerebral arteries. Given the unique pathogenesis of anterior circulation FCA, it stands to reason that dissections of the posterior arterial circulation should be distinctly classified, particularly since these usually occur in the setting of a generalized or diffuse arteriopathy. Additionally, although the strictly pattern-based CASCADE criteria also recognize congenital anomalies as a potential form of FCA, neurocristopathies expressing a monofocal anterior circulation dysplasia rarely mimic the vascular imaging findings of FCA and can usually be differentiated on the basis of clinical presentation and ancillary neuroimaging findings.

The incidence of AIS has been reported to be 2.4 per 100,000 person-years.[4–6] On a population basis, FCA accounts for up to 25% of childhood stroke—[1,2]most commonly in patients aged 5 to 9 y old.[7]

Although AIS typically has a male predominance across all types, there is a 50/50 male to female distribution in FCA.[8]

b. Pathophysiology

The underlying etiology of many cases of FCA remains uncertain, but most cases of FCA are thought to be inflammatory in nature, termed FCA-i. In FCA-i, it is postulated that an episode of arterial inflammation leads to narrowing of vessels with secondary thrombus formation within the arterial lumen surrounded by inflamed or damaged endothelium.[9] Wintermark and colleagues note that FCA-i tends to be restricted to the territory of the distal intradural ICA and its terminal branches.[2] There is increasing evidence that many cases of FCA, specifically FCA-i, are secondary to previous infection.[2] Black blood vessel wall imaging (VWI) has shown promise in directly imaging mural inflammation in FCA through detection of vessel wall thickening and enhancement, discussed further in the following section.[10] Black blood VWI may also reveal intramural blood products that cause T1 shortening in the case of arterial dissection.

Post-varicella arteriopathy (PVA) is an important subtype of FCA-i occurring following primary varicella zoster virus (VZV) infection, with an average latency interval of 2 mo from infection to stroke.[2,11,12] PVA occurs when varicella virus infection involving the cutaneous distribution of the ophthalmic division of the trigeminal nerve results in retrograde transport of virus through dendritic processes to cell bodies in the trigeminal ganglion where virus remains latent. Subsequent reactivation of virus enables viral spread through trigeminal axons to the adventitia of the intradural ICA and its terminal branches.[13] Vascular imaging features of PVA are indistinguishable from other etiologies of FCA-i.[14] PVA may present in patients who are positive for VZV without cutaneous stigmata, or many months after known VZV infection, which can cloud the clinical picture.[15] If PVA is suspected as a potential cause of FCA, there should be a low threshold to obtain cerebrospinal fluid (CSF) to test for VZV-DNA, especially in unvaccinated patients.[16] In general, increasing rates of vaccination against VZV have been associated with a decreasing incidence of PVA.[17,18] Although PVA is a well-described cause of FCA-i in pediatric populations, other potential infectious etiologies are increasingly recognized. Other common infections, including Parvovirus-B19, cytomegalovirus and herpes viruses specifically have also been found to be potential triggers of AIS, even if initial infectious symptoms are subclinical.[2,12,19] Recent case studies also suggest the novel virus COVID-19 as a potential infectious trigger of FCA-i.[20]

Isolated intracranial arterial dissections involving the intradural ICA and/or M1-middle cerebral artery (MCA) are regarded as FCA-d subtype in the most recent VIPS classification (see **Fig. 5**).[2] Most reported cases are associated with head and neck trauma, most commonly due to mechanical forces resulting from rapid acceleration-deceleration injuries (whiplash), or from the shock wave effects of intracranial penetrating injuries. The forces of such injuries may produce tears in the tunica intima of intracranial arteries that are subjected to traction forces near fixation points (ie, petrolingual ligament, petroclival ligament, and paraclinoid dural rings encircling ICA).[2,21] Nonetheless, many cases of intracranial arterial dissection are often spontaneous or follow minor trauma. While generalized or diffuse arteriopathies (ie, Ehlers Danlos type 4, Marfan's Syndrome, Loeys Dietz Syndrome, and Arterial Tortuosity Syndrome) may be associated with intracranial arterial dissections, FCA-d, which is a monofocal process, is by definition distinct from these entities. Intracranial stenoses involving the intradural ICA are frequently difficult to diagnose and distinguish as purely inflammatory or dissecting processes. Moreover, overlap between arterial wall inflammation and arterial dissection likely exists. Inflammation, as a form of vessel wall injury can lead to arterial dissection, and arterial dissection as a distinct form of vessel wall injury can lead to vessel wall inflammation. When dissections form, exposure of the thrombogenic subendothelial tissue to circulating blood can lead to in-situ thrombosis, false lumen expansion with reciprocal collapse of the true lumen, and downstream embolization of thrombus. Any or all of these processes can serve as a mechanism of AIS. Notably, intracranial arterial dissection can be complicated by dissecting aneurysm formation when the false lumen of the dissection undergoes intramural expansion or by subarachnoid hemorrhage when the false lumen extends completely across the arterial wall from the adluminal side to the abluminal side. Consequently, close monitoring by vascular imaging is recommended.[21]

c. Presentation, symptoms, diagnosis

The typical presentation of FCA is in a previously healthy school age child with an acute onset of neurologic symptoms, most commonly acute hemiplegia, headache, and variable sensorimotor findings.[22–24] Symptoms may progress over hours to days, with faster progression of symptoms associated with an increased risk of recurrent ischemic stroke.[23–25] In pediatric AIS patients found to have arteriopathy, the risk of recurrent stroke within 1 y is up to 21%, a much higher rate of recurrence than for cardioembolic or cryptogenic stroke.[26] The mortality rate from AIS in FCA is 2.6%.[27,28] Survivors have high rates of permanent neurologic morbidity, up to 50% having disabling sensorimotor deficits and/or cognitive deficits at 1 y.[29,30]

Accurate diagnostic evaluation of FCA relies on prompt recognition of neurologic symptoms, demonstration of characteristic neuroimaging findings and the results of laboratory testing. Relevant laboratory results include C-reactive protein, erythrocyte sedimentation rate, D-dimer, and CSF indices. CSF studies should include polymerase chain reaction to look for underlying infectious etiologies.[9,26,31] Inflammatory markers commonly used to diagnose adult stroke can also be collected to help clarify the diagnosis, including interleukin (IL)-6, IL-10, IL-1Ra, and granulocyte macrophage colony-stimulating factor.[9,26,31] D-dimer may also be used as a biomarker of prognosis since elevated levels have been associated with poor outcomes.[32]

As discussed, vascular imaging manifestations of FCA include steno-occlusion and/or luminal irregularity of the distal intradural ICA and contiguous proximal anterior cerebral artery and MCA segments.[2,33,34] A banded pattern of luminal irregularity involving the intradural ICA and M1 on catheter-directed cerebral angiography has long been considered pathognomonic for FCA-i (Fig. 1B), although the finding can also be suggested on computed tomography (CT) angiography and MR angiography (MRA) (with or without contrast).[2] Imaging features strongly suggestive of the FCA-d subtype include intimal flap, intramural hematoma, segmental corkscrew tortuosity (caused by dissections with a spiral intramural trajectory), segmental ectasia, aneurysm, and pseudoaneurysm.[35–37] Segmental ectasias, aneurysms, pseudoaneurysms, and some intimal flaps are adequately shown by MRI, MRA, and computed tomography angiography (CTA) techniques. MRA has been shown to be concordant with CTA in up to 100% of cases when localizing vascular lesions in large to medium size intracranial arteries.[38] MRA is also as reliable as CTA in detecting stenotic or occlusive disease of the ICA and MCA, and so can help in determination of the many causes of AIS, including cardioembolic disease, MMA, FCA-d, and FCA-i.[38] Some pediatric patients with an isolated striatocapsular infarction and no detectable arterial narrowing at presentation will go on to develop arterial stenosis typical of FCA-i. Thus, early repeat vascular imaging should be undertaken in such cases if initial angiography is negative (Fig. 2). Rapid MRA protocols that reduce the need for sedation can also be employed by decreasing coverage and spatial resolution, and by leveraging modern acceleration techniques such as compressed SENSE (Fig. 3).[39]

Isolated striatocapsular infarction is an early and specific brain imaging finding in patients presenting with FCA (regardless of subtype). It is most likely to be demonstrated by MRI, highlighting the importance of obtaining MRI acutely whenever possible.[40–42] In contrast to

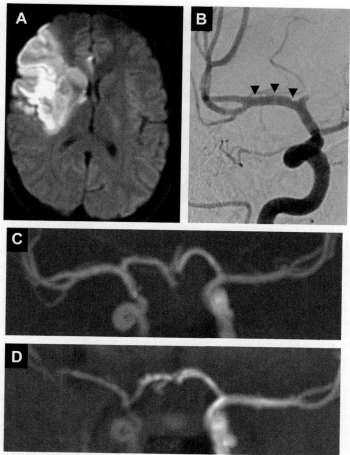

Fig. 1. Focal cerebral arteriopathy. 17-year-old boy presenting with acute onset left sided weakness and headache. (*A*) Axial diffusion weighted MRI h after presentation showing acute infarct within right basal ganglia, insula and anterior cortical MCA territory. (*B*) Frontal projection of catheter-directed angiogram in the right internal carotid artery (ICA) performed immediately after MRI showing banded pattern of luminal irregularity primarily involving proximal MCA (*arrowheads*) typical of FCA-i. (*C*) Coronal MIP image of TOF MRA performed at the same time as (*A*) shows narrowing and irregularity of proximal right MCA and intradural ICA, although it is less apparent than on catheter-directed angiogram. (*D*) Follow-up MRA performed 2 months later shows marked progression of stenosis.

other vascular imaging techniques, which exclusively depict the vascular lumen, black blood VWI highlights the vessel wall, and is uniquely able to show vessel wall thickening and enhancement. Black Blood VWI without contrast will reveal intramural hematomas in cases of FCA-d. Multiple studies have noted the utility of MRI intracranial Black Blood VWI in the evaluation of steno-occlusive intracranial large vessel arteriopathies, as this modality directly images the arterial wall where the pathology is found, in contradistinction to luminal techniques like CTA, MRA, and catheter angiography (CA).[43] Recommendations for how to acquire Black Blood VWI have been outlined elsewhere.[44] Research into pediatric populations is still limited to small case series and case reports. Stence and colleagues demonstrated strong vessel wall enhancement at stroke onset was associated with arteriopathy progression over time in both FCA and MMA (see **Fig. 2**; **Fig. 4**).[45] Dlamini and colleagues showed that mural enhancement of intracranial vessels on Black Blood VWI in pediatric populations is more concentric than seen in adults, and is associated with a range of diagnoses including FCA-i,

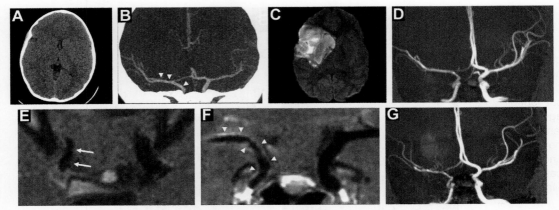

Fig. 2. Focal cerebral arteriopathy. 7-year-old girl presenting with acute left sided weakness and confusion. (A) Initial axial non-contrast head CT without evidence of infarction. (B) Coronal CTA demonstrating subtle decrease in caliber of intradural right ICA and M1 segment (*arrowheads*). (C) Axial DWI obtained 12 h later demonstrating a large infarction involving right basal ganglia, internal capsule, insula and opercular cortex with parenchymal edema. (D) Coronal MIP MRA showing more obvious decreased caliber of right intradural ICA, A1 and M1 segments, with mild irregularity of the intradural ICA. E & F) Small field of view, post-contrast axial (E) and coronal (F) black-blood vessel wall imaging of internal carotid arteries demonstrates stenosis and luminal irregularity involving the intradural right ICA (*arrows*), with a banded pattern of vessel wall thickening and enhancement involving the intradural right ICA and M1 segment (*arrowheads*). (G) Repeat coronal MIP MRA obtained 2 days after (D) demonstrates worsened stenosis and luminal irregularity involving the intradural right ICA and M1 segment in the region of vessel wall thickening and enhancement.

vasculitis, vasospasm, and cryptogenic AIS.[46] It is important to note that mural enhancement on Black Blood VWI is not present in all cases of FCA-i.[47]

Catheter-directed angiography, although less utilized than in the past for diagnostic evaluation of childhood AIS, remains an important diagnostic modality for the assessment of intracranial large vessel occlusion (LVO) of indeterminate etiology. Very small intimal flaps or other findings associated with subtle dissections (ie, prolonged retention of contrast media within the false lumen) may only be detected by catheter-directed angiography.

In addition to initial diagnostic imaging, repeat vascular imaging is important to document early worsening and eventual improvement or resolution of many cases of FCA (see Figs. 1 and 2).[33]

d. Management and treatment

Early diagnosis of FCA is important to guide treatment and avoid complications. In

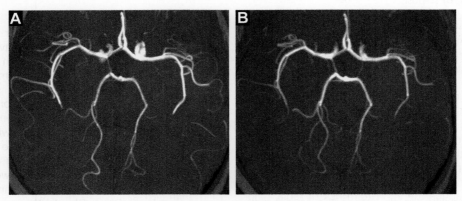

Fig. 3. (A) Axial MIP from a routine, non-contrast TOF MRA with voxel size of 0.5 mm and compressed SENSE factor of 4, acquisition time 3.5 minutes. (B) Axial MIP from a fast, non-contrast TOF MRA with voxel size of 0.8 mm and compressed SENSE factor of 7, acquisition time 30 seconds. The central arteries are equally conspicuous on both acquisitions, although detail of peripheral arteries is superior on the routine acquisition.

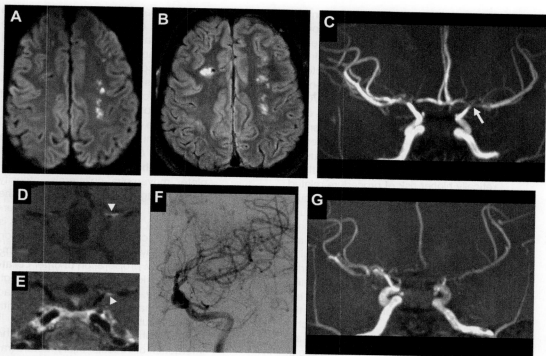

Fig. 4. Moyamoya arteriopathy. 12-year-old girl with a history of a posterior fossa juvenile pilocytic astrocytoma treated with surgery several years prior, presenting acutely with right arm weakness. (*A*) Axial DWI demonstrating several small foci of acute infarction in the left periventricular white matter watershed territory, while an axial FLAIR at the same level (*B*) demonstrates additional foci of more chronic infarction. (*C*) Coronal MIP of a TOF MRA demonstrates moderate to marked narrowing of the left ICA terminus, proximal M1 and A1 (*arrow*), as well as moderate narrowing of the right A1 and M1. Axial (*D*) and coronal (*E*) post-contrast small field of view black-blood VWI over the terminal ICAs shows asymmetric wall thickening and mural enhancement involving the distal left ICA and proximal A1 and M1 (*arrowheads*). Frontal projection of left ICA injection from catheter-directed angiogram (*F*) confirms narrowing of the left carotid terminus, proximal A1 and M1, and prominent moyamoya collaterals. TOF MRA performed 2 years later (*G*) shows marked progression of bilateral ICA termini, M1 and A1 narrowing, worse on the left.

general, FCA is acutely treated with antiplatelet therapy, avoiding hypotension, and bed-rest with 15° Trendelenberg position to reduce risk of recurrent stroke.[48] Although data are limited, one study demonstrated that the addition of corticosteroid treatment in FCA-i may be associated with better clinical outcomes for behavior and cognitive domains.[49] As such, corticosteroids and acyclovir are increasingly utilized in cases of FCA-i, especially those with early progressive arterial stenosis or recurrent stroke events. To better determine the best use of steroids in FCA-i, the FOCAS trial has begun enrollment in North America and will compare the use of immediate treatment of all patients with FCA-i to delayed steroid administration in children with progressive FCA or recurrent

stroke within the first week.[50] Other options for treatment of recurrent or progressive disease include escalation of antithrombotic management, blood pressure augmentation, and/or more prolonged bed-rest in a supine position. The use of intravenous thrombolytic drugs and catheter-directed revascularization techniques in selected children with AIS is an area of active research and was examined in both the TIPS-ER study and Save ChildS study, respectively.[51–53] Preliminary results from the Save ChildS study indicate that mechanical thrombectomy performed for intracranial LVO (intracranial ICA, M1, vertebral artery, basilar artery, and posterior cerebral artery) within 6 to 24 h of symptom onset in a small cohort of children (N = 20) with a variety of LVO mechanisms (only 5% FCA) had comparable or better functional outcomes compared to adult patients who received the same treatment, and had a similar safety profile.[54] Whether thrombectomy should have a role in the management of FCA patients with intracranial LVO is, however, not yet settled. Several concerns remain regarding the use of endovascular thrombectomy techniques in pediatric AIS patients with FCA, including a lack of high-level evidence, and a theoretically higher risk of procedure related vessel trauma (de novo dissection, acute mural perforation, acute or delayed mural rupture, and delayed traumatic aneurysm formation). These concerns are centered around the increased fragility of the acutely inflamed or dissected arterial wall, the increased frailty, smaller vessel diameters, and propensity to severe vasospasm that characterizes the developing cerebral arteries of children.[55,56] Although the numbers are small, TIPS-ER suggests that the use of intravenous tPA in children with FCA may be safe.[53] Confirmation with larger numbers is needed to be certain.

2. MMA
   a. Definition, epidemiology, and pathophysiology

   MMA are chronic and progressively occlusive vascular diseases that affect terminal intracranial ICA bifurcation unilaterally or bilaterally, resulting in the sequential development and eventual exhaustion of specific unique collateral arteries, thus expressing a distinct clinical and neuroimaging phenotype.[57] The patterns of collateral vessel development that are unique to MMA include: (1) moyamoya collaterals (hypertrophied lenticulostriate collateral vessels that vascularize striatum and internal capsule), (2) choroidal collaterals involving anastomoses between the anterior choroidal artery and perforating arteries, (3) transdural collaterals from the external carotid artery, which extend across intact dura matter and provide cerebral vascularization. Although leptomeningeal collaterals involving anastomoses between arterial tributaries in the cortical watershed zones are also a prominent feature of MMA, this pattern of collateral vessel development is not unique to MMA. All the collateral patterns that form in MMA reflect the distribution of steno-occlusive disease at the intracranial ICA terminus and within the anterior circle of Willis, which precludes collateral flow through the circle of Willis and forces collateral networks to form distal to the circle of Willis. In most cases, MMA begins with progressive occlusion of the intracranial ICA terminus, and initiation of true moyamoya collaterals (Suzuki stages 1 and 2). As the occlusion becomes complete, moyamoya collaterals intensify (Suzuki stage 3). As the lumen of the M1 and A1 segments become obliterated, inflow to moyamoya collaterals is eliminated causing a gradual involution of moyamoya collaterals that is accompanied by a proliferation of other collateral networks (Suzuki stages 4 through 6). Notably, this proliferation can lead to the formation of fragile vessels with angiomatous features.

The MMA phenotype results from the interaction of vascular injury factors (radiation, mycobacterial/viral infection, and rheometric shear stress caused by sickled erythrocytes) with genetically programmed permissivity traits (mutations in neurofibromin, JAG1, and RNF213) expressed by arteries that are segmentally vulnerable because of their positional identity in the cerebrovascular tree (terminal carotid artery bifurcation and anterior circle of Willis). Segmental vulnerability is conferred by variable exposure to hemodynamic stimuli driving vascular remodeling processes, and by genetic programs that are differentially executed by vascular cells according to metameric location. Consequently, the moyamoya phenotype can be expressed in many different clinical settings and is variably associated with a variety of syndromic conditions. In contrast to FCA, which has been defined in part by the monophasic clinical course and sometimes resolving nature of the index vascular lesion, MMAs are progressive and chronic with no expectation of resolution of symptoms and with more frequent episodes of stroke recurrence over time.[2,58] Notably, the initial early-stage presentation of bilateral MMA, may occasionally be mild and inapparent on one side, resulting in the misdiagnosis of FCA. Progression from unilateral to bilateral disease with will usually differentiate the patient with MMA from FCA.[59] In contrast to FCA, truly unilateral or early-stage bilateral MMA does not typically present with focal striatocapsular infarction as an early initial manifestation. Moreover, true moyamoya collaterals found in MMA directly vascularize the striatum and internal capsule, in contrast to the lenticulostriate collaterals of FCA, which form anastomotic networks that bridge an M1 or A1 occlusion. In MMA, the involvement of the anterior circulation is predominant, with basilar terminus and posterior circle of Willis affected in about 20% of cases later in the disease and less often associated with symptomatic presentation.[2]

When MMA is associated with recognizable systemic pathologic traits, the condition is referred to as a Moyamoya syndrome (MMS). Examples of MMS include Down syndrome, neurofibromatosis, and sickle cell disease.[60] When not associated with any recognizable physical or pathologic traits affecting tissues beyond the circle of Willis vessels, it is referred to Moyamoya disease (MMD). In general, there is a much higher incidence of MMD in Asian countries, but MMD is increasingly prevalent in the United States.[57,61] It is unclear if the higher incidence of MMD in Asian countries is accounted for by genetic factors, environmentally based injury factors (ie, endemic mycobacterial infection), or some combination of these.

Although MMD was originally described as idiopathic, MMD has long been known to harbor an inherited predisposition. Recently, mutations in the *RNF213* gene have been shown to cause susceptibility to the isolated development of MMA in otherwise normal individuals.[62] Although it was once believed that MMD represents a single disease process, it is likely that the genetic factors contributing to the development of MMD are a diverse and heterogenous group with population dependent variability, and future studies will reveal additional susceptibility genes.

b. Presentation, symptoms, and diagnosis
   In the pediatric population, the first onset of MMA is most often seen between ages 5 to 9 y old (school age children).[58] MMA most often presents acutely with ischemic events, seen in 51% of pediatric patients.[58] However, prior to an acute onset of AIS, patients often report a long history of mild to severe headaches.[63]

Diagnosis of MMA relies on neuroimaging with brain MRI, CT, CTA, MRA, and/or CA (see **Fig. 4**). In acutely symptomatic pediatric patients, brain imaging studies most often show infarcts in cerebral watershed zones and deep white matter watershed zones, often varying in age from acute to chronic. Brain MRI studies obtained in children with MMA will frequently reveal prominent moyamoya collaterals on T2 weighted imaging sequences, and angiomatous leptomeningeal collaterals in the form of sulcal hyperintensity ('ivy sign') on FLAIR images. Vascular imaging studies reveal the presence of stenosis or occlusion involving the terminal ICA, M1 or A1 with moyamoya collaterals depicted as abnormal vascular networks in the basal subarachnoid cisterns, corpus striatum, and internal capsule.[59,64] The changes are most often bilateral, though asymmetry is often present. CA is often performed for surgical treatment planning because the uniquely superior spatial and temporal resolution of CA enables detailed characterization of collateral circulation patterns and external carotid branch anatomy. In MMA patients undergoing cerebral revascularization surgery, preservation of transdural collaterals is particularly important for prevention of ischemic surgical complications, and CA provides neurosurgeons with the vascular roadmap that is necessary to avoid interruption of such collaterals during craniotomy.[62] Many grading systems for MMA have been proposed, the most well-known of which is the Suzuki system, which is based on CA (see above).[65] Black Blood VWI has also been studied as an imaging modality in MMA. Black Blood VWI can depict the constrictive remodeling that typifies MMD,[62] and some series have associated strong concentric mural enhancement on Black Blood VWI with a poor prognosis.[66]

c. Management and treatment
   In MMA, revascularization surgery reduces recurrent stroke risk, and is therefore

indicated for clinical symptoms of transient ischaemic attack, cognitive decline, or neuroimaging showing evidence of progression.[58] Surgical treatment in asymptomatic patients is controversial, although revascularization is reportedly associated with decreased progression of symptoms including headaches, and ischemic strokes.[61,67] The FLAIR 'ivy sign' has been used as surrogate for slow flow in angiomatous leptomeningeal collaterals indicating a need for revascularization, although it is subject to variation from differences in imaging and sedation techniques.[68] Other modalities of treatment include anti-platelet therapy, salt, blood pressure augmentation, and rehydration to improve cerebral blood flow.[69-78] Intravenous thrombolysis, while used in other types of pediatric AIS, is relatively contraindicated in MMA due to the high risk of hemorrhage from the fragile collateral vasculature.[67] In

MMA due to sickle cell disease, exchange transfusion plays a critical role in AIS treatment and stroke prevention. Reversal of the MMA phenotype by hematopoietic stem cell transplant in pediatric Sickle cell disease has been reported.[79]

3. Multi-focal arteriopathy (MFA)

Multi-focal cerebral arteriopathy is the least common pattern of steno-occlusive intracranial large vessel arteriopathy phenotype encountered in children. It is characterized by involvement of the anterior circulation bilaterally, and/or the posterior circulation and is often accompanied by involvement of small to medium size intracranial arteries. In contrast to MMA, multi-focal cerebral arteriopathy often involves the posterior circulation and may be driven by immunoinflammatory processes (infectious and autoimmune forms of CNS vasculitis, including the cerebral arteriopathy expressed by bacterial meningitis

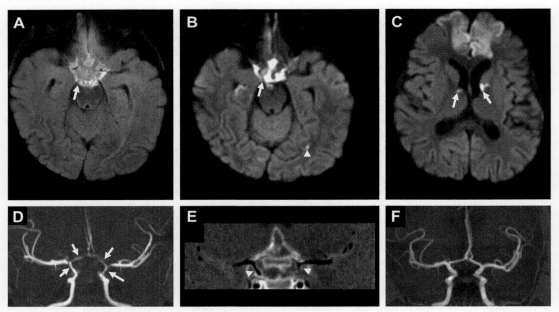

Fig. 5. Intracranial arteriopathy secondary to bacterial meningitis. 18-month-old male presenting with fever of unknown origin, malaise and altered mental status. (A) Axial FLAIR image showing hyperintense material in the suprasellar cisterns surrounding the distal ICAs and optic chiasm (arrow). (B) Axial DWI showing this material is diffusion restricting (arrow), suggestive of purulence. Small amount of intraventricular purulence is also seen (arrowhead). (C) More superior axial DWI image demonstrating restricted diffusion in the bilateral anterior medial frontal lobes corresponding to ACA territory infarctions, as well as small foci of infarction in the right anterior thalamus and left caudate head (arrows). (D) Coronal MIP from TOF MRA showing marked narrowing of the bilateral intradural ICAs and A1 segments (arrows). (E) Coronal post-contrast vessel wall image showing wall enhancement involving these vessels (arrowheads), as well as leptomeningeal enhancement surrounding the optic chiasm and suprasellar cistern. (F) Coronal MRA MIP 1-year later after treatment showing complete resolution of arterial narrowing.

[Figure 5]), maladaptive responses to endothelial injury (reversible cerebral vasoconstriction syndrome) or genetic defects that corrupt mechanical integrity of the arterial wall in diffuse or mosaic fashion (Arterial Tortuosity Syndrome, Ehlers Danlos Syndrome, Loeys Dietz Syndrome, Marfan's Syndrome, Menke's Syndrome, Neurocristopathies). A diverse and heterogenous group of conditions with varied mechanisms express this phenotype, and thus a comprehensive discussion of pathophysiology, diagnosis, management and treatment is beyond the scope of this review. This steno-occlusive intracranial large vessel arteriopathy phenotype is primarily included to differentiate it from the more common patterns covered in detail above.**Fig. 5**

SUMMARY

a. Neuroimaging points

i. FCA-i characteristically presents acutely with isolated striatocapsular infarction, but often variably associated with geographic infarctions of cerebral cortex and subcortical white matter in the distribution of the MCA and anterior cerebral artery. The associated stenosis of the intradural ICA ranges from very subtle to severe on initial vascular imaging. Early repeat vascular imaging is indicated, particularly if no stenosis is detected at the time of initial vascular imaging. Collaterals are typically horizontally-oriented bridging lenticulostriate arteries.

ii. Fast MRI and MRA brain sequences can increase the chances of obtaining images in young children without sedation.

iii. Intracranial arterial dissection is an important cause of AIS in children. Monofocal intracranial dissection with isolated involvement of the intradural ICA and/or M1 is sometimes referred to as FCA-d and it may or may not be preceded by significant trauma.

MMA are caused by the interaction of vascular injury factors with genetically determined susceptibilities in segmentally vulnerable vessels. Progressive stenosis and occlusion of the intracranial ICA terminus accompanied by formation of moyamoya, transdural, choroidal, and leptomeningeal collaterals is characteristic. The process is bilateral in most cases. Revascularization procedures are a vital treatment modality for patients with MMA.

DISCLOSURE

The authors have nothing to disclose.

REFERENCES

1. Fullerton HJ, Wu YW, Sidney S, et al. Risk of recurrent childhood arterial ischemic stroke in a population-based cohort: the importance of cerebrovascular imaging. Pediatrics 2007;119(3):495–501.
2. Wintermark M, Hills NK, DeVeber GA, et al. Clinical and imaging characteristics of arteriopathy subtypes in children with arterial ischemic stroke: results of the VIPS study. Am J Neuroradiol 2017;38(11):2172–9.
3. Bernard TJ, Manco-Johnson MJ, Lo W, et al. Towards a consensus-based classification of childhood arterial ischemic stroke. Stroke 2012;43(2):371–7.
4. Agrawal N, Johnston SC, Wu YW, et al. Imaging data reveal a higher pediatric stroke incidence than prior US estimates. Stroke 2009;40(11):3415–21.
5. Giroud M, Lemesle M, Gouyon JB, et al. Cerebrovascular disease in children under 16 years of age in the city of Dijon, France: a study of incidence and clinical features from 1985 to 1993. J Clin Epidemiol 1995;48(11):1343–8.
6. Beslow LA, Agner SC, Santoro JD, et al. International prevalence and mechanisms of SARS-CoV-2 in childhood arterial ischemic stroke during the COVID-19 pandemic. Stroke 2022;53(8):2497–503.
7. Mackay MT, Wiznitzer M, Benedict SL, et al. Arterial ischemic stroke risk factors: the international pediatric stroke study. Ann Neurol 2011;69(1):130–40.
8. Golomb MR, Fullerton HJ, Nowak-Gottl U, et al. Male predominance in childhood ischemic stroke. Stroke 2009;40(1):52–7.
9. Buerki SE, Grandgirard D, Datta AN, et al. Inflammatory markers in pediatric stroke: an attempt to better understanding the pathophysiology. Eur J Paediatr Neurol 2016;20(2):252–60.
10. Arnett N, Pavlou A, Burke MP, et al. Vessel wall MR imaging of central nervous system vasculitis: a systematic review. Neuroradiology 2022;64(1):43–58.
11. Amlie-Lefond C, Bernard TJ, Sébire G, et al. Predictors of cerebral arteriopathy in children with arterial ischemic stroke. Circulation 2009;119(10):1417–23.
12. Sébire G, Meyer L, Chabrier S. Varicella as a risk factor for cerebral infarction in childhood: a case-control study. Ann Neurol 1999;45(5):679–80.
13. Nagel MA, Cohrs RJ, Mahalingam R, et al. The varicella zoster virus vasculopathies: clinical, CSF, imaging, and virologic features. Neurology 2008;70(11):853–60.
14. Chabrier S, Sébire G, Fluss J. Transient cerebral arteriopathy, postvaricella arteriopathy, and focal

cerebral arteriopathy or the unique susceptibility of the M1 segment in children with stroke. Stroke 2016;47(10):2439–41.

15. Nagel MA, Traktinskiy I, Azarkh Y, et al. Varicella zoster virus vasculopathy. Analysis of virus-infected arteries 2011;77(4):364–70.

16. Persa L, Shaw DW, Amlie-Lefond C. Why would a child have a stroke? J Child Neurol 2022;37(12–14):907–15.

17. Fullerton HJ, Hills NK, Elkind MSV, et al. Infection, vaccination, and childhood arterial ischemic stroke. Results of the VIPS study 2015;85(17):1459–66.

18. Vora SB, Amlie-Lefond Catherine, Perez Francisco A, et al. Varicella-associated stroke. J Pediatr 2018;199.

19. Elkind MSV, Hills NK, Glaser CA, et al. Herpesvirus infections and childhood arterial ischemic stroke. Circulation 2016;133(8):732–41.

20. Mirzaee SMM, Gonçalves FG, Mohammadifard M, et al. Focal cerebral arteriopathy in a pediatric patient with COVID-19. Radiology 2020;297(2):E274–5.

21. Nash M, Rafay MF. Craniocervical arterial dissection in children: pathophysiology and management. Pediatr Neurol 2019;95:9–18.

22. Chabrier S, Rodesch G, Lasjaunias P, et al. Transient cerebral arteriopathy: a disorder recognized by serial angiograms in children with stroke. J Child Neurol 1998;13(1):27–32.

23. Oesch G, Perez FA, Wainwright MS, et al. Focal cerebral arteriopathy of childhood. Stroke 2021;52(7):2258–65.

24. Bulder MMM, Braun KPJ, Leeuwis JW, et al. The course of unilateral intracranial arteriopathy in young adults with arterial ischemic stroke. Stroke 2012;43(7):1890–6.

25. Braun KPJ, Bulder MMM, Chabrier S, et al. The course and outcome of unilateral intracranial arteriopathy in 79 children with ischaemic stroke. Brain 2008;132(2):544–57.

26. Fullerton HJ, deVeber GA, Hills NK, et al. Inflammatory biomarkers in childhood arterial ischemic stroke. Stroke 2016;47(9):2221–8.

27. Steinlin M, O'callaghan F, Mackay MT. Planning interventional trials in childhood arterial ischaemic stroke using a Delphi consensus process. Dev Med Child Neurol 2017;59(7):713–8.

28. Beslow LA, Dowling MM, Hassanein SMA, et al. Mortality after pediatric arterial ischemic stroke. Pediatrics 2018;141(5).

29. Fullerton HJ, Stence N, Hills NK, et al. Focal cerebral arteriopathy of childhood. Stroke 2018;49(11):2590–6.

30. Kitchen L, Westmacott R, Friefeld S, et al. The pediatric stroke outcome measure. Stroke 2012;43(6):1602–8.

31. Mineyko A, Narendran A, Fritzler ML, et al. Inflammatory biomarkers of pediatric focal cerebral arteriopathy. Neurology 2012;79(13):1406–8.

32. Goldenberg NA, Jenkins S, Jack J, et al. Arteriopathy, D-dimer, and risk of poor neurologic outcome in childhood-onset arterial ischemic stroke. J Pediatr 2013;162(5):1041–6.e1.

33. Danchaivijitr N, Cox TC, Saunders DE, et al. Evolution of cerebral arteriopathies in childhood arterial ischemic stroke. Ann Neurol 2006;59(4):620–6.

34. Twilt M, Benseler SM. Childhood inflammatory brain diseases: pathogenesis, diagnosis and therapy. Rheumatology 2013;53(8):1359–68.

35. Wintermark M, Hills NK, deVeber GA, et al. Arteriopathy diagnosis in childhood arterial ischemic stroke. Stroke 2014;45(12):3597–605.

36. Mackay MT, Chua ZK, Lee M, et al. Stroke and non-stroke brain attacks in children. Neurology 2014;82(16):1434–40.

37. Lehman LL, Beslow LA, Steinlin M, et al. What will improve pediatric acute stroke care? Stroke 2019;50(2):249–56.

38. Husson B, Rodesch G, Lasjaunias P, et al. Magnetic resonance angiography in childhood arterial brain infarcts. Stroke 2002;33(5):1280–5.

39. Ding J, Duan Y, Zhuo Z, et al. Acceleration of brain TOF-MRA with compressed sensitivity encoding: a multicenter clinical study. AJNR Am J Neuroradiol 2021;42(7):1208–15.

40. Christy A, Murchison C, Wilson JL. Quick brain magnetic resonance imaging with diffusion-weighted imaging as a first imaging modality in pediatric stroke. Pediatr Neurol 2018;78:55–60.

41. De Jong G, Kannikeswaran N, DeLaroche A, et al. Rapid sequence MRI protocol in the evaluation of pediatric brain attacks. Pediatr Neurol 2020;107:77–83.

42. Hernandez-Garcia L, Lahiri A, Schollenberger J. Recent progress in ASL. Neuroimage 2019;187:3–16.

43. Vranic JE, Hartman JB, Mossa-Basha M. High-resolution magnetic resonance vessel wall imaging for the evaluation of intracranial vascular pathology. Neuroimaging Clin N Am 2021;31(2):223–33.

44. Mandell DM, Mossa-Basha M, Qiao Y, et al. Intracranial vessel wall MRI: principles and expert consensus recommendations of the american society of neuroradiology. AJNR Am J Neuroradiol 2017;38(2):218–29.

45. Stence NV, Pabst LL, Hollatz AL, et al. Predicting progression of intracranial arteriopathies in childhood stroke with vessel wall imaging. Stroke 2017;48(8):2274–7.

46. Dlamini N, Yau I, Muthusami P, et al. Arterial wall imaging in pediatric stroke. Stroke 2018;49(4):891–8.

47. Perez FA, Oesch G, Amlie-Lefond CM. MRI vessel wall enhancement and other imaging biomarkers in pediatric focal cerebral arteriopathy-inflammatory subtype. Stroke 2020;51(3):853–9.

48. Tolani AT, Yeom KW, Elbers J. Focal cerebral arteriopathy: the face with many names. Pediatr Neurol 2015;53(3):247–52.

49. Steinlin M, Bigi S, Stojanovski B, et al. Focal cerebral arteriopathy: do steroids improve outcome? Stroke 2017;48(9):2375–82.

50. Park Y, Fullerton HJ, Elm JJ. A pragmatic, adaptive clinical trial design for a rare disease: the FOcal Cerebral Arteriopathy Steroid (FOCAS) trial. Contemp Clin Trials 2019;86:105852.

51. Braun KP, van der Worp HB. Thrombolysis in childhood ischaemic stroke: still a bridge too far. Lancet Neurol 2009;8(6):503–5.

52. Sporns PB, Sträter R, Minnerup J, et al. Feasibility, safety, and outcome of endovascular recanalization in childhood stroke: the save childs study. JAMA Neurol 2020;77(1):25–34.

53. Amlie-Lefond C, Shaw DWW, Cooper A, et al. Risk of intracranial hemorrhage following intravenous tPA (tissue-type plasminogen activator) for acute stroke is low in children. Stroke 2020;51(2):542–8.

54. Sporns PB, Psychogios MN, Straeter R, et al. Clinical diffusion mismatch to select pediatric patients for embolectomy 6 to 24 hours after stroke: an analysis of the save childs Study. Neurology 2021;96(3):e343–51.

55. Chabrier S, Ozanne A, Naggara O, et al. Hyperacute recanalization strategies and childhood stroke in the evidence age. Stroke 2021;52(1):381–4.

56. Sun LR, Harrar D, Drocton G, et al. Mechanical thrombectomy for acute ischemic stroke. Stroke 2020;51(10):3174–81.

57. Ghaffari-Rafi A, Ghaffari-Rafi S, Leon-Rojas J. Socioeconomic and demographic disparities of moyamoya disease in the United States. Clin Neurol Neurosurg 2020;192:105719.

58. Lee S, Rivkin MJ, Kirton A, et al. Moyamoya disease in children: results from the international pediatric stroke study. J Child Neurol 2017;32(11):924–9.

59. Elbers J, Armstrong D, Benseler SM, et al. The utility of collaterals as a biomarker in pediatric unilateral intracranial arteriopathy. Pediatr Neurol 2018;78:27–34.

60. Kim JE, Jeon JS. An update on the diagnosis and treatment of adult Moyamoya disease taking into consideration controversial issues. Neurol Res 2014;36(5):407–16.

61. Guzman R, Lee M, Achrol A, et al. Clinical outcome after 450 revascularization procedures for moyamoya disease. Clinical article. J Neurosurg 2009;111(5):927–35.

62. Ihara M, Yamamoto Y, Hattori Y, et al. Moyamoya disease: diagnosis and interventions. Lancet Neurol 2022;21(8):747–58.

63. Ibrahimi DM, Tamargo RJ, Ahn ES. Moyamoya disease in children. Childs Nerv Syst 2010;26(10):1297–308.

64. Kuroda S, Fujimura M, Takahashi J, et al. Diagnostic criteria for moyamoya disease - 2021 revised version. Neurol Med -Chir 2022;62(7):307–12.

65. Liu ZW, Han C, Zhao F, et al. Collateral circulation in moyamoya disease: a new grading system. Stroke 2019;50(10):2708–15.

66. Hao F, Han C, Lu M, et al. High-resolution MRI vessel wall enhancement in moyamoya disease: risk factors and clinical outcomes. Eur Radiol 2024;34(8):5179–89.

67. Sun LR, Lynch JK. Advances in the diagnosis and treatment of pediatric arterial ischemic stroke. Neurotherapeutics 2023;20(3):633–54.

68. Scott RM, Smith ER. Moyamoya disease and moyamoya syndrome. N Engl J Med 2009;360(12):1226–37.

69. Sporns PB, Fullerton HJ, Lee S, et al. Childhood stroke. Nat Rev Dis Primers 2022;8(1):12.

70. Sébire G, Fullerton H, Riou E, et al. Toward the definition of cerebral arteriopathies of childhood. Curr Opin Pediatr 2004;16(6).

71. Rawanduzy CA, Earl E, Mayer G, et al. Pediatric stroke: a review of common etiologies and management strategies. Biomedicines 2022;11(1).

72. Baltensperger A, Mirsky D, Maloney J, et al. Cost and utility of routine contrast-enhanced neck MRA in a pediatric MRI stroke evaluation protocol. AJNR Am J Neuroradiol 2019;40(12):2143–5.

73. Stence NV, Fenton LZ, Goldenberg NA, et al. Craniocervical arterial dissection in children: diagnosis and treatment. Curr Treat Options Neurol 2011;13(6):636–48.

74. Uohara MY, Beslow LA, Billinghurst L, et al. Incidence of recurrence in posterior circulation childhood arterial ischemic stroke. JAMA Neurol 2017;74(3):316–23.

75. Debette S, Compter A, Labeyrie MA, et al. Epidemiology, pathophysiology, diagnosis, and management of intracranial artery dissection. Lancet Neurol 2015;14(6):640–54.

76. Lucas MJ, Brouwer MC, van de Beek D. Neurological sequelae of bacterial meningitis. J Infect 2016;73(1):18–27.

77. Zainel A, Mitchell H, Sadarangani M. Bacterial meningitis in children: neurological complications, associated risk factors, and prevention. Microorganisms 2021;9(3).

78. Sun LR, Cooper S. Neurological complications of the treatment of pediatric neoplastic disorders. Pediatr Neurol 2018;85:33–42.

79. Booth N, Ngwube A, Appavu B, et al. Reversal of cerebral arteriopathy post-hematopoietic stem cell transplant for sickle cell disease. Pediatrics 2024;153(2). e2023062643.

Imaging of Hemorrhagic Stroke in Children

James L. Leach, MD[a,*], Betul E. Derinkuyu, MD[a], John Michael Taylor, MD[b],
Sudhakar Vadivelu, DO[c]

KEYWORDS

- Children • Hemorrhagic • Stroke • Computed tomography • MR imaging • Brain • Angiography
- DSA

KEY POINTS

- Nearly half of pediatric stroke cases are hemorrhagic, in contrast to adults where most stroke presentations are ischemic.
- There are substantial differences in etiology of hemorrhagic stroke in the preterm neonate, term neonate, and older child.
- Vascular malformations predominate as a cause of hemorrhagic stroke in children and adolescents while germinal matrix-intraventricular hemorrhage, venous thrombosis, and coagulopathies are more common in neonates.
- Neuroimaging plays the key role in diagnosis. Identification of hemorrhage patterns associated with common etiologies in each age group and application of rapid vascular imaging is critical for directing patient management.

INTRODUCTION

This study aims to provide a practical overview of the causes and imaging findings in childhood hemorrhagic stroke (HS). HS is a clinical term, which typically refers to an acute, nontraumatic, neurologic presentation associated with intracranial hemorrhage (ICH). It traditionally encompasses spontaneous intraparenchymal hemorrhage (IPH) with or without intraventricular extension, isolated intraventricular hemorrhage (IVH), and nontraumatic subarachnoid hemorrhage (SAH). Despite its common usage, the term "hemorrhagic stroke" remains confusing. It has occasionally been used to imply hemorrhagic transformation of arterial ischemic stroke and is often used to describe hemorrhagic cerebral venous thrombosis (CVT).

Notably, some authors exclude one or both conditions under the general "hemorrhagic stroke" definition.[1] For the purposes of this review, HS will be defined as those acute clinical scenarios where nontraumatic spontaneous ICH is the dominant feature. Since a broadening spectrum of CVT is an increasingly recognized underlying cause of IPH and HS across the pediatric age cohort (particularly in neonates), it will be reviewed in this article. Hemorrhagic transformation of arterial ischemic stroke and hypoxic ischemic encephalopathy typically does not present with ICH as the dominant or sole imaging finding[2] and is not specifically discussed in this study.

Although stroke (ischemic and hemorrhagic) in childhood is uncommon compared to stroke in adults (estimated incidence of 2–13 per 100,000

[a] Division of Pediatric Neuroradiology, Department of Radiology, Cincinnati Children's Hospital Medical Center, University of Cincinnati College of Medicine, Cincinnati, OH, USA; [b] Division of Neurology, Department of Pediatrics, Cincinnati Children's Hospital Medical Center, University of Cincinnati College of Medicine, Cincinnati, OH, USA; [c] Division of Pediatric Neurosurgery, Department of Neurosurgery, Cincinnati Children's Hospital Medical Center, University of Cincinnati College of Medicine, Cincinnati, OH, USA
* Corresponding author. Cincinnati Children's Hospital Medical Center, University of Cincinnati College of Medicine, 3333 Burnet Avenue, Cincinnati, OH 45229.
E-mail address: james.leach@cchmc.org

Neuroimag Clin N Am 34 (2024) 615–636
https://doi.org/10.1016/j.nic.2024.08.023
1052-5149/24/© 2024 Elsevier Inc. All rights are reserved, including those for text and data mining, AI training, and similar technologies.

children per year), pediatric stroke can result in significant long-term disability and mortality.[3,4] In contrast to adults where ischemic stroke predominates (85%), nearly half of all pediatric stroke is hemorrhagic.[4–6] Notably, the importance of HS relative to ischemic stroke varies across different age groups within the pediatric population. While ischemic stroke predominates in the first year of life, hemorrhagic stroke is more common between the ages of 1 and 14 years. In the latter half of the second decade of life, as adult physiology and stroke risk factors set in, ischemic stroke predominates. Most patients with HS are critically ill with up to 73% requiring intensive care unit admission.[7] Delayed diagnosis or misdiagnosis of HS negatively affects outcome due to the potential for progressive bleeding over time and increased risk of rebleeding with rapid clinical deterioration and neurologic injury.[8] Early and accurate neuroimaging assessment with prompt diagnosis is crucial for guiding interdisciplinary management and informing acute treatment.

ETIOLOGY OF HEMORRHAGIC STROKE IN CHILDREN

Multiple clinical studies have addressed the underlying causes of HS in children[9,10] with marked variability between cohorts and definitions. Most studies have excluded neonates, and many exclude CVT. Moreover, some studies only include IPH, while others include all subtypes of ICH.[9–14] What is clear from these studies is that etiologies and imaging patterns are quite different in the neonatal period versus older children and that preterm neonates differ significantly from term neonates (Box 1).[1,10,13] In preterm neonates, HS is more commonly related to venous thrombosis, coagulopathy, and the spectrum of hemorrhagic germinal matrix pathologies, which includes germinal matrix-intraventricular hemorrhage (GM-IVH) and periventricular hemorrhagic infarction (PVHI). In term neonates CVT, medullary venous thrombosis (MVT), subpial hemorrhage (SPH), coagulopathies, and hemorrhagic transformation of arterial ischemic stroke are more common causes of nontraumatic ICH, with vascular malformations and aneurysms much less commonly seen. In many cases of neonatal HS, no cause can be identified.[13,16] In older children and adolescents, vascular malformations strongly predominate as a cause of ICH (60%), most commonly cerebral arteriovenous malformations (AVM) and cerebral cavernous malformations (CCM).[9,10] Importantly, cerebral arteriovenous shunt lesions, including cerebral AVM and pial arteriovenous

fistulae (pAVFs), are the leading cause of hemorrhagic stroke in the first two decades of life. Since these high-flow vascular lesions are surgically or endovascularly treatable and carry a high risk of life-threatening recurrent hemorrhage, they should be recognized early in the diagnostic evaluation of children with HS. Cerebral aneurysms have similar implications, though these are significantly less common as a cause of HS in children.

IMAGING EVALUATION

When a child presents with an abrupt onset of a neurologic deficit, ischemic or hemorrhagic stroke is often the presumed diagnosis. While stroke mimics (postictal state or migraine) are more common in children than in adults,[17] rapid neuroimaging is essential to guide therapy and to exclude ICH as a cause.

The choice of imaging modality for children with an acute neurologic deficit should be driven by clinical presentation, age, modality availability, and likely cause. Many pediatric stroke guidelines recommend brain MR imaging as an initial imaging modality especially in suspected arterial ischemic stroke, as computed tomography (CT) is less sensitive for the detection of early ischemic abnormalities.[18,19] Round-the-clock availability for MR imaging in pediatric patients is not universal; MR imaging often requires sedation or anesthesia in young children and entails longer preparation and imaging times. Given the higher prevalence of HS in children compared to adults, exclusion of ICH as an etiology of stroke symptoms is a critical first step in evaluating these patients.

Noncontrast head CT is the initial study of choice in emergency settings (particularly in unstable patients) because of its near universal availability, rapid image acquisition, high sensitivity for acute hemorrhage[20,21] and ability to perform in almost all patients without sedation (particularly important in the pediatric population).[22,23] CT angiography (CTA) and/or CT-venography (CTV) can be performed immediately after the identification of spontaneous ICH. CTA has a high sensitivity and specificity (90%–100%) in identifying vascular malformations and other potential causes of ICH[24] although as discussed later may be negative in the acute stage because of local mass effect and/or vasospasm. CT utilizes ionizing radiation, and even with modern dose reduction techniques, there is concern for use in children.[25] In the acute clinical scenario, time is of the essence and rapid diagnosis of a vascular cause is of paramount clinical importance. Head CT followed by CTA/CTV (if indicated) should be considered as the first-choice examination.

Box 1
Common etiologies of hemorrhagic stroke by age group in children

Neonatal: Preterm (0–28 days, < 34–36 week gestation)

- Germinal matrix-intraventricular hemorrhage-periventricular hemorrhagic infarction spectrum (GMH-IVH-PVHI)
- Cerebellar hemorrhage
- Cerebral venous thrombosis with associated parenchymal hemorrhage
  - Medullary Vein Thrombosis (MVT)
- Hematologic/coagulopathy
  - Coagulopathy (iatrogenic/ECMO), hemophilia, and vitamin K deficiency, thrombocytopenia
- Diffuse hypoxic ischemic injury with associated parenchymal hemorrhage
- Arterial ischemic infarction with associated parenchymal hemorrhage
- Unknown

Neonatal: Term/near term (0–28 days, >34–36 week gestation)

- Cerebral venous thrombosis with associated parenchymal hemorrhage
  - Dural sinus thrombosis without or with cortical, deep, or MVT
  - Isolated cortical venous thrombosis
  - MVT
- Arterial ischemic infarction with associated parenchymal hemorrhage
- GMH-IVH-PVHI
- SPH
- Hematologic/coagulopathy
  - Coagulopathy (iatrogenic and ECMO), hemophilia, vitamin K deficiency, and thrombocytopenia
- Unknown

Childhood

- Vascular
  - Arteriovenous malformation
  - Cavernous malformation
  - Aneurysm
  - Arteriovenous fistula
- Hematologic/cardiac
  - Coagulopathy (iatrogenic and ECMO), hemophilia, and thrombocytopenia
- Cerebral venous thrombosis with associated parenchymal hemorrhage
  - Dural sinus thrombosis without or with cortical, deep, or MVT
  - Isolated cortical venous thrombosis
- Arterial ischemic infarction with associated parenchymal hemorrhage
- Neoplastic

Etiologies are listed in rough order as most common to least common in each age group based upon published data.[9,10,12–15] More cases of HS are of unknown etiology in neonates than in older children. Details regarding the estimated etiology prevalence in each group is provided in the text.

In a clinically stable patient, as an initial follow-up examination when a cause is not identified by CT/CTA/CTV, or when the findings of CT/CTA/CTV require further clarification, MR imaging is very useful given its higher sensitivity for brain parenchymal abnormalities and ability to differentiate high flow from low flow vascular pathology. Besides conventional noncontrast sequences, additional MR imaging techniques are helpful. Gradient-recalled echo (GRE) or susceptibility-weighted imaging (SWI) should always be performed given high sensitivity for hemorrhage (particularly subacute and chronic hemorrhage)[26] as well as sensitivity for intraluminal thrombus (arterial and venous). Noncontrast time-of-flight (TOF), contrast-enhanced magnetic resonance angiography (MRA), and MR venography (MRV) should also be considered. MRA coverage should be tailored to cover the hemorrhagic area and surrounding regions. Contrast-enhanced MR imaging (optimally using volumetric-isotropic techniques that allow multiplanar reformations) is important to assess vascular malformations with complex flow and to optimally assess for venous thrombus. Time-resolved 4 dimensional contrast-enhanced MRA (4D MRA) can be very useful to detect arteriovenous shunt lesions, but often it has limitations related to spatial resolution and temporal resolution depending upon the sequence and magnet field strength and may be more limited in sensitivity in the acute setting.[27] Arterial spin labeling (ASL) is a more recent technique that can detect focal areas that characterize arteriovenous shunt lesions. ASL has shown excellent sensitivity for high-flow vascular lesions in the initial workup of IPH in children. In one report of 121 children with nontraumatic IPH studied by catheter-directed digital subtraction angiography (DSA), ASL imaging showed a high sensitivity (90%), specificity (97%), and accuracy (92%) for the detection of arteriovenous shunt lesions.[27] Its performance was better than conventional contrast-enhanced MR imaging without ASL, 4D MRA, and CTA for the detection of an arteriovenous shunt lesion. Incorporation of ASL (always performed precontrast administration) is highly recommended in the MR imaging workup of children with spontaneous ICH. It is important to note that MR imaging and CT/CTA/CTV can provide complementary information regarding causes of HS and are often both performed in the pediatric cohort.[23]

Catheter-directed DSA remains the reference standard imaging technique for intracranial vascular evaluation, with superior sensitivity and specificity for the detection of vascular etiology in children with HS,[1] and an excellent safety profile when performed by experienced operators in specialized pediatric centers.[28] Catheter-directed DSA can detect subtle arteriovenous shunt lesions or aneurysms that escape detection by CT and MR imaging given its unsurpassed temporal and spatial resolution, and it is, therefore, an essential diagnostic study in children with HS. Moreover, detailed angioarchitectural and hemodynamic data uniquely available from catheter-directed DSA analysis are vital for guiding the formulation and execution of a definitive treatment plan in children with HS.[29] The timing of performing catheter-directed DSA performance in a child with ICH depends upon the clinical stability of the patient, intracranial pressure, neurologic status, results of previous noninvasive imaging, and timing of planned endovascular or surgical therapy. If imaging evaluations are negative in the acute phase of HS, delayed imaging including repeat catheter-directed DSA should be strongly considered, as well as comprehensive hematologic workup. Vasospasm, transient thrombosis, and compression of blood vessels by adjacent hematoma may transiently mask the underlying vascular lesion in the acute setting.[30,31] The timing of the follow-up evaluation depends upon the suspected etiology but is typically performed within 1 to 3 months.

In neonates, head ultrasound (HUS) is a useful and easily performed screening study for the diagnosis of GM-IVH or a large IPH that is typically associated with PVHI.[32,33] HUS is often the first screening test obtained in preterm neonates and in term neonates with neurologic deficits or seizures. While MR imaging is more sensitive for the detection of ICH and brain parenchymal ischemia, HUS can identify clinically significant GMH-IVH, PVHI, and ventriculomegaly without the need for patient transport from the neonatal intensive care unit or sedation.[32] Commonly, serial HUS are performed in preterm infants to identify clinically significant hemorrhagic and ischemic injuries, with brain MR imaging performed at term equivalent age (TEA) for more detailed brain parenchymal assessment or to answer clinically relevant questions (eg, suspected CVT in a term neonate).[34,35]

The imaging patterns and findings of the more common causes of spontaneous (nontraumatic) ICH in children are reviewed.

Neonatal Hemorrhagic Stroke

The majority of spontaneous ICH cases with identifiable cause in this age group are related to GMH-IVH and PVHI in the preterm neonate, and CVT or coagulopathy in the term neonate.[15] As stated, in many neonates with HS no definite cause can be found.[12,13] Neonatal HS is distinct from HS in any other period of life due to specific developmental risk factors, unique developmentally specific pathophysiologic mechanisms, and lifelong consequences.[15] The common HS etiologies of preterm and term neonates are listed in **Box 1**.

Germinal matrix-intraventricular hemorrhage
GMH-IVH is a multifactorial brain injury seen predominantly in preterm newborns before the

germinal matrix completely involutes (approximately the 34th week of gestation). It is especially common in those younger than 32 weeks of gestation (very preterm). GMH is thought to occur when perinatal stress triggers a sudden or marked alteration of blood flow or venous pressure in the rich, immature, and fragile vascular network of the subependymal germinal matrix. GMH may secondarily disrupt the ependyma and extend into the lateral ventricles, resulting in IVH. Most cases occur within the first week of life of preterm neonates, particularly in the first 72 hours.[15,36,37] The main risk factors for GMH-IVH are low gestational age, low birth weight, and perinatal distress. GMH can occur anywhere along the germinal matrix, most common in the caudothalamic groove region. GM-IVH has traditionally been graded using the Papile system (Grade I—isolated GMH, Grade II—GMH and IVH without ventriculomegaly, Grade III—GMH and IVH with ventriculomegaly, and Grade IV—associated IPH [now termed PVHI]).[38] High-grade GMH-IVH is usually symptomatic and associated with abnormal neurodevelopmental outcomes such as posthemorrhagic hydrocephalus, cerebral palsy, epilepsy, and severe cognitive impairment.[15] While HUS is the most common imaging study performed to assess GMH-IVH, MR imaging is more sensitive and specific.[39] In a recent study, up to 50% of neonates with a normal HUS show mild GMH-IVH (Grades I–II) on MR imaging at TEA. Conversely, up to 60% of neonates with a normal brain MR imaging had grade I or II GMH-IVH identified on HUS.[40] While MR imaging may have higher sensitivity and specificity, GMH-IVH is typically diagnosed by HUS, which is routinely done at birth in premature neonates and then through the first few weeks of life. HUS has excellent sensitivity for higher grades of GM-IVH and clinically important ventriculomegaly. The characteristic findings of subependymal hyperechoic globular thickening detected during the first week of life (usually remaining visible for a few weeks) and mixed echogenicity within the lateral ventricles (with or without enlargement) have been well described[34,41,42] (Fig. 1). Imaging findings of GMH-IVH on MR imaging are best delineated using SWI, which is highly sensitive for IVH, IPH, and SAH.[40]

Periventricular hemorrhagic infarction
Grade IV GMH-IVH is currently termed PVHI and is thought to be a type of hemorrhagic periventricular venous infarction precipitated by impairment of deep medullary venous drainage resulting from compression of the terminal (thalamostriate) vein distributions by adjacent subependymal germinal matrix hemorrhage.[43,44] Notably, deep medullary

vein thrombosis (MVT) may also occur without GMH (see later discussion). PVHI can occur in any grade (I–III) of GMH-IVH but is most common with grade III.[41] The critical venous structures involved in the pathogenesis of PVHI are the superior thalamostriate vein (superior terminal vein) tributary of the internal cerebral vein (ICV), which drains the internal capsule and corpus striatum, and the inferior thalamostriate vein (inferior terminal vein) tributary of the basal vein of Rosenthal, which drains the periventricular temporal lobe.[45] The unusual "U-shaped" morphology of the superior thalamostriate vein in the caudothalamic groove region, near the foramen of Monro, is believed to predispose to venous obstruction by adjacent subependymal hemorrhage resulting in thrombosis and the ensuing complications that result from impairment of deep medullary venous drainage.[46]

PVHI occurs in 4% to 11% of preterm newborns, is most commonly unilateral (90%), adjacent to regions of GMM-IVH (84% grade III), and typically within the periventricular white matter of the parietal and posterior frontal regions.[47,48] PVHI continues to have a high mortality (40%) with over two-thirds of survivors having severe motor and cognitive deficits.[47,49,50] The location of the PVHI correlates well with functional outcome. Those neonates with PVHI involving the superior and middle terminal vein territory (caudate and central corona radiata in the parietal/posterior frontal regions) are more likely to have severe hemiplegia.[45] Diffusion tensor imaging (DTI) of the internal capsule can be useful for the prediction of motor outcomes.[51] When a GMH or PVHI-like pattern is identified after 32 weeks, it is more likely to be an epiphenomenon of other injuries such as primary venous thrombosis.[42]

PVHI has a very typical imaging pattern (see Fig. 1). On HUS, PVHI is typically diagnosed as a focal unilateral or less commonly asymmetric bilateral fan-shaped periventricular white matter hyperechogenicity often extending from a region of GMH.[41,42] Over time, the echogenicity decreases and the resulting periventricular encephalomalacia results in a porencephalic cyst communicating with the ventricle. On MR imaging, PVHI signal depends upon the age of the hemorrhage with typical marked susceptibility effect on SWI. In the acute stage, surrounding edema is common with variable diffusion restriction. Engorged and/or thrombosed medullary veins can be identified on SWI but may be obscured by adjacent IPH.[14] As on HUS, evolution of the IPH occurs often with resultant typical porencephaly.

Medullary vein thrombosis
MVT is an increasingly recognized cause of IPH and brain injury in preterm and term neonates[52-55]

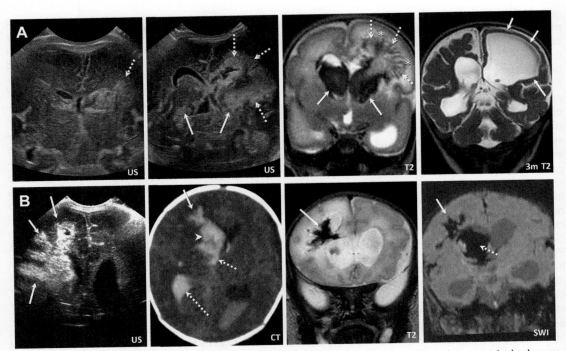

Fig. 1. Hemorrhagic germinal matrix spectrum pathology (germinal matrix hemorrhage-intraventricular hemorrhage [GMH-IVH]-periventricular hemorrhagic infarction [PVHI]). (*A*) A 28 week gestation premature neonate. Initial head ultrasound (US) at day of life (DOL) 1 demonstrates mixed echogenicity IVH and a large area of hyperechogenicity compatible with PVHI in the left periventricular white matter (dashed *arrows*). Brain MR imaging performed the next day. Coronal T2-weighted image (T2) demonstrates predominantly hypointense intraventricular hemorrhage (*solid arrows*) and fan-shaped intraparenchymal hemorrhage extending along thrombosed medullary veins (*dashed arrows*). Adjacent edema in the brain parenchyma is noted (*). Coronal T2-weighted image 3 months later (3m T2) demonstrates typical porencephaly related to PVHI (*solid arrows*). (*B*) Former 34 week gestational neonate, DOL 5 with increased irritability and difficulty feeding. US demonstrates large flame-shaped echogenicity in the right periventricular white matter consistent with PVHI (*solid arrows*). Head CT (CT) demonstrates extensive IVH (*dashed arrows*), GMH (*arrowhead*), and irregular PVHI (*solid arrow*). Thrombosed medullary veins with adjacent parenchymal hemorrhage are well demonstrated on T2-weighted coronal (T2) and susceptibility-weighted coronal (SWI) brain MR imaging performed the next day (*solid arrows*). Large GMH and adjacent IVH are noted (*dashed arrow*).

and can occur in isolation, with GM-IVH (PVHI, described in earlier discussion), with dural sinus thrombosis or with SPH (as described in later discussion). The medullary venous system can be divided into the *superficial ventriculofugal system* (draining the subcortical white matter toward cortical veins on the brain surface) and the *deep ventriculopetal system* (draining toward the subependymal and deep veins). Anastomotic veins can bridge these 2 systems, and drainage patterns can overlap.[53] The deep medullary veins are a part of the deep venous system draining the white matter and striatum and originate 1 to 2 cm deep to the pial surface.[53] They have radial orientation perpendicular to the lateral ventricles with drainage to the subependymal veins and subsequently via the ICV and basal vein of Rosenthal to the vein of Galen. Imaging findings of MVT are best identified on

MR imaging. MVT should be considered in the setting of a fan-shaped area of edema and hemorrhagic signal extending from the ventricular margin into the deep white matter and/or basal ganglia (Fig. 2A). IPH (petechial, small punctate, and larger hematomas) can be seen in most cases. Multifocal deep white matter and corpus callosum edema/infarction can also be present depending on the drainage territory of the involved vein(s).[52,53] The SWI sequence outlines the engorged/thrombosed medullary veins in a typical radial pattern extending into the deep white matter. As the medullary veins are not typically identified with venographic techniques or contrast administration, confirmation of occlusion of the medullary veins is often not possible.[56] Because of this some authors have used the term medullary vein engorgement to describe this appearance.[53] MRV and contrast

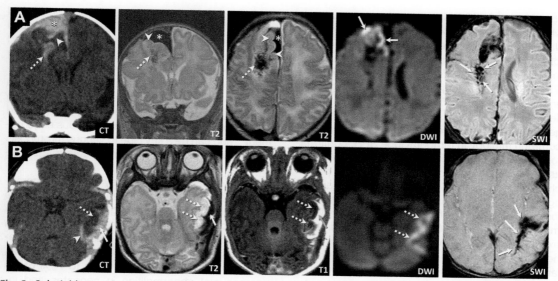

Fig. 2. Subpial hemorrhage (SPH) and medullary venous congestion/thrombosis (MVT). (*A*) A 2 day old male infant, 38 weeks' gestation age at delivery. Left arm and leg jerking consistent with seizure. Head CT demonstrates a sizable hemorrhage along the surface of the right frontal lobe (*) focally distorting the adjacent brain parenchyma. Irregular subcortical hemorrhage is present (*dashed arrow*). Intervening cortex is hypodense consistent with edema (*arrowhead*). Coronal and axial T2-weighted images (T2) show similar superficial hemorrhage (*) displacing the brain parenchyma with cortical edema (*arrowhead*) and irregular subcortical hemorrhage with morphology consistent with engorged or thrombosed medullary veins (*dashed arrows*). Localized cortical diffusion restriction of the cortex is noted (DWI, *arrows*). Thrombosed ependymal and medullary veins are more readily demonstrated on SWI (SWI *arrows*). CTA was performed without evidence of vascular malformation, DVA, or cortical venous thrombosis. Hematologic workup documented a prothrombotic Factor V Leiden mutation. (*B*) A 2 day old male infant, term gestation with prolonged traumatic delivery followed by seizure activity postnatally. Localized superficial subpial hemorrhage noted along left temporal lobe on CT (*arrow*), with displaced edematous cortex (*dashed arrows*), and subcortical hemorrhage (*arrowhead*). On MR imaging (T1 and T2), the subpial hemorrhage was T2 hypointense, and T1 hyperintense (*arrows*), compatible with early subacute hemorrhage with displaced edematous brain (*dashed arrows*). Diffusion restriction compatible with cortical infarction is noted (DWI, *dashed arrows*). On SWI, adjacent thrombosed/engorged medullary veins were noted (SWI, *arrows*).

administration, however, are important to identify any associated CVT in these cases. Edema (cytotoxic and vasogenic) and IPH are seen in most cases (98%) with resultant encephalomalacia on follow-up imaging.[52,53]

Subpial hemorrhage

SPH is a form of ICH more commonly seen in term neonates, characterized by bleeding into a potential space between the glia limitans (outermost layer of the astrocytic foot processes in the neocortex) and the pia mater, distinct from the subarachnoid space.[57,58] SPH is thought to represent up to 15% of ICH in the neonatal period.[59] Many risk factors (birth trauma, neonatal asphyxia, fetal head molding with venous compression, and venous thrombosis) have been suggested but the exact pathophysiology is still uncertain. It has been proposed that a primary injury to the glia limitans with rupture of intracortical vessels results in

subpial pooling of hemorrhage and elevation of the pia mater, which secondarily causes mechanical compression of traversing venous structures resulting in venous thrombosis, venous hypertension, and focal cortical infarction.[58,60] While HUS and CT can identify the characteristic hemorrhage pattern, MR imaging can more completely characterize SPH and associated brain injuries.[58] Localized hemorrhagic signal is identified closely opposed to the superficial cortex, often elliptical in shape with the long axis tangential to the brain surface. A key feature is that the cortex is deformed and displaced away from the elevated layer of pia mater by the hemorrhagic collection[58] (see **Fig. 2**). There is often cortical and subcortical injury identified as increased T2/FLAIR (fluid-attenuated inversion recovery) signal and associated cortical diffusion restriction complicated by parenchymal hemorrhage (up to 67%).[61] The intense susceptibility effect on SWI images can mask the characteristic subpial location of the hemorrhage, which is better assessed on T2-weighted images. Notably, SAH may coexist with SPH.[61] Temporal lobe involvement is the most common location for SPH (52%–82% of cases).[61,62] In many cases (76%–100%), imaging findings suggesting deep and/or superficial MVT or congestion are identified[53,62] (see **Fig. 2**B). While earlier reports suggested that cortical vein thrombosis might be a common etiology in temporal lobe SPH, confirmatory evidence of this is rare.[56,61] In the absence of associated parenchymal infarction and/or parenchymal hemorrhage, SPH can resolve without imaging sequelae.[61] Neurologic deficits relate to the location and extent of parenchymal injury. While many patients (60%–70%) have normal neurologic examination at discharge and generally good neurologic outcomes, long-term effects such as language delays, mild hemiparesis, and epilepsy can result.[61,62]

Cerebral Venous Thrombosis

Thrombosis of the dural venous sinuses and/or cortical veins (CVT) is a common cause of spontaneous ICH in children. Also, as noted earlier, venous thrombosis or hypertension is thought to be at least a contributory factor in the pathogenesis of GM-IVH, the likely cause of PVHI, and an important pathogenic factor in some cases of neonatal SPH. Its incidence is probably underestimated but is approximately 0.4 to 1.1 cases/100,000/y in children overall, 6.4/100,000/y in neonates and infants, 0.6 to 0.8/100,000/y in younger children, and 1.2/100,000/y in adolescents.[63–68] There is a high prevalence (up to 43% of pediatric HS cases) in the neonatal period.[63] In neonates and younger children, there is a male predominance.[64–68] Conversely, in adolescents and adults, CVT is much more common in female individuals.[68,69]

Clinical presentation is variable and often nonspecific including seizures, encephalopathy, and altered levels of consciousness. Focal neurologic findings are more common in patients with parenchymal sequelae of CVT (localized edema, venous infarction, or IPH).[70] As in adults, CVT in neonates, infants, and children is often multifactorial in etiology. A predisposing condition can be identified in up to 95% of cases including febrile illness, dehydration, head and neck infection (sinusitis and oto-mastoiditis), genetic and acquired prothrombotic states, bacterial meningitis, anemia, and L-asparaginase therapy for acute lymphocytic leukemia (ALL).[63,70,71]

Imaging findings of CVT are well documented[56,72–74] (**Figs. 3** and **4**). Clues to the diagnosis of CVT as a cause of IPH include hyperdense (thrombus-filled) dural venous sinuses or cortical veins on noncontrast CT, filling defects in dural venous sinuses and cortical veins on CTV and postcontrast MR imaging sequences (including postcontrast MRV), and absent or decreased flow-related enhancement of dural venous sinuses on noncontrast MRV. SWI sequences are critical on MR imaging for directly identifying thrombosed venous segments and associated venous engorgement[75] and can be a key clue to venous thrombosis as an etiology for parenchymal hemorrhage (see **Fig. 3**B).

While imaging studies may show no parenchymal abnormality, parenchymal sequelae are commonly found on imaging, occurring in 30% to 60% of cases, with an increased prevalence in neonates.[64,76] Parenchymal changes can represent vasogenic edema, parenchymal infarction, and parenchymal hemorrhage. Up to 76% of the parenchymal abnormalities in neonates and infants and 33% of those in older children are hemorrhagic.[76] Thalamic, basal ganglia, deep white matter, and IVHs (related to deep venous occlusion) are more common in neonates than in older children and adults with CVT.[55,77,78] Multiple patterns may coexist.

The pathophysiology of parenchymal abnormalities in CVT is thought to be related to venous hypertension, which causes a secondary decrease in local perfusion pressure resulting in cellular energy depletion (potentially complicated by parenchymal infarction), and blood–brain barrier disruption that features vasogenic edema, and varying degrees of mural integrity failure affecting microvascular networks in the brain parenchyma.[76–79] Recruitment of collaterals after venous occlusion is thought to be critical in preventing parenchymal sequelae. Adaptive collateral venous drainage can be achieved through microvascular anastomoses[80] or variations in cortical venous anatomy.[81] Cortical venous or medullary venous involvement[82,83] limits access of affected brain parenchyma to collateral venous drainage pathways. Consequently, parenchymal sequelae (including parenchymal hemorrhage) are more common with cortical vein involvement (associated with dural sinus thrombosis or isolated cortical venous thrombosis).[82,84–86]

Common parenchymal hemorrhage patterns include lobar hemorrhage (particularly involving the frontal and temporal lobes) with a multilobular or flame-shaped morphology, hemorrhage associated with venous infarction manifesting cortical diffusion restriction, and localized subcortical hemorrhage.[72] Multiple patterns can be seen in the same patient. Bilateral frontal parenchymal hemorrhages (superior sagittal sinus thrombosis

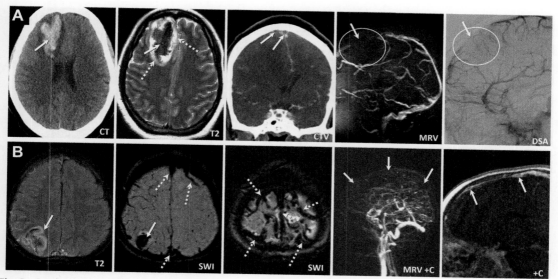

Fig. 3. Cerebral venous thrombosis. (*A*) An 18 year old female patient with aplastic anemia presenting with headache. Focal parenchymal hemorrhage noted in the right frontal lobe on the initial CT (*arrows*) with mild surrounding edema. On MR imaging, T2-weighted images (T2) demonstrate localized T2 hypointense hemorrhage (*arrow*) with moderate surrounding edema (*dashed arrows*). CT venogram (CTV) was performed documenting filling defects within the superior sagittal sinus (SSS) and superficial cortical veins (*arrows*). TOF MR-venogram (MRV) demonstrates the lack of flow-related enhancement in the SSS (*arrow*) and the lack of visualization of cortical veins (outlined by circle) consistent with thrombosis. Because of the size of the hemorrhage, a catheter-directed digital subtraction angiogram was performed to exclude an arteriovenous shunt lesion. This documented segmental occlusion of the SSS (*arrow*) and associated cortical veins (outlined by circle) consistent with thrombosis. (*B*) A 2 year old male patient with focal seizures. MR imaging of the brain was performed. On T2-weighted images (T2), a focal area of cortical and subcortical edema is noted in the right parietal lobe (*arrow*). On SWI, a focal area of susceptibility effect is noted consistent with focal parenchymal hemorrhage in the immediate subcortical region (*arrow*). The SSS and enlarged cortical veins exhibit extensive magnetic susceptibility blooming compatible with dural sinus and cortical vein thrombosis (*dashed arrows*). Absence of enhancement of the SSS and cortical veins noted on postcontrast MRV (MRV +C, *arrows*), with cortical vein filling defects on postcontrast sagittal T1 images (+C, *arrows*). Hematologic workup revealed a prothrombin G20210A mutation.

pattern); lateral temporal lobe parenchymal hemorrhage and edema (transverse sinus thrombosis pattern); unilateral or bilateral thalamic, caudate, and/or deep white matter edema with associated hemorrhage (deep venous system pattern) should prompt strong consideration of CVT as an etiology and should be evaluated with contrast administration and/or venographic techniques[56,72] (see **Figs. 3 and 4**).

Vascular Malformations

Vascular malformations, including cerebral AVMs, pAVFs, and cavernous malformations, are the most common overall cause of HS (particularly IPH) in children beyond the neonatal period.[9,10] Vascular malformations are identified as the underlying cause of nontraumatic ICH in 44% to 87% of nonperinatal pediatric cases.[4,10,11,87–91] In a child presenting with nontraumatic IPH, imaging exclusion of a vascular malformation as a cause should be a top priority. A separate article is devoted to vascular malformations; here, we discuss their HS implications.

Cerebral arteriovenous malformations

Cerebral AVMs are thought to be the cause of up to 50% of cases of spontaneous IPH in children.[10] In comparison to adults, hemorrhagic presentation (75% vs 60%) and deep location (38% vs 18%) are more common in children.[4,92,93] Adjusting for the increased hemorrhagic presentation in children, the long-term cumulative risk of brain AVM hemorrhage in children is similar to adults (approximately 2%–4% per year)[4] but mortality related to brain AVMs is higher in children.[92] Brain AVM hemorrhage patterns can be variable depending upon nidus location, venous drainage pattern, and associated aneurysms. Deep venous drainage (most common with deep AVM location), single draining vein and infratentorial location have been shown to correlate with an increased risk of hemorrhage in pediatric brain AVMs.[94] A recent study found that

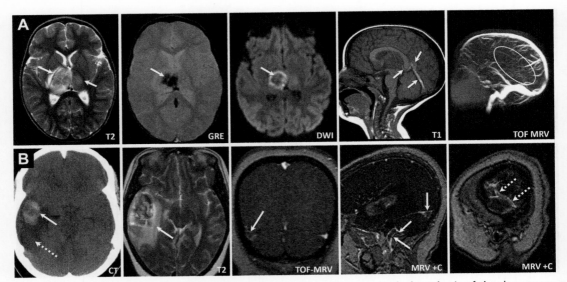

Fig. 4. Cerebral venous thrombosis. (*A*) Thalamic edema and hemorrhage with thrombosis of the deep venous system. Three year old female patient with lethargy and altered mental status. T2-weighted axial MR image (T2) at the level of foramen of Monro demonstrates marked edema and swelling of the right thalamus, with milder edema in the left thalamus (*arrows*). On gradient recalled echo (GRE) sequence, marked ill-defined feathery blooming effect is noted in the medial right thalamus (*arrow*), consistent with hemorrhage. Peripheral diffusion restriction is noted on DWI (*arrow*). T1 hyperintense thrombus noted in the straight sinus, vein of Galen, and proximal internal cerebral veins (*arrows*) consistent with thrombus. TOF MRV demonstrates lack of any flow-related enhancement in the deep venous system consistent with thrombosis (region outlined by circle). (*B*) Thrombosis of the transverse sinus and vein of Labbe'. A 14 year old female patient with headache and new onset seizure. CT demonstrated focal hemorrhage in the right temporal lobe (*arrow*) with moderate surrounding edema (*dashed arrows*). On MR imaging, edema with central mixed signal consistent with hemorrhage is noted (*arrows*). On TOF-MRV, thrombosis of the right transverse sinus is noted (*arrow*). On postcontrast MRV (MRV+C), extensive filling defects are noted throughout the transverse sinus, sigmoid sinus and jugular bulb (*arrows*) as well as the vein of Labbe' (*dashed arrows*).

AVM with associated flow-related aneurysms (perinidal and intranidal) were more likely hemorrhagic at presentation (94% vs 59%), have smaller nidal size, and have a higher annual hemorrhage risk if not obliterated compared to those AVMs without associated aneurysms.[95]

ICH occupying multiple intracranial compartments (IPH, IVH, and SAH) is common with AVM rupture. Approximately 50% of AVM-associated ICHs are isolated IPH, 30% to 38% are IPH with IVH or SAH, and 20% are isolated SAH.[96] Noncontrast CT findings suggesting AVM as a source of hemorrhage include dilated blood density tubular structures. IPH is typically oblong within the brain parenchyma suggesting a high-pressure vascular rupture. On CTA, AVM nidus morphology/location, dilated supplying arteries, and venous drainage pattern can be identified with high sensitivity[97] (**Fig. 5**). In the acute setting, the AVM nidus may not be readily visible on CTA (related to hematoma compression, vasospasm, and transient thrombosis), especially if small and compact, but enlarged feeding arteries and draining veins can

be identified and are an important clue to AVM diagnosis. Intranidal, perinidal, and feeding (afferent) artery aneurysms, while detectable by CTA (and should be searched for), are better seen by catheter-directed DSA.[97] MR imaging (particularly with the use of ASL flow techniques) should be considered in stable patients. As described earlier, focal increase in ASL signal has a high sensitivity for arteriovenous shunt lesions in the setting of IPH, outperforming CTA in some studies.[27] Flow-related enhancement of ectatic vessels near the location of hemorrhage and/or draining veins on TOF MRA suggests an underlying arteriovenous shunt lesion. If no vascular cause is found on imaging, delayed imaging follow up is important.[30,31]

Pial arteriovenous fistulae

pAVFs consist of a monofocal arteriovenous shunt zone constituted by a solitary pial vein or venous pouch that is arterialized by one or more pial arterial feeders, predisposing it to marked degrees of venous ectasia, variceal dilatation, and hemorrhage. The vast majority of pAVFs is congenital

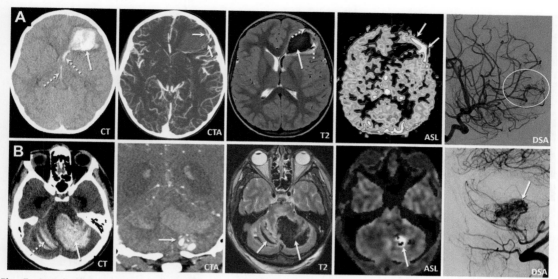

Fig. 5. Arteriovenous malformation with associated hemorrhage. (*A*) A 7 year old female patient with acute onset of headache, confusion, and vomiting. CT demonstrated a left frontal lobe parenchymal hemorrhage (*arrow*) tapering toward the ventricle with intraventricular extension (*dashed arrow*). Minimal surrounding edema. Immediately performed CTA demonstrated splaying of normal cerebral vascularity with an asymmetrically enlarged vessel along the lateral margin of the hemorrhage suspicious for an arteriovenous shunt lesion (*arrows*). MR imaging was performed and T2-weighted images demonstrated a T2-hypointense hemorrhage (*arrow*) with prominent vessels along the left frontal lobe surface (*dashed arrows*). ASL images demonstrated focal increased ASL signal in superficial vessels along the lateral margin of the hemorrhage consistent with high flow arteriovenous shunting (*arrows*). Catheter-directed digital subtraction angiogram (DSA) revealed arteriovenous shunting through a nidal AVM along the dorsal lateral aspect of the hematoma (*outline*), supplied by frontal branches of the left middle cerebral artery, with venous drainage to a frontal cortical vein (corresponding to the enlarged vascularity seen by CTA and high flow on ASL). (*B*) A 15 year old male patient with sudden headache, vomiting, and unresponsiveness, glasgow coma scale 3/15 on arrival to hospital. CT revealed a large cerebellar hemorrhage (*arrow*) with intraventricular extension, and extensive subarachnoid hemorrhage (*dashed arrows*). Immediately performed CTA demonstrated abnormally ectatic vessels (*arrows*) localized along the inferior margin of the hematoma suggesting a nidal AVM. The hemorrhage was hypointense on MR (T2, *arrows*) with localized high flow signal on ASL along the inferior hematoma consistent with shunting (ASL, *arrow*). Catheter-directed DSA demonstrated a nidus supplied by branches of the left posterior inferior cerebellar artery (*arrow*). Despite emergency posterior fossa decompression and embolization, the patient did not regain neurologic function and expired.

and present in infancy or early childhood, in contradistinction to cerebral AVMs that typically present in older children. Although some angioarchitectural features of pAVFs overlap with vein of Galen malformations (VOGM), intracranial hemorrhagic complications are exceedingly rare in patients with VOGM prior to adolescence. Consequently, VOGM is generally not considered in the differential diagnosis of pediatric hemorrhagic stroke.

pAVFs are predisposed to rupture, making them an important cause of pediatric HS. The markedly elevated pial venous pressures associated with pAVFs leads to secondary complications of venous hypertension including subependymal white matter injury, cortical atrophy, parenchymal calcification, encephaloclastic changes, high-flow occlusive venopathy, and communicating hydrocephalus.[98,99] Hemorrhage can occur at presentation in approximately 20% to 25% of cases.[100,101]

Hemorrhagic presentation is more common in older children/adults but can occur at any age. Hemorrhage patterns are often mixed, with varying degrees of IPH, IVH, and SAH depending upon the location of the shunt and bleeding point (**Fig. 6**). Successful endovascular treatment has been reported in up to 90% of cases.[100] There is a common (25%–30%) association with hereditary hemorrhagic telangiectasia and RASA1 gene mutations.[100,102]

Cavernous malformation
Up to 25% of all CCM manifest in childhood and are thought to be the cause of up to 9% of HS presentations in children.[9,10] Approximately 20% of all CCMs are associated with developmental venous anomaly (DVA), more commonly within the posterior fossa.[103,104] When multiple CCMs are identified on imaging in a patient not previously

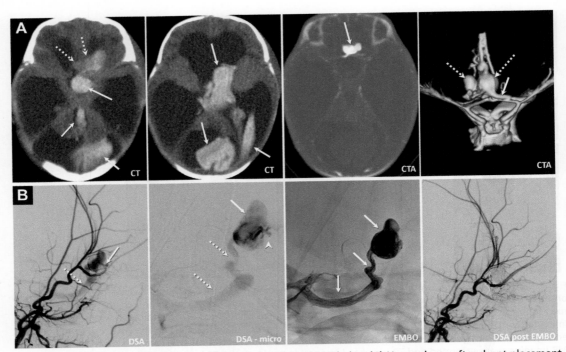

Fig. 6. Pial arteriovenous fistula. A 2 day old infant with hydrocephalus. (*A*) Hemorrhage after shunt placement. CT demonstrates large amount of intraventricular hemorrhage (*arrows*). Subtle lobular regions of mild hyperdensity seen along the inferior frontal lobe adjacent to the hemorrhage concerning for a vascular lesion (*dashed arrows*). Immediate CTA demonstrates a lobular venous aneurysm (*arrows*) in the inferior frontal region corresponding to the areas of mild hyperdensity seen on CT. 3D reconstruction (3D-CTA) demonstrates a single arterial feeder arising from the left anterior cerebral artery (*arrow*) and associated lobular venous aneurysm (*dashed arrows*). (*B*) Catheter-directed DSA documents the feeder artery originating from the anterior cerebral artery (*arrow*) with rapid venous drainage into the right superficial middle cerebral vein on the right (dashed *arrow*). Microcatheter injection (DSA-micro) at the fistulous point (*arrowhead*) demonstrates direct connection to the venous aneurysm (*arrow*) and rapid flow into middle cerebral vein (dashed *arrow*). Embolization (EMBO) was performed with onyx (onyx cast-arrows), totally occluding the fistula and venous drainage (post-EMBO).

treated with cranial radiotherapy, a genetic cause (familial CCM) should be considered.[105]

On CT imaging, CCM appearance depends upon internal hemorrhagic product evolution, associated extralesional hemorrhage, and associated calcification. On MR imaging, CCM have a typical pattern of a multilobular circumscribed lesion with a T2 hypointense rim that blooms on SWI/GRE sequences. Centrally the sinusoidal spaces have differing signal intensities depending upon the stage of internal blood products[106] (**Fig. 7**). Often definitive diagnosis on CT is not possible with the imaging differential being localized parenchymal hemorrhage, AVM, or tumor. Recognizing the typical MR imaging appearance of a CCM, associated DVA (if present), and additional CCM (suggesting a familial CM syndrome) is often a useful finding when diagnosing CCM as a cause for ICH. With extensive intralesional or extralesional hemorrhage, the typical imaging features may not be present and may only become manifest on delayed

imaging, or as a diagnosis of exclusion when careful repeat MR imaging and catheter-directed DSA fail to identify another cause.

Hemorrhage related to CCM is a major cause of clinical symptoms and can occur within the CCM (intralesional) or outside the CCM in the adjacent brain parenchyma (extralesional). IVH can occur if the CCM is in a subependymal location. The most widely accepted definition of CCM hemorrhage is an acute or subacute onset of lesion referable symptoms in the context of imaging, pathologic, surgical, or CSF evidence of recent extralesional or intralesional hemorrhage.[107] Given that symptoms are lesion location dependent and that criteria for intralesional and extralesional hemorrhage are poorly defined, some authors have expanded this definition to include more detailed imaging-based criteria. Nikoubashman[108] in a study of pediatric CCM defined acute CCM hemorrhage on MR imaging as *intralesional*: acute or subacute internal hemorrhagic signal accompanied by lesion growth,

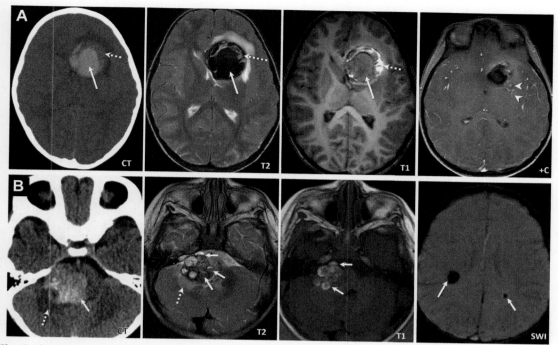

Fig. 7. Cavernous malformation. (*A*) A 5 year old female patient with increasing headache and lethargy. CT demonstrated a large (4 cm) hemorrhagic lesion in the left frontal lobe with surrounding edema (*dashed arrows*). The hemorrhage was lobular with high density centrally and medially and lower density laterally. Immediate CTA was performed, which did not demonstrate a shunting lesion or aneurysm. Subsequent MR imaging was performed to differentiate between cerebral cavernous malformation (CCM) and neoplasm. T2-weighted and T1-weighted images show a multilobular hemorrhagic lesion with central acute blood products (*arrows*) corresponding to the hyperdensity on CT and more peripheral, less-circumscribed subacute hemorrhage (*dashed arrows*) compatible with extralesional hemorrhage. An adjacent developmental venous anomaly was seen on postcontrast images (*arrowheads*). Findings were consistent with CCM complicated by intralesional and extralesional hemorrhage (documented surgically). (*B*) A 10 month old male patient with vomiting, right eye deviation, and lethargy. Head CT demonstrates a hyperdense lesion (*arrow*) in the right pons with mild surrounding edema (*dashed arrows*), and small calcifications. Immediate CTA did not show a shunting lesion or aneurysm. MR imaging demonstrates a multilobular popcorn like mass with dark T2 signal surrounding multiple circumscribed internal spaces (some with fluid levels, *arrows*). On T1, many of the areas exhibit isointense and hyperintense signal consistent with a mix of acute and subacute blood products. There is adjacent edema (*dashed arrow*). Imaging findings consistent with CCM. Multiple additional small CCM identified (*arrows*) in both cerebral hemispheres on SWI suggesting a familial CCM syndrome.

mass effect, or surrounding edema and *extralesional*: gross extralesional hemorrhage manifested as acute or subacute blood degradation products outside the confines of the CCM. Because of varying criteria and differences in cohorts, hemorrhage rates in CCM have been variably reported. In children, the overall annual hemorrhage rate of CCM is approximately 3%[109] or 4.5%/lesion/year,[108] with much higher annual rates in CCM initially presenting with hemorrhage (11%).[108] Prior CCM hemorrhage and brainstem location have universally been reported as the most significant risk factors for subsequent CCM hemorrhage.[109,110]

Imaging appearance has also been shown to correlate with annual hemorrhage risk: CCM with acute or subacute internal blood products—23%,

CCM without acute or subacute blood products—3.4%, and dot-sized SWI or GRE lesions—1.3%.[108] Hemorrhage risk is highest in the first 3 years after initial hemorrhage.[109,110] While an associated DVA has been suggested as a risk factor for hemorrhage by some authors,[109] others have not found this association.[110–113] Lesions located within the brainstem or near eloquent cortex are more often symptomatic related to CCM expansion and extralesional hemorrhage.[113,114]

Intracranial Arterial Aneurysms

While intracranial arterial aneurysms (IAAs) rupture is a less common clinical presentation in children than in adults, they are responsible for 10% to

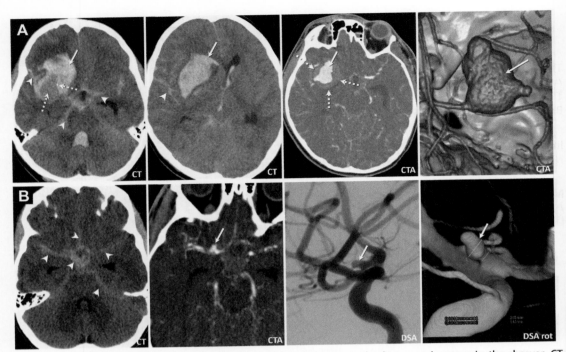

Fig. 8. Intracranial arterial aneurysm. (*A*) A 15 year old male patient who lost consciousness in the shower. CT shows a large parenchymal hemorrhage in the right frontal lobe (*arrow*) extending into the right lateral ventricle, extensive subarachnoid hemorrhage in the right sylvian fissure, basal cisterns, and cerebral sulci (*arrowheads*). In the right sylvian region, an area of intermediate-to-high density noted within the hemorrhage with an associated tiny calcification (*dashed arrows*). CTA demonstrates a giant (26 mm) lobular fusiform aneurysm arising from the right middle cerebral artery bifurcation intrinsically involving the superior M2 division (*arrow*), surrounded by hemorrhage (*dashed arrows*). (*B*) A 13 year old male patient with history of aortic coarctation presented with vomiting and acute headache. Head CT reveals diffuse SAH, more prominent in the right suprasellar cistern (*arrowheads*). Immediate CTA demonstrates a small aneurysm from the right carotid terminus at the origin of the right A1 segment. Catheter-directed DSA confirms the aneurysm and its angioarchitecture is further elucidated by reconstructed 3D images generated with rotational angiography (DSA rot).

15% of childhood HS and up to 60% of isolated spontaneous SAH in children.[6] Overall, pediatric IAAs present with ICH in 35% to 50% of identified cases.[115,116] Aneurysm rupture typically causes isolated SAH (80%) but can also cause IVH and IPH (20%).[6] Although flow-related mechanical stresses caused by arteriovenous shunt lesions often lead to aneurysm formation and rupture, in such cases, the underlying arteriovenous shunt lesion usually dominates the diagnostic picture.

Noncontrast CT is highly sensitive for SAH (93%–100%) particularly in the first 6 hours after headache onset.[117] Typically immediate CTA is performed after identification of nontraumatic SAH,[118] and it can identify the cause in 80% to 95% of patients.[119] When negative, catheter-directed DSA should be performed and can identify vascular pathology in up to 13% of CTA-negative cases. If both CTA and DSA are negative, follow-up CTA and or DSA are recommended (additional yield of 4%).[119] Pediatric IAAs arise more commonly in the posterior

circulation and from the internal carotid artery terminus compared to adults (**Fig. 8**B). Giant (>25 mm) and fusiform aneurysms are more common in young children and infants[116,120,121] (**Fig. 8**A). While idiopathic IAAs are the most common type identified in children (as in adults), infectious and traumatic aneurysms are more common in children. The presence of multiple cerebral aneurysms (particularly when located distal to the circle of Willis) in a febrile patient (particularly if immunocompromised or with cardiac valve vegetations) should be considered highly suspicious for infectious aneurysms.

Coagulopathy-related Hemorrhagic Stroke

Disorders of coagulation (iatrogenic, hematologic, or hereditary) are a cause of pediatric HS in 12% to 30% of cases depending upon the age cohort evaluated, being more common in children aged less than 2 years.[9,10,12–14] Coagulopathy related to the treatment of congenital cardiac disease or

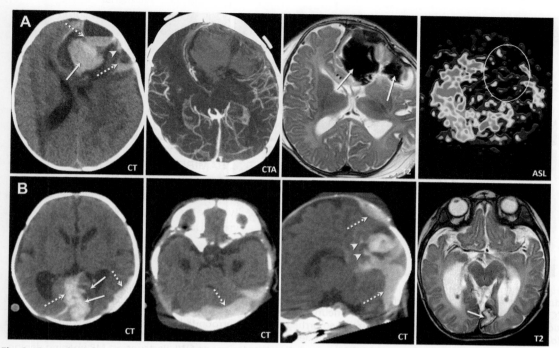

Fig. 9. Coagulopathy-related hemorrhage. (*A*) A 3 month old male patient with increased fussiness and vomiting. Head CT demonstrates a huge lobular left frontal lobe IPH (*arrow*) and adjacent subarachnoid hemorrhage (*arrowhead*). Multiple fluid–fluid levels are identified consistent with nonclotting blood products (*dashed arrows*). CTA was performed, which shows no evidence of shunting lesion, aneurysm, or dural sinus thrombosis. MR imaging performed after hemicraniectomy demonstrates T2 hypointense hemorrhage (*arrows*) with surrounding edema. MRA (not shown) and ASL images show no evidence of shunting (ASL, region outlined by circle). Detailed hematological studies identified a profound coagulopathy secondary to acquired vitamin K deficiency in the setting of autosomal recessive progressive familial intrahepatic cholestasis-type 4. Follow-up MR imaging/MRA/MRV as the clot retracted showed no vascular abnormalities. (*B*) An 11 day old female infant (38 weeks' gestation) with congenital diaphragmatic hernia and pulmonary hypoplasia, on ECMO for pulmonary hypertension and respiratory arrest. Dramatic hematocrit drop triggered imaging, which revealed a large left hemothorax and ICH on head CT. Head CT demonstrates extensive multicompartment ICH with localized parenchymal hemorrhage and adjacent edema in the left occipital lobe (*arrows*), extensive subdural hemorrhage (*dashed arrows* on axial and sagittal CT images) and adjacent subarachnoid hemorrhage (*arrowheads* on sagittal CT image). Follow-up MR (T2) 3 months later showed residual encephalomalacia with hemosiderin staining in the left occipital lobe, which is likely the sequelae of infarction with hemorrhagic transformation (T2, *arrow*). No abnormality on MRA, MRV, or ASL (not shown).

severe pulmonary disease (including therapeutic anticoagulation and extracorporeal membrane oxygenation [ECMO]) is more common in younger children, particularly in infants.[10] When HS is associated with congenital cardiac disease, up to 70% have a coagulation deficit, usually iatrogenic.[10] In neonates, alloimmune thrombocytopenia and vitamin K deficiency are also important causes of coagulopathy leading to HS.[122] Routine vitamin K supplementation for neonates has dramatically decreased vitamin K deficiency-related ICH; however, it remains a substantial cause (up to 50% of cases) in countries where supplementation is not standard.[123]

Coagulopathy-related ICH is often multicompartmental and dramatic on imaging. Fluid levels (indicating nonclotted blood products) can be seen both with IPH and extra-axial hemorrhage (Fig. 9). In a cardiac patient, on either anticoagulation or ECMO therapy with a new neurologic deficit or change in mental status, ICH is the diagnosis of exclusion and should be immediately assessed by CT imaging. In the setting of coagulopathy, usually, no vascular cause is identified by CTA or MR imaging/MRA. Nonetheless, it may be important to evaluate the possibility of an anatomic/vascular cause in the acute phase and with delayed follow-up imaging depending upon the clinical scenario. Detailed hematologic/coagulation studies are warranted when no cause of ICH can be documented by comprehensive imaging evaluation.

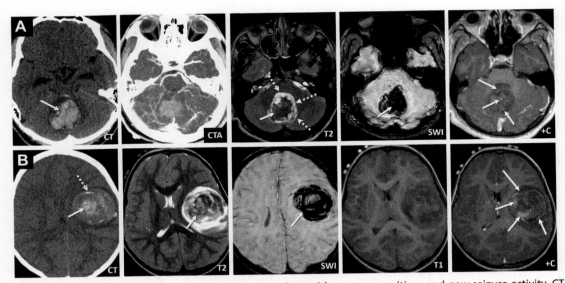

Fig. 10. Hemorrhagic tumor. (*A*) A 15 year old male patient with nausea, vomiting, and new seizure activity. CT demonstrates a localized hemorrhage in the central cerebellum (*arrow*) with minimal surrounding low density (CT). CTA was normal without evidence of aneurysm or shunting lesion (CTA). Follow-up MR imaging examination (T2, SWI, +C) demonstrates a localized hemorrhage (*arrow*) surrounded by irregular T2 hyperintense tissue (*dashed arrow*) suggesting hemorrhage into an underlying mass. There was an extensive susceptibility effect that obscures detail within the lesion on SWI (SWI, *arrow*). No other lesions on SWI. Postcontrast MR imaging demonstrates a small linear area of enhancement within the hemorrhagic region and along its periphery, which may represent vasculature or possibly tumor enhancement (+C, *arrows*). The typical lobular morphology of CCM was not present. ASL was negative for high flow (not shown). Hemorrhagic tumor was felt to be most likely. Low-grade glioneuronal neoplasm (BRAF–) was found on surgical resection. (*B*) An 8 year old female patient with vomiting and seizure activity. Noncontrast CT demonstrates localized hemorrhagic lesion in the left frontal parietal region (CT). Ill-defined intraparenchymal hemorrhage with more prominent hyperdensity centrally is seen on CT (*arrow*). A small calcification present along the ventral margin (*dashed arrow*). T2-weighted images on MR imaging demonstrate extensive T2 hypointense hemorrhage (T2, *arrow*) with blooming susceptibility on SWI images (SWI, *arrow*). The hemorrhage is very heterogeneous suggesting hemorrhage in an underlying lesion, and there is moderate surrounding edema (CT, *dashed arrows*). Postcontrast images demonstrate irregular enhancement within and along the margins of the lesion strongly supporting neoplasm (+C, *arrows*). Resection confirmed pilomyxoid astrocytoma.

Neoplasia

Neoplastic disorders presenting with ICH or having hemorrhage as a predominant imaging finding occurs in 3% to 18% of children with HS.[9,10] Up to 10% of intracranial tumors in children can present with ICH.[124] Tumor-related ICH has most commonly been reported with embryonal tumors and metastatic tumors (neuroblastoma, hepatoblastoma, rhabdomyosarcoma, leukemic infiltration, melanoma, and thyroid origin tumors), but it can also be seen with low-grade (pilocytic, pilomyxoid) and higher grade glial neoplasms.[124–128] In higher grade primary tumors and metastatic lesions, rapid tumor cell proliferation, vascular invasion, tumor neovascularization with fragile blood vessels, and tumor necrosis are likely causative. In pilocytic astrocytomas, dysplastic capillaries with "glomeruloid" morphology, vessel hyalinization, and intratumoral microaneurysms have been described.[129] When intratumoral hemorrhage

involves only a part of the tumor, imaging diagnosis of tumor-related hemorrhage is typically straightforward. When intratumoral hemorrhage is diffusely noted throughout the tumor with the disruption of tumor architecture, the diagnosis may be more challenging. Tumoral hemorrhage may mimic CCM or bland IPH. A large amount of edema surrounding the hematoma, patchy hemorrhage occupying only a portion of an identified lesion, and internal "tumor like" enhancement or signal may provide clues (**Fig. 10**). Careful imaging follow-up as the hemorrhage resolves may sometimes be the only way to make the diagnosis.

Other conditions

Other conditions can be associated with HS in children, though less commonly than those entities covered thus far. These include a variety of noninflammatory steno-occlusive arteriopathies (moyamoya arteriopathies), inflammatory arteriopathies

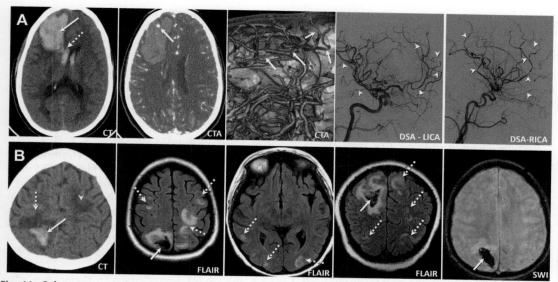

Fig. 11. Other causes. (A) Secondary central nervous system (CNS) vasculitis and pseudoaneurysm. A 15 year old female patient, newly diagnosed systemic lupus erythematosus (SLE) with acute onset of severe headache. CT demonstrates an IPH in the left frontal lobe (CT, *arrow*) with intraventricular extension (*dashed arrow*). CTA demonstrates a focal area of collection of extravascular contrast within the ventral margin of the hematoma without direct continuity to other vessels (CTA, *arrow*). The finding suggests a pseudoaneurysm or localized contrast extravasation ("spot-sign"). Luminal irregularity involving multiple vessels suggests vasculitis and/or vasospasm (*arrows* on 3D volume reconstruction image). Decompressive craniotomy was performed with clipping/exclusion of the pseudoaneurysm and partial hematoma evacuation. Subsequent catheter directed-DSA shows widespread, multifocal, segmental luminal constriction irregularly involving cortical branch arteries throughout the left internal carotid artery distribution (DSA-LICA) and right internal carotid artery distribution (DSA-RICA) (*arrowheads*) as well as posterior cerebral arteries (not shown) consistent with CNS vasculitis. Follow-up angiogram 4 months after immunosuppressive treatment (not shown) for presumed SLE-related vasculitis showed improvement in vessel narrowing with mild irregularity remaining. (B) Hemorrhagic posterior reversible encephalopathy syndrome (PRES). A 12 year old male patient with relapsed ALL after bone marrow transplant. Two seizures in the setting of marked hypertension. CT demonstrated localized hemorrhage within the right parietal lobe (CT, *arrow*) with moderate surrounding edema (CT, dashed *arrow*) and edema in the left frontal lobe (CT, *arrowhead*). MR imaging showed localized subcortical hemorrhage in the right parietal lobe with moderate surrounding edema. Axial and coronal T2 FLAIR images (FLAIR) show multifocal regions of cortical and subcortical edema throughout the brain parenchyma in a pattern consistent with PRES (*dashed arrows*) and focal T2 hypointensity indicative of hemorrhage (*arrow*). Localized marked susceptibility effect on SWI in the area of T2 FLAIR signal hypointensity (SWI, *arrow*) consistent with hemorrhage. No evidence of venous thrombosis on MRV, SWI, or postcontrast MR imaging (not shown). No abnormal flow-related enhancement on ASL imaging (not shown).

(primary and secondary central nervous system angiitis), and arteriopathies resulting from maladaptive responses to endothelial injury (posterior reversible encephalopathy syndrome and reversible cerebral vasoconstriction syndrome). These conditions typically present in school-age children and adolescents. The clinical context, MR imaging findings and catheter-directed DSA features aid in the differential diagnosis[87,130–134] **(Fig. 11).**

SUMMARY

HS is an important cause of neurologic morbidity and mortality in children and is more common than ischemic stroke between the ages of 1 and 14 years, a notable contradistinction relative to adult stroke epidemiology. Rapid neuroimaging is of the utmost importance in making the diagnosis of HS, identifying a likely etiology, and directing acute care. In the neonatal period, HS is usually due to GMH, PVHI, CVT (including MVT), SPH, and coagulopathy. In older children, HS is usually caused by vascular malformations, and less commonly IAA. The differential diagnosis of HS at any age is strongly guided by the pattern of hemorrhage within specific intracranial compartments. CT and MR imaging with flow-sensitive MR imaging (ASL, TOF MRA) and other noninvasive vascular imaging studies (CTA, MRA, and 3D-CEMRI) play a primary role in the initial diagnostic evaluation. Catheter-directed DSA is critical for definitive diagnosis and treatment planning.

CLINICS CARE POINTS

- Vascular malformations are the most common cause of hemorrhagic stroke in children after the neonatal period. When non-traumatic spontaneous intraparenchymal hemorrhage is identified in a child, immediate vascular imaging utilizing CTA (first choice given availability and speed) and/or MRI/MRA (if patient is stable and MRI immediately available) should be performed to exclude a shunting lesion and identify the likely cause. Catheter-directed DSA can be performed for more detailed assessment or if no cause is initially identified on non-invasive imaging given its high spatial and temporal resolution for vascular lesions.

- Cerebral venous thrombosis is an increasingly recognized cause of hemorrhagic stroke throughout childhood. Highest prevalence is in neonates with periventricular hemorrhagic infarction (PVHI), medullary vein thrombosis (MVT), and subpial hemorrhage all likely having venous occlusion as the underlying etiology. In older children, sequelae of infection and prothrombotic states are common causes for CVT.

- In pre-term neonates, most cases of spontaneous intracranial hemorrhage with identified cause are related to germinal matrix hemorrhage and associated pathology (intraventricular hemorrhage, PVHI). While head ultrasound is the primary initial diagnostic tool for initial diagnosis and to inform clinical care, MRI is often used for definitive diagnosis and for prognostic information, often at term equivalent age.

- When isolated non-traumatic subarachnoid hemorrhage occurs in a child, intracranial arterial aneurysm rupture is the diagnosis of exclusion. Immediate CTA is the diagnostic test of choice in this scenario and can identify a cause in 80-95% of patents. Digital subtraction angiography can be performed for further characterization and can identify vascular pathology in up to 13% of CTA negative cases.

REFERENCES

1. Ferriero DM, Fullerton HJ, Bernard TJ, et al. Management of stroke in neonates and children: a scientific statement from the American heart association/American stroke association. Stroke 2019;50(3):e51–96.

2. Beslow LA, Smith SE, Vossough A, et al. Hemorrhagic transformation of childhood arterial ischemic stroke. Stroke 2011;42(4):941–6.

3. Hollist M, Au K, Morgan L, et al. Pediatric stroke: overview and recent updates. Aging Dis 2021;12(4):1043–55.

4. Fullerton HJ, Wu YW, Zhao S, et al. Risk of stroke in children: ethnic and gender disparities. Neurology 2003;61(2):189–94.

5. Broderick J, Talbot GT, Prenger E, et al. Stroke in children within a major metropolitan area: the surprising importance of intracerebral hemorrhage. J Child Neurol 1993;8(3):250–5.

6. Jordan LC, Hillis AE. Hemorrhagic stroke in children. Pediatr Neurol 2007;36(2):73–80.

7. Fox CK, Johnston SC, Sidney S, et al. High critical care usage due to pediatric stroke: results of a population-based study. Neurology 2012;79(5):420–7.

8. Romero JM, Rojas-Serrano LF. Current evaluation of intracerebral hemorrhage. Radiol Clin North Am 2023;61(3):479–90.

9. Ciochon UM, Bindslev JBB, Hoei-Hansen CE, et al. Causes and risk factors of pediatric spontaneous intracranial hemorrhage-A systematic review. Diagnostics (Basel) 2022;12(6). https://doi.org/10.3390/diagnostics12061459.

10. Boulouis G, Stricker S, Benichi S, et al. Etiology of intracerebral hemorrhage in children: cohort study, systematic review, and meta-analysis. J Neurosurg Pediatr 2021;27(3):357–63.

11. Boulouis G, Blauwblomme T, Hak JF, et al. Nontraumatic pediatric intracerebral hemorrhage. Stroke 2019;50(12):3654–61.

12. Bruno CJ, Beslow LA, Witmer CM, et al. Haemorrhagic stroke in term and late preterm neonates. Arch Dis Child Fetal Neonatal Ed 2014;99(1):F48–53.

13. Cole L, Dewey D, Letourneau N, et al. Clinical characteristics, risk factors, and outcomes associated with neonatal hemorrhagic stroke: a population-based case-control study. JAMA Pediatr 2017;171(3):230–8.

14. Sandoval Karamian AG, Yang QZ, Tam LT, et al. Intracranial hemorrhage in term and late-preterm neonates: an institutional perspective. AJNR Am J Neuroradiol 2022;43(10):1494–9.

15. Srivastava R, Mailo J, Dunbar M. Perinatal stroke in fetuses, preterm and term infants. Semin Pediatr Neurol 2022;43:100988.

16. Armstrong-Wells J, Johnston SC, Wu YW, et al. Prevalence and predictors of perinatal hemorrhagic stroke: results from the kaiser pediatric stroke study. Pediatrics 2009;123(3):823–8.

17. Shellhaas RA, Smith SE, O'Tool E, et al. Mimics of childhood stroke: characteristics of a prospective cohort. Pediatrics 2006;118(2):704–9.

18. Pangprasertkul S, Borisoot W, Buawangpong N, et al. Comparison of arterial ischemic and hemorrhagic pediatric stroke in etiology, risk factors, clinical manifestations, and prognosis. Pediatr Emerg Care 2022;38(9):e1569–73.

19. Gerstl L, Weinberger R, Heinen F, et al. Arterial ischemic stroke in infants, children, and adolescents: results of a Germany-wide surveillance study 2015-2017. J Neurol 2019;266(12):2929–41.

20. Morgenstern LB, Hemphill JC 3rd, Anderson C, et al. Guidelines for the management of spontaneous intracerebral hemorrhage: a guideline for healthcare professionals from the American Heart Association/American Stroke Association. Stroke 2010;41(9):2108–29.

21. Dubosh NM, Bellolio MF, Rabinstein AA, et al. Sensitivity of early brain computed tomography to exclude aneurysmal subarachnoid hemorrhage: a systematic review and meta-analysis. Stroke 2016;47(3):750–5.

22. Sporns PB, Psychogios MN, Fullerton HJ, et al. Neuroimaging of pediatric intracerebral hemorrhage. J Clin Med 2020;9(5). https://doi.org/10.3390/jcm9051518.

23. Srinivasan VM, Gressot LV, Daniels BS, et al. Management of intracerebral hemorrhage in pediatric neurosurgery. Surg Neurol Int 2016;7(Suppl 44):S1121–6.

24. Jain A, Malhotra A, Payabvash S. Imaging of spontaneous intracerebral hemorrhage. Neuroimaging Clin N Am 2021;31(2):193–203.

25. Mirsky DM, Beslow LA, Amlie-Lefond C, et al. Pathways for neuroimaging of childhood stroke. Pediatr Neurol 2017;69:11–23.

26. Kidwell CS, Chalela JA, Saver JL, et al. Comparison of MRI and CT for detection of acute intracerebral hemorrhage. JAMA 2004;292(15):1823–30.

27. Hak JF, Boulouis G, Kerleroux B, et al. Arterial spin labeling for the etiological workup of intracerebral hemorrhage in children. Stroke 2022;53(1):185–93.

28. Lin N, Smith ER, Scott RM, et al. Safety of neuroangiography and embolization in children: complication analysis of 697 consecutive procedures in 394 patients. J Neurosurg Pediatr 2015;16(4):432–8.

29. Harrar DB, Sun LR, Goss M, et al. Cerebral digital subtraction angiography in acute intracranial hemorrhage: considerations in critically ill children. J Child Neurol 2022;37(8–9):693–701.

30. Hino A, Fujimoto M, Yamaki T, et al. Value of repeat angiography in patients with spontaneous subcortical hemorrhage. Stroke 1998;29(12):2517–21.

31. Ogilvy CS, Heros RC, Ojemann RG, et al. Angiographically occult arteriovenous malformations. J Neurosurg 1988;69(3):350–5.

32. Intrapiromkul J, Northington F, Huisman TA, et al. Accuracy of head ultrasound for the detection of intracranial hemorrhage in preterm neonates: comparison with brain MRI and susceptibility-weighted imaging. J Neuroradiol 2013;40(2):81–8.

33. Elkhunovich M, Sirody J, McCormick T, et al. The utility of cranial ultrasound for detection of intracranial hemorrhage in infants. Pediatr Emerg Care 2018;34(2):96–101.

34. Dudink J, Jeanne Steggerda S, Horsch S. State-of-the-art neonatal cerebral ultrasound: technique and reporting. Pediatr Res 2020;87(Suppl 1):3–12.

35. Hinojosa-Rodríguez M, Harmony T, Carrillo-Prado C, et al. Clinical neuroimaging in the preterm infant: diagnosis and prognosis. Neuroimage Clin 2017;16:355–68.

36. Roy B, Walker K, Morgan C, et al. Epidemiology and pathogenesis of stroke in preterm infants: a systematic review. J Neonatal Perinat Med 2022;15(1):11–8.

37. Elgendy MM, Puthuraya S, LoPiccolo C, et al. Neonatal stroke: clinical characteristics and neurodevelopmental outcomes. Pediatr Neonatol 2022;63(1):41–7.

38. Papile LA, Burstein J, Burstein R, et al. Incidence and evolution of subependymal and intraventricular hemorrhage: a study of infants with birth weights less than 1,500 gm. J Pediatr 1978;92(4):529–34.

39. Buchmayer J, Kasprian G, Giordano V, et al. Routine use of cerebral magnetic resonance imaging in infants born extremely preterm. J Pediatr 2022;248:74–80.e1.

40. Nataraj P, Svojsik M, Sura L, et al. Comparing head ultrasounds and susceptibility-weighted imaging for the detection of low-grade hemorrhages in preterm infants. J Perinatol 2021;41(4):736–42.

41. You SK. Neuroimaging of germinal matrix and intraventricular hemorrhage in premature infants. J Korean Neurosurg Soc 2023;66(3):239–46.

42. Parodi A, Govaert P, Horsch S, et al. Cranial ultrasound findings in preterm germinal matrix haemorrhage, sequelae and outcome. Pediatr Res 2020;87(Suppl 1):13–24.

43. Gould SJ, Howard S, Hope PL, et al. Periventricular intraparenchymal cerebral haemorrhage in preterm infants: the role of venous infarction. J Pathol 1987;151(3):197–202.

44. Volpe JJ. Intracranial hemorrhage: germinal matrix-Intraventircular hemorrhage of the premature infant. Neurology of the Newborn. 5th edition. Philadelphia, PA: Saunders/Elsevier; 2008. chap 11.

45. Dudink J, Lequin M, Weisglas-Kuperus N, et al. Venous subtypes of preterm periventricular haemorrhagic infarction. Arch Dis Child Fetal Neonatal Ed 2008;93(3):F201–6.

46. Tortora D, Severino M, Malova M, et al. Differences in subependymal vein anatomy may predispose preterm infants to GMH-IVH. Arch Dis Child Fetal Neonatal Ed 2018;103(1):F59–65.

47. Cizmeci MN, de Vries LS, Ly LG, et al. Periventricular hemorrhagic infarction in very preterm infants:

characteristic sonographic findings and association with neurodevelopmental outcome at age 2 years. J Pediatr 2020;217:79–85.e1.

48. Soltirovska Salamon A, Groenendaal F, van Haastert IC, et al. Neuroimaging and neurodevelopmental outcome of preterm infants with a periventricular haemorrhagic infarction located in the temporal or frontal lobe. Dev Med Child Neurol 2014;56(6):547–55.

49. Bassan H, Feldman HA, Limperopoulos C, et al. Periventricular hemorrhagic infarction: risk factors and neonatal outcome. Pediatr Neurol 2006;35(2): 85–92.

50. Bassan H, Limperopoulos C, Visconti K, et al. Neurodevelopmental outcome in survivors of periventricular hemorrhagic infarction. Pediatrics 2007; 120(4):785–92.

51. Roze E, Benders MJ, Kersbergen KJ, et al. Neonatal DTI early after birth predicts motor outcome in preterm infants with periventricular hemorrhagic infarction. Pediatr Res 2015;78(3):298–303.

52. Pin JN, Leonardi L, Nosadini M, et al. Deep medullary vein thrombosis in newborns: a systematic literature review. Neonatology 2023;120(5):539–47.

53. Khalatbari H, Wright JN, Ishak GE, et al. Deep medullary vein engorgement and superficial medullary vein engorgement: two patterns of perinatal venous stroke. Pediatr Radiol 2021;51(5):675–85.

54. Benninger KL, Benninger TL, Moore-Clingenpeel M, et al. Deep medullary vein white matter injury global severity score predicts neurodevelopmental impairment. J Child Neurol 2021;36(4):253–61.

55. Christensen R, Krishnan P, deVeber G, et al. Cerebral venous sinus thrombosis in preterm infants. Stroke 2022;53(7):2241–8.

56. Lai LM, Sato TS, Kandemirli SG, et al. Neuroimaging of neonatal stroke: venous focus. Radiographics 2024;44(2):e230117.

57. Pinto C, Cunha B, Pinto MM, et al. Subpial hemorrhage : a distinctive neonatal stroke pattern. Clin Neuroradiol 2022;32(4):1057–65.

58. Barreto ARF, Carrasco M, Dabrowski AK, et al. Subpial hemorrhage in neonates: what radiologists need to know. AJR Am J Roentgenol 2021;216(4): 1056–65.

59. Friede RL. Subpial hemorrhage in infants. J Neuropathol Exp Neurol 1972;31(3):548–56.

60. Marín-Padilla M. Developmental neuropathology and impact of perinatal brain damage. I: hemorrhagic lesions of neocortex. J Neuropathol Exp Neurol 1996;55(7):758–73.

61. Zhuang X, Jin K, Li J, et al. Subpial hemorrhages in neonates: imaging features, clinical factors and outcomes. Sci Rep 2023;13(1):3408.

62. Cain DW, Dingman AL, Armstrong J, et al. Subpial hemorrhage of the neonate. Stroke 2020;51(1): 315–8.

63. Heller C, Heinecke A, Junker R, et al. Cerebral venous thrombosis in children: a multifactorial origin. Circulation 2003;108(11):1362–7.

64. deVeber G, Andrew M, Adams C, et al. Cerebral sinovenous thrombosis in children. N Engl J Med 2001;345(6):417–23.

65. Carvalho KS, Bodensteiner JB, Connolly PJ, et al. Cerebral venous thrombosis in children. J Child Neurol 2001;16(8):574–80.

66. Lynch JK, Nelson KB. Epidemiology of perinatal stroke. Curr Opin Pediatr 2001;13(6):499–505.

67. Devianne J, Legris N, Crassard I, et al. Epidemiology, clinical features, and outcome in a cohort of adolescents with cerebral venous thrombosis. Neurology 2021;97(19):e1920–32.

68. Otite FO, Vanguru H, Anikpezie N, et al. Contemporary incidence and burden of cerebral venous sinus thrombosis in children of the United States. Stroke 2022;53(12):e496–9.

69. Ferro JM, Canhão P, Stam J, et al. Prognosis of cerebral vein and dural sinus thrombosis: results of the international study on cerebral vein and dural sinus thrombosis (ISCVT). Stroke 2004;35(3): 664–70.

70. Dlamini N, Billinghurst L, Kirkham FJ. Cerebral venous sinus (sinovenous) thrombosis in children. Neurosurg Clin N Am 2010;21(3):511–27.

71. Cornelius LP, Elango N, Jeyaram VK. Clinico-etiological factors, neuroimaging characteristics and outcome in pediatric cerebral venous sinus thrombosis. Ann Indian Acad Neurol 2021;24(6): 901–7.

72. Leach JL, Fortuna RB, Jones BV, et al. Imaging of cerebral venous thrombosis: current techniques, spectrum of findings, and diagnostic pitfalls. Radiographics 2006;26(Suppl 1):S19–41. discussion S42-3.

73. Bracken J, Barnacle A, Ditchfield M. Potential pitfalls in imaging of paediatric cerebral sinovenous thrombosis. Pediatr Radiol 2013;43(2):219–31.

74. Canedo-Antelo M, Baleato-González S, Mosqueira AJ, et al. Radiologic clues to cerebral venous thrombosis. Radiographics 2019;39(6):1611–28.

75. Idbaih A, Boukobza M, Crassard I, et al. MRI of clot in cerebral venous thrombosis: high diagnostic value of susceptibility-weighted images. Stroke 2006;37(4):991–5.

76. Teksam M, Moharir M, Deveber G, et al. Frequency and topographic distribution of brain lesions in pediatric cerebral venous thrombosis. AJNR Am J Neuroradiol 2008;29(10):1961–5.

77. Berfelo FJ, Kersbergen KJ, van Ommen CH, et al. Neonatal cerebral sinovenous thrombosis from symptom to outcome. Stroke 2010;41(7):1382–8.

78. Wu YW, Hamrick SE, Miller SP, et al. Intraventricular hemorrhage in term neonates caused by sinovenous thrombosis. Ann Neurol 2003;54(1):123–6.

79. Usman U, Wasay M. Mechanism of neuronal injury in cerebral venous thrombosis. J Pakistan Med Assoc 2006;56(11):509–12.

80. Kanaiwa H, Kuchiwaki H, Inao S, et al. Changes in the cerebrocortical capillary network following venous sinus occlusion in cats. Surg Neurol 1995; 44(2):172–9. discussion 179-80.

81. Dinç Y, Özpar R, Hakyemez B, et al. The relationship between early neurological deterioration, poor clinical outcome, and venous collateral score in cerebral venous sinus thrombosis. Neurological Sciences and Neurophysiology 2021;38(3):158–65.

82. Ritchey Z, Hollatz AL, Weitzenkamp D, et al. Pediatric cortical vein thrombosis: frequency and association with venous infarction. Stroke 2016;47(3): 866–8.

83. Cervós-Navarro J, Kannuki S, Matsumoto K. Neuropathological changes following occlusion of the superior sagittal sinus and cerebral veins in the cat. Neuropathol Appl Neurobiol 1994;20(2):122–9.

84. Liu L, Zhou C, Jiang H, et al. Cortical vein involvement and its influence in a cohort of adolescents with cerebral venous thrombosis. Thromb J 2023; 21(1):78.

85. Coutinho JM, Gerritsma JJ, Zuurbier SM, et al. Isolated cortical vein thrombosis: systematic review of case reports and case series. Stroke 2014;45(6): 1836–8.

86. Liang J, Chen H, Li Z, et al. Cortical vein thrombosis in adult patients of cerebral venous sinus thrombosis correlates with poor outcome and brain lesions: a retrospective study. BMC Neurol 2017; 17(1):219.

87. Liu J, Wang D, Lei C, et al. Etiology, clinical characteristics and prognosis of spontaneous intracerebral hemorrhage in children: a prospective cohort study in China. J Neurol Sci 2015;358(1–2):367–70.

88. Meyer-Heim AD, Boltshauser E. Spontaneous intracranial haemorrhage in children: aetiology, presentation and outcome. Brain Dev 2003;25(6):416–21.

89. Jordan LC, Johnston SC, Wu YW, et al. The importance of cerebral aneurysms in childhood hemorrhagic stroke: a population-based study. Stroke 2009;40(2):400–5.

90. Kumar R, Shukla D, Mahapatra AK. Spontaneous intracranial hemorrhage in children. Pediatr Neurosurg 2009;45(1):37–45.

91. El-Ghanem M, Kass-Hout T, Kass-Hout O, et al. Arteriovenous malformations in the pediatric population: review of the existing literature. Interv Neurol 2016;5(3–4):218–25.

92. Oulasvirta E, Koroknay-Pál P, Hafez A, et al. Characteristics and long-term outcome of 127 children with cerebral arteriovenous malformations. Neurosurgery 2019;84(1):151–9.

93. Pepper J, Lamin S, Thomas A, et al. Clinical features and outcome in pediatric arteriovenous malformation: institutional multimodality treatment. Childs Nerv Syst 2023;39(4):975–82.

94. Ai X, Ye Z, Xu J, et al. The factors associated with hemorrhagic presentation in children with untreated brain arteriovenous malformation: a meta-analysis. J Neurosurg Pediatr 2018;23(3):343–54.

95. Lu A, Winkler E, Morshed R, et al. 196 increased hemorrhage risk with brain AVM-associated aneurysms in children. Neurosurgery 2023;69:32.

96. Dinc N, Won SY, Quick-Weller J, et al. Prognostic variables and outcome in relation to different bleeding patterns in arteriovenous malformations. Neurosurg Rev 2019;42(3):731–6.

97. Zwanzger C, López-Rueda A, Campodónico D, et al. Usefulness of CT angiography for characterizing cerebral arteriovenous malformations presenting as hemorrhage: comparison with digital subtraction angiography. Radiologia (Engl Ed) 2020;62(5):392–9. Utilidad de la angio-TC para la caracterización de malformaciones arteriovenosas cerebrales con presentación hemorrágica comparada con la angiografía por sustracción digital.

98. Li J, Ji Z, Yu J, et al. Angioarchitecture and prognosis of pediatric intracranial pial arteriovenous fistula. Stroke Vasc Neurol 2023;8(4):292–300.

99. Requejo F, Jaimovich R, Marelli J, et al. Intracranial pial fistulas in pediatric population. Clinical features and treatment modalities. Childs Nerv Syst 2015;31(9):1509–14.

100. Lim J, Kuo CC, Waqas M, et al. A systematic review of non-galenic pial arteriovenous fistulas. World Neurosurg 2023;170:226–35.e3.

101. Hetts SW, Keenan K, Fullerton HJ, et al. Pediatric intracranial nongalenic pial arteriovenous fistulas: clinical features, angioarchitecture, and outcomes. AJNR Am J Neuroradiol 2012;33(9):1710–9.

102. Walcott BP, Smith ER, Scott RM, et al. Pial arteriovenous fistulae in pediatric patients: associated syndromes and treatment outcome. J Neurointerventional Surg 2013;5(1):10–4.

103. Linscott LL, Leach JL, Jones BV, et al. Developmental venous anomalies of the brain in children – imaging spectrum and update. Pediatr Radiol 2016;46(3):394–406. quiz 391-3.

104. Abdulrauf SI, Kaynar MY, Awad IA. A comparison of the clinical profile of cavernous malformations with and without associated venous malformations. Neurosurgery 1999;44(1):41–6. discussion 46-7.

105. Jaman E, Abdallah HM, Zhang X, et al. Clinical characteristics of familial and sporadic pediatric cerebral cavernous malformations and outcomes. J Neurosurg Pediatr 2023;32(4):506–13.

106. Zabramski JM, Wascher TM, Spetzler RF, et al. The natural history of familial cavernous malformations: results of an ongoing study. J Neurosurg 1994; 80(3):422–32.

107. Al-Shahi SR, Berg MJ, Morrison L, et al. Hemorrhage from cavernous malformations of the brain: definition and reporting standards. Angioma Alliance Scientific Advisory Board. Stroke 2008;39(12):3222–30.

108. Nikoubashman O, Di Rocco F, Davagnanam I, et al. Prospective hemorrhage rates of cerebral cavernous malformations in children and adolescents based on MRI appearance. AJNR Am J Neuroradiol 2015; 36(11):2177–83.

109. Gross BA, Du R, Orbach DB, et al. The natural history of cerebral cavernous malformations in children. J Neurosurg Pediatr 2016;17(2):123–8.

110. Gross BA, Du R. Hemorrhage from cerebral cavernous malformations: a systematic pooled analysis. J Neurosurg 2017;126(4):1079–87.

111. Flemming KD, Kumar S, Brown RD, et al. Predictors of initial presentation with hemorrhage in patients with cavernous malformations. World Neurosurg 2020;133:e767–73.

112. Jeon JS, Kim JE, Chung YS, et al. A risk factor analysis of prospective symptomatic haemorrhage in adult patients with cerebral cavernous malformation. J Neurol Neurosurg Psychiatry 2014;85(12): 1366–70.

113. Santos AN, Rauschenbach L, Saban D, et al. Natural course of cerebral cavernous malformations in children: a five-year follow-up study. Stroke 2022;53(3):817–24.

114. Paddock M, Lanham S, Gill K, et al. Pediatric cerebral cavernous malformations. Pediatr Neurol 2021;116:74–83.

115. Hetts SW, Narvid J, Sanai N, et al. Intracranial aneurysms in childhood: 27-year single-institution experience. AJNR Am J Neuroradiol 2009;30(7): 1315–24.

116. Xu R, Xie ME, Yang W, et al. Epidemiology and outcomes of pediatric intracranial aneurysms: comparison with an adult population in a 30-year, prospective database. J Neurosurg Pediatr 2021; 28(6):685–94.

117. Perry JJ, Stiell IG, Sivilotti ML, et al. Sensitivity of computed tomography performed within six hours of onset of headache for diagnosis of subarachnoid haemorrhage: prospective cohort study. BMJ 2011;343:d4277.

118. Levinson S, Pendharkar AV, Gauden AJ, et al. Modern imaging of aneurysmal subarachnoid hemorrhage. Radiol Clin North Am 2023;61(3):457–65.

119. Heit JJ, Pastena GT, Nogueira RG, et al. Cerebral angiography for evaluation of patients with CT angiogram-negative subarachnoid hemorrhage: an 11-year experience. AJNR Am J Neuroradiol 2016;37(2):297–304.

120. Aeron G, Abruzzo TA, Jones BV. Clinical and imaging features of intracranial arterial aneurysms in the pediatric population. Radiographics 2012;32(3): 667–81.

121. Clarke JE, Luther E, Oppenhuizen B, et al. Intracranial aneurysms in the infant population: an institutional case series and individual participant data meta-analysis. J Neurosurg Pediatr 2022;1–11.

122. Tan AP, Svrckova P, Cowan F, et al. Intracranial hemorrhage in neonates: a review of etiologies, patterns and predicted clinical outcomes. Eur J Paediatr Neurol 2018;22(4):690–717.

123. Xie LL, Jiang L. Arterial ischemic stroke and hemorrhagic stroke in Chinese children: a retrospective analysis. Brain Dev 2014;36(2):153–8.

124. Laurent JP, Bruce DA, Schut L. Hemorrhagic brain tumors in pediatric patients. Childs Brain 1981; 8(4):263–70.

125. Teshigawara A, Kimura T, Ichi S. Critical cerebellar hemorrhage due to pilocytic astrocytoma in a child: a case report. Surg Neurol Int 2021;12:448.

126. Yadav SS, Lawande MA, Patkar DA, et al. Rare case of hemorrhagic brain metastasis from hepatoblastoma. J Pediatr Neurosci 2012;7(1):73–4.

127. Sidi-Fragandrea V, Hatzipantelis E, Panagopoulou P, et al. Isolated central nervous system recurrence in a child with stage IV neuroblastoma. Pediatr Hematol Oncol 2010;27(5):387–92.

128. Gokce M, Aytac S, Altan I, et al. Intracerebral metastasis in pediatric acute lymphoblastic leukemia: a rare presentation. J Pediatr Neurosci 2012; 7(3):208–10.

129. Donofrio CA, Gagliardi F, Callea M, et al. Pediatric cerebellar pilocytic astrocytoma presenting with spontaneous intratumoral hemorrhage. Neurosurg Rev 2020;43(1):9–16.

130. Ge P, Zhang Q, Ye X, et al. Clinical features, surgical treatment, and long-term outcome in children with hemorrhagic moyamoya disease. J Stroke Cerebrovasc Dis 2018;27(6):1517–23.

131. Maldonado-Soto AR, Fryer RH. Reversible cerebral vasoconstriction syndrome in children: an update. Semin Pediatr Neurol 2021;40:100936.

132. Ducros A, Fiedler U, Porcher R, et al. Hemorrhagic manifestations of reversible cerebral vasoconstriction syndrome: frequency, features, and risk factors. Stroke 2010;41(11):2505–11.

133. Hefzy HM, Bartynski WS, Boardman JF, et al. Hemorrhage in posterior reversible encephalopathy syndrome: imaging and clinical features. AJNR Am J Neuroradiol 2009;30(7):1371–9.

134. Chen TH. Childhood posterior reversible encephalopathy syndrome: clinicoradiological characteristics, managements, and outcome. Front Pediatr 2020;8:585.

Pediatric Spinal Vascular Abnormalities
Overview, Diagnosis, and Management

Ali Shaibani, MD[a],*, Anas S. Al-Smadi, MD[a,b]

KEYWORDS

- Hemangioblastomas • Spinal cord hemangioblastomas • Tumors
- Pediatric spinal vascular abnormalities • Syringomyelia • Hemorrhage • Spinal AVM • Spinal AVF

KEY POINTS

- Spinal vascular malformations (SVMs) are broadly categorized into shunting and non-shunting types (e.g., cavernous malformations, ischemia, and aneurysms). Arteriovenous shunts are further classified based on their location, angioarchitecture, and flow patterns.
- Certain SVMs, like spinal dural arteriovenous fistulas, are acquired later in adulthood due to environmental factors, while others, such as Anson-Spetzler Type II and IV malformations, develop in early childhood and are often linked to hereditary conditions.
- SVMs can cause progressive neurological deterioration involving the spinal cord and/or spinal nerves, leading to sensory and motor deficits, pain, and issues with bowel and bladder function.
- MRI is the primary imaging modality for diagnosing SVMs, and this chapter details its role in identifying the specific characteristics of each malformation.
- Treatment strategies for SVMs vary based on the type of vascular malformation and clinical presentation and may include conservative management, endovascular intervention, surgical approaches, or a combination of these methods.

INTRODUCTION

Spinal vascular abnormalities in children are a category of neurovascular conditions that present unique challenges.[1] These abnormalities encompass a diversity of conditions which range from vascular malformations and tumors to spinal cord ischemia and aneurysms (Table 1). Vascular complications caused by these abnormalities can lead to the deterioration of neurologic function involving the spinal cord and/or spinal nerves, resulting in sensory and motor impairments, pain, and difficulties with bowel and bladder control.[2,3] It is therefore crucial for clinicians to have a high level of suspicion and promptly identify spinal vascular abnormalities in children so that permanently disabling neurologic injuries can be prevented. This article aims to provide an overview of spinal vascular disorders by summarizing their presenting clinical symptoms, diagnostic methods, and treatment approaches. Fundamentals of etiology, pathophysiology, and epidemiology that pertain to neuroimaging diagnosis and contemporary treatment strategies will also be discussed.

Vascular malformations account for a significant share of spinal vascular abnormalities encountered in the pediatric population. Similar to intracranial vascular malformations, vascular malformations

[a] Department of Radiology, Neurology & Neurosurgery, Northwestern University Feinberg School of Medicine, Chicago, IL, USA; [b] Section of Interventional Neuroradiology, Department of Radiology, Northwestern Memorial Hospital, 676 North Street, Clair street, Suite 1400, Chicago, IL 60611, USA
* Corresponding author. Department of Medical Imaging, Lurie Childrens Hospital, 225 East Chicago Avenue, Chicago, IL 60611.
E-mail addresses: ashaibani@luriechildrens.org; anas.alsmadi@nm.org

Neuroimag Clin N Am 34 (2024) 637–663
https://doi.org/10.1016/j.nic.2024.08.014
1052-5149/24/© 2024 Elsevier Inc. All rights are reserved, including those for text and data mining, AI training, and similar technologies.

Table 1
Classification of spinal vascular abnormalities

Spinal Vascular Pathology	Etiology	Possible Genetic/Hereditary Association	Pathophysiology	Presentation	Common Presenting Age (years)	Diagnostic Tests
Hemangioblastoma	Hereditary neoplastic lesion	VHL syndrome	Slowly progressive cord compression and acute hemorrhage from aneurysms in the tumor and on tumor feeding arteries	Acute and progressive myelopathy	20–50	CTA, MRI/MRA, DSA
Cavernous malformation	Sporadic or familial vascular malformation	(Table 2)	Repetitive intramedullary bleeding and cord compression	Acute and progressive myelopathy	Adult: 20–50 Pediatric: <18	MRI
Anson-Spetzler Type I; spinal DAVF	Sporadic or acquired vascular malformation	N/A	Spinal cord venous hypertension	Progressive myelopathy, pain	50–70	MRI/MRA, DSA
Anson-Spetzler Type II; Intramedullary glomus AVM	Sporadic or hereditary developmental	RASA1(CM-AVM1) ENG, ACVRL1, and SMAD4 (HHT)	Spinal cord hemorrhage, compression, perfusion steal	Acute myelopathy (hemorrhage), pain, progressive myelopathy	< 25	MRI/MRA, DSA
Anson-Spetzler Type III; Spinal juvenile AVM/Spinal Arteriovenous Metameric Syndrome (SAMS)	Sporadic developmental	Unknown	Spinal cord compression, hemorrhage, perfusion steal, spinal cord venous hypertension	Progressive myelopathy, acute myelopathy (hemorrhage), pain	< 15	MRI/MRA, CTA, DSA
Anson-Spetzler Type IV; Intradural Perimedullary AVF	Hereditary or sporadic developmental	RASA1(CM-AVM1 and PWS); ENG, ACVRL1, and SMAD4 (HHT); PIK3CA (CLOVES); AKT1 (Proteus syndrome)	Spinal cord compression, vascular steal, hemorrhage (SAH, IPH)	Progressive myelopathy, acute myelopathy (hemorrhage)	Pediatric: <18 Adult: 20–50	MRI/MRA, DSA

Anson-Spetzler Type V; Extradural AVF	Sporadic developmental and acquired	Spinal cord venous hypertension, spinal cord and nerve root compression, hemorrhage (EDH)	Progressive myelopathy, pain	Pediatric: <18 Adult: 60s	MRI/MRA, DSA
Vertebral hemangioma	Sporadic developmental	Spinal cord and nerve root compression, hemorrhage (EDH)	Pain, myelopathy, radiculopathy	Incidence increases with age	CT, MRI
Spinal artery aneurysm	Acquired due to hemodynamic stress, trauma, infection or arteriopathy which may be sporadic or hereditary	SAH, spinal cord compression, ASA syndrome	Headache (*most common*), myelopathy	Etiology dependent	CTA, MRI/MRA, DSA
Spinal hemorrhage	Etiology dependent	SAH, EDH, SDH, hematomyelia	Acute headache, cervical pain, acute myelopathy, radiculopathy	Etiology dependent	CT/CTA, MRI/MRA, DSA
Spinal cord ischemia	Etiology dependent	ASA syndrome	Acute myelopathy (lower > upper limbs)	Etiology dependent	CTA, MRI/MRA, DSA

of the spine and spinal cord are broadly differentiated into shunting (arteriovenous) malformations and nonshunting malformations (cavernous malformations, venous anomalies). The vast majority of pediatric spinal vascular malformations (SVMs), whether they are shunting or nonshunting, result from developmental errors affecting the formation of blood vessels within and around the spinal canal. While the exact cause of specific forms of SVM remains largely unknown, the mechanisms have been shown to involve an interaction of environmental factors, anatomic susceptibility, age-related temporal vulnerability, and genetic factors.[4] While some SVMs are acquired late in adulthood with a pathogenesis that is driven primarily by environmental factors (eg, spinal dural arteriovenous fistula), others (Anson-Spetzler Type II and IV) develop in early childhood and are strongly under the influence of genetic factors such as the loss of function mutations expressed in hereditary hemorrhagic telangiectasia (HHT) or the capillary malformation-arteriovenous malformation (CM-AVM) syndrome.[4–7] The genes that are altered in these syndromes play vital roles in angiogenesis and vascular development. On the other hand, Anson-Spetzler type III SVM (A.K.A. juvenile type SVM or spinal arteriovenous metameric syndrome) is a nonhereditary condition related to somatic activating mutations arising in neural crest cells before migration is initiated in the 3rd to 4th weeks of gestation.[8,9] Although our understanding of the interplay between genetics, environment, and development in SVMs is rapidly advancing, further research is necessary to develop targeted therapies for improved patient outcomes.

SPINAL ARTERIO-VENOUS SHUNTS

Spinal arteriovenous shunts (SAVSs) are rare vascular lesions with direct connections between arteries and veins that may be congenital or acquired. Although numerous classification systems for SAVSs have been described, this article will primarily rely on the Anson-Spetzler classification system, which is based on lesion angioarchitecture and flow pattern. In adults, the most common spinal vascular malformation is the spinal dural AVF (A.K.A. Anson-Spetzler type 1 spinal vascular malformation) which is an acquired lesion. In contradistinction to what is observed in adults, a significant majority of pediatric SAVSs are found to be associated with a germline loss-of-function mutation in one of the genes responsible for HHT or CM-AVM syndrome (ACVRL1, ENG, RASA1, EphB4, RASA1).[7] Therefore, genetic screening in children with SAVSs is recommended unless the clinical and neuroimaging findings strongly favor

a nongenetic basis. In particular, spinal epidural AVF may be post-traumatic (see **Fig. 11**). On the other hand, the paraspinal subgroup of parachordal arteriovenous fistulae (AVF) [vertebra-vertebral arteriovenous fistulae], which present in young children, may be congenital or acquired, and acquired lesions may be the result of a genetic arteriopathy such as Ehlers Danlos type IV or Neurofibromatosis type 1.

With the advancements in endovascular therapy, classifications were refined to consider the suitability of treatments based on complexity and location.[10,11] A more recent system proposed by Takai and colleagues considers both location (dural, intradural, extradural) and type (AVF, AVM) and aligns with the widely used Anson-Spetzler classification system (I - IV).[11] This article will focus on the most prevalent forms of SAVSs, emphasizing epidemiology, clinical presentation, imaging, and management approaches (see **Table 1**).

Anson-Spetzler Type I; Spinal Dural Arteriovenous Fistulae

Spinal Dural arteriovenous fistulas (DAVFs) develop when an abnormal connection develops between one or more radiculomeningeal arteries and a radicular vein within the dural sleeve of a nerve root, resulting in retrograde drainage through peri medullary veins and spinal cord venous congestion due to leptomeningeal venous hypertension.[11–13]

Epidemiology and etiology

Spinal DAVFs account for approximately 70% of all spinal vascular malformations in adults presenting between 40 and 70 years of age, with a mean presenting age of 55 years.[10,14,15] Spinal DAVF have a strong predilection for the male sex (4–5:1), and are exceptionally rare in the pediatric population barring extraordinary circumstances.[10,14,15] DAVFs are widely considered to be acquired through a variety of mechanisms with overlapping pathophysiology. Leading models are centered around the concept of the thrombosis and inflammation of radicular veins due to trauma, degenerative disc disease, or infection followed by maladaptive reactive angiogenesis.[13,16] There is only one reported case in the English language literature of pediatric spinal DAVF. The report describes a 16-year-old male with a spinal DAVF arising from nodular fasciitis (myofibroblastic tumor) centered in the right L1-L2 intervertebral neural foramen.[17]

Pathophysiology and clinical features

Arterialization of a radicular vein resulting from direct communication with a radicular artery increases pressure within the affected radicular vein, resulting in a pressure gradient that causes retrograde flow from the arterialized vein into the valveless coronal perimedullary venous plexus and longitudinal spinal veins. This leads to venous congestion, edema, and hypoxemia of the spinal cord. While estimates vary slightly, studies indicate that most spinal DAVFs involve the thoracolumbar spine.[12,14] This could be explained by the relative scarcity of venous channels compared with more rostral spinal segments. This anatomic feature also aggravates the severity of medullary venous congestion in the caudocranial distribution of the radicular vein and explains why myelopathy symptoms correspond to the spinal cord territory drained by the arterialized radiculomedullary vein rather than the territory supplied by the feeding artery of the spinal DAVF.[10,13,18] Hemorrhage is an extremely unusual manifestation of spinal DAVF.[19]

Myelopathy symptoms resulting from venous congestion are typically gradual, progressive, aggravated with physical activity or maneuvers that increase the central venous pressure, and often ascending. These neurologic symptoms commonly include sensory deficits, numbness, and weakness. Back pain with radicular distribution is also common. Aminoff and colleagues reported 19% and 50% of the patients develop severe disability within 6 months and 3 years, respectively. Depending on the extent of cord involvement, individuals may also experience bowel and bladder dysfunction.[13,16,20,21]

Diagnostic imaging

MR imaging is the first-line modality in patients with known or suspected spinal vascular malformations. MRI provides detailed images of the spinal cord and surrounding blood vessels with high soft tissue contrast. On T2-weighted images (T2WI), spinal DAVFs are usually associated with central ill-defined intramedullary hyperintensity and cord expansion related to congestive edema, which involves multiple segments with surrounding prominent and serpentine flow voids that represent engorged perimedullary veins (dorsal > ventral). 3D T2-weighted sequences (CISS or FIESTA) decrease CSF flow artifacts and are better at depicting the congested perimedullary veins compared with standard T2-TSE.[13,22–24] Intramedullary enhancement depicted on contrast-enhanced T1-weighted sequences might be observed in cases of associated arterial or venous ischemia due to the disruption of the blood-cord barrier.[13,23] Contrast enhancement of dilated perimedullary blood vessels may be observed.[23,24] It is important to note that the location of spinal cord signal abnormality and distribution of perimedullary vascular flow voids does not correlate with the level of spinal DAVF. Advanced MRA techniques, including 3D contrast-enhanced MRA (CE-MRA) and 4D time-resolved MRA (TR-MRA), using a large field of view, can provide specific information about shunt localization, directing catheter-directed spinal angiography and guiding treatment planning.[24–26] Time-resolved CTA is another noninvasive method that can aid the localization of larger shunts; however, it is limited for smaller shunts or those with subtle flow abnormalities.[3,26]

Catheter-directed spinal angiography is considered the gold standard for definitive diagnosis of spinal DAVF. This method allows for a real-time imaging of blood flow through the spinal cord vasculature, and is highly sensitive, even for very small or slow-flow fistulae. Catheter-directed spinal angiography accurately identifies feeders and delineates the details of venous drainage, which is essential for planning endovascular or surgical treatments.[3,27] Furthermore, recent advances in 3D rotational angiography (3DRA) and cone beam CT angiography allow for the precise localization of the fistulous communication (arteriovenous shunt zone) and detailed evaluation of the shunt angioarchitecture. This level of structural detail significantly facilitates treatment success for all types of SAVSs.[28–30]

Treatment

For uncomplicated spinal DAVF, the microneurosurgical ligation of the radicular draining vein is very effective. This approach has a success rate of 98% and carries minimal risks of complications.[27] Endovascular embolization offers a minimally invasive alternative with varying success rates (75%–100%).[9]

Anson-Spetzler Type II; Intramedullary or Glomus Type Arteriovenous Malformation

Intramedullary or glomus-type spinal cord AVM (glomus malformations) are rare AVMs that occur within the spinal cord parenchyma and are usually small. They are characterized by multiple feeders from anterior or posterior spinal artery branches with drainage into perimedullary veins (**Fig. 1**).[11,31]

Epidemiology and etiology

Glomus-type AVM accounts for 10% to 20% of SAVSs.[8,12,31] Intradural SAVS is more common in children, contrary to spinal DAVF in the adult population, with glomus type AVM being the most common.[1] These lesions have no sex predominance, with 50% to 65% presenting before age 25 years.[8,19] Glomus-type AVM is associated with hereditary monogenic syndromes such as

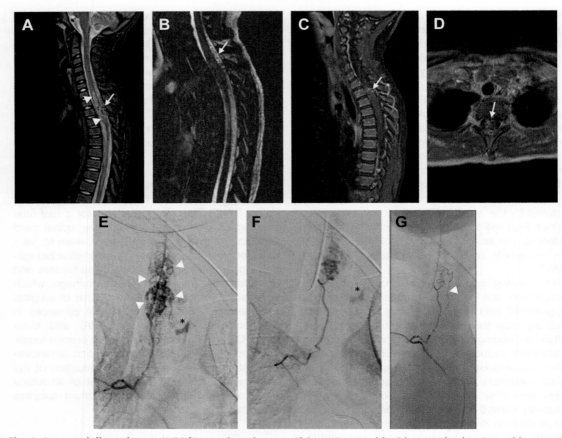

Fig. 1. Intramedullary glomus AVM (Anson Spetzler type II) in a 10-year-old with acute back pain and lower extremity weakness. (*A*) Sagittal T2 weighted image demonstrates a heterogeneously hyperintense lesion in the dorsal aspect of the spinal cord with few intramedullary and perimedullary vascular flow voids (*arrow*) indicative of hematomyelia surrounding an AVM nidus. Note the cord expansion and adjacent cord hyperintensity, which indicates vasogenic edema and/or gliosis/ischemia (*arrowheads*). (*B*) Sagittal high-resolution 3D T2 image shows prominent flow voids at the dorsal aspect of the cord (*arrow*) consistent with prominent draining perimedullary venous plexus. (*C, D*) A sagittal and axial contrast-enhanced T1-weighted image shows the serpentine enhancement of the right eccentric intramedullary nidus (*arrow*). (*E*) Selective right T5 posterior intercostal artery angiogram demonstrating supply to the intramedullary AVM. Additional supply was seen from 2 other pedicles (not shown). The nidus is well-delineated (*arrowheads*). Venous drainage is into perimedullary (*arrow*) and radicular (*asterisk*) veins. (*F*) Selective right T5 posterior intercostal artery angiogram before particle embolization again shows the nidus and an intranidal aneurysm (*arrow*) suspected to be the site of hemorrhage (*asterisk*). (*G*) Repeated right T5 posterior intercostal artery angiogram after particle embolization (500–700 um) demonstrates the good devascularization of the nidus and occlusion of hemorrhagic intranidal aneurysm. Backfilling of a second arterial pedicle is noted (*arrowhead*).

HHT and CM-AVM syndrome in 15% to 20% of the cases.[4,8]

Pathophysiology and clinical features

Glomus-type AVM are true intraparenchymal nidal-type pial AVM characterized by rapid arteriovenous shunting through an angiomatous nidus. The nidus is typically eccentric, partially or completely intramedullary, with multiple feeders and drainage into perimedullary veins.[11,15,31] Associated flow-related aneurysms are seen in 5% to 10% of cases,

which increases the risk of hemorrhage.[32,33] These lesions can also be located in the conus medullaris and along the filum terminale.[34]

Glomus-type AVMs have the highest risk of rupture and hemorrhage among the various SAVS with an estimated risk of 4% per year. Bleeding from a glomus-type AVM is characterized by severe focal pain described as a "dagger stab" and is responsible for 50% to 75% of symptoms, which could be acute or subacute.[8,34] Rebleeding risk after the initial hemorrhage is estimated at 10%

within the first month and 40% within the first year.[10,34] Venous thrombosis is another less common complication of glomus-type AVM. Affected patients present with intermittent or progressive neurologic symptoms, including sensory and motor disturbances, which can be due to vascular steal, or venous hypertension.[10] An overlying cutaneous capillary malformation or "port-wine stain" suggests CM-AVM syndrome. Notably, CM-AVM syndrome may express Anson-Spetzler type II or type IV lesions.[8]

Diagnostic imaging

MR imaging is the cornerstone for the diagnostic evaluation of intramedullary glomus type AVM. T2WI depicts a network of tangled serpentine flow voids consisting of the intramedullary nidus, the feeding artery, and enlarged perimedullary veins. Increased perilesional T2 signal intensity within the spinal cord parenchyma may reflect edema and/or gliosis in the adjacent cord segment. Depending on the size and location of the AVM and the chronicity of parenchymal injury, the involved spinal cord segment may show expansion or myelomalacia which can be appreciated on T2WI and T1WI.[8,12,15] Contrast-enhanced T1WI exhibits variable enhancement of the nidus. Hematomyelia demonstrates varying signal intensities depending on the age of the bleeding.[12] Similar to DAVF, MRA techniques are helpful in evaluating the feeding artery, the nidus, and draining perimedullary venous plexus as well as associated venous ectasias.[22,23]

Catheter-directed spinal angiography remains the gold standard for evaluating spinal cord AVM. It accurately depicts AVM feeding arteries, AVM nidus, AVM venous drainage, spinal cord circulation, and associated hemodynamic derangements, as well as associated flow-related aneurysms and varicosities.[15,35]

Treatment

In cases with a favorable risk-benefit profile, the early treatment of glomus-type spinal cord AVM is favored to mitigate the risk of future hemorrhage and spinal cord injury due to venous hypertension and ischemia. In many cases, however, curative treatment is not feasible due to the high risk of severe treatment-related neurologic morbidity. Consequently, the indications for treatment are often limited to palliative goals, and conservative management by observation is frequently advised. Treatment modalities include endovascular embolization, stereotactic radiosurgery, microneurosurgical resection, or a combination of these. Endovascular embolization is usually considered the primary approach either as a stand-alone or adjunctive presurgical intervention. Collin and colleagues reported in a retrospective analysis that in contradistinction to brain AVM, particle embolization of the spinal cord AVM can be safe and may effectively reduce the subsequent rerupture risk in patients with a prior history of AVM bleeding.[36] In this setting, the goal of endovascular embolization is to minimize the shunt volume rather than accomplish complete angiographic obliteration of the AVM nidus (Fig. 1).[8,9,34]

Anson Spetzler Type III; Spinal Juvenile Arteriovenous Malformation

Juvenile AVM, also known as spinal arteriovenous metameric syndrome (SAMS), are complex extradural-intradural arteriovenous shunts of the spine involving multiple tissue components derived from different primary germ layers of the same embryonic metamere, including spinal cord, nerve root, bone, muscle, and skin. If all components of the metamere are involved, it is referred to as Cobb's syndrome. Different tissue components in discrete AVM compartments receive blood flow from the related division of the spinal segmental artery supplying the affected metamere, with regional differences in venous drainage for different tissue components (Fig. 2).[11,15,31] AVM of the paraspinal tissues and vertebral column are considered a subset of this entity and may drain into paravertebral, epidural, or intradural venous systems (Fig. 3).[37,38]

Epidemiology and etiology

Juvenile AVM are the least common type of SAVS accounting for 5% to 9% of SAVSs overall.[8,15] Similar to cerebrofacial metameric vascular malformations, the somatic activating mutation that leads to the SAMS phenotype is acquired between the 3rd and 4th weeks of gestation.[8,35] Owing to its early developmental origins, Type III lesions are most commonly present in the pediatric population, typically younger than 15 years of age, with slight male predominance (1.7:1).[15] In most cases of SAMS, there is mosaic expression of vascular malformation in affected tissues because some cells carry the index somatic mutation responsible for the SAVS phenotype while others do not. Parks Weber Syndrome (PWS), which involves limb overgrowth, AVM of the extremity, and associated cutaneous capillary malformation also involves mosaic expression of somatic activating mutations, and up to a third of pediatric cases present with SAVS. The SAVS expressed in PWS are Anson Spetzler type II in 50%, Anson-Spetzler type IV in 30%, and paraspinal AVM in 20%. Similarly, CLOVES syndrome, which is a PIK3CA-Related Overgrowth Syndrome (PROS) involves

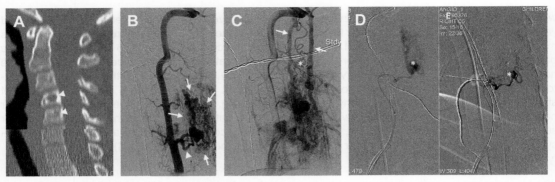

Fig. 2. Juvenile spinal AVM or spinal arteriovenous metameric syndrome (Anson Spetzler type III). A 16-year-old child presented with SAH and hematomyelia. (A) A sagittally reconstructed CT image of the cervical spine shows the bony involvement of the C4 and C5 vertebral bodies (*arrowheads*). (B, C) Lateral view of selective vertebral artery angiogram, arterial phase (B), and venous phase (C), showing the supply of the intramedullary portion of the AVM (*arrows*) by an enlarged radiculomedullary branch of the C6 segmental branch of the vertebral artery (*arrowhead*). Venous drainage extends to the perimedullary venous plexus (*asterisk*), as well as dorsal and ventral median spinal veins (*arrows*). (D) Selective microcatheter angiogram of the radiculomedullary artery shows an intranidal aneurysm (*asterisk*). (D) Selective embolization of the aneurysm with n-butyl cyanoacrylate/ethiodol mixture (n-BCA cast is marked by *asterisk*).

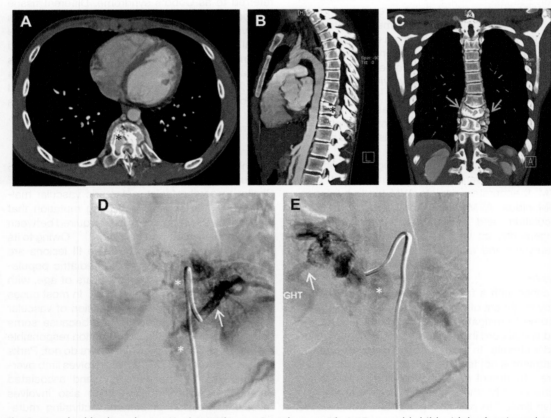

Fig. 3. Vertebral body and paraspinal AVM (Anson Spetzler type V). A 15-year-old child with back pain and radiculopathy. (A, B) Axial and sagittal CTA of the thoracic spine demonstrates prominent intravertebral veins of T8 and T9 vertebral bodies (*asterisk*) and prominent distended epidural venous plexus (anterior internal vertebral venous plexus) (*orange arrow*) causing severe spinal canal and foraminal stenoses. (C) Coronal CTA of the thoracic spine shows enlarged paraspinal draining segmental veins, left more than right (*green arrows*). (D, E) Selective bilateral T8 posterior intercostal artery angiograms demonstrate enlarged segmental feeding arteries and extensive epidural (*asterisk*) and paravertebral (*white arrow*) venous drainage.

mosaic expression of somatic activating mutations and variable expression of SAVS in affected patients (Anson Spetzler type II and Anson Spetzler type IV).

Pathophysiology and clinical features

Juvenile AVM are high-flow lesions, usually located in the cervical and upper thoracic spine, and can be associated with flow-related or intranidal aneurysms.[8,10,19] Symptoms might arise from cord compression, vascular steal, or hemorrhage. The most common clinical presentation is progressive myelopathy in 35%, acute hemorrhage in 31%, and less commonly nonhemorrhagic acute deficits (22%).[15]

Diagnostic imaging

MRI plays a vital role in the initial evaluation of SAMS. T2WI depicts the prominent flow voids of the intramedullary nidus as well as the serpentine ectatic vascular flow voids in the surrounding subarachnoid space, epidural space, and paraspinal soft tissues. Contrast-enhanced T1WI also demonstrates the enhancement of these vascular structures. T2 and T1 weighted sequences also depict compression of the cord by distended extramedullary vascular structures.[8,15,23,35] MRA techniques, including CEMRA and TR-MRA, can better visualize these vascular structures.[23,25] CT angiography is helpful in further detailing the involvement of paraspinal soft tissues and bony spinal elements.[15] Numerous high-flow shunts with rapid drainage into dilated draining veins are characteristic of catheter-directed digital subtraction spinal angiography.[8,15]

Treatment

Juvenile AVM are complex disorders that require detailed treatment planning and a multidisciplinary approach. Achieving complete obliteration is difficult and usually associated with excessive morbidity. Surgery is reserved for decompression of the neural elements and may require multilevel laminectomy for sufficient lesion access. Palliative endovascular interventions are the mainstay for the management of these complex lesions. These interventions are usually directed at the symptomatic component of the malformation with the goal of slowing or halting symptom progression and minimizing neurologic sequelae.[9,15,31,34]

Anson Spetzler Type IV: Intradural Perimedullary Arteriovenous Fistulae

Perimedullary AVFs are pial-based lesions with a monofocal shunt zone involving a spinal cord pial vein supplied by one or more pial feeders originating from the anterior and/or posterior spinal arteries

and drained through perimedullary veins. The characteristic angioarchitecture of the arteriovenous shunt zone is a single-hole or multi-hole arteriovenous macrofistula. There are 3 angioarchitectural subtypes with varying degress of flow[8,11,15,31,39,40].

- *IV-A; represents a small shunt with a single normal-sized or minimally enlarged ASA feeder and only the minimal dilatation of the draining vein. The location of the arteriovenous shunt zone can be difficult to detect angiographically but is generally characterized by the vessel caliber change between the smaller artery and the larger draining vein. This type is typically located at the anterior aspect of the conus medullaris or proximal filum terminale and usually presents in adults (Fig. 4).*
- *IV-B; represents a medium-sized shunt with the moderate enlargement of the feeding artery/arteries and draining veins. The location of the arteriovenous shunt zone is marked by venous ectasia. Associated flow-related arterial or venous aneurysms may be present (Fig. 5). This type is typically but not exclusively located at the conus level.*
- *IV-C; represents a giant shunt with multiple enlarged feeders draining directly into a giant ectatic venous pouch. which secondarily drains into the local efferent veins, which are also dilated. These lesions are typically at the cervical or thoracic levels (Fig. 6).*

Epidemiology and etiology

Anson Spetzler Type IV accounts for 10% to 25% of SAVS shunts among adults and children. These lesions can present at any age with generally no sex predominance; however, slight male predominance was noted for type IVA (1.4:1) and a peak presentation age of 20 to 50 years.[8,15] There is a strong association with HHT and CM-AVM and a reported association with CLOVES syndrome, Proteus syndrome, Down syndrome, and PWS.[4,8,41]

Pathophysiology and clinical features

These lesions, namely types B and C, are high-flow shunts commonly associated with flow-related aneurysms. Symptoms may arise from subarachnoid hemorrhage, spinal cord compression, venous congestive myelopathy, or vascular steal phenomenona. In the pediatric population, the majority of these lesions present with subarachnoid hemorrhage, and a significant minority present with venous congestive myelopathy.[8,15,19,42]

Diagnostic imaging

T2WI depicts the prominent perimedullary venous flow voids typically at the ventral cord surface,

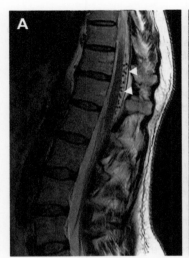
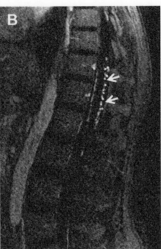
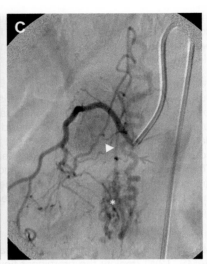

Fig. 4. Intradural perimedullary AVF (Anson Spetzler IV-B). (*A*) T2-weighted image of the thoracic spine shows prominent perimedullary leptomeningeal veins on the dorsal surface of the cord (*arrowheads*). There is no abnormal cord signal. (*B*) Contrast-enhanced T1-weighted image shows the enhancement of the leptomeningeal veins (*arrows*). (*C*) Selective angiogram of the right T12 posterior intercostal artery shows a mildly prominent radiculomedullary artery (*orange arrow*) supplying the ASA (*arrowhead*), which descends in the midline to supply the arteriovenous sunt zone (*asterisk*) which has to ascend venous drainage through an ectatic and tortuous arterialized posterior median spinal vein (*green arrow*).

which contrasts with spinal DAVF. Less frequently observed is hyperintense cord signal and cord expansion related to congestive edema, gliosis, and/or ischemia. Cord compression may be observed due to enlarged, tense perimedullary arterialized venous structures.[8,15,34,35] CTA and MRA may depict single or multiple arterial feeders and delineate the shunt size that aids in shunt classification and management planning.[15,22,25] Catheter-directed spinal angiography is the optimal technique to depict the arterial supply, venous drainage, and arteriovenous shunt zone (usually seen as a point of distinct caliber transition between the artery and recipient vein), possible associated extra-axial nidus, and flow-related aneurysms. The magnitude of arteriovenous shunting increases with subtype order.[15] Arterioectatic spinal angiopathy of childhood, which presents with progressive multi-segmental myelopathy in preschool children, resembles intradural perimedullary AVF complicated by venous congestive myelopathy on the MR imaging of the spine.[43] Definitive diagnosis is made by catheter-directed spinal angiography which shows diffuse enlargement and tortuosity of spinal cord arteries, spinal cord hyperemia, and spinal cord edema in the absence of arteriovenous shunting or venous ectasia.

Treatment

The subtype encountered dictates the preferred management approach. A small AVF with a small solitary feeder (IV-A) is preferably treated by a surgical approach. On the other hand, an endovascular approach is favored for the treatment of larger AVF with larger arterial feeders and larger recipient venous pouches (IV-B and IV-C) (see **Figs. 5** and **6**).[8,9,15,34,44]

Anson Spetzler Type V; Extradural Arteriovenous Fistulae

Spinal epidural AVFs occur primarily inside the spinal canal but may have paraspinal foci of arteriovenous shunting as well. These lesions have one or multiple feeders and can drain into the epidural, vertebral, or paravertebral veins. The arterial supply varies and may arise from radiculomeningeal, radiculomedullary, and bony or epidural branches.[45] Epidural AVFs are divided into subtypes based on venous drainage[11,46].

- *V-A; This subtype has intradural venous drainage, characterized by a vein that travels intradurally and drains into the perimedullary venous plexus (***Fig. 7***).[46]*
- *V-B; This subtype does not have direct intradural venous drainage and is characterized by limited venous drainage into the extradural venous plexus. This can be further subdivided into B1 if there is associated compression and myelopathy by the epidural venous plexus and B2 if there is no radiologic evidence of spinal cord compression.[46]*

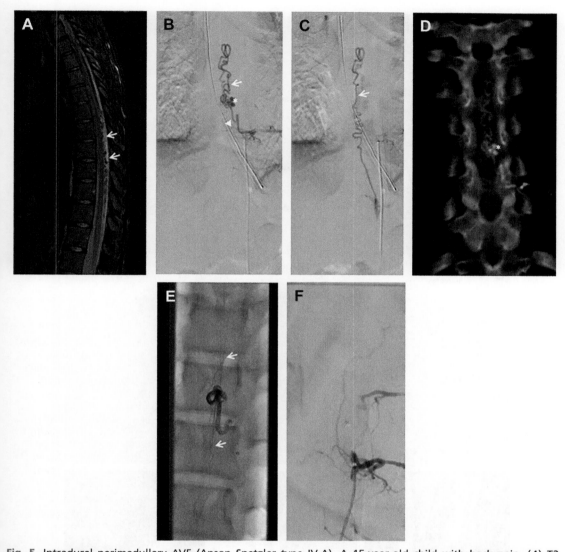

Fig. 5. Intradural perimedullary AVF (Anson Spetzler type IV-A). A 15-year-old child with back pain. (*A*) T2-weighted image of the thoracic spine shows prominent perimedullary leptomeningeal veins on the dorsal surface of the cord (*white arrow*). The spinal cord is normal. *B, C*) Selective angiogram of the left T9 posterior intercostal artery in early arterial (*B*) and late arterial (*C*) phases shows arteriovenous shunt zone (marked by an *asterisk* in *B*) supplied by radiculopial artery (*arrowhead* in *B*) drained by ascending (*arrow* in *B*) and descending (*arrow* in *C*) perimedullary venous segments. There are multiple flow-related aneurysms at the shunt site (*asterisk* in *B* and *D*). (*D*) Coronal reformatted images reconstructed from a 3D rotational angiogram better delineate the shunt zone and the flow-related aneurysms (*asterisk*). The AVF was treated by catheter-directed transarterial embolization with ethylene vinyl alcohol copolymer containing micronized tantalum (EvOH). (*E*) Frontal radiograph of the thoracic spine showing radio-opaque EvOH cast filling the shunt zone, arterial feeder, and proximal draining vein with the obliteration of flow-related aneurysms. Note the small amount of nontarget embolic agent in the left posterior spinal artery (*arrows*). Fortunately, due to the extensive collateral network of the posterior spinal arteries afforded by the arterial vasocorona, the patient's procedure-related foot numbness resolved completely in 3 months. (*F*) Follow-up catheter-directed spinal angiography shows persistent AVF obliteration.

Epidemiology and etiology

Epidural SAVS remains elusive since the literature is primarily based on case reports and limited case series. While these lesions typically present in the 6th decade of life, they are also seen in toddlers, school-age children, and adolescents.[11,46] In the pediatric population, epidural SAVS may be post-traumatic but are frequently idiopathic.

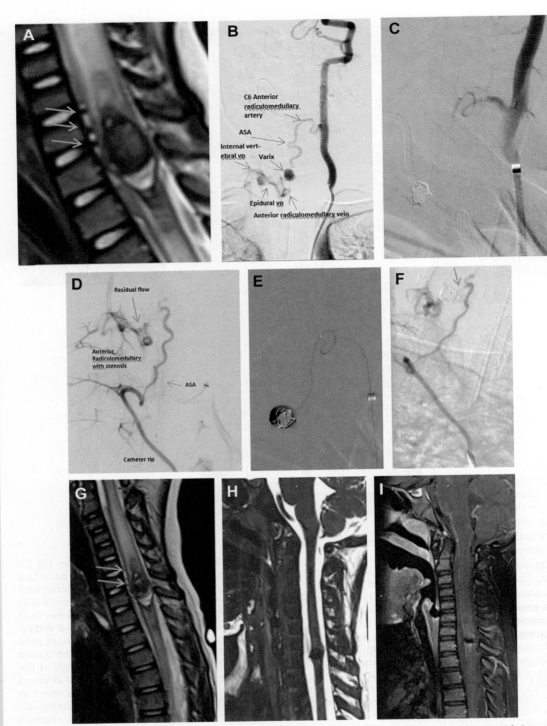

Fig. 6. Intradural perimedullary AVF (Anson-Spetzler type IV-C). A 4-year-old left-handed patient with 2 weeks of progressive lower extremity weakness (3/5) and back pain. The patient had scattered cutaneous capillary malformations and proved CM-AVM hereditary association. (*A*) Sagittal T2-weighted MR of the cervical spine shows intramedullary hemorrhage with edematous expanded cord. Note prominent perimedullary venous plexus flow voids on the ventral pial surface (*Orange arrows*). (*B*) Selective angiogram of the left vertebral artery in frontal projection shows a prominent C6 radiculomedullary feeder artery and shunting into the internal vertebral and ventral epidural venous plexuses. Also, note a prominent varix at the arteriovenous junction. (*C*) Following the

Vertebro-vertebral arteriovenous fistulae (VVAVF), thoracolumbar spinal epidural AVF, and sacral spinal epidural AVF belong to the paraspinal subgroup of parachordal arteriovenous fistulae. The angioarchitectural features of paraspinal parachordal AVF are most similar to type spinal epidural AVF type V-B. In contrast to the branchial subgroup of parachordal arteriovenous fistulae, which are associated with HHT and SAMS, these lesions are frequently associated with arteriopathies characterized by arterial wall fragility including Ehlers Danlos type IV, Marfan syndrome, and Neurofibromatosis type I. Such cases are believed to be related to spontaneous arterial rupture into the peri-arterial venous plexus (Fig. 8).[47–50]

Pathophysiology and clinical features
The majority of type A spinal epidural AVF are encountered in the lower thoracic and lumbar regions. Thoracolumbar spinal epidural AVF may be associated with myelopathic symptoms due to intradural venous drainage and venous congestive myelopathy (see Fig. 7). Type B spinal epidural AVF is more commonly encountered in the cervical and upper thoracic regions. Symptoms vary depending on the presence of mass effect caused by ectatic epidural venous pouches (type B1) (see Fig. 8). Depending on the spinal segments involved, symptoms may include sensory impairment, radiculopathy, motor weakness, bladder, and bowel dysfunction.[11,46] Subjective bruit is the most common presenting symptom of VVAVF, though these may be asymptomatic (30%) or present with neurologic symptoms such as vertigo and paresthesias.[50]

Diagnostic imaging
Type A spinal epidural AVF is often associated with T2 hyperintense cord signal abnormality related to vasogenic edema. Cord expansion and enhancement may be encountered on CE T1-weighted sequence in chronic venous congestion associated with the disruption of the blood cord barrier. Mass effect on the cord is typically demonstrated in type B1 spinal epidural AVF. While type B2 may be difficult to confirm on MR imaging it is well depicted on catheter-directed spinal angiography.[11,46,48] A VVAVF is revealed on MRI imaging

studies as a massively dilated vertebral venous plexus enveloping a vertebral artery that has poor antegrade flow beyond the arteriovenous shunt zone on TOF-MRA.

Treatment
The endovascular approach is the mainstay for the treatment of spinal epidural AVF. For type A spinal epidural AVF, occluding the intradural draining vein is critical to achieving the durable obliteration of the lesion and successful relief of symptoms. Trans arterial and transvenous approaches have been described with a complete resolution obtained in 59% of cases after endovascular therapy compared with 56% with surgical treatment.[11,45,46,48,49]

CAVERNOUS MALFORMATIONS

Spinal cord cavernous malformations (SCCM) are congenital or acquired focal lesions comprising cystic, thin-walled sinusoids partitioned by collagenous stroma, lined by endothelial cells and filled with blood in various stages of thrombus formation and organization, without intervening spinal cord parenchyma or blood vessels. These lesions are primarily located within the spinal cord parenchyma but are occasionally found in the dura mater. This entity is not common and is estimated to represent about 1% of spinal vascular anomalies in children.[51,52]

Determining the prevalence and incidence of SCCM in pediatric patients poses several challenges. The fact that patients often do not exhibit symptoms makes diagnosis difficult. In some cases, symptoms may only become noticeable when there is bleeding, which can lead to underdiagnosis in less severe instances.[53] The presence of an underestimation bias likely contributes to the discrepancies that have been observed across various studies. It is important to note that pediatric patients diagnosed with familial cavernous malformations (FCCMs) have a significantly higher chance of also having spinal cord lesions with an estimated prevalence as high as 72.4% in some studies.[54] Hence, taking into account family history, presentation, and age becomes crucial when evaluating children for SCCM.

---

coil embolization of the varix there is no residual supply from the C6 feeding artery. However, microcatheter injection in the varix (not shown) revealed residual flow. (D) Selective angiogram of the right 3rd segmental artery shows residual flow to varix. (E) Microcatheter placed in the varix followed by controlled EvOH embolization. (F) Postembolization angiogram shows EvOH proximal to the varix (green arrow) with no residual flow. (G) Sagittal T2-weighted MRI of the cervical spine postembolization shows diminished flow voids on the ventral pial surface of the spinal cord (orange arrows). Follow-up MRI after 2 years (H, I) shows residual intramedullary hemosiderin deposition, resolved cord edema, and interval resolution of the previously noted prominent flow voids.

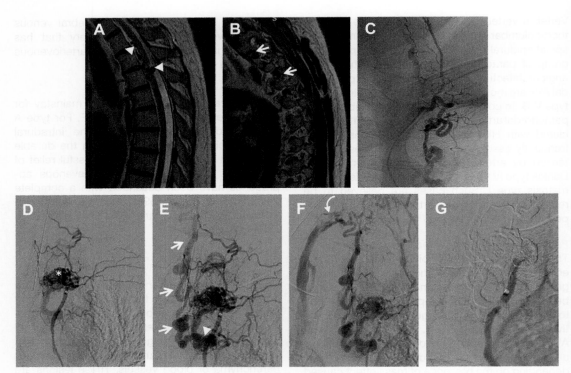

Fig. 7. Paraspinal AVM with perimedullary venous drainage (Anson Spetzler Type V-A). A 56-year-old with back pain and thoracic radiculopathy. (*A, B*) Sagittal T2WI image of the upper thoracic spine shows dilated vessels ventrally and dorsal to the spinal cord (*arrowheads*) and some mass effect on the dorsal cord. Also, note large flow voids in several neural foramina (*arrows*). (*C*) Selective angiogram of left T2 posterior intercostal artery shows markedly enlarged dorsal muscular branch coursing caudally to supply the left paravertebral AVM. (*D–F*) Selective angiogram of left T5 posterior intercostal artery demonstrating supply to the left paravertebral AVM nidus (*asterisk*) which drains into a large radiculomedullary vein (*arrowhead*) which in turn drains to a longitudinal perimedullary vein (*arrows*). This in turn drains out of the spinal canal via a cranially located radicular vein (curved *arrow*). (*G*) Repeat selective angiogram of left T5 posterior intercostal artery post-EvOH embolization demonstrates no residual angiographic filling of AVM.

The annual frequencies of bleeding in SCCM, both in children and adults, vary between 1.4% and 8.2%.[52,55] However, the exact link between these frequencies and the detection of SCCM cases in pediatric patients is still uncertain.

Classification

SCCMs have been categorized based on factors such as their location, appearance, clinical presentation, flow characteristics, and genetic background (as shown in **Table 2**).[56–60]

Clinical Features

Although uncommon, SCCM can present a range of clinical symptoms that are often influenced by the specific location and extent of hemorrhage associated with the lesion. The prevalent manifestations include motor and sensory deficits.[52,58,59] Weakness, clumsiness, and abnormal sensations are frequently observed symptoms.

Pain has been observed in a number of children, either radicular, myelopathic, or a combination of both. Around one-fourth of cases involve bowel and bladder dysfunction, which can manifest as constipation, urinary retention, or incontinence.[59] In instances where there is cervical cord involvement, respiratory failure may occur but at a rate as low as 0.5%. Hemorrhage and rehemorrhage rates are higher in children—8.2% and 30.7%, respectively, compared with 2.8% and 7.4% in adults.[52,61]

Diagnostic Imaging

Magnetic resonance imaging (MRI) is widely considered the gold standard for evaluating SCCM.[62] When viewed on an MRI, blood products at various stages of breakdown often have heterogeneous signal intensities with a "popcorn" appearance on T1WI and[62] well-defined multilobulated appearance on gradient echo sequences.[63] T2 weighted images frequently show a hypointense

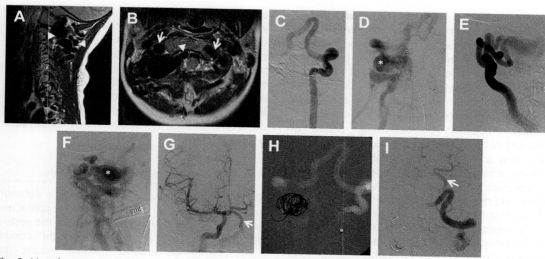

Fig. 8. Vertebrovertebral arteriovenous fistula (VVAVF). An 8-year-old with neck bruit. (*A*) Sagittal and (*B*) axial T2WI images of the cervical spine demonstrating enlarged flow voids in the right perivertebral, posterior paraspinal, and epidural venous structures (*arrowheads*) and enlarged vertebral arteries bilaterally (*arrows*). (*C, D*) Selective left vertebral artery angiogram, frontal projection early arterial phase (*C*) demonstrates diffuse ectasia of the left vertebral artery without the antegrade filling of the basilar artery. The same angiogram shows delayed retrograde flow through the right vertebral artery (*D*) supplying the VVAVF via a shunt zone that features a large recipient venous pouch (*asterisk*). (*E, F*) Lateral projection angiograms of the right (*E*) and left (*F*) deep cervical arteries demonstrating supply to the VVAVF through the same large recipient venous pouch (*asterisk*). (*G*) Right internal carotid artery angiogram shows the retrograde filling of the basilar artery (*arrow*). (*H*) Coils were placed in the recipient's venous pouch via a retrograde transvenous approach. (*I*) Repeat left vertebral artery angiogram postcomplete embolization of the VVAVF, now demonstrating antegrade basilar artery flow (*arrow*).

rim surrounding the lesion, indicating the presence of hemosiderin from prior bleeding.[52,63] While not as common in children as in adults, calcifications can appear as focal signal hypointensities.[63,64] Panda and colleagues described adjacent intramedullary hemorrhage as a frequently associated feature with SCCM, observed in 58% of cases, often with the eccentric and bidirectional distribution.[63]

Susceptibility-weighted imaging (SWI) is highly sensitive for the detection of SCCM and occult bleeding due to its ability to detect subtle traces of extravascular blood products..[65] In some cases, MR angiography (MRA) and Gadolinium contrast may be necessary to rule out other vascular abnormalities.

Treatment

The management of SCCM in children requires a delicate balance between addressing symptoms

---

Table 2
Categories of spinal cavernous malformations

Category	Sub-category	
Morphology	Typical	Homogeneous, single cavity with well-defined borders
	Multilobular	Multiple interconnected cavities with irregular borders
	Mixed	Combination of typical and multilobular features
Location		Most commonly found within the spinal cord tissue itself.
		Situated outside the cord. Within the dura mater.
		Rare cases involving both the dural sac and spinal cord.
Clinical manifestation	Symptomatic	
	Asymptomatic	
Genetic	Sporadic	Most common
	Familial [10%–20%]	Associated with mutations in CCM1 (*KRIT1*), CCM2
	(*mutated gene*)	(*Malcavernin*), or CCM3 (*PDCD10*)

and minimizing the risks associated with micro-neurosurgical procedures. Asymptomatic lesions are managed nonoperatively with periodic MR imaging obtained at intervals according to surgeon preference with the primary goal of detecting asymptomatic disease progression.[66] On the other hand, symptomatic SCCM calls for a nuanced strategy. The main treatment method is microneurosurgical resection or debulking, aimed at removing as much malformation as possible while preserving and prioritizing spinal cord function. Several factors come into play when making treatment decisions, including the location, size, accessibility, and hemorrhage status of the lesion.[67,68] it is important to consider that complete resection may not always be possible, and there is a potential for term neurologic sequelae.[55,68] Ongoing research exploring antiangiogenic medications shows promise and may offer an alternative option in the future for patients who are considered high-risk candidates for surgery.[69]

SPINAL CORD ISCHEMIA

Spinal cord ischemia is relatively rare in children. It is estimated to account for 1% of all ischemic strokes and 5% to 8% of all myelopathies in children and adults.[70,71] In contrast to the epidemiologic patterns observed in adults, whereby spinal cord injury incidence reaches its highest point during young adulthood as a result of trauma, the pediatric population displays a broader range of age groups affected, with the possibility of occurrences even in newborns.[72] This varied the presentation of spinal cord ischemia indicates a wide range of potential causes in pediatric patients, including congenital vascular malformations, cardiac disease, decompression sickness, aortic dissection (type 4 Ehlers Danlos, Marfans, Loeys Dietz) trauma, thoracoabdominal/retroperitoneal surgery (particularly when aortic cross-clamping is involved), anesthetic procedures (epidural anesthesia, intercostal nerve blocks and celiac blocks), fibrocartilaginous emboli, hypotensive shock, Sickle Cell Disease and occasionally infectious or inflammatory processes including but not limited to vasculitides.[72–74] Surfer's myelopathy is increasingly recognized as an important cause of spinal cord ischemia in young athletes who participate in gymnastics, ballet, surfing, trampoline play, and other recreational activities in which the prone spine is subjected to marked hyperextension forces that are capable of stretching the ASA or a major radiculomedullary artery thus causing severe spasm or dissection of the affected vessel. The Gailloud-von Haller syndrome, which results from compression of the artery of von Haller by endothoracic fascia, may theoretically present with spinal cord ischemia in children.[75] Also in theory, an artery of the conus medullaris, which typically arises from a lumbar segmental artery at the L1 through L3 levels may be compromised by the median arcuate ligament. Though there is no sex predilection in the incidence of spinal cord ischemia among children younger than 5 year old, it is noted to be more common in males in older groups[76,77]

Pathophysiology and Clinical Features

The spinal cord is supplied by a midline anterior spinal artery (ASA) and paired posterior spinal arteries (PSA). The ASA arises at or near the vertebrobasilar junction and extends to the conus medullaris in the anterior median fissure. Its caudad flow is reinforced at variable levels by radiculomedullary arteries, which arise from radicular arteries. In the cervical region, these segmental arteries arise from the vertebral and cervical arteries (ascending and deep), with a relatively consistent "artery of the cervical enlargement" at the C4-C6 spinal level. In the thoracic and lumbar regions, segmental arteries arise from posterior intercostal and lumbar arteries. Two large segmental arteries, the artery of von Haller (upper thoracic) and the artery of Adamkiewicz (thoracolumbar) are also consistently noted. The paired PSA shows bidirectional flow, and with the ASA, forms a pial arterial plexus (vasacorona) around the spinal cord, from which perforating arteries penetrate centripetally (penetrating radial arteries) to supply the periphery of the spinal cord. In addition, multilevel sulcocommisural arteries from the ASA penetrate at the anterior median fissure to the center of the cord and supply the gray matter in a centrifugal manner. The ASA essentially supplies the anterior two-thirds of the spinal cord. The pediatric spinal cord has numerous ASA radiculomedullary contributors, which reduce with age to about 7 to 10 in the adult. This abundance of reinforcements to the ASA provides protection against rostro-caudal watershed ischemia or spinal cord ischemia caused by the loss of individual radiculomedullary arteries.

Occlusion of a major radiculomedullary artery or of the ASA results in anterior spinal artery (ASA) syndrome, which is characterized by motor paralysis (corticospinal tracts) with loss of pain and temperature sensation (spinothalamic and spinocerebellar tracts) and occasional autonomic dysfunction (involvement of lateral horns T1 to L2), with the relative sparing of proprioception and vibratory sense (dorsal columns) below the lesion level. Central cord syndrome is a specific type of spinal cord injury pattern, often due to cervical spine hyperextension that causes direct mechanical compression of the spinal cord by the ligamentum flavum and stretching of the ASA. It mainly results in upper extremity paralysis and bladder dysfunction. Posterior cord syndrome, which is rarer, affects the dorsal columns of the spinal cord resulting in ipsilateral loss of fine touch, vibration, and proprioception with or without loss of sensation. This syndrome can result from a compromise of the posterior spinal arteries. Although Brown Sequard syndrome, or hemicord syndrome, can result from occlusion of a central sulcal penetrating artery, it is extremely rare as a manifestation of spinal cord ischemia. Cauda equina syndrome due to vascular compromise presents as severe pain with exercise-induced leg numbness and weakness is also rare.

Although spinal cord ischemia in children is rare, its presentation differs from that in adults. Children with spinal cord ischemia due to major trauma often have delayed diagnosis, up to 4 days after symptom onset in patients without abnormality on spine radiographs.[76] This is compared with adults whose symptoms develop within a few minutes and in whom the diagnosis is usually established early[8,76]. Notably, spinal cord injury without radiographic abnormality (SCIWORA) or obvious spinal disruption is more common among children. This could be attributed to the more elastic spine and more flexible facet joint capsules and ligaments compared with adults.[76,78] The most common site of spinal injury in the pediatric population is the cervical spine (87%), followed by the thoracic spine and the lumbar spine.[76,79] It is important to note that children have a narrower spinal canal, making the anterior spinal artery or radiculomedullary artery more susceptible to compression caused by disc herniation in the setting of trauma.[80] Sensory deficits are less frequent manifestations of spinal cord ischemia in children. Other common symptoms in children include transient "clumsiness" and paresthesias.[76]

Diagnostic Imaging

Diagnosing spinal cord ischemia in children can be challenging since it is rare, and its symptoms as well as neuroimaging features may overlap with those of other neurologic disorders. The primary method used for diagnosis is high-resolution spinal MRI which has high sensitivity and specificity. ASA syndrome is the most common presentation of spinal cord ischemia and is characterized by hyperintensity of the anterior two-thirds of the spinal cord on axial T2-weighted and diffusion-weighted images. The distribution of signal abnormality corresponds to the vascular territory supplied by the ASA (Fig. 9).[72] CT angiography or magnetic resonance angiography may be useful for assessing vasculitis or aortitis. On T1 weighted imaging sequences obtained in the acute phase, the ischemic cord shows expansion and decreased signal intensity. Myelomalacia is a feature of chronic or late-stage ischemia. On T2 weighted imaging, the affected spinal cord is hyperintense more so centrally and anteriorly than peripherally and posteriorly. Typically, the cord lesion is present more than more than one vertebral level. When infarction is predominantly in the watershed zone of the anterior horn gray matter on T2 weighted axial MR images, an "Owl's eyes" appearance has been described. Hyperintense T2 weighted signal abnormality in the medullary bone of vertebral bodies adjacent to the affected spinal cord is a relatively specific feature of spinal cord ischemia. The affected spinal cord will usually demonstrate diffusion restriction in the acute phase and contrast enhancement in the subacute phase. Gadolinium-enhanced sequences are also useful to rule out associated infectious or inflammatory etiologies.[71,72,81,82] Demyelinating lesions are distinguished by a distribution in the peripheral white matter of the spinal cord, a length that extends more than less than 2 vertebral segments, and a width that covers less than half of the cross-section area of the cord. Moreover, the vast majority of demyelinating spinal cord lesions are also associated with intracranial demyelinating lesions. Transverse myelitis is also considered in the neuroimaging differential diagnosis of spinal cord ischemia. Transverse myelitis is centrally distributed and characteristically involves more than two-thirds of the cross-sectional area of the spinal cord, extending more than 3 to 4 vertebral segments. Venous congestive myelopathy should be considered in the differential diagnosis of spinal cord ischemia. The absence of spinal cord diffusion restriction and the presence of dilated perimedullary vascular flow voids related to the underlying vascular malformation helps to distinguish this entity. Finally, spinal cord neoplasm should also be considered in the neuroimaging differential diagnosis of spinal cord ischemia. Spinal cord neoplasia will typically display spinal cord expansion with diffuse or nodular contrast enhancement. Cystic changes and/or peritumoral edema may also be present.

Treatment

The current treatment approach to spinal cord ischemia mainly involves supportive care. The

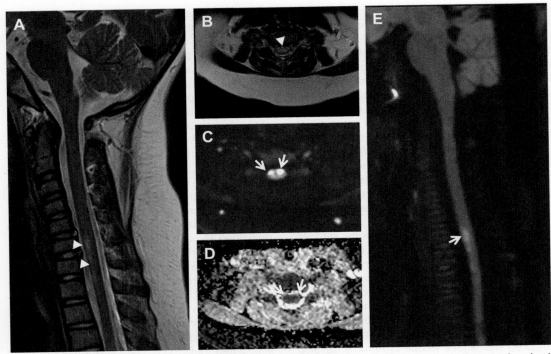

Fig. 9. Spinal cord infarction. A 10-year-old child with sudden-onset neurologic deficit. (*A*, *B*) Sagittal and axial T2-weighted images show long-segment hyperintensity in the ventral cervicothoracic spinal cord (*arrowheads*). (*C*, *E*) Axial and sagittal b1000 DWI images show hyperintense signal in the anterior horns (*arrows*) of the central gray matter of the spinal cord with low signal on corresponding ADC map (*D*), demonstrating the classic "owl's eyes" sign. The pattern of spinal cord infarction is diagnostic of anterior spinal artery syndrome.

medical management strategy focuses on maintaining blood pressure and tissue oxygenation.[76,83] Anticoagulation with heparin or aspirin may be considered in cases with underlying embologenic vascular lesions or coagulation disorders.[72,84] The use of corticosteroids is still debated. They may have some potential to reduce secondary injury; however, there is limited evidence of their effectiveness in pediatric patients.[83] Early surgical intervention is crucial for cases involving neural compression or spinal instability due to trauma. However, it is important to note that there is no robust evidence supporting surgery for cases of pure spinal cord ischemia.[76] Perioperative CSF diversion has been performed to decrease intrathecal pressure and augment spinal cord perfusion during aortic cross-clamping in patients undergoing vascular surgery.[85,86] This has been performed in other settings, though evidence of benefit is lacking. An intensive rehabilitation approach that includes physical and occupational therapy can substantially improve outcomes in patients who have experienced spinal cord ischemia. This approach aims to optimize recovery and address persistent impairments.[72]

SPINAL ARTERIAL ANEURYSMS

Spinal arterial aneurysms (SAA) are rare but serious vascular abnormalities arising on radiculomeningeal, radiculomedullary, radiculopial, or spinal arteries (anterior or posterior).[8,87,88] The actual incidence of SAA in children is not known as the literature is limited to a small number of case reports and case series.[88,89] Venkatesh and colleagues suggested a simple dichotomous classification system that differentiates between Type 1 SAA due to high flow arteriovenous shunts, more commonly found in children (see **Figs. 2** and **5**), and Type 2 SAAs, which are not associated with arteriovenous shunts.[90] In terms of etiology and mechanism, a more comprehensive and inclusive classification system considers six categories of SAA due to: (1) noninfectious/noninflammatory arteriopathy, (2) infection, (3) noninfectious inflammatory vasculitis, (4) trauma, (5) flow-related stress that is either due to aortic coarctation with collateral flow loading or arteriovenous shunting with the flow loading of arterial feeders (**Fig. 10**), and (6) neoplastic aneurysms.[8,33,88,90] Underlying noninfectious/noninflammatory arteriopathies reported in patients with SAA include type 4 Ehlers-Danlos

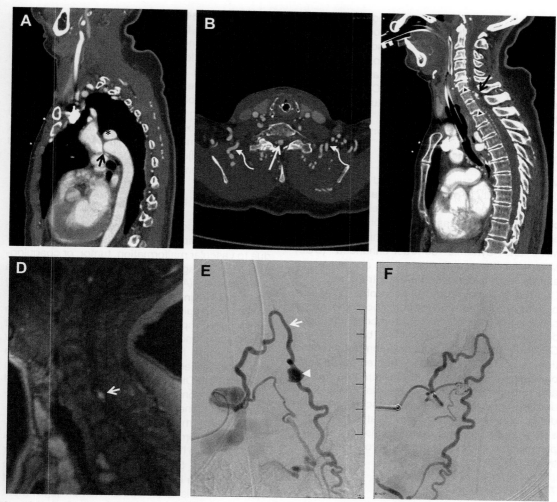

Fig. 10. Spinal arterial aneurysm. A 59-year-old presented with severe neck pain and headache with evidence of SAH and IVH (not shown). (*A*) Oblique CTA chest shows the severe postductal coarctation of the aorta (*arrow*) and adjacent intercostal arterial aneurysmal dilatation (*asterisk*). (*B*) Axial and sagittal (*C*) CTA chest images show the spinal arterial aneurysm at C7 level (*arrow*) with prominent ASA above and below the aneurysm (*arrowheads*). Also, note arterial collaterals to compensate for the coarctation (curved *arrows*). (*D*) CE-MRA of the spine shows the spinal arterial aneurysm (*arrow*). (*E*) Selective angiogram of the right supreme intercostal artery shows an enlarged anterior spinal artery (*arrow*) with a fusiform aneurysm (*arrowhead*). (*F*) Repeat selective angiogram following the coil embolization of the aneurysm while preserving the spinal artery.

and fibromuscular dysplasia. Notably, in cases of idiopathic SAA, undefined arteriopathies lacking recognizable disease markers are presumed to be present. Neoplastic SAA is most commonly associated with hemangioblastoma.

Detecting SAA in children can be challenging due to their unusual location, small size, lack of conspicuity, and technical imaging challenges. These aneurysms are typically smaller than 3 mm and have fusiform morphology.[87,88,90] In patients with noninfectious/noninflammatory arteriopathy, SAA is often found on the proximal intradural segment of radiculomedullary and radiculopial

arteries, whereby these arteries pierce dura. SAA is presumed to have a dissecting mechanism of pathogenesis.

Pathophysiology and Clinical Features

SAA in children, while rare, presents a spectrum of clinical manifestations that may exhibit differences depending on whether they are isolated or associated with an SAVS. Notably, in patients with SAVS, the SAVS dominates the clinical and neuroimaging picture. The vast majority of SAA which are unrelated to SAVS present with SAH in older adult patients.[88,90] Children with isolated SAA tend to experience aneurysmal hemorrhage at a higher rate (92.2%) than those with underlying SAVS (79.2%).[90,91] The location of hemorrhage is predominantly (78%) subarachnoid and less likely intramedullary (hematomyelia).[90] Cranial SAH is reported in 33% of those with ruptured SAA, predominantly in the posterior fossa.[90] Headache is the predominant accompanying symptom.[8]

Diagnostic Imaging

MRI is the primary modality used for diagnosis due to its ability to provide the excellent visualization of the spinal cord, blood vessels, and related complications such as bleeding or parenchymal edema. High-resolution gadolinium-enhanced MRA and dynamic contrast-enhanced (DCE) MRA offer the visualization of the aneurysm sac and its relationship with nearby structures.[8,25,33] Computed tomography angiography (CTA) can provide additional information about the spinal canal, aorta, possible associated conditions, and collateral circulation.[92] However, both CTA and CE-MRA do not offer adequate temporal resolution comparable to catheter-directed spinal angiography. Therefore, catheter-directed spinal angiography is considered the diagnostic standard as it provides unmatched vascular anatomic detail, superior temporal and spatial resolution, and uniquely enables comprehensive treatment planning for endovascular or microneurosurgical treatment.[8,90]

Treatment

Given their complex structure and intimate relationship to critical spinal cord blood supply, SAA poses a major treatment challenge. Treatment may be microneurosurgical, endovascular, or conservative. Some flow-related SAA may resolve after the eradication of the related SAVS, and some infectious SAA may resolve after the underlying infection is resolved. Microneurosurgical clip ligation is usually the approach for aneurysms that are easily accessible, particularly when endovascular strategies involve a high risk of compromising the spinal cord blood supply. Fusiform aneurysms not amenable to clip reconstruction are sometimes treated by wrapping the aneurysm with gauze, or autologous tissue. An endovascular approach may be recommended for some complex fusiform aneurysms.[89,92,93] Both microneurosurgical and endovascular methods aim to exclude the aneurysm from the circulation to prevent bleeding. The choice of treatment approach depends on numerous factors which include the size of the aneurysm, the morphology of the aneurysm (fusiform, circumferential, saccular, combined), the territorial distribution of the parent artery, the diameter of the parent artery, the precise aneurysm location, the aneurysm relationship to surrounding blood vessels, and most importantly, the presence or absence of radiculomedullary or radiculopial supply from the parent artery or its neighboring segmental arteries above and below the index segment. For some aneurysms, conservative management involving monitoring and lifestyle adjustments (ie, blood pressure control) may be considered.[92]

SPINAL HEMORRHAGE

In children, spontaneous nontraumatic hemorrhage in the spinal column is most commonly due to vascular malformation, tumor, or coagulopathy. Hemorrhagic vascular malformations include both shunting (Anson Spetzler types II through V) and nonshunting lesions (cavernous malformations). Hemangioblastoma is the most common hemorrhagic spinal cord tumor. Anticoagulant therapy is the most common form of coagulopathy causing spinal hemorrhage. Spinal hemorrhages can be classified according to anatomic location as epidural (EDH), subdural (SDH), subarachnoid (SAH) (most common), or intramedullary (hematomyelia)[8,94] Spinal hemorrhage related to coagulopathy is most commonly subarachnoid. Vascular malformations may cause hematomyelia (type II through IV), SAH/SDH (type II through V), or EDH (type V). Spontaneous spinal EDH due to bone infarction is also a reported complication of Sickle Cell Disease. Spinal hemorrhage most commonly presents with an acute onset of pain and myelopathy or radiculopathy, but a more insidious course may occur. SDH and SAH may also present with cranial symptoms due to meningeal irritation. EDH may present with radiculopathy due to mass effect.

MR imaging is the first-line neuroimaging study to reveal the distribution of hemorrhage, completed spinal cord/nerve injury, and ongoing potential for additional neural injury, as well as to illuminate the underlying cause of hemorrhage. CT and CTA may play a supportive role in the diagnostic evaluation, as may catheter-directed spinal angiography. EDH is typically lentiform in shape and outlined by epidural fat on MRI (see **Fig. 11**). SDH usually appears as a clumped or lobulated lesion that conforms to the dural sac and which may encase nerve roots. Hematomyelia demonstrates varying signal intensities depending on the bleeding age (see **Fig. 6**).[8,12] Catheter-directed DSA better delineates underlying SAVS, active bleeding following trauma, and hemorrhagic

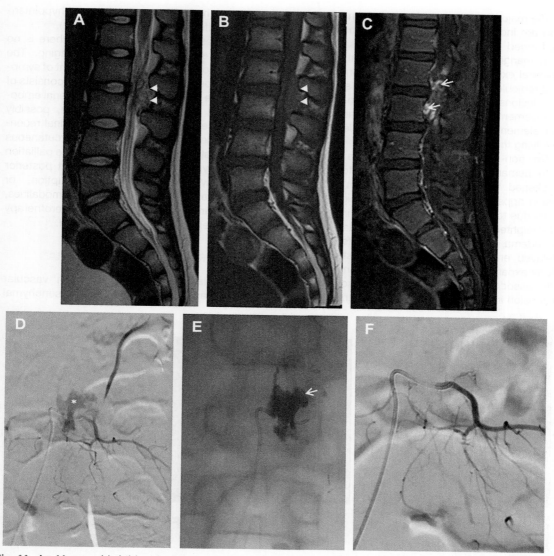

Fig. 11. An 11-year-old child with spinal epidural hematoma following trauma. (*A*) Sagittal T2-weighted image shows heterogenous dorsal epidural collection at L2-L3 level causing the effacement of the thecal sac and severe spinal canal stenosis (*arrowheads*). (*B*) Sagittal T1-weighted image shows epidural collection hypointense to bone marrow consistent with acute hematoma (*arrowheads*). (*C*) Postcontrast T1-weighted image demonstrates heterogenous enhancement surrounding the hematoma and serpentine enhancement within the hematoma concerning active bleeding (*arrows*). (*D*) Selective angiogram of the left L3 lumbar segmental artery shows a fistula between the dorsal epidural tributary of the spinal artery branch and the posterior internal vertebral venous plexus with active extravasation from the venous plexus (*asterisk*). (*E*) Frontal fluoroscopic image of the thoracic spine shows the n-BCA cast following catheter-directed transarterial embolization (*arrow*). (*F*) Selective left L3 lumbar artery angiogram following embolization demonstrates the interval elimination of the hemorrhagic arteriovenous fistula.

tumor blood supply, all of which aid in endovascular and/or microneurosurgical treatment planning.

VERTEBRAL HEMANGIOMA

Vertebral hemangiomas are benign venous malformations of the vertebral bone related to postcapillary vascular dys-embryogenesis.[95] The incidence of hemangiomas is variable, though rare in children and found with increasing age in adults. Around 30% of affected patients have multiple lesions. Vertebral hemangiomas are most commonly present in the thoracic spine.[95,96]

The majority of these lesions are asymptomatic and are incidental findings on MRI examinations performed for other reasons, with less than 1% of hemangiomas becoming symptomatic due to epidural extension resulting in cord compression and radiculopathy.[95–97] The majority of symptomatic lesions are characterized by holo-vertebral involvement, followed by partial body and posterior element/pedicle involvement, and least likely involving the vertebral body alone.[95]

On non-contrast-enhanced CT, the vertebra with hemangioma typically appears to have a thickened trabecula interspersed with fat. The lesion appears hyperintense on T1-weighted images due to high-fat content and hyperintense on T2-weighted images due to fat, vascularity, and/or edema. These lesions demonstrate uniform delayed enhancement on postcontrast images. Bony expansion of the posterior elements is usually associated with extraosseous soft tissue extension into the spinal canal. The extraosseous

soft tissue shows T2 hyperintensity, T1 hypointensity, and uniform enhancement (**Fig. 12**).[96,98,99]

If these lesions are asymptomatic, there is no need for treatment or follow-up imaging. The most common approach to the treatment of symptomatic lesions with epidural extension consists of preoperative catheter-directed transarterial embolization and operative decompression, possibly with the resection of the lesion and spinal reconstruction and stabilization.[97,100,101] Percutaneous vertebroplasty can be considered for the palliation of painful symptomatic lesions without posterior element involvement, cortical disruption, or epidural extension.[102] Other treatment modalities, including direct ethanol injection sclerotherapy and radiotherapy, have been described.[101,103]

SPINAL CORD HEMANGIOBLASTOMA

Hemangioblastomas are true benign vascular neoplasms arising from pluripotent mesenchymal

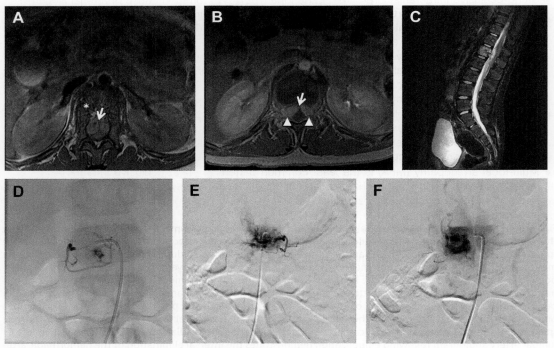

Fig. 12. Vertebral hemangioma with extraosseous extension. (*A*) Axial T1 weighted image of the thoracic spine shows mildly hyperintense vertebral hemangioma with typical prominent trabeculation (asterisk). The lesion involves the pedicles and has extraosseous hypointense soft tissue extension causing spinal cord compression. The posterior longitudinal ligament of the vertebral column causes the typical midline indentation of the epidural mass (*arrow* in *A* and *B*). (*B*) Contrast-enhanced axial T1 weighted image shows the homogenous enhancement of the epidural soft tissue component (*arrowheads*). (*C*) Sagittal T2 weighted image shows a hyperintense vertebral hemangioma lesion centered within the vertebral body with exophytic epidural soft tissue component causing severe spinal canal stenosis. (*D–F*) Selective bilateral L1 lumbar segmental artery angiograms show hypervascular L1 vertebral body with supply from ventral epidural tributaries of the spinal branches. Preoperative embolization was performed.

stem cells that give rise to vascular endothelial cells, and are most commonly found in the cerebellum, spinal cord, brainstem and retina. These tumors may be isolated sporadic lesions or may be associated with hereditary genetic factors in the case of von Hippel-Lindau (VHL) syndrome. Spinal cord hemangioblastomas constitute 1.1% to 2.4% of all central nervous system tumors,[104] with the majority being single tumors that present in the fourth decade of life.[105] In the pediatric population, sporadic spinal cord hemangioblastomas are exceedingly rare. The prevalence of spinal cord hemangioblastomas in children is increased among those with VHL syndrome. The thoracic cord is the most common site for spinal cord hemangioblastomas, followed by the cervical cord. Although these tumors are benign, they cause disabling symptoms due to spinal cord compression, syringomyelia, or hemorrhage from the tumor itself or from aneurysms that form on tumor-feeding arteries or intratumoral vessels.

On MRI studies, hemangioblastomas typically appear as an expansile intramedullary mass lesion that has cystic and solid components. The cystic component of the tumor may be unilocular or multilocular, and the solid component arises from the cyst wall appearing as a mural nodule. On T2 weighted images, the cystic and solid components of the tumor are both hyperintense. Vasogenic edema of the adjacent spinal cord, syrinx formation, and exophytic extension may also be well demonstrated on T2 weighted images. On T1 weighted images enhanced with gadolinium, the cyst walls and mural nodule demonstrate intense homogenous contrast enhancement and are well differentiated from the nonenhancing hypointense cystic component. Additional tumors of the spinal cord, cerebellum, brainstem, and retina should be sought and may be a clue to underlying VHL syndrome.

The primary treatment for these lesions is microneurosurgical resection with curative intent. If it can be performed safely, preoperative embolization may reduce the risk of resection.[104–107]

REFERENCES

1. Song D, Garton HJL, Fahim DK, et al. Spinal cord vascular malformations in children. Neurosurg Clin N Am. 2010;21(3):503–10.
2. Spinal vascular lesions an historical perspective.
3. Da Ros V, Picchi E, Ferrazzoli V, et al. Spinal vascular lesions: anatomy, imaging techniques and treatment. Eur J Radiol Open 2021;8.
4. Hong T, Yan Y, Li J, et al. High prevalence of KRAS/BRAF somatic mutations in brain and spinal cord arteriovenous malformations. Brain 2019;142(1): 23–34.
5. Ustaszewski A, Janowska-Głowacka J, Wołyńska K, et al. Genetic syndromes with vascular malformations - Update on molecular background and diagnostics. Arch Med Sci 2021;17(4):965–91.
6. ISSVA Classification of Vascular Anomalies ©2018 International Society for the Study of Vascular Anomalies Available at: issva.org/classification, Accessed March 14, 2024.
7. Saliou G, Eyries M, Iacobucci M, et al. Clinical and genetic findings in children with central nervous system arteriovenous fistulas. Ann Neurol 2017; 82(6):972–80.
8. Vuong SM, Jeong WJ, Morales H, et al. Vascular diseases of the spinal cord: infarction, hemorrhage, and venous congestive myelopathy. Seminars Ultrasound, CT MRI 2016;37(5):466–81.
9. Endo T, Endo H, Sato K, et al. Surgical and endovascular treatment for spinal arteriovenous malformations. Neurol Med -Chir 2016;56(8):457–64.
10. Lizana J, Aliaga N, Marani W, et al. Spinal vascular shunts: single-center series and review of the literature of their classification. Neurol Int 2022;14(3): 581–99.
11. Takai K. Spinal arteriovenous shunts: angioarchitecture and historical changes in classification. Neurol Med -Chir 2017;57(7):356–65.
12. Saliou G, Krings T. Vascular diseases of the spine.; 2016.
13. Krings T, Geibprasert S. Spinal dural arteriovenous fistulas. Am J Neuroradiol 2009;30(4):639–48.
14. Hiramatsu M, Ishibashi R, Suzuki E, et al. Incidence and clinical characteristics of spinal arteriovenous shunts: hospital-based surveillance in Okayama. Japan. J Neurosurg Spine 2022;36(4): 670–7.
15. Kona MP, Buch K, Singh J, et al. Spinal vascular shunts: a patterned approach. In: Am J Neuroradiol 2021;42:2110–8.
16. Koch C. Spinal dural arteriovenous fistula.
17. Chu CL, Lu YJ, Lee TH, et al. Concomitant spinal dural arteriovenous fistula and nodular fasciitis in an adolescent: case report. BMC Pediatr 2022;22(1).
18. Aminoff MJ, Barnard RO, Logue V. The pathophysiology of spinal vascular malformations. J Neurol Sci 1974;23.
19. Rosenblum B, Oldfield EH, Doppman JL, et al. Spinal arteriovenous malformations: a comparison of dural arteriovenous fistulas and intradural AVM's in 81 Patients. J Neurosurg 1987;67.
20. Ma Y, Chen S, Peng C, et al. Clinical outcomes and prognostic factors in patients with spinal dural arteriovenous fistulas: a prospective cohort study in two Chinese centres. BMJ Open 2018;8(1).
21. Aminoff MJ, Logue V. Clinical features of spinal vascular malformations. Brain 1974;97. Available

at: https://academic.oup.com/brain/article/97/1/197/314990.

22. Condette-Auliac S, Boulin A, Roccatagliata L, et al. MRI and MRA of spinal cord arteriovenous shunts. J Magn Reson Imag 2014;40(6):1253–66.

23. Condette-Auliac S, Gratieux J, Boulin A, et al. Imaging of vascular diseases of the spinal cord. Rev Neurol (Paris) 2021;177(5):477–89.

24. Gilbertson JR, Miller GM, Goldman MS, et al. Spinal dural arteriovenous fistulas: mr and myelographic findings. AJNR Am J Neuroradiol 1995;16.

25. Amarouche M, Hart JL, Siddiqui A, et al. Time-resolved contrast-enhanced MR angiography of spinal vascular malformations. Am J Neuroradiol 2015;36(2):417–22.

26. Mascalchi M, Bianchi MC, Quilici N, et al. MR angiography of spinal vascular malformations. AJNR Am J Neuroradiol 1995;16(2):289–97.

27. Kalani MYS, Ahmed AS, Martirosyan NL, et al. Surgical and endovascular treatment of pediatric spinal arteriovenous malformations. World Neurosurg 2012;78(3–4):348–54.

28. Jiang L, Huang CG, Liu P, et al. 3-Dimensional rotational angiography for the treatment of spinal cord vascular malformations. Surg Neurol 2008;69(4):369–73.

29. Li ZF, Hong B, Xv Y, et al. Using DynaCT rotational angiography for angioarchitecture evaluation and complication detection in spinal vascular diseases. Clin Neurol Neurosurg 2015;128:56–9.

30. Sivakumar W, Zada G, Yashar P, et al. Endovascular management of spinal dural arteriovenous fistulas. A review. Neurosurg Focus 2009;26(5).

31. Kim LJ, Spetzler RF. Classification and surgical management of spinal arteriovenous lesions: arteriovenous fistulae and arteriovenous malformations. Neurosurgery 2006;59(5 Suppl 3).

32. Rodesch G, Hurth M, Alvarez H, et al. Angio-architecture of spinal cord arteriovenous shunts at presentation. Clinical correlations in adults and children: the Bicêtre experience on 155 consecutive patients seen between 1981-1999. Acta Neurochir 2004;146(3):217–27.

33. Kramer CL. Vascular disorders of the spinal cord. Continuum 2018. https://doi.org/10.1212/CON.0000000000000595.

34. Causin F, Gabrielli J, Orrù E. Classification and treatment of vascular malformations of the spinal cord. In: interventional neuroradiology of the spine: clinical features, diagnosis and therapy. Springer-Verlag Milan 2013;231–48.

35. Krings T, Lasjaunias PL, Hans FJ, et al. Imaging in spinal vascular disease. Neuroimaging Clin N Am. 2007;17(1):57–72.

36. Collin A, Labeyrie MA, Lenck S, et al. Long term follow-up of endovascular management of spinal cord arteriovenous malformations with emphasis on particle embolization. J Neurointerv Surg 2018;10(12):1183–7.

37. Kitagawa RS, Mawad M, Whitehead WE, et al. Paraspinal arteriovenous malformations in children: case report. J Neurosurg Pediatr 2009;3(5):425–8.

38. Cognard C, Semaan H, Bakchine S, et al. Paraspinal arteriovenous fistula with perimedullary venous drainage. AJNR Am J Neuroradiol 1995;16(10):2044–8.

39. Bao YH. Classification and therapeutic modalities of spinal vascular malformations in 80 patients. Neurosurgery 1997;40. Available at: https://ovidsp-dc2-ovid-com.turing.library.northwestern.edu/ovid-new-a/ovidweb.cgi.

40. Author Information JJ, Mourier KL, Gobin P. Intradural perimedullary arteriovenous fistulae: results of surgical and endovascular treatment in a series of 35 cases the current address for. Neurology 1993;32. Available at: https://ovidsp-dc2-ovid-com.turing.library.northwestern.edu/ovid-new-a/ovidweb.cgi.

41. Abdalla RN, Shokuhfar T, Hurley MC, et al. Metachronous spinal pial arteriovenous fistulas: case report. J Neurosurg Spine 2021;34(2):310–5.

42. Consoli A, Smajda S, Trenkler J, et al. Intradural spinal cord arteriovenous shunts in the pediatric population: natural history, endovascular management, and follow-up. Childs Nerv Syst 2019;35:945–55.

43. Abruzzo T, van den Berg R, Vadivelu S, et al. Arterioectatic spinal angiopathy of childhood: clinical, imaging, laboratory, histologic, and genetic description of a novel CNS vascular pathology. AJNR Am J Neuroradiol 2022 Jul;43(7):1060–7.

44. Lv X, Li Y, Yang X, et al. Endovascular embolization for symptomatic perimedullary AVF and intramedullary AVM: a series and a literature review. Neuroradiology 2012;54(4):349–59.

45. Kiyosue H, Tanoue S, Okahara M, et al. Spinal ventral epidural arteriovenous fistulas of the lumbar spine: angioarchitecture and endovascular treatment. Neuroradiology 2013;55(3):327–36.

46. Rangel-Castilla L, Holman PJ, Krishna C, et al. Spinal extradural arteriovenous fistulas: a clinical and radiological description of different types and their novel treatment with Onyx: clinical article. J Neurosurg Spine 2011;15(5):541–9.

47. Ashour R, Orbach DB. Lower vertebral-epidural spinal arteriovenous fistulas: a unique subtype of vertebrovertebral arteriovenous fistula, treatable with coil and penumbra occlusion device embolization. J Neurointerv Surg 2016;8(6):643–7.

48. Patro SN, Gupta AK, Arvinda HR, et al. Combined transarterial and percutaneous coiling of a spontaneous vertebrovertebral fistula associated with neurofibromatosis Type 1: case report. J Neurosurg 2009;111(1):37–40.

49. Walcott BP, Berkhemer OA, Leslie-Mazwi TM, et al. Multimodal endovascular treatment of a vertebro-vertebral fistula presenting with subarachnoid hemorrhage and hydrocephalus. J Clin Neurosci 2013;20(9):1295–8.

50. Aljobeh A, Sorenson TJ, Bortolotti C, et al. Vertebral arteriovenous fistula: a review article. World Neurosurg 2019;122:e1388–97.

51. Khalatbari MR, Hamidi M, Moharamzad Y. Pediatric intramedullary cavernous malformation of the conus medullaris: case report and review of the literature. Child's Nerv Syst 2011;27(3):507–11.

52. Fiani B, Reardon T, Jenkins R, et al. Intramedullary spinal cord cavernous malformations in the pediatric population. Surg Neurol Int 2020;11.

53. Al-Holou WN, O'Lynnger TM, Pandey AS, et al. Natural history and imaging prevalence of cavernous malformations in children and young adults. Clinical article. J Neurosurg Pediatr 2012;9(2):198–205.

54. Mabray MC, Starcevich J, Hallstrom J, et al. High prevalence of spinal cord cavernous malformations in the familial cerebral cavernous malformations type 1 cohort. Am J Neuroradiol 2020;41(6):1126–30.

55. Badhiwala JH, Farrokhyar F, Alhazzani W, et al. Surgical outcomes and natural history of intramedullary spinal cord cavernous malformations: a single-center series and meta-analysis of individual patient data. J Neurosurg Spine 2014;21(4):662–76.

56. Petersen TA, Morrison LA, Schrader RM, et al. Familial versus sporadic cavernous malformations: differences in developmental venous anomaly association and lesion phenotype. Am J Neuroradiol 2010;31(2):377–82.

57. Liu T, Wang L, Zhang S, et al. Prediction of outcomes for symptomatic spinal cavernous malformation surgery: a multicenter prospective clinical study. Eur Spine J 2023;32(4):1326–33.

58. Tong X, Deng X, Li H, et al. Clinical presentation and surgical outcome of intramedullary spinal cord cavernous malformations: clinical article. J Neurosurg Spine 2012;16(3):308–14.

59. Goyal A, Rinaldo L, Alkhataybeh R, et al. Clinical presentation, natural history and outcomes of intramedullary spinal cord cavernous malformations. J Neurol Neurosurg Psychiatry 2019;90(6):695–703.

60. Cosri~ove GR, Bertrand G, Fontaine S, et al. Cavernous angiomas of the spinal cord. J Neurosurg 1988;68(1).

61. Ren J, Hong T, Zeng G, et al. Characteristics and long-term outcome of 20 children with intramedullary spinal cord cavernous malformations. Neurosurgery 2020;86(6):817–24.

62. Ren J, Jiang N, Bian L, et al. Natural history of spinal cord cavernous malformations: a multicenter cohort study. Neurosurgery 2022;90(4):390–8.

63. Panda A, Diehn FE, Kim DK, et al. Spinal cord cavernous malformations: MRI commonly shows adjacent intramedullary hemorrhage. J Neuroimaging 2020;30(5):690–6.

64. Hegde A, Mohan S, Tan KK, et al. Spinal cavernous malformations: magnetic resonance imaging and associated findings. Singapore Med 2012;53(9):582–6.

65. Ozanne A, Krings T, Facon D, et al. MR diffusion tensor imaging and fiber tracking in spinal cord arteriovenous malformations: a preliminary study. Am J Neuroradiol 2007;28(7):1271–9.

66. Santos AN, Rauschenbach L, Gull HH, et al. Natural course of cerebral and spinal cavernous malformations: a complete ten-year follow-up study. Sci Rep 2023.

67. Ohnishi YI, Nakajima N, Takenaka T, et al. Conservative and surgical management of spinal cord cavernous malformations. World Neurosurg X 2020;5.

68. Lu DC, Lawton MT. Clinical presentation and surgical management of intramedullary spinal cord cavernous malformations. Neurosurg Focus 2010;29(3):1–6.

69. Wüstehube J, Bartol A, Liebler SS, et al. Cerebral cavernous malformation protein CCM1 inhibits sprouting angiogenesis by activating DELTA-NOTCH signaling. Proc Natl Acad Sci U S A 2010;107(28):12640–5.

70. Han JJ, Massagli TL, Jaffe KM. Fibrocartilaginous embolism–an uncommon cause of spinal cord infarction: a case report and review of the literature. Arch Phys Med Rehabil 2004;85(1):153–7.

71. Vargas MI, Gariani J, Sztajzel R, et al. Spinal cord ischemia: practical imaging tips, pearls, and pitfalls. Am J Neuroradiol 2015;36(5):825–30.

72. Nance JR, Golomb MR. Ischemic spinal cord infarction in children without vertebral fracture. Pediatr Neurol 2007;36(4):209–16.

73. Sheikh A, Warren D, Childs AM, et al. Paediatric spinal cord infarction—a review of the literature and two case reports. Child's Nerv Syst 2017;33(4):671–6.

74. Han JJ, Massagli TL, Jaffe KM. Fibrocartilaginous embolism - an uncommon cause of spinal cord infarction: a case report and review of the literature. Arch Phys Med Rehabil 2004;85(1):153–7.

75. Gailloud P, Ponti A, Gregg L, et al. Focal compression of the upper left thoracic intersegmental arteries as a potential cause of spinal cord ischemia. AJNR Am J Neuroradiol 2014 Jun;35(6):1226–31.

76. Wang JZ, Yang M, Meng M, et al. Clinical characteristics and treatment of spinal cord injury in children

and adolescents. Chinese Journal of Traumatology - English Edition 2023;26(1):8–13.

77. Bravar G, Luchesa Smith A, Siddiqui A, et al. Acute myelopathy in childhood. Children 2021;8(11).

78. Bosch PP, Vogt MT, Ward WT. Pediatric spinal cord injury without radiographic abnormality (sciwora) the absence of occult instability and lack of indication for bracing. Spine 2002;27(24): 2788–800.

79. Carroll T, Smith CD, Liu X, et al. Spinal cord injuries without radiologic abnormality in children: a systematic review. Spinal Cord 2015;53(12): 842–8.

80. Weidauer S, Nichtweiß M, Hattingen E, et al. Spinal cord ischemia: aetiology, clinical syndromes and imaging features. Neuroradiology 2015;57(3): 241–57.

81. Morshid A, Al Jadiry H, Chaudhry U, et al. Pediatric spinal cord infarction following a minor trauma: a case report. Spinal Cord Ser Cases 2020;6(1).

82. Kuker W, Weller M, Klose U, et al. Diffusion-weighted MRI of spinal cord infarction. J Neurol 2004;251(7).

83. Bracken MB, Shepard J, Collins WF, et al. Methyl-prednisolone or naloxone treatment after acute spinal cord injury: i-year follow-up data results of the second national acute spinal cord injury study clinical material and methods. J Neurosurg 1992; 76(1).

84. Ramelli GP, Wyttenbach R, San O, et al, Axial Tl-weighted Spin echo (TR 500 Ms; TE 11 Ms) contrast-enhanced magnetic resonance image shows an anterior intramedullary enhancement at the Th5 level consistent with an anterior spinal.

85. Kelly H, Herman D, Loo K, et al. Recognition of significantly delayed spinal cord ischemia following thoracic endovascular aortic repair: a case report and review of the literature. Cureus 2024. https://doi.org/10.7759/cureus.51522.

86. Epstein N. Cerebrospinal fluid drains reduce risk of spinal cord injury for thoracic/thoracoabdominal aneurysm surgery: a review. Surg Neurol Int 2018;9(1).

87. Aoun SG, El Ahmadieh TY, Soltanolkotabi M, et al. Ruptured spinal artery aneurysm associated with coarctation of the aorta. World Neurosurg 2014; 81(2):441. e17-441.e22.

88. Romero DG, Batista AL, Gentric JC, et al. Ruptured isolated spinal artery aneurysms: report of two cases and review of the literature. Intervent Neuroradiol 2014;20(6):774–80.

89. Berlis A, Scheufler KM, Schmahl C, et al. Solitary spinal artery aneurysms as a rare source of spinal subarachnoid hemorrhage: potential etiology and treatment strategy. AJNR Am J Neurosurg 2005; 26(2):405–10.

90. Madhugiri VS, Ambekar S, Roopesh Kumar VR, et al. Spinal aneurysms: clinicoradiological features and management paradigms A systematic review. J Neurosurg Spine 2013;19(1):34–48.

91. Biondi A, Merland JJ, Hodes JE, et al. Aneurysms of spinal arteries associated with intramedullary arteriovenous malformations. I. angiographic and clinical aspects. AJNR Am J Neurosurg 1992; 13(3):913–22.

92. Abdalkader M, Samuelsen BT, Moore JM, et al. Ruptured spinal aneurysms: diagnosis and management paradigms. World Neurosurg 2021;146: e368–77.

93. Tenorio A, Holmes BB, Abla AA, et al. An isolated ruptured spinal aneurysm presents with a thalamic Infarct: case report. BMC Neurol 2021; 21(1).

94. Shaban A, Moritani T, Al Kasab S, et al. Spinal cord hemorrhage. J Stroke Cerebrovasc Dis 2018;27(6): 1435–46.

95. Jayakumar PN, Vasudev MK, Srikanth SG. Symptomatic vertebral haemangioma: endovascular treatment of 12 patients. Spinal Cord 1997;35(9): 624–8.

96. Sekar A, Datta D, Parameshwar Gulla KM, et al. Aggressive vertebral hemangiomas in children. Child's Nerv Syst 2022. https://doi.org/10.1007/s00381-022-05760-9.

97. De Marco R, Piatelli G, Rossi A, et al. Stepwise approach for vertebral hemangioma in children: case-reports and treatment algorithm proposal. Eur Spine J 2022;31(12):3748–58.

98. Sahajwalla D, Vorona G, Tye G, et al. Aggressive vertebral hemangioma masquerading as neurological disease in a pediatric patient. Radiol Case Rep 2021;16(5):1107–12.

99. Cloran FJ, Pukenas BA, Loevner LA, et al. Aggressive spinal haemangiomas: imaging correlates to clinical presentation with analysis of treatment algorithm and clinical outcomes. Br J Radiol 2015; 88(1055).

100. Eichberg DG, Starke RM, Levi AD. Combined surgical and endovascular approach for treatment of aggressive vertebral haemangiomas. Br J Neurosurg 2018;32(4):381–8.

101. Doppman JL, Oldfield EH, Heiss JD. Vascular and interventional radiology symptomatic vertebral hemangiomas: treatment by means of direct intralesional injection of ethanol 1. Radiology 2000; 214(2):341–8.

102. Fox MW, Onofrio BM. The natural history and management of symptomatic and asymptomatic vertebral hemangiomas. J Neurosurg 1993; 78(1):36–45.

103. Bremnes RMMD;, Hauge HNMD;, Sagsveen RMD;, Bremnes RM. Radiotherapy in the treatment of symptomatic vertebral hemangiomas: technical

case report. Neurosurgery 1996;39. Available at: https://ovidsp-dc2-ovid-com.turing.library.north western.edu/ovid-new-a/ovidweb.cgi.

104. Tampieri DMD, Leblanc RMD, Terbrugge KMD, et al. Preoperative embolization of brain and spinal hemangioblastomas. Neurosurgery 1993;33. Available at: https://ovidsp-dc2-ovid-com.turing.library.north western.edu/ovid-new-a/ovidweb.cgi.

105. Ueba T, Hiroshi ABE, Matsumoto J, et al. Efficacy of indocyanine green videography and real-time evaluation by FLOW 800 in the resection of a spinal cord hemangioblastoma in a child: case report. J Neurosurg Pediatr 2012;9(4):428–31.

106. Eskridge JM, Mcauliffe W, Harris B, et al. Preoperative endovascular embolization of craniospinal hemangioblastomas. AJNR Am J Neuroradiol 1996; 17(3):525–31.

107. Anson JA, Spetzler RF. Interventional neuroradiology for spinal pathology. Clin Neurosurg 1992; 39:388–417.

UNITED STATES POSTAL SERVICE®

Statement of Ownership, Management, and Circulation (All Periodicals Publications Except Requester Publications)

1. Publication Title
NEUROIMAGING CLINICS OF NORTH AMERICA

2. Publication Number
010 – 548

3. Filing Date
9/18/2024

4. Issue Frequency
FEB, MAY, AUG, NOV

5. Number of Issues Published Annually
4

6. Annual Subscription Price
$430.00

7. Complete Mailing Address of Known Office of Publication (Not printer) (Street, city, county, state, and ZIP+4®)
ELSEVIER INC.
230 Park Avenue, Suite 800
New York, NY 10169

Contact Person
Malathi Samayan

Telephone (Include area code)
91-44-4299-4507

8. Complete Mailing Address of Headquarters or General Business Office of Publisher (Not printer)
ELSEVIER INC.
230 Park Avenue, Suite 800
New York, NY 10169

9. Full Names and Complete Mailing Addresses of Publisher, Editor, and Managing Editor (Do not leave blank)

Publisher (Name and complete mailing address)
DOLORES MELONI, ELSEVIER INC.
1600 JOHN F KENNEDY BLVD. SUITE 1800
PHILADELPHIA, PA 19103-2899

Editor (Name and complete mailing address)
JOHN VASSALLO, ELSEVIER INC.
1600 JOHN F KENNEDY BLVD. SUITE 1800
PHILADELPHIA, PA 19103-2899

Managing Editor (Name and complete mailing address)
PATRICK MANLEY ELSEVIER INC.
1600 JOHN F KENNEDY BLVD. SUITE 1800
PHILADELPHIA, PA 19103-2899

10. Owner (Do not leave blank. If the publication is owned by a corporation, give the name and address of the corporation immediately followed by the names and addresses of all stockholders owning or holding 1 percent or more of the total amount of stock. If not owned by a corporation, give the names and addresses of the individual owners. If owned by a partnership or other unincorporated firm, give its name and address as well as those of each individual owner. If the publication is published by a nonprofit organization, give its name and address.)

Full Name	Complete Mailing Address
WHOLLY OWNED SUBSIDIARY OF REED/ELSEVIER, US HOLDINGS	1600 JOHN F KENNEDY BLVD. SUITE 1800 PHILADELPHIA, PA 19103-2899

11. Known Bondholders, Mortgages, and Other Security Holders Owning or Holding 1 Percent or More of Total Amount of Bonds, Mortgages, or Other Securities. If none, check box ▶ ☐ None

Full Name	Complete Mailing Address
N/A	

12. Tax Status (For completion by nonprofit organizations authorized to mail at nonprofit rates) (Check one)
The purpose, function, and nonprofit status of this organization and the exempt status for federal income tax purposes:
☒ Has Not Changed During Preceding 12 Months
☐ Has Changed During Preceding 12 Months (Publisher must submit explanation of change with this statement)

PS Form 3526, July 2014 [Page 1 of 4 (see instructions page 4)] PSN: 7530-01-000-9931   PRIVACY NOTICE: See our privacy policy on www.usps.com.

---

13. Publication Title
NEUROIMAGING CLINICS OF NORTH AMERICA

14. Issue Date for Circulation Data Below
MAY 2024

15. Extent and Nature of Circulation

		Average No. Copies Each Issue During Preceding 12 Months	No. Copies of Single Issue Published Nearest to Filing Date
a. Total Number of Copies (Net press run)		394	371
b. Paid Circulation (By Mail and Outside the Mail)	(1) Mailed Outside-County Paid Subscriptions Stated on PS Form 3541 (Include paid distribution above nominal rate, advertiser's proof copies, and exchange copies)	293	276
	(2) Mailed In-County Paid Subscriptions Stated on PS Form 3541 (Include paid distribution above nominal rate, advertiser's proof copies, and exchange copies)	0	0
	(3) Paid Distribution Outside the Mails Including Sales Through Dealers and Carriers, Street Vendors, Counter Sales, and Other Paid Distribution Outside USPS®	63	49
	(4) Paid Distribution by Other Classes of Mail Through the USPS (e.g., First-Class Mail®)	0	0
c. Total Paid Distribution (Sum of 15b (1), (2), (3), and (4)) ▶		356	325
d. Free or Nominal Rate Distribution (By Mail and Outside the Mail)	(1) Free or Nominal Rate Outside-County Copies Included on PS Form 3541	22	31
	(2) Free or Nominal Rate In-County Copies Included on PS Form 3541	0	0
	(3) Free or Nominal Rate Copies Mailed at Other Classes Through the USPS (e.g., First-Class Mail)	0	0
	(4) Free or Nominal Rate Distribution Outside the Mail (Carriers or other means)	0	0
e. Total Free or Nominal Rate Distribution (Sum of 15d (1), (2), (3) and (4)) ▶		22	31
f. Total Distribution (Sum of 15c and 15e) ▶		378	356
g. Copies not Distributed (See Instructions to Publishers #4 (page #3)) ▶		16	15
h. Total (Sum of 15f and g) ▶		394	371
i. Percent Paid (15c divided by 15f times 100)		94.17%	91.29%

* If you are claiming electronic copies, go to line 16 on page 3. If you are not claiming electronic copies, skip to line 17 on page 3.

PS Form 3526, July 2014 (Page 2 of 4)

16. Electronic Copy Circulation

	Average No. Copies Each Issue During Preceding 12 Months	No. Copies of Single Issue Published Nearest to Filing Date
a. Paid Electronic Copies ▶		
b. Total Paid Print Copies (Line 15c) + Paid Electronic Copies (Line 16a) ▶		
c. Total Print Distribution (Line 15f) + Paid Electronic Copies (Line 16a) ▶		
d. Percent Paid (Both Print & Electronic Copies) (16b divided by 16c × 100) ▶		

☒ I certify that 50% of all my distributed copies (electronic and print) are paid above a nominal price.

17. Publication of Statement of Ownership
☒ If the publication is a general publication, publication of this statement is required. Will be printed in the NOVEMBER 2024 issue of this publication. ☐ Publication not required.

18. Signature and Title of Editor, Publisher, Business Manager, or Owner

Malathi Samayan - Distribution Controller

Malathi Samayan

Date 9/18/2024

I certify that all information furnished on this form is true and complete. I understand that anyone who furnishes false or misleading information on this form or who omits material or information requested on the form may be subject to criminal sanctions (including fines and imprisonment) and/or civil sanctions (including civil penalties).

PS Form 3526, July 2014 (Page 3 of 4)   PRIVACY NOTICE: See our privacy policy on www.usps.com.

Moving?

Make sure your subscription moves with you!

To notify us of your new address, find your **Clinics Account Number** (located on your mailing label above your name), and contact customer service at:

Email: journalscustomerservice-usa@elsevier.com

800-654-2452 (subscribers in the U.S. & Canada)
314-447-8871 (subscribers outside of the U.S. & Canada)

Fax number: 314-447-8029

Elsevier Health Sciences Division
Subscription Customer Service
3251 Riverport Lane
Maryland Heights, MO 63043

*To ensure uninterrupted delivery of your subscription, please notify us at least 4 weeks in advance of move.

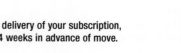

Printed and bound by CPI Group (UK) Ltd, Croydon, CR0 4YY

08/05/2025

01864751-0020

INTERVENTIONAL CARDIOLOGY CLINICS

www.interventional.theclinics.com

Consulting Editor

MARVIN H. ENG

Antiplatelet and Anticoagulation Therapy in Cardiovascular and Pulmonary Embolism Transcatheter Interventions

October 2024 • Volume 13 • Number 4

Editor

Luis Ortega-Paz

ELSEVIER

1600 John F. Kennedy Boulevard • Suite 1800 • Philadelphia, Pennsylvania, 19103-2899

http://www.theclinics.com

INTERVENTIONAL CARDIOLOGY CLINICS Volume 13, Number 4
October 2024 ISSN 2211-7458, ISBN-13: 978-0-443-29672-7

Editor: Joanna Gascoine
Developmental Editor: Akshay Samson

Interventional Cardiology Clinics (ISSN 2211-7458) is published quarterly by Elsevier Inc., 360 Park Avenue South, New York, NY 10010-1710. Months of issue are January, April, July, and October. Subscription prices are USD 224 per year for US individuals, USD 100 per year for US students, USD 224 per year for Canadian individuals, USD 100 per year for Canadian students, USD 317 per year for international individuals, and USD 150 per year for international students. For institutional access pricing please contact Customer Service via the contact information below. To receive student/resident rate, orders must be accompanied by name of affiliated institution, date of term, and the *signature* of program/residency coordinator on institution letterhead. Orders will be billed at individual rate until proof of status is received. Foreign air speed delivery is included in all *Clinics* subscription prices. All prices are subject to change without notice. Orders, claims, and journal inquiries: Please visit our Support Hub page https://service.elsevier.com for assistance.

Reprints. For copies of 100 or more of articles in this publication, please contact the Commercial Reprints Department, Elsevier Inc., 360 Park Avenue South, New York, NY 10010-1710. Tel.: 212-633-3874; Fax: 212-633-3820; E-mail: reprints@elsevier.com.

CONTRIBUTORS

CONSULTING EDITOR

MARVIN H. ENG, MD
Medical Director, Structural Heart Program, Banner University Medical Center, Phoenix, Arizona, USA

EDITOR

LUIS ORTEGA-PAZ, MD, PhD, FESC
Division of Cardiology, Assistant Professor, UF Health Cardiovascular Center, University of
Florida College of Medicine–Jacksonville, Jacksonville, Florida, USA

AUTHORS

DOMINICK J. ANGIOLILLO, MD, PhD
Distinguished Professor, Chair, Division of Cardiology, University of Florida College of Medicine, Jacksonville, Florida, USA

BEHNOOD BIKDELI, MD, MS
Associate Physician, Cardiovascular Medicine Division and the Thrombosis Research Group, Brigham and Women's Hospital, Harvard Medical School, Boston, Massachusetts, USA; Center for Outcomes Research and Evaluation, Yale New Haven Hospital, New Haven, Connecticut, USA; Cardiovascular Research Foundation, New York, New York, USA

MARC P. BONACA, MD, MPH
Executive Director, CPC Clinical Research, Division of Cardiology, Professor, Department of Medicine, University of Colorado School of Medicine, Aurora, Colorado, USA

SALVATORE BRUGALETTA, MD, PhD
Interventional Cardiologist, Hospital Clínic, Cardiovascular Clinic Institute, Institut d'Investigacions Biomèdiques August Pi i Sunyer (IDIBAPS), University of Barcelona, Barcelona, Spain

FEDERICA BUONGIORNO, MD
Senior Researcher, Department of Advanced Biomedical Sciences, Federico II University of Naples, Naples, Italy

MARIO ENRICO CANONICO, MD, PhD
Clinician Scientist, CPC Clinical Research, Post Doctoral Fellow, Division of Cardiology, Department of Medicine, University of Colorado School of Medicine, Aurora, Colorado, USA

DAVIDE CAPODANNO, MD, PhD
Professor, Division of Cardiology, Azienda Ospedaliero-Universitaria Policlinico "G. Rodolico – San Marco", University of Catania, Catania, Italy

DOMENICO SIMONE CASTIELLO, MD
Physician, Department of Advanced Biomedical Sciences, Federico II University of Naples, Naples, Italy

LARISA H. CAVALLARI, PharmD
Professor, Department of Pharmacotherapy and Translational Research, Center for Pharmacogenomics and Precision Medicine, University of Florida, Gainesville, Florida, USA

CALVIN CHOI, MD
Professor, Director of the Cardiac Catheterization Laboratory, Division of Cardiology, University of Florida College of Medicine, Jacksonville, Florida, USA

PLINIO CIRILLO, MD, PhD
Professor, Department of Advanced Biomedical Sciences, Federico II University of Naples, Naples, Italy

JAMES C. COONS, PharmD
Professor, Department of Pharmacy and
Therapeutics, Center for Clinical
Pharmaceutical Sciences, University of
Pittsburgh, Pittsburgh, Pennsylvania, USA

FRANCESCO COSTA, MD, PhD
Professor, Área del Corazón, Hospital
Universitario Virgen de la Victoria, CIBERCV,
IBIMA Plataforma BIONAND, Departamento
de Medicina UMA, Malaga, Spain;
Department of Biomedical and Dental
Sciences and of Morphological and Functional
Images, University of Messina, Messina, Italy

DOMENICO D'AMARIO, MD, PhD
Associate Professor, Dipartimento di
MedicinaTraslazionale, Università del
Piemonte Orientale, Novara, Italy

ÁLVARO DUBOIS-SILVA, MD
Internal Medicine Specialist, Venous
Thromboembolism Unit, Department of
Internal Medicine, Complexo Hospitalario
Universitario de A Coruña (CHUAC),
Universidade da Coruña (UDC), Hospital at
Home and Palliative Care Department,
Complexo Hospitalario Universitario de A
Coruña (CHUAC), A Coruña, Spain

GIOVANNI ESPOSITO, MD, PhD
Associate Professor, Department of Advanced
Biomedical Sciences, Federico II University of
Naples, Naples, Italy

DOMENICO FLORIMONTE, MD
Department of Advanced Biomedical
Sciences, Federico II University of Naples,
Naples, Italy

IMMA FORZANO, MD
Cardiology Resident, Department of
Advanced Biomedical Sciences, Federico II
University of Naples, Naples, Italy

ROBERTO GALEA, MD
Research Associate, Department of
Cardiology, Inselspital, Bern University
Hospital, University of Bern, Consultant
Interventional Cardiologist, Research
Associate, Cardiology Department, Bern
University Hospital, Bern, Switzerland

MATTIA GALLI, MD, PhD
Interventional Cardiologist, Maria Cecilia
Hospital, GVM Care & Research, Cotignola,
Ravenna, Italy

GIUSEPPE GARGIULO, MD, PhD
Associate Professor of Cardiology,
Department of Advanced Biomedical
Sciences, Federico II University of Naples,
Naples, Italy

TOBIAS GEISLER, MD
Professor, Vice Head of the Department,
Department of Cardiology and Angiology,
University Hospital Tübingen, Tübingen,
Germany

DANIELE GIACOPPO, MD, PhD
Interventional Cardiologist, Department of
General Surgery and Medical-Surgical
Specialties, University of Catania, Catania,
Italy

GIUSEPPE GIUGLIANO, MD, PhD
Associate Professor, Department of Advanced
Biomedical Sciences, Federico II University of
Naples, Naples, Italy

TOBIAS HARM, MD
Resident Physician, Department of Cardiology
and Angiology, University Hospital Tübingen,
Tübingen, Germany

CONNIE N. HESS, MD, MHS
Clinician Scientist, CPC Clinical Research,
Division of Cardiology, Associate Professor,
Department of Medicine, University of
Colorado School of Medicine, Aurora,
Colorado, USA

JOSE IGNACIO LARRUBIA VALLE, MD
Cardiologist, Unidad de Gestión Clínica de
Cardiología, Hospital Regional Universitario
de Malaga, Malaga, Spain

MADELINE K MAHOWALD, MD
Assistant Professor of Medicine, Division of
Cardiology, University of Florida College of
Medicine, Jacksonville, Florida, USA

LINA MANZI, MD
Department of Advanced Biomedical
Sciences, Federico II University of Naples,
Naples, Italy

PLACIDO MARIA MAZZONE, MD
Division of Cardiology, Azienda Ospedaliero-
Universitaria Policlinico "G. Rodolico – San
Marco" University of Catania, Catania, Italy

KARIN ANNE LYDIA MUELLER, MD
Managing Senior Physician of the
Department, Department of Cardiology and

Angiology, University Hospital Tübingen,
Tübingen, Germany

ROBERTA PAOLILLO, PhD
Department of Advanced Biomedical
Sciences, Federico II University of Naples,
Naples, Italy

LORENZ RÄBER, MD, PhD
Director Catheterization Laboratory,
Extraordinary Professor, Department of
Cardiology, Inselspital, Bern University
Hospital, University of Bern, Professor,
Cardiology Department, Bern University
Hospital, Bern, Switzerland

RICCARDO RINALDI, MD
Cardiologist, Hospital Clínic, Cardiovascular
Clinic Institute, Institut d'Investigacions
Biomèdiques August Pi i Sunyer (IDIBAPS),
University of Barcelona, Barcelona, Spain;
Department of Cardiovascular and Pulmonary
Sciences, Catholic University of the Sacred
Heart, Rome, Italy

ANDREA RUBERTI, MD
Interventional Cardiology Fellow, Hospital
Clínic, Cardiovascular Clinic Institute, Institut
d'Investigacions Biomèdiques August Pi i
Sunyer (IDIBAPS), University of Barcelona,
Barcelona, Spain

ALESSANDRO SCIAHBASI, MD, PhD
Interventional Cardiology, Sandro Pertini
Hospital, Rome, Italy

ERIC A. SECEMSKY, MD, MSc
Director of Vascular Intervention,
Section Head, Richard A. and Susan
F. Smith Center for Outcomes Research in
Cardiology, Division of Cardiovascular
Medicine, Beth Israel Deaconess Medical
Center, Associate Professor of Medicine,
Harvard Medical School, Boston,
Massachusetts, USA

MARCO SPAGNOLO, MD
Division of Cardiology, Azienda Ospedaliero-
Universitaria Policlinico "G. Rodolico – San
Marco" University of Catania, Catania, Italy

LUCA SPERANDEO, MD
Department of Advanced Biomedical
Sciences, Federico II University of Naples,
Naples, Italy

CRISTÓBAL A. URBANO-CARRILLO, MD
Cardiologist, Unidad de Gestión Clínica de
Cardiología, Hospital Regional Universitario
de Malaga, Malaga, Spain

CONTENTS

> Antiplatelet and anticoagulant therapies are cornerstones of secondary prevention in high-risk cardiovascular patients. Whereas in former days the focus was set on effective antithrombotic effects, more recent trials and guidelines placed emphasis on a more balanced approach, thus including the bleeding risk for an individualized therapy. Type, strength, combination, and duration are important components to modify the individual bleeding risk. Novel antiplatelet and anticoagulant agents have shown promising results that might offer safer options in the future for high-risk cardiovascular patients. This review aims to give an overview about established drug target and pharmacologic approaches that are currently in the pipeline.

> The CYP2C19 enzyme metabolizes clopidogrel, a prodrug, to its active form. Approximately 30% of individuals inherit a loss-of-function (LoF) polymorphism in the *CYP2C19* gene, leading to reduced formation of the active clopidogrel metabolite. Reduced clopidogrel effectiveness has been well documented in patients with an LoF allele following an acute coronary syndrome or percutaneous coronary intervention. Prasugrel or ticagrelor is recommended in those with an LoF allele as neither is affected by *CYP2C19* genotype. Although data demonstrate improved outcomes with a *CYP2C19*-guided approach to P2Y$_{12}$ inhibitor selection, genotyping has not yet been widely adopted in clinical practice.

> Percutaneous coronary and structural heart interventions are increasingly preferred over cardiac surgery due to reduced rates of periprocedural complications and faster recovery but often require postprocedural antithrombotic therapy for the prevention of local thrombotic events. Antithrombotic therapy is inevitably associated with increased bleeding, the extent of which is proportional to the number, duration, and potency of the antithrombotic agents used. Bleeding complications have important clinical implications, which may outweigh the expected benefit of reducing thrombotic events. Herein, we provide a comprehensive description of the classification and clinical relevance of high bleeding risk in patients undergoing coronary and structural heart interventions.

The antithrombotic management of chronic coronary syndrome (CCS) involves a 6-month course of dual antiplatelet therapy (DAPT), followed by chronic aspirin therapy. In patients with a baseline indication for anticoagulation, a variable duration of triple antithrombotic therapy is administered, followed by dual antithrombotic therapy until the sixth month post-percutaneous coronary intervention (PCI), and ultimately a transition to chronic anticoagulation. However, advancements in stent technology reducing the risk of stent thrombosis and a growing focus on the impact of bleeding on prognosis have prompted the development of new therapeutic strategies. These strategies aim to enhance protection against ischemic events in the initial stages after PCI while mitigating the risk of bleeding in the long term. This article delineates the therapeutic strategies outlined in European and American guidelines for CCS management, with special attention to investigational strategies.

Early mechanical reperfusion, primarily via percutaneous coronary intervention, combined with timely antithrombotic drug administration, constitutes the main approach for managing acute coronary syndrome (ACS). Clinicians have access to a variety of antithrombotic agents, necessitating careful selection to balance reducing thrombotic events against increased bleeding risks. This review offers a comprehensive update on current antithrombotic therapy in ACS, emphasizing the need for individualized treatment strategies.

Managing antithrombotic therapy in patients undergoing complex and high-risk in indicated patients, including those treated with complex percutaneous coronary intervention (PCI) or presenting with cardiogenic shock (CS), is challenging. This review highlights the critical role of antithrombotic therapy, during and after PCI, to optimize the efficacy while minimizing risks. Unfractionated heparin remains the mainstay anticoagulant for complex PCI and CS, with bivalirudin as a potential safer alternative. Cangrelor offers consistent antiplatelet effects, especially when timely absorption of oral agents is uncertain.

Dual antiplatelet therapy with aspirin and a P2Y12 inhibitor is fundamental in all patients undergoing percutaneous coronary intervention (PCI) to prevent coronary thrombosis. In patients with atrial fibrillation (AF), an oral anticoagulant gives protection against ischemic stroke or systemic embolism. AF-PCI patients are at high bleeding risk and decision-making regarding the optimal antithrombotic therapy remains challenging. Dual antithrombotic therapy (DAT) has been shown to reduce bleeding events but at the cost of a higher risk of stent thrombosis. Further studies are needed to clarify the optimal duration of triple antithrombotic therapy (TAT) or DAT and the role of more potent antiplatelet drugs.

Percutaneous left atrial appendage closure (LAAC) is a valid alternative to oral anticoagulation to prevent ischemic stroke in patients with atrial fibrillation. The devices approved in Europe and United States for percutaneous LAAC contain metal and temporary antithrombotic therapy is strongly recommended following implantation to prevent thrombus formation on the atrial device surface. There is still uncertainty regarding to the optimal antithrombotic drug regimen after device implantation for several reasons. Thus, this review aims at summarizing the available evidence and the remaining challenges related to the management of antithrombotic therapy in the context of LAAC procedure.

Patients with peripheral artery disease (PAD) who undergo lower extremity revascularization (LER) are at high risk for cardiovascular and limb-related ischemic events. The role of antithrombotic therapy is to prevent thrombotic complications, but this requires balancing increased risk of bleeding events. The dual pathway inhibition (DPI) strategy including aspirin and low-dose rivaroxaban after LER has been shown to reduce major adverse cardiovascular and limb-related events without significant differences in major bleeding. There is now a need to implement the broad adoption of DPI therapy in PAD patients who have undergone LER in routine practice.

Catheter-based interventions and surgical embolectomy represent alternatives to systemic fibrinolysis for patients with high-risk pulmonary embolism (PE) or those with intermediate-high-risk PE who deteriorate hemodynamically. They are indicated when systemic fibrinolysis is contraindicated or ineffective, or if obstructive shock is imminent. Extracorporeal membrane oxygenation can be added to reperfusion therapies or used alone for severe right ventricular dysfunction and cardiogenic shock. These advanced therapies complement but do not replace anticoagulation, which remains the cornerstone in PE management. This review summarizes the evidence and shares practical recommendations for the use of anticoagulant therapy before, during, and after acute PE interventions.

Antiplatelet therapy is integral to reduce the risk of future ischemic events following acute coronary syndrome (ACS) or percutaneous coronary intervention (PCI); this aim must be balanced by limiting the risk of bleeding. Women with ACS or undergoing PCI have distinct platelet physiology, vascular anatomy, and clinical profiles that can influence the selection of an appropriate regimen. There are procedural techniques that can enhance safety in women. The poor inclusion of women in ACS and PCI trials limits our understanding of the ideal antiplatelet regimen in women, and future studies must find ways to increase the participation of female patients.

ANTIPLATELET AND ANTICOAGULATION THERAPY IN CARDIOVASCULAR AND PULMONARY EMBOLISM TRANSCATHETER INTERVENTIONS

THE CLINICS ARE NOW AVAILABLE ONLINE!

Access your subscription at:
www.theclinics.com

FOREWORD

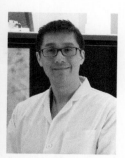

Marvin H. Eng, MD
Consulting Editor

This issue of *Interventional Cardiology Clinics* provides the latest update in the clinical science of using antithrombotic pharmacology in cardiology interventions. Advances in molecular science have pushed clinical pharmacology to new frontiers; however, the classic challenge of balancing the risks of thrombosis with bleeding remains central in treating patients.

The accumulated knowledge from decades of clinical research in antiplatelets, antithrombotics, and interventional patients has produced very nuanced risk models and algorithms for intensity, duration, and combinations of therapies. Beginning with estimating individualized patient risk for bleeding or thrombosis pre-intervention, further estimates must occur during the intervention and afterward. This issue provides a detailed review for this process in chronic stable angina, acute coronary syndromes, peripheral arterial disease, venous thromboembolism, and atrial fibrillation. Risks are further compounded when antiplatelets and oral anticoagulation are combined, and this issue provides the most current clinical science to provide guidance in decision making.

With great pride, we congratulate Dr. Luis Ortega-Paz on completing this comprehensive collection of reviews on interventional pharmacology. This compendium is of the highest caliber and will inform both trainees and experts.

Marvin H. Eng, MD
Banner University Medical Center
1111 East McDowell Road
Phoenix, AZ 85006, USA

E-mail address:
marvin.eng@bannerhealth.com

Intervent Cardiol Clin 13 (2024) xi
https://doi.org/10.1016/j.iccl.2024.07.006
2211-7458/24/© 2024 Published by Elsevier Inc.

PREFACE

Antiplatelet and Anticoagulation Therapy in Cardiovascular and Pulmonary Embolism Transcatheter Interventions

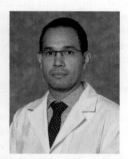

Luis Ortega-Paz, MD, PhD, FESC
Editor

Antiplatelet and anticoagulation therapies are crucial for improving immediate and long-term outcomes in cardiovascular and pulmonary embolism transcatheter interventions. This issue, titled "Antiplatelet and Anticoagulation Therapy in Cardiovascular and Pulmonary Embolism Transcatheter Interventions," explores the evolving understanding of high-bleeding and gender-specific risks, influencing therapeutic decisions. In addition, advancements in transcatheter techniques for structural heart disease, peripheral artery disease, and pulmonary embolism have prompted the development of innovative antithrombotic therapies.

Understanding the mechanisms regulating platelet activation and coagulation is crucial for developing effective and safe therapies. Drs Tobias Harm and colleagues analyzed current concepts and novel targets in this field, highlighting potential new therapeutic options. The genetic determinants of response to P2Y$_{12}$ inhibitors, mainly clopidogrel, are vital for precision antiplatelet management. Drs Larisa H. Cavallari and James C. Coons explore these genetic factors and their clinical implications, offering insights into tailoring treatments to individual patient profiles.

High-bleeding risk has become the major driver of the decision-making process for selecting antiplatelet and anticoagulant therapy in patients undergoing coronary and structural heart interventions. Drs Mattia Galli and Domenico D'Amario discuss the balance between ischemic risk and bleeding complications, emphasizing strategies to mitigate bleeding risks while maintaining antithrombotic efficacy.

Patients with chronic coronary syndromes require tailored antithrombotic therapy to balance benefits and risks. Drs Placido Maria Mazzone and Davide Capodanno discuss the complexities of long-term therapy, integrating the latest data and guidelines. For acute coronary syndrome (ACS), specific timing, selection, modulation, and duration of antithrombotic therapy are crucial. Drs Riccardo Rinaldi and Salvatore Brugaletta provide an overview of current and emerging practices. Patients undergoing complex percutaneous coronary interventions (PCI) and those in cardiogenic shock face unique challenges, including poor gastrointestinal absorption and high-ischemic risk. Drs Jose Ignacio Larrubia Valle and Francesco Costa detail the specialized strategies for these high-risk patients, addressing the limitations of oral medications and available intravenous options.

The intersection of antiplatelet therapy and oral anticoagulation in patients undergoing PCI requires careful consideration of patient bleeding and ischemic risks, alongside a thorough understanding of the pharmacologic profiles of antiplatelet and

Intervent Cardiol Clin 13 (2024) xiii–xiv
https://doi.org/10.1016/j.iccl.2024.07.007
2211-7458/24/© 2024 Published by Elsevier Inc.

anticoagulant agents. Drs Lina Manzi and Giuseppe Gargiulo review the best strategies for managing these patients, emphasizing the importance of minimizing bleeding and ischemic complications. Moreover, percutaneous left atrial appendage occlusion (LAAO) is increasingly utilized to prevent stroke and bleeding in patients with atrial fibrillation. Drs Roberto Galea and Lorenz Räber examine the antithrombotic therapy protocols for patients undergoing LAAO, ensuring effective stroke prevention while reducing bleeding complications.

Peripheral artery disease and pulmonary embolism interventions are rapidly increasing as a less-invasive strategy for the treatment of these frequent conditions, requiring the development of new specialized antithrombotic management. Drs Mario Enrico Canonico and Marc P. Bonaca discuss the therapeutic approaches in peripheral artery disease procedures, balancing efficacy and safety. In addition, Drs Álvaro Dubois-Silva and Behnood Bikdeli explore the latest anticoagulant strategies for acute pulmonary embolism interventions, which are critical for patient outcomes and require prompt anticoagulation therapy.

Antiplatelet therapy considerations in women undergoing treatment for ACS or PCI are essential for addressing gender-specific risks and outcomes. Drs Madeline K. Mahowald, Calvin Choi, and Dominick J. Angiolillo provide a detailed analysis of these considerations, promoting optimized care for women.

This issue of *Interventional Cardiology Clinics* serves as a comprehensive resource for interventional cardiologists, bridging the gap between thorough review articles and cutting-edge clinical practices. It offers valuable insights and guidance on managing antiplatelet and anticoagulation therapy in cardiovascular and pulmonary embolism transcatheter interventions, fulfilling its objective to be an essential tool for our readers.

Luis Ortega-Paz, MD, PhD, FESC
Division of Cardiology
UF Health Cardiovascular Center
University of Florida College
of Medicine–Jacksonville
ACC Building, 5th Floor
655 West 8th Street
Jacksonville, FL 32209, USA

E-mail address:
Luis.Ortega@jax.ufl.edu

Regulation of Platelet Activation and Coagulation
Current Concepts, Novel Targets, and Therapies

Tobias Harm, MD, Karin Anne Lydia Mueller, MD, Tobias Geisler, MD*

KEYWORDS

- Coagulation • Antiplatelet therapy • Anticoagulants • Thrombosis • Bleeding
- Personalized treatment • Cardiovascular disease

KEY POINTS

- Antiplatelet and anticoagulant therapies improve outcome in patients with cardiovascular disease.
- Bleeding is the major limitation of antithrombotic treatment regimens and is associated with an increased risk of death.
- Novel targets of anticoagulants and antiplatelet drugs offer compelling perspectives to attenuate both, the thromboischemic and bleeding risk.
- Personalized antithrombotic therapy aims to counterbalance the individual risk of ischemic and bleeding events.

INDIVIDUAL RISK ASSESSMENT OF BLEEDING VERSUS THROMBOSIS, NEED FOR NEW CONCEPTS AND NOVEL TARGETS

Pharmacologic antithrombotic strategies have undergone tremendous advances during the last decade to reduce the thromboischemic as well as the bleeding risk. Antiplatelet therapy is the cornerstone of primary and secondary prevention in atherosclerosis and has been proven to reduce coronary, cerebrovascular, and peripheral atheroprogression and the occurrence of thrombotic events. However, the beneficial, protective effect of antithrombotic agents is counterbalanced by an increase of bleeding risk that impacts the prognosis of cardiovascular patients. Albeit all these advances in clinical standard of care, there still is an unmet clinical need for individual antithrombotic approaches to address bleeding, thromboinflammatory, and ischemic risks. The development of practical and easily accessible risk scores, establishment of consensus definitions to standardize effective treatment, and innovative artificial intelligence (AI) stratification tools could improve current treatment strategies tremendously (**Fig. 1**). Furthermore, the assessment of platelet function (ie, platelet activity, aggregation, and responsiveness) and genetic testing has been evaluated intensively and could be useful for tailored antithrombotic approaches. Moreover, novel strategies also consider the intensity of dual antiplatelet therapy (DAPT) by varying combinations of agents and dose adjustments as well as therapy duration, especially in patients undergoing percutaneous coronary intervention (PCI) or in patients with critical peripheral artery

---

Funding: T. Harm receives research funding from the German Cardiac Society, Germany (DGK) Clinical Scientist Program.

Department of Cardiology and Angiology, University Hospital Tübingen, Germany

* Corresponding author. Department of Cardiology and Angiology, University Hospital Tübingen, Eberhard Karls University Tübingen, Otfried-Müller-Str. 10, Tübingen 72076, Germany.

E-mail address: tobias.geisler@med.uni-tuebingen.de

Intervent Cardiol Clin 13 (2024) 451–467
https://doi.org/10.1016/j.iccl.2024.06.001
2211-7458/24/© 2024 Elsevier Inc. All rights are reserved, including those for text and data mining, AI training, and similar technologies.

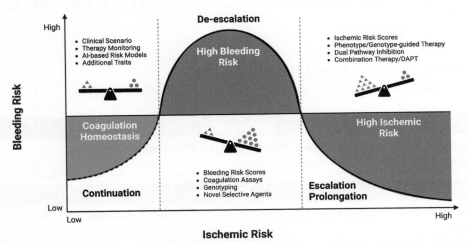

Fig. 1. Risk-stratification tools and personalized antithrombotic strategies in patients with cardiovascular diseases. Importance of integrating characteristics of patients with cardiovascular diseases, an individual risk stratification, and the optimal treatment regimen to defy both, the thromboischemic and bleeding risk.

disease (PAD). Here, the adaption of mono and combination therapy, the implementation of parenteral antiplatelet agents in high-ischemic risk clinical settings, and the combination of antiplatelet agents with low-dose factor Xa inhibition has changed the standard clinical care approach over the last years. This review summarizes currently available evidence and provides an overview of risk-stratification tools and personalized antithrombotic strategies in cardiovascular diseases (see **Fig. 1**).

ROLE OF PERSONALIZED ANTITHROMBOTIC THERAPY

Various tools to establish a risk-associated personalized antithrombotic therapy have been assessed over the years and intensively evaluated in clinical trials comprising platelet activity and aggregation test, or genotyping. Especially individual therapy regimens have been investigated in patients with coronary artery disease (CAD) and acute coronary syndrome (ACS). DAPT, consisting of aspirin plus a potent $P2Y_{12}$-receptor inhibitor, has been recommended for at least 6 to 12 months after PCI/ACS for the last years. Primarily, this recommendation was driven by concerns about the risk of stent thrombosis with drug-eluting stents (DES) rather than addressing pathomechanisms of thromboinflammation and atheroprogression but also did not consider the

individual characteristics and risk profile. More recently, several randomized trials have evaluated the safety and effectiveness of other DAPT strategies regarding the length and/or intensity of DAPT. These strategies comprise short duration of DAPT followed by $P2Y_{12}$ inhibitor monotherapy or platelet function or genotype-guided de-escalation or escalation of $P2Y_{12}$ inhibition. Procedural and technical features in the setting of PCI also play an important role in determining the subsequent ischemic or bleeding risks and should be taken into consideration. De-escalation of DAPT intensity, for example, downgrading from potent $P2Y_{12}$ inhibitor at conventional doses to either clopidogrel or reduced-dose prasugrel/ticagrelor may reduce bleeding without increasing ischemic risk and can be guided by platelet function testing or genotyping. Foreshortening of DAPT duration after 1 to 6 months, followed by monotherapy with acetylsalicylic acid (ASA) or a $P2Y_{12}$ inhibitor could be another approach in patients with high bleeding risk (HBR) but low risk for recurrent ischemia.

To stratify bleeding and thrombotic risk, several risk calculators, prediction tools and assessment models have been proposed over the years (**Table 1**). The PARIS risk model consists of 2 different prediction models, 1 for coronary thrombotic events and another to assess relevant bleeding by Bleeding Academic Research Consortium (BARC). Accordingly, patients can be

Table 1
Bleeding risk scores in patients receiving antiplatelet therapy

	BleeMACS	DAPT	Dutch ASA Score	PARIS	PRECISE-DAPT	Reach
Year	2018	2016	2014	2016	2017	2010
Follow-Up	1 y	30 mo	530 d	2 y	552 d	2 y
Population	ACS patients undergoing PCI	CAD patients 12–30 mo after PCI	New low-dose ASA users	Patients with CAD	CAD patients undergoing PCI	Patients with CAD, CVD, PAD
Cohort	BleeMACS registry (n = 15,401)	DAPT randomized trial (n = 11,648)	Dutch ASA registry (n = 235,531)	PARIS registry (n = 4190)	Pooled analysis of 8 RCTs (n = 14,963)	REACH registry (n = 56,616)
Ischemic Endpoint	-	Myocardial infarction or likely/definite stent thrombosis	-	Myocardial infarction or likely/definite stent thrombosis	-	-
Bleeding Endpoint	Protocol-defined major bleeding	GUSTO moderate/severe bleeding	Upper GI bleeding	BARC 3 or 5 major bleeding	Out-of-hospital TIMI minor or major bleeding	Non-fatal ICH or bleeding necessitating hospitalization/transfusion
Discrimination (AUC)	0.71	0.70 (Ischemic EP) 0.68 (Bleeding EP)	0.64	0.72	0.73	0.68
Validation Cohort	SWEDEHEART (n = 96,239)	PROTECT (n = 8136)	Dutch health insurance cohort (n = 32,613)	ADAPT-DES (n = 8130)	PLATO (n = 8595) Bern PCI registry (n = 6172)	CHARISMA (n = 15,603)
Validation Discrimination (AUC)	0.65	0.64 (Ischemic EP) 0.64 (Bleeding EP)	0.63	0.64	0.70 (PLATO) 0.66 (Bern PCI registry)	0.64
Score Range	0–80	–2 to 10	0–15	0–14	0–100	0–23

categorized into 3 risk groups (low risk: <3, moderate risk: 3–7, and high risk: ≥8 points). Independent predictors of recurrent thrombotic complications included ACS, prior revascularization, diabetes mellitus, renal impairment among others. Most relevant independent predictors of major bleeding included older age, body mass index, concomitant use of anticoagulants, and renal dysfunction.[1] The ARC criteria classify patients to HBR according to minor and major criteria. 2 prognostic models have been developed to identify individual patients' risk of major coronary thrombotic and bleeding events (trade-off).[2,3] Another well-defined, feasible tool is the PRECISE-DAPT score, a 5-item risk score that incorporates age, creatinine clearance, hemoglobin levels, white blood cell count, and previous spontaneous bleeding.[4] This score provides a tool for the prediction of thrombolysis in myocardial infarction (TIMI) major or minor bleeding during DAPT in PCI patients and has been endorsed by current guidelines. The DAPT score was developed from the DAPT trial in patients who completed DAPT for 1 year post PCI without major adverse cardiovascular events or bleeding. Initially, the DAPT score aimed to identify patients who might benefit from extended DAPT up to 30 months without major bleedings. The DAPT score comprises age, present heart failure/low left ventricular ejection fraction, vein graft stenting, recent myocardial infarction (MI), prior MI or PCI, diabetes mellitus type 2, stent diameter less than 3 mm, smoking, and the use of paclitaxel-eluting stents.[5] There are various other alternative scores assessing the long-term bleeding or thrombotic/ischemic risk given in Table 1. Another current AI based approach suggests the establishment of the PRAISE score that aims to predict 1-year all-cause death, MI, and major bleeding derived from large patient cohorts (BleeMACS and RENAMI).[6]

However, there are limitations when using and interpreting these risk scores. One must keep in mind that they are all intrinsically influenced by the characteristics of the study populations used for their development and may not be applicable to the general population or all cardiovascular patients. In addition, there is a large overlap of bleeding and thrombotic risk factors and their validity in real world patients exhibiting both a high thrombotic and HBR remains uncertain. AI learning tools hold the promise to improve predictive model performance and could represent another future game changer in the field of precision medicine.

CURRENT CONCEPTS OF ANTIPLATELET THERAPY

De-escalation (Guided/Unguided) and Abbreviation of Antiplatelet Therapy

Strategies to decrease the bleeding risk comprise guided or unguided de-escalation of DAPT and the duration of antiplatelet therapy can be adjusted and shortened in special occasions.

Short DAPT followed by ASA monotherapy has been extensively explored in large clinical trials regarding risks and benefits in contrast to standard DAPT (Table 2).

Most of these studies revealed that early discontinuation of the P2Y$_{12}$ inhibitor reduces bleeding without a significant increase of ischemic events. However, these studies analyzed predominantly patients with low risk of recurrent ischemic/thrombotic complications and statistical analysis lacked power for major adverse cardiac events (MACE). In clinical perspectives patients with stable atherosclerotic disease without complex interventions and low clinical risk can be treated by short DAPT duration followed by ASA monotherapy to improve prognosis and compliance. Here, we need to mention that also "ultra-short" DAPT durations have been mainly investigated in patients with HBR. These participants received a newer-generation DES platform (Ultimaster, Terumo) in the MASTER DAPT trial among others (see Table 2). In this trial, a 1-month DAPT regimen was non-inferior to standard DAPT.[7] Another strategy proposes short DAPT followed by P2Y$_{12}$ inhibitor monotherapy. For example, clopidogrel monotherapy after 1 to 3 months DAPT was investigated as an alternative to standard 12-month DAPT in patients undergoing PCI in SMART-CHOICE, STOPDAPT-2, and STOPDAPT-2 ACS (see Table 2). Here, clopidogrel monotherapy was non-inferior to 12-month DAPT but a numerical increase in MACE could be a clinically relevant safety issue. Based on current evidence, P2Y$_{12}$ inhibitor monotherapy after an initial short DAPT can be considered as an alternative to standard DAPT, especially when bleeding risk is a concern. In ACS patients, however, early DAPT discontinuation followed by clopidogrel monotherapy may not provide sufficient antithrombotic protection; thus, potent P2Y$_{12}$ inhibitors should remain the agent of choice. The GLOBAL LEADERS trial analyzed a 1-month DAPT followed by 23-month ticagrelor monotherapy versus 12-month DAPT followed by aspirin monotherapy among a large cohort of CAD/ACS patients. However, GLOBAL LEADERS failed to significantly reduce all-cause death and non-fatal Q-wave MI (see Table 2). The TWILIGHT trial

Table 2
Randomized clinical trials evaluating abbreviation or de-escalation of DAPT in CAD patients undergoing PCI

Study Cohort	Year	DAPT Strategy	Patients	Follow-Up	Primary Endpoint (EP)	Results
Abbreviation to ASA monotherapy						
DAPT STEMI	2018	6 vs 12 mo DAPT (ASA + P2Y12 inhibitor)	n = 870	18 mo	All-cause mortality, MI, revascularization, stroke, TIMI major bleeding	Non-inferior for primary EP (4.8% vs 6.6%, P = .004; P = .26 for superiority). No significant reduction of bleeding (0.2% vs 0.5%, P = .49).
EXCELLENT	2012	6 vs 12 mo DAPT (ASA + clopidogrel)	n = 1443	1 y	Cardiac death, MI, ischemia-driven target-lesion revascularization	Non-inferior for primary EP (4.8% vs 4.3%, P = .004; P = .60 for superiority). No significant reduction of bleeding (0.3% vs 0.6%, P = .64).
I-LOVE-IT 2	2016	6 vs 12 mo DAPT (ASA + P2Y12 inhibitor)	n = 1829	1 y	Cardiac death, target-vessel MI, clinically indicated target-lesion revascularization, BARC ≥3 bleeding	Non-inferior for primary EP (6.8% vs 5.9%, P = .007). No significant reduction of bleeding (1.2% vs 0.7%, P = .21).
ISAR-SAFE	2015	6 vs 12 mo DAPT (ASA + clopidogrel)	n = 4000	9 mo	Cardiac death, MI, ST, stroke, BARC ≥3 bleeding	Non-inferior for primary EP (1.5% vs 1.6%, P<.001). No significant reduction of bleeding (0.2% vs 0.3%, P = .74).
IVUS-XPL	2016	6 vs 12 mo DAPT (ASA + P2Y12 inhibitor)	n = 1400	1 y	Cardiac death, MI, stroke, TIMI major bleeding	No differences for primary EP (2.2% vs 2.1%, P = .85 for superiority). No significant reduction of bleeding (0.7% vs 1%, P = .56).
OPTIMCA-C	2018	6 vs 12 mo DAPT (ASA + P2Y12 inhibitor)	n = 1368	1 y	Cardiac death, MI, ischemia-driven target-lesion revascularization	Non-inferior for primary EP (1.2% vs 0.6%, P<.05, P = .24 for superiority).

(continued on next page)

Table 2
(continued)

Study Cohort	Year	DAPT Strategy	Patients	Follow-Up	Primary Endpoint (EP)	Results
REDUCE	2019	3 vs 12 mo DAPT (ASA + P2Y12 inhibitor)	n = 1496	1 y	All-cause mortality, MI, ST, stroke, target-vessel revascularization, BARC ≥2 bleeding	Non-inferior for primary EP (8.2% vs 8.4%, $P<.001$; $P = .80$ for superiority). No significant reduction of bleeding (2.5% vs 3%, $P = .54$)
RESET	2012	3 vs 12 mo DAPT (ASA + clopidogrel)	n = 2117	1 y	Cardiovascular death, MI, ST, target-vessel revascularization, bleeding	Non-inferior for primary EP (4.7% vs 4.7%, $P<.001$; $P = .84$ for superiority). No significant reduction of bleeding (0.2% vs 0.6%, $P = .16$)
SMART DATE	2018	6 vs 12 mo DAPT (ASA + P2Y12 inhibitor)	n = 2117	18 mo	All-cause death, MI, stroke	Non-inferior for primary EP (4.7% vs 4.2%, $P = .03$; $P = .51$ for superiority). Significant increase of MI (1.8% vs 0.8%, $P = .02$). No significant reduction of bleeding (2.7% vs 3.9%, $P = .09$)
Abbreviation to P2Y$_{12}$ monotherapy						
GLOBAL LEADERS ACS subgroup	2018	1 mo DAPT (ASA + ticagrelor) followed by 23 mo ticagrelor vs 12 mo DAPT followed by ASA	n = 7487	2 y	All-cause mortality, non-fatal new Q-wave MI	No differences for primary EP (3.9% vs 4.5%, $P = .19$ for superiority). Reduction of bleeding (2% vs 2.7%, $P = .04$)
MASTER DAPT	2021	1 vs 3–12 mo DAPT (ASA + P2Y$_{12}$ inhibitor)	n = 4434	1 y	Net adverse events (all-cause death, MI, stroke, BARC ≥3 bleeding); Composite EP (all-cause death, MI, stroke); BARC ≥2 bleeding	Non-inferior for net adverse events (7.5% vs 7.7%, $P<.001$), and composite EP (6.1% vs 5.9%, $P<.001$). Reduction of bleeding (6.5% vs 9.4%, $P<.001$)
SMART-CHOICE	2019	3 vs 12 months DAPT (ASA + P2Y$_{12}$ inhibitor)	n = 2993	1 y	All-cause death, MI, stroke	Non-inferior for primary EP (2.9% vs 2.5%, $P = .007$). Reduction of bleeding (2% vs 3.4%, $P = .02$)

Trial	Year	n	Duration	Intervention	Endpoints	Results
STOPDAPT-2 ACS	2022	n = 4169	1 y	1-2 mo DAPT (ASA + clopidogrel/prasugrel 3.75 mg) followed by clopidogrel vs 1-2 mo DAPT (ASA + clopidogrel or prasugrel 3.75 mg) followed by DAPT	Cardiovascular death, MI, ischemic, hemorrhagic stroke, definite ST, major or minor bleeding	Failed to reach non-inferiority for primary EP (3.2% vs 2.8%, $P = .06$).
TICO	2020	n = 3056	1 y	3 vs 12 mo DAPT (ASA + ticagrelor)	Death, MI, ST, stroke, target-vessel revascularization, TIMI major bleeding	Superior for primary EP (3.9% vs 5.9%, $P = .01$) Reduction of bleeding (1.7% vs 3%, $P = .02$)
TWILIGHT-ACS	2020	n = 4614	1 y	3 mo DAPT (ASA + ticagrelor) followed by 12 mo ticagrelor vs 15 mo DAPT (ASA + ticagrelor)	BARC ≥ 2 bleeding	Superior for primary EP (3.6% vs 7.6%, $P<.001$) Reduction of bleeding (0.8% vs 2.1%, $P<.001$)
Guided de-escalation						
ANTARCTIC	2016	n = 877	1 y	12 mo ASA + 2 wk prasugrel 5 mg followed by 2 wk PFT-guided therapy (continuation, prasugrel 10 mg if HPR, clopidogrel 75 mg if LPR) followed by PFT-guided adjustment (continuation, prasugrel 5 mg if LPR with prasugrel 10 mg, or HPR with clopidogrel 75 mg) for 11 mo vs 12 mo ASA + prasugrel 5 mg	Cardiovascular death, MI, stroke, ST, urgent revascularization, BARC ≥ 2 bleeding	No significant differences in ischemic endpoints (28% vs 28%, $P = .98$). No significant reduction of bleeding (20% vs 21%, $P = .77$)
POPular Genetics	2019	n = 2488	1 y	12 mo ASA + genotype-guided $P2Y_{12}$ inhibitor (prasugrel or ticagrelor if CYP2C19 loss-of-function allele, clopidogrel in non-carriers) vs 12 mo aspirin + ticagrelor or prasugrel	Composite endpoint (all-cause death, MI, definite ST, stroke, PLATO major bleeding); PLATO major or minor bleeding	No significant differences in ischemic endpoints (5.1% vs 5.9%, $P<.001$ for non-inferiority, $P = .40$ for superiority). Reduction of bleeding (9.8% vs 12.5%, $P = .04$)

(continued on next page)

Table 2
(continued)

Study Cohort	Year	DAPT Strategy	Patients	Follow-Up	Primary Endpoint (EP)	Results
TROPICAL-ACS	2017	12 mo ASA + 1 wk prasugrel 5/10 mg (age/weight-based) followed by 1 wk clopidogrel 75 mg and 11.5 mo PFT-guided maintenance (continuation, prasugrel if HPR) vs 12 mo ASA + prasugrel 5/10 mg (age/weight-based)	n = 2610	1 y	Cardiovascular death, MI, stroke, ST, urgent revascularization, BARC ≥2 bleeding	No significant differences in ischemic endpoints (7% vs 9%, $P<.001$ for non-inferiority, $P = .12$ for superiority). No significant reduction of bleeding (5% vs 6%, $P = .23$)
Unguided de-escalation						
HOST-REDUCE-POLYTHEC-ACS	2020	12 mo ASA + 1 mo prasugrel 10 mg followed by 11 mo prasugrel 5 mg vs 12 mo ASA + prasugrel 10 mg	n = 3429	1 y	All-cause death, non-fatal MI, ST, repeat revascularization, stroke, BARC ≥2 bleeding	No significant differences in ischemic EP but reduction of primary EP (7.2% vs 10.1, $P<.001$ for non-inferiority, $P = .012$ for equivalence) Reduction of bleeding (2.9% vs 5.9%, $P<.001$)
TALOS-AMI	2021	12 mo ASA + 1 mo ticagrelor 90 mg twice daily followed by 11 mo clopidogrel 75 mg vs 12 mo ASA + ticagrelor 90 mg twice daily	n = 2697	1–12 mo	Cardiovascular death, MI, stroke, BARC ≥2 bleeding	No significant differences in ischemic EP but reduction of primary EP (4.6% vs 8.2, $P<.001$ for non-inferiority, $P<.001$ for superiority). Reduction of bleeding (3% vs 5.6%, $P = .001$)
TOPIC	2017	12 mo ASA + 1 mo ticagrelor/prasugrel followed by 11 mo clopidogrel 75 mg vs 12 mo ASA + ticagrelor/prasugrel	n = 646	1 y	Cardiovascular death, urgent revascularization, stroke, BARC ≥2 bleeding	No significant differences in ischemic EP but reduction of primary EP (13.4% vs 26.3, $P<.01$). Reduction of bleeding (4% vs 14.9%, $P<.01$).

enrolled high-risk patients undergoing PCI who completed an initial course of DAPT with ticagrelor for 3 months without adverse events. Here, ticagrelor monotherapy was compared to ticagrelor plus ASA for an additional 12 months. Ticagrelor monotherapy significantly reduced the primary outcome of relevant BARC bleeding, and the ischemic endpoint met the non-inferiority criterion (see Table 2).

Phenotype-guided or genotype-guided antiplatelet strategies are another approach to adapt antiplatelet therapy because clopidogrel is a prodrug and requires conversion to an active metabolite by the hepatic cytochrome P450 enzyme CYP2C19. In up to 30% of patients inadequate response to clopidogrel has been found due to loss-of-function polymorphisms of CYP2C19 alleles which leads to high platelet reactivity (HPR) with an increased risk of cardiovascular events under antiplatelet agents. These genetic polymorphisms do not alter the pharmacokinetics of prasugrel and ticagrelor and therefore, their use might be beneficial in these patients. Thus, prasugrel and ticagrelor were shown to reduce MACE in CYP2C19 loss-of-function carriers (see Table 2).

These findings suggest that the determination of HPR may optimize antithrombotic treatment. Therefore, platelet function tests predict the response to clopidogrel and have been shown to correlate with the bleeding and ischemic risk. Thereby, DAPT can be modulated toward a more potent $P2Y_{12}$ inhibitor in the setting of HPR on clopidogrel. However, randomized trials assessing the clinical utility of standardized platelet function tests or point of care tests have generated contradictory results. Therefore, phenotyping of platelet hyperreactivity is not part of the risk screening in clinical routine, but rather an exception in challenging patient scenarios. The TROPICAL-ACS trial propagated a platelet functional guided de-escalation strategy which resulted in a non-inferior performance compared with conventional DAPT including prasugrel in ACS patients (see Table 2). The POPULAR GENETICS trial reported a reduction of bleeding risk in patients with a genotype-guided DAPT strategy (see Table 2). The TAILOR PCI trial in PCI patients randomized to standard treatment or use of a point-of-care genotyping test for the selection of ticagrelor or clopidogrel did not show significant reduction of cardiovascular events. The ABCD-GENE (age, body mass index, chronic kidney disease, diabetes mellitus, and genotyping) risk score was generated from this analysis to identify patients with HPR on clopidogrel at increased risk for adverse ischemic events,

who may benefit from escalation of DAPT.[8] Overall, a strategy of guided selection of antiplatelet therapy by means of genotyping or phenotyping platelet function tests was associated with improved clinical outcome, however routine phenotype-guided or genotype-guided antithrombotic therapies in clinical practice remain limited.

Prolonging Dual Antiplatelet Therapy
Strategies for thrombotic risk reduction comprise extended DAPT as safety concerns about the risk of late stent thrombosis were raised over years. However, recent data prove that newer-generation DES are associated with a very-low incidence of stent thrombosis (<1%/year). Nonetheless, the observation that certain patients with CAD remain at high risk for recurrent ischemic events provides another rationale for prolonged DAPT duration, even beyond 1 year. To date, several well-designed randomized clinical trials have compared extended DAPT up to 48 months with standard 6 to 12 months DAPT. Most trials failed to demonstrate a clear benefit of extended DAPT. It was shown that the reduction in MI and stent thrombosis did not result in improved survival. The DAPT study compared a 30-month DAPT versus standard 12-month DAPT among participants with either stable CAD or ACS. Extended DAPT significantly reduced the incidence of adverse cardiovascular events but at the expense of increased bleeding and mortality. Extended DAPT may be applied to selected patients in whom the thrombotic risk outweighs the bleeding risk. However, careful clinical use, especially in older patients is necessary to avoid potential harm.

Long-Term Single Antiplatelet Therapy for Secondary Prevention
ASA is well established for life-long secondary prevention and remains the drug of choice after discontinuation of DAPT. Albeit all benefits, long-term ASA use involves potential negative effects like gastrointestinal bleeding. Thus, $P2Y_{12}$ inhibitors may offer an alternative for a protective antiplatelet therapy. The benefit of long-term strategies in high-risk ACS patients was investigated in the PEGASUS-TIMI 54 trial where patients with a history of prior MI were randomized to ticagrelor 90 mg twice daily, ticagrelor 60 mg twice daily, or placebo, on top of ASA. At 3 years, ticagrelor 60 mg on top of aspirin was associated with an overall benefit in patients with a recent MI and patients without HBR.[9] Adding a second antithrombotic agent to aspirin for extended long-term secondary prevention should be considered in

patients with high ischemic risk (eg, patients with diabetes mellitus, recurrent MI, multivessel disease, or chronic kidney disease) and without HBR.[10] There is growing evidence that $P2Y_{12}$ inhibitor monotherapy may be a safe and effective alternative for secondary prevention in patients with established atherosclerosis cardiovascular disease. The HOST-EXAM trial showed that clopidogrel monotherapy was associated with a significant reduction in both thrombotic and bleeding events up to 5 years as compared to low-dose aspirin in PCI.[11] A recent meta-analysis showed a significant risk reduction in MI with $P2Y_{12}$ inhibitor versus aspirin monotherapy, with no differences in mortality, stroke, and major bleeding. Considered for cost-effectiveness, $P2Y_{12}$ inhibitor monotherapy represents a valid alternative to aspirin, in patients who do not tolerate ASA or have recurrent adverse events.

Need for Novel Targets of Antiplatelet Therapy

The ongoing trends of clinical studies aiming for an early de-escalation of antiplatelet regimen and the search for tailorized therapies reflect the major limitation of current antiplatelet treatment strategies due to an increased bleeding risk. On the other hand, the need for novel targets to selectively inhibit platelet activation and prevent thrombus formation is accompanied by the aim to maintain coagulation homeostasis and attenuate the bleeding risk in patients with antiplatelet treatment. Therefore, in the last decade outstanding efforts were made to unveil new pharmacologic targets of antiplatelet treatment. Beyond conventional activators and platelet surface receptors, downstream signaling cascades have been recognized in the search of novel treatment options for cardiovascular diseases (Fig. 2).

Inhibition of the Adenosine Diphosphate-Receptor

Among others, platelet activation is predominantly governed by surface receptors $P2Y_1$ and $P2Y_{12}$. Recently, various antagonists of the $P2Y_1$ and $P2Y_{12}$ receptors have been described and tested in preclinical studies. Lately, the selective $P2Y_{12}$ receptor antagonist selatogrel was demonstrated to lower the bleeding risk at the same level of antithrombotic efficacy in an animal model of carotid artery thrombosis.[12] Likewise, autoinjection of selatogrel disclosed substantial platelet inhibition in 2 phase II clinical trials.[13,14] Currently, the promising results are scrutinized in a large-scale phase III study powered to investigate the clinical outcome of patients with ACS.

Thus, the SOS-AMI study investigates the efficacy of symptom-based self-reliant administration of selatogrel in patients with history of MI at elevated risk for recurring ACS.[15]

Inhibition of Protease-Activated Receptors

Protease-activated receptors (PAR) represent a family of G protein-coupled receptors promoting thrombin-induced platelet activation. In the past decade, distinct PAR inhibitors have been developed and exhibited substantial antiplatelet effects. Above all, in a large randomized controlled trial (RCT), the irreversible PAR1 inhibitor vorapaxar, in addition to standard antiplatelet treatment, was proven to reduce the risk of cardiovascular death or ischemic events when compared to SAPT, but at the expense of an increased bleeding risk.[16] In patients with PAD, diabetes, or a prior history of MI, vorapaxar further reduced the risk of major atherothrombotic ischemic events. An increased bleeding risk was predominant in older, low-weight patients and in those with a history of stroke. Therefore, vorapaxar was approved for restricted use in the United States of America in patients with PAD or a prior history of MI.

Fibrinogen Receptor Blockers, RUC-4

The interaction of fibrinogen and αIIbβ3 integrin strongly boosts platelet-dependent thrombus formation. Abciximab, a monoclonal chimeric antibody was the first integrin inhibitor but has been discontinued and replaced by other important αIIbβ3 inhibitors (ie, eptifibatide, tirofiban), commonly used to defy uncontrolled intracoronary thrombus formation. However, due to the restricted scope as bail-out regimen and increased bleeding risk, there is an ongoing need for novel integrin inhibitors. The point-of-care treatment RUC-4 (Zalunfiban) attaches to the metal ion-binding domain of β3integrin and thus, inhibits binding of fibrinogen unaccompanied by an intrinsic activation.[17] Further, promising novel and highly specific single-chain antibodies allow the inhibition of only activated αIIbβ3 integrin and thus, might reduce the bleeding risk by disregarding resting platelets. RUC-4 is undergoing investigation in a phase 3 trial (NCT04825743).

Inhibition of Collagen Receptor

The glycoprotein VI (GPVI) serves as platelet surface receptor and binds to collagen exposed by the subendothelium and at site of plaque rupture GPVI promotes platelet adhesion and thrombus formation. Interestingly, preclinical research suggests that inhibition of GPVI

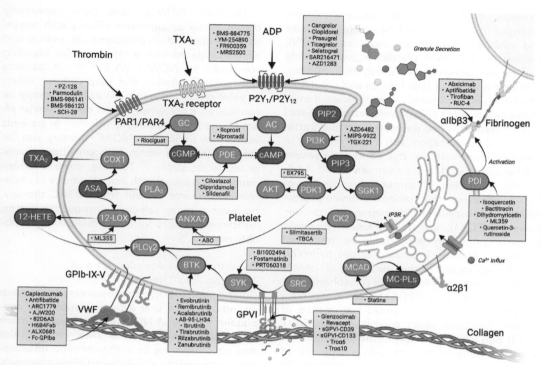

Fig. 2. Synopsis of targets for novel antiplatelet treatment strategies. Alongside conventional surface receptors (ie, purinergic $P2Y_{12}$ receptor, glycoprotein VI (GPVI) and GPIb, thrombin protease-activated receptor, thromboxane A_2 receptor (TXA_2R)), antiplatelet agents modulate downstream signaling cascades critical for platelet activation. 12-HETE, 12-hydroxyeicosatetraenoic acid; 12-LOX, 12-lipoxygenase; AC, adenylyl cyclase; ADP, adenosine diphosphate; AKT, RAC-alpha serine/threonine-protein kinase; ANXA7, annexin A7; BTK, Bruton's tyrosine kinase; CK2, casein kinase 2; COX1, cyclooxygenase 1; GC, guanylyl cyclase; MC-PLs, medium-chain phospholipids; MCAD, medium-chain acyl-CoA dehydrogenase; PDE, phosphodiesterase; PDI, protein disulfide isomerase; PDK1, 3-phosphoinositide-dependent protein kinase 1; PIP2/3, phosphatidylinositol bisphosphate/triphosphate; PLCγ2, phospholipase γ2; PKA, protein kinase A; PLA$_2$, phospholipase A_2; SGK1, serine/threonine-protein kinase SGK1; SRC, tyrosine kinase SRC; SYK, tyrosine kinase SYK; TXA_2, thromboxane A_2.

critically attenuates atherothrombosis while only marginally augmenting the bleeding severity. In contrast to conventional inhibitors, soluble GPVI (sGPVI) binds to exposed collagen upon rupture of a vulnerable plaque and blocks the site for platelet—GPVI interaction. Thus, the clinically validated soluble GPVI receptor revacept serves as a vascular band aid that temporarily inhibits platelet adhesion and thrombus formation.[18] In an animal model mimicking ischemic stroke, revacept reduced infarction size and improved functional outcomes without increasing bleeding events.[19] Moreover, revacept in addition to standard antiplatelet therapy led to an improved combined endpoint (eg, bleeding events, ischemic stroke, ACS) in patients with carotid stenosis.[20] Likewise, in a placebo controlled RCT that included patients with chronic coronary syndrome (CCS) undergoing PCI, revacept in addition to DAPT did not enhance the bleeding risk compared to DAPT.[21] Further, glenzocimab, a monoclonal antibody fragment substantially inhibits platelet GPVI but did not improve clinical outcome as SAPT in patients with ischemic stroke.[22] However, a current clinical trial investigates the efficacy of glenzocimab in addition to standard APT in patients with ischemic stroke.[23]

Other Targets

Von Willebrand factor (vWF) promotes platelet-dependent thrombus formation via the GPIb-GPV-GPIX axis. Hitherto, various agents with inhibiting potential of vWF fell short of expectations mainly due to an increased bleeding risk. Novel intracellular signaling cascades downstream of platelet receptors are promising pharmacologic targets for developing effective antiplatelet treatment regimens. Here, a spleen tyrosine kinase inhibitor approved for patients with idiopathic immune cytopenia was shown to prevent atherothrombosis in preclinical trials.

Likewise, Bruton's tyrosine kinase inhibitors emerged from oncological treatment strategies and inhibited downstream cascades of GPVI, leading to decreased platelet activation while slightly increasing the bleeding risk. Further, PI3Ks are a family of lipid kinases and regulators of αIIbβ3 integrin. Recently, the efficacies of small molecule inhibitors of PI3K were tested in phase I and II clinical trials and unveiled suppressed arterial thrombus formation with a mild increase of bleeding complications, but concluding results will be anticipated in the next years.[24–26] Additionally, inhibition of targets downstream of PI3K, including the serine/threonine-protein kinase, 3-phosphoinositide-dependent protein kinase 1 (PDK1), and casein kinase 2, might become promising antithrombotic treatment strategies. Another promising target to inhibit platelet activation is the elevation of cAMP/cGMP through the inhibition of phosphodiesterases (PDE). Inhibition of PDE3 following cilostazol treatment resulted in sustained suppression of platelet functions when combined with SAPT and is non-inferior to ASA in the prevention of adverse events in patients with a high risk of ischemic stroke.[27,28] Likewise, inhibition of PDE3 and PDE5 has been approved as a secondary prevention strategy in patients with ischemic stroke.

Ultimately, bioactive lipids, including phospholipids and arachidonic acid derivates, promote platelet activation and are associated with disease severity in patients with ACS.[29,30] Interestingly, distinct lipid species are susceptible to statin treatment and downregulation of phospholipids as well as inhibition of 12-lipoxygenase (LOX), leading to decreased 12-hydroxyeicosatetraenoic acid (12-HETE) concentrations are associated with a decreased platelet aggregation.[31] Further, inhibition of annexin A7, a regulator of 12-HETE and GPVI downstream signaling, using ABO in a mouse model significantly reduced atherothrombosis while maintaining coagulation homeostasis.[32] Thus, a combined antiplatelet and lipid-lowering therapy in patients with cardiovascular diseases might go hand in hand to improve clinical outcomes.

CURRENT CONCEPTS OF ANTICOAGULATION

Vitamin K antagonist (VKA) remain standard of therapy in patients with mechanical heart valves, valvular atrial fibrillation, recurrent thromboembolic events under novel oral anticoagulant drugs (NOACs) therapy, and impaired renal function/dialysis.

However, NOACs have been repeatedly shown similar or improved efficacy with regard to prevention of thromboembolic events and were associated with a lower risk for bleeding compared to NOACs (VKA).[33–35] In patients with atrial fibrillation and bioprosthetic valves or valve repair including TAVR, NOACs may be considered a preferred option due to similar efficacy and lower bleeding risk.[36,37] In patients with atrial fibrillation, NOAC therapy can be safely re-initiated within 48 hours after a minor or moderate stroke.[38] To date, there is no evidence that patients with embolic stroke of undetermined source benefit from NOAC therapy, however a more selective approach including enrichment factors for atrial fibrillation is probably needed.[39]

Combination of Antiplatelet and Anticoagulant Therapy

Combination therapy is necessary in patients with an indication for oral anticoagulation and antiplatelet therapy. A NOAC-based dual approach with clopidogrel has led to lower bleeding risk and no differences in antithrombotic effectiveness compared to a VKA-based triple approach, including ASA.[40] In the only RCT that randomized NOAC and VKA, apixaban resulted in significantly fewer major bleeding and similar mortality or ischemic events compared to VKA. In the latter trial, triple therapy was given at a median of 1 week.[41] Thus, after up to 1 week of triple NOAC-based antithrombotic therapy following the ACS/PCI event, dual antithrombotic therapy using a NOAC at the recommended dose for stroke prevention and a single oral antiplatelet agent (preferably clopidogrel) for up to 12 months is recommended according to current guidelines.[10] In patients at high risk for ischemic events/stent thrombosis, triple therapy may be prolonged for up to 30 days.[10,42] The use of more potent $P2Y_{12}$ inhibitors in combination with NOAC therapy in patients with ACS/PCI and atrial fibrillation is currently being investigated in a clinical trial (NCT04981041).

Dual Pathway Inhibition

Dual pathway inhibition (DPI) consisting of very-low dose rivaroxaban plus aspirin shows similar effects on platelet-mediated global thrombogenicity but reduced thrombin generation compared to DAPT. DPI was shown superior for the prevention of MACE in patients with CAD and multiple risk factors and for the prevention of major adverse limb events in patients with PAD at the cost of an increased risk for major bleeding.[43–45] Therefore, DPI should be considered for patients with atherosclerotic disease in the chronic phase at high ischemic and low bleeding risk or after lower-extremity revascularization.

Novel Targets of Anticoagulation

Anticoagulation is a cornerstone in acute treatment and prevention of venous and cardiac thromboembolism.[35] Over the past decades, oral anticoagulants simplified the management and safety of pharmacologic treatment strategies in cardiovascular diseases.[46] Hitherto, an increased bleeding risk remains a major concern and reflects the demand for novel agents.

Inhibition of Factor XI/XIa

Hypercoagulability, endothelial activation, and reduced blood flow often trigger signaling cascades involving the secretion of cytokines and recruitment of inflammatory cells, which promote thrombosis. The final common pathways include expression tissue factor (TF) and

initiation of the extrinsic or intrinsic coagulation cascade to promote aggregation of platelets and clotting. Factor XI (FXI, plasma thromboplastin antecedent) is an important enzyme of the coagulation cascade promoting thrombus formation independent of the initial pathway. At first, TF binds to factor VII or IIa and triggers activation of FX to FXa, resulting in cleavage of prothrombin. Thereafter, thrombin induces fibrin formation and feedback activation of FXI to promote additional thrombus formation, stability, and resistance against fibrinolysis.

Preliminary Trial Evidence

Recently, several studies suggested a direct association between FXI levels and thrombosis and an inverse correlation with bleeding events.[47–49] However, there are only preliminary data investigating the relevance of FXI in coagulation and thrombosis.[50] Thus, research data mostly represent evidence from epidemiologic studies and animal models.[50] Nonetheless,

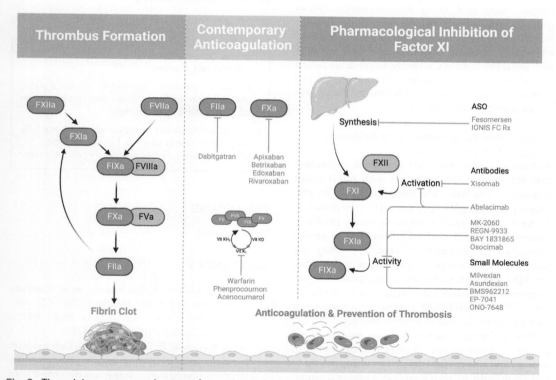

Fig. 3. Tissue injury promotes the tissue factor-dependent pathway essential for hemostasis. This extrinsic pathway is does not usually need FXI activation for hemostatic plug formation. Contrarily, contact activation initiates the intrinsic pathway leading to thrombus formation. Further, plaque rupture or thromboinflammation trigger thrombin generation and fibrin formation leading to adverse thrombotic events. Contemporary treatment options with non-vitamin K antagonist oral anticoagulants (NOAC) bind factor IIa (ie, dabigatran) to inhibit thrombin activity, or factor Xa (ie, apixaban, betrixaban, edoxaban, and rivaroxaban) to inhibit thrombin generation. Novel and selective blockade of the contact pathway via inhibition of factor XIa is a promising strategy to reduce thrombus formation without inhibiting physiologic hemostasias.

several treatment strategies have been developed to inhibit FXI-dependent coagulation (**Fig. 3**). They comprise monoclonal antibodies against FXI activation and FXIa activity, small molecules blocking the active site of FXIa, and antisense oligonucleotides (ASOs) that reduce FXI synthesis (see **Fig. 3**).

Antibody Therapies

Phase II studies that enrolled patients undergoing knee or hip replacement investigated the efficacy of abelacimab, a monoclonal antibody that prevents activation of FXI, and osocimab (ie, an inhibitor of FXIa) to prevent venous thromboembolism (VTE) in contrast to enoxaparin.[51,52] Additionally, osocimab was compared to apixaban, but there are insufficient data comparing the efficacy of FXI inhibitors to established oral anticoagulants.[52,53] Meta-analyses unveiled a significant 50% reduction of VTE alongside an even stronger reduction in bleeding events in patients receiving FXI inhibitors when compared to those with enoxaparin treatment.[53] Only recently, the United States Food and Drug Administration (FDA) granted abelacimab fast-track designation for the treatment of cancer-associated VTE as well as for the prevention of embolic stroke in patients with atrial fibrillation. Currently, large-scale phase III studies compare the safety of monthly-injected abelacimab in contrast to apixaban or dalteparin in this collective of patients.[54–56]

Small Molecule Inhibitors and Antisense Oligonucleotides

Asundexian and milvexian are small molecules that act as oral FXI inhibitors with rapid onset and offset. The latter was investigated for its efficacy in preventing VTE compared to enoxaparin.[57] Phase II trials showed a tolerable safety profile in patients with ACS, atrial fibrillation, and stroke compared to standard of care.[58–61] They are currently tested in a phase III study program after the FDA granted fast-track designation for patients with ischemic Stroke, ACS, and atrial fibrillation.[62] The OCEANIC-AF trial for asundexian was recently stopped due to inferior efficacy.

The ASOs fesomersen reduces the synthesis of FXI by binding the distinct mRNA and acts with a slow onset and offset. Likewise, the ASO was compared to enoxaparin in a phase II study, and further clinical trials are yet to be started.[63]

SUMMARY AND FUTURE PERSPECTIVES

Due to changes in patient populations (eg, by demographic change) and safer cardiovascular procedures and due to the recognition of bleeding as a main driver for mortality, there are growing efforts to individualize antithrombotic therapy in different stages of cardiovascular disease. Thus, there has been a paradigm change from "the more, the better" to "the less, the better." This is particularly true for the elderly patient population and patients at increased bleeding risk. However, more data and inclusion of these vulnerable patient populations in clinical trials are needed. Novel antiplatelet and anticoagulant strategies all follow this principle to further reduce bleeding while maintaining antithrombotic efficacy. On the other hand, there are patients in whom a high thrombotic risk persists despite guideline adherent therapy. A better understanding of the mechanisms and a comprehensive approach to inhibit platelet activation upstream in case of acute thrombotic events and to target atheroprogression (eg, by combined antithrombotic and novel anti-inflammatory therapies) in the chronic phase will be essential to improve prognosis in the future.

CLINICS CARE POINTS

- Assess bleeding and thrombotic risk and take it into consideration for personalized antiplatelet therapy.
- Current concepts comprise de-escalation, abbreviaton and escalation and prolongation of dual antiplatelet therapy.
- Novel antitplatelet compounds will hopefully target the sweet spot to further reduce bleeding while not promote thrombotic risk.

DISCLOSURE

None declared.

REFERENCES

1. Baber U, Mehran R, Giustino G, et al. Coronary Thrombosis and Major Bleeding After PCI With Drug-Eluting Stents: Risk Scores From PARIS. J Am Coll Cardiol 2016;67(19):2224–34.
2. Urban P, Mehran R, Colleran R, et al. Defining high bleeding risk in patients undergoing percutaneous coronary intervention: a consensus document from the Academic Research Consortium for High Bleeding Risk. Eur Heart J 2019;40(31):2632–53.
3. Urban P, Gregson J, Owen R, et al. Assessing the Risks of Bleeding vs Thrombotic Events in Patients at High Bleeding Risk After Coronary Stent Implantation: The ARC-High Bleeding Risk Trade-off Model. JAMA Cardiol 2021;6(4):410–9.

4. Costa F, van Klaveren D, James S, et al. Derivation and validation of the predicting bleeding complications in patients undergoing stent implantation and subsequent dual antiplatelet therapy (PRECISE-DAPT) score: a pooled analysis of individual-patient datasets from clinical trials. Lancet 2017; 389(10073):1025–34.

5. Yeh RW, Kereiakes DJ, Steg PG, et al. Benefits and Risks of Extended Duration Dual Antiplatelet Therapy After PCI in Patients With and Without Acute Myocardial Infarction. J Am Coll Cardiol 2015; 65(20):2211–21.

6. D'Ascenzo F, De Filippo O, Gallone G, et al. Machine learning-based prediction of adverse events following an acute coronary syndrome (PRAISE): a modelling study of pooled datasets. Lancet 2021; 397(10270):199–207.

7. Valgimigli M, Frigoli E, Heg D, et al. Dual Antiplatelet Therapy after PCI in Patients at High Bleeding Risk. N Engl J Med 2021;385(18):1643–55.

8. Angiolillo DJ, Capodanno D, Danchin N, et al. Derivation, Validation, and Prognostic Utility of a Prediction Rule for Nonresponse to Clopidogrel: The ABCD-GENE Score. JACC Cardiovasc Interv 2020;13(5):606–17.

9. Bonaca MP, Im K, Magnani G, et al. Patient selection for long-term secondary prevention with ticagrelor: insights from PEGASUS-TIMI 54. Eur Heart J 2022;43(48):5037–44.

10. Byrne RA, Rossello X, Coughlan JJ, et al. 2023 ESC Guidelines for the management of acute coronary syndromes: Developed by the task force on the management of acute coronary syndromes of the European Society of Cardiology (ESC). Eur Heart J 2023;44(38):3720–826.

11. Koo BK, Kang J, Park KW, et al. Aspirin versus clopidogrel for chronic maintenance monotherapy after percutaneous coronary intervention (HOST-EXAM): an investigator-initiated, prospective, randomised, open-label, multicentre trial. Lancet 2021; 397(10293):2487–96.

12. Rey M, Kramberg M, Hess P, et al. The reversible P2Y(12) antagonist ACT-246475 causes significantly less blood loss than ticagrelor at equivalent antithrombotic efficacy in rat. Pharmacol Res Perspect 2017;5(5). https://doi.org/10.1002/prp2.338.

13. Storey RF, Gurbel PA, Ten Berg J, et al. Pharmacodynamics, pharmacokinetics, and safety of single-dose subcutaneous administration of selatogrel, a novel P2Y12 receptor antagonist, in patients with chronic coronary syndromes. Eur Heart J 2020;41(33):3132–40.

14. Sinnaeve P, Fahrni G, Schelfaut D, et al. Subcutaneous Selatogrel Inhibits Platelet Aggregation in Patients With Acute Myocardial Infarction. J Am Coll Cardiol 2020;75(20):2588–97.

15. US National Library of Medicine. ClinicalTrials.gov, Available at: https://ClinicalTrials.gov/show/NCT04957719, Study Start 2021-08-14, Study Completion (Estimated) 2025-08-13, (Accessed July 30 2024).

16. Morrow DA, Braunwald E, Bonaca MP, et al. Vorapaxar in the Secondary Prevention of Atherothrombotic Events. N Engl J Med 2012;366(15): 1404–13.

17. Bor WL, Zheng KL, Tavenier AH, et al. Pharmacokinetics, pharmacodynamics, and tolerability of subcutaneous administration of a novel glycoprotein IIb/IIIa inhibitor, RUC-4, in patients with ST-segment elevation myocardial infarction. EuroIntervention 2021;17(5):e401–10.

18. Ungerer M, Rosport K, Bültmann A, et al. Novel Antiplatelet Drug Revacept (Dimeric Glycoprotein VI-Fc) Specifically and Efficiently Inhibited Collagen-Induced Platelet Aggregation Without Affecting General Hemostasis in Humans. Circulation 2011; 123(17):1891–9.

19. Goebel S, Li Z, Vogelmann J, et al. The GPVI-Fc Fusion Protein Revacept Improves Cerebral Infarct Volume and Functional Outcome in Stroke. PLoS One 2013;8(7):e66960.

20. Uphaus T, Richards T, Weimar C, et al. Revacept, an Inhibitor of Platelet Adhesion in Symptomatic Carotid Stenosis: A Multicenter Randomized Phase II Trial. Stroke 2022;53(9):2718–29.

21. Mayer K, Hein-Rothweiler R, Schüpke S, et al. Efficacy and Safety of Revacept, a Novel Lesion-Directed Competitive Antagonist to Platelet Glycoprotein VI, in Patients Undergoing Elective Percutaneous Coronary Intervention for Stable Ischemic Heart Disease: The Randomized, Double-blind, Placebo-Controlled ISAR-PLASTER Phase 2 Trial. JAMA Cardiol 2021;6(7):753–61.

22. Wichaiyo S, Parichatikanond W, Rattanavipanon W. Glenzocimab: A GPVI (Glycoprotein VI)-Targeted Potential Antiplatelet Agent for the Treatment of Acute Ischemic Stroke. Stroke 2022;53(11):3506–13.

23. US National Library of Medicine. ClinicalTrials.gov, Available at: https://ClinicalTrials.gov/show/NCT05070260, Study Start 2021-09-23, Study Completion (Actual) 2024-04-30, (Accessed July 30 2024).

24. Nylander S, Kull B, Björkman JA, et al. Human target validation of phosphoinositide 3-kinase (PI3K)β: effects on platelets and insulin sensitivity, using AZD6482 a novel PI3Kβ inhibitor. J Thromb Haemost 2012;10(10):2127–36.

25. Nylander S, Wågberg F, Andersson M, et al. Exploration of efficacy and bleeding with combined phosphoinositide 3-kinase β inhibition and aspirin in man. J Thromb Haemost 2015;13(8):1494–502.

26. US National Library of Medicine. ClinicalTrials.gov, Available at: https://ClinicalTrials.gov/show/NCT05363397, Study Start 2023-09-27, Study Completion (Estimated) 2025-05-01, (Accessed July 30 2024).

27. Sun B, Li H, Shakur Y, et al. Role of phosphodiesterase type 3A and 3B in regulating platelet and cardiac function using subtype-selective knockout mice. Cell Signal 2007;19(8):1765–71.

28. Toyoda K, Uchiyama S, Yamaguchi T, et al. Dual antiplatelet therapy using cilostazol for secondary prevention in patients with high-risk ischaemic stroke in Japan: a multicentre, open-label, randomised controlled trial. Lancet Neurol 2019;18(6):539–48.

29. Harm T, Bild A, Dittrich K, et al. Acute coronary syndrome is associated with a substantial change in the platelet lipidome. Cardiovasc Res 2022;118(8):1904–16.

30. Harm T, Dittrich K, Brun A, et al. Large-scale lipidomics profiling reveals characteristic lipid signatures associated with an increased cardiovascular risk. Clin Res Cardiol 2023. https://doi.org/10.1007/s00392-023-02260-x.

31. Harm T, Frey M, Dittrich K, et al. Statin Treatment Is Associated with Alterations in the Platelet Lipidome. Thromb Haemost 2023. https://doi.org/10.1055/s-0043-1764353.

32. Li H, Huang S, Wang S, et al. Targeting annexin A7 by a small molecule suppressed the activity of phosphatidylcholine-specific phospholipase C in vascular endothelial cells and inhibited atherosclerosis in apolipoprotein E−/− mice. Cell Death Dis 2013;4(9):e806.

33. Joglar JA, Chung MK, Armbruster AL, et al. 2023 ACC/AHA/ACCP/HRS Guideline for the Diagnosis and Management of Atrial Fibrillation: A Report of the American College of Cardiology/American Heart Association Joint Committee on Clinical Practice Guidelines. Circulation 2024;149(1):e1–156.

34. Hindricks G, Potpara T, Dagres N, et al. 2020 ESC Guidelines for the diagnosis and management of atrial fibrillation developed in collaboration with the European Association for Cardio-Thoracic Surgery (EACTS): The Task Force for the diagnosis and management of atrial fibrillation of the European Society of Cardiology (ESC) Developed with the special contribution of the European Heart Rhythm Association (EHRA) of the ESC. Eur Heart J 2021;42(5):373–498.

35. Konstantinides SV, Meyer G, Becattini C, et al. 2019 ESC Guidelines for the diagnosis and management of acute pulmonary embolism developed in collaboration with the European Respiratory Society (ERS): The Task Force for the diagnosis and management of acute pulmonary embolism of the European Society of Cardiology (ESC). Eur Heart J 2019;41(4):543–603.

36. Guimarães HP, Lopes RD, de Barros e Silva PGM, et al. Rivaroxaban in Patients with Atrial Fibrillation and a Bioprosthetic Mitral Valve. N Engl J Med 2020;383(22):2117–26.

37. Vahanian A, Beyersdorf F, Praz F, et al. 2021 ESC/EACTS Guidelines for the management of valvular heart disease. Eur Heart J 2022;43(7):561–632.

38. Fischer U, Koga M, Strbian D, et al. Early versus Later Anticoagulation for Stroke with Atrial Fibrillation. N Engl J Med 2023;388(26):2411–21.

39. Geisler T, Keller T, Martus P, et al. Apixaban versus Aspirin for Embolic Stroke of Undetermined Source. NEJM Evidence 2024;3(1). EVIDoa2300235.

40. Lopes RD, Hong H, Harskamp RE, et al. Optimal Antithrombotic Regimens for Patients With Atrial Fibrillation Undergoing Percutaneous Coronary Intervention: An Updated Network Meta-analysis. JAMA Cardiol 2020;5(5):582–9.

41. Lopes RD, Heizer G, Aronson R, et al. Antithrombotic Therapy after Acute Coronary Syndrome or PCI in Atrial Fibrillation. N Engl J Med 2019;380(16):1509–24.

42. Lopes RD, Leonardi S, Wojdyla DM, et al. Stent Thrombosis in Patients With Atrial Fibrillation Undergoing Coronary Stenting in the AUGUSTUS Trial. Circulation 2020;141(9):781–3.

43. Galli M, Capodanno D, Benenati S, et al. Efficacy and safety of dual-pathway inhibition in patients with cardiovascular disease: a meta-analysis of 49 802 patients from 7 randomized trials. Eur Heart J Cardiovasc Pharmacother 2022;8(5):519–28.

44. Eikelboom JW, Connolly SJ, Bosch J, et al. Rivaroxaban with or without Aspirin in Stable Cardiovascular Disease. N Engl J Med 2017;377(14):1319–30.

45. Bonaca MP, Bauersachs RM, Anand SS, et al. Rivaroxaban in Peripheral Artery Disease after Revascularization. N Engl J Med 2020;382(21):1994–2004.

46. Chen A, Stecker E, Warden BA. Direct Oral Anticoagulant Use: A Practical Guide to Common Clinical Challenges. J Am Heart Assoc 2020;9(13):e017559.

47. Sharman Moser S, Chodick G, Ni YG, et al. The Association between Factor XI Deficiency and the Risk of Bleeding, Cardiovascular, and Venous Thromboembolic Events. Thromb Haemost 2022;122(5):808–17.

48. Preis M, Hirsch J, Kotler A, et al. Factor XI deficiency is associated with lower risk for cardiovascular and venous thromboembolism events. Blood 2017;129(9):1210–5.

49. Meijers JCM, Tekelenburg WLH, Bouma BN, et al. High Levels of Coagulation Factor XI as a Risk Factor for Venous Thrombosis. N Engl J Med 2000;342(10):696–701.

50. Chan NC, Weitz JI. New Therapeutic Targets for the Prevention and Treatment of Venous Thromboembolism With a Focus on Factor XI Inhibitors. Arterioscler Thromb Vasc Biol 2023;43(10):1755–63.

51. Verhamme P, Yi BA, Segers A, et al. Abelacimab for Prevention of Venous Thromboembolism. N Engl J Med 2021;385(7):609–17.

52. Weitz JI, Bauersachs R, Becker B, et al. Effect of Osocimab in Preventing Venous Thromboembolism Among Patients Undergoing Knee Arthroplasty: The FOXTROT Randomized Clinical Trial. JAMA 2020;323(2):130–9.

53. Galli M, Laborante R, Ortega-Paz L, et al. Factor XI Inhibitors in Early Clinical Trials: A Meta-analysis. Thromb Haemost 2023;123(6):576–84.

54. US National Library of Medicine. ClinicalTrials.gov, Available at: https://ClinicalTrials.gov/show/NCT05171049, Study Start 2022-05-05, Study Completion (Estimated) 2025-09, (Accessed July 30 2024).

55. US National Library of Medicine. ClinicalTrials.gov, Available at: https://ClinicalTrials.gov/show/NCT05171075, Study Start 2022-09-27, Study Completion (Estimated) 2025-09, (Accessed July 30 2024).

56. US National Library of Medicine. ClinicalTrials.gov Available at: https://ClinicalTrials.gov/show/NCT05712200, Study Start 2022-12-27, Study Completion (Estimated) 2025-03, (Accessed July 30 2024).

57. Weitz JI, Strony J, Ageno W, et al. Milvexian for the Prevention of Venous Thromboembolism. N Engl J Med 2021;385(23):2161–72.

58. Shoamanesh A, Mundl H, Smith EE, et al. Factor XIa inhibition with asundexian after acute non-cardioembolic ischaemic stroke (PACIFIC-Stroke): an international, randomised, double-blind, placebo-controlled, phase 2b trial. Lancet 2022;400(10357):997–1007.

59. Rao SV, Kirsch B, Bhatt DL, et al. A Multicenter, Phase 2, Randomized, Placebo-Controlled, Double-Blind, Parallel-Group, Dose-Finding Trial of the Oral Factor XIa Inhibitor Asundexian to Prevent Adverse Cardiovascular Outcomes After Acute Myocardial Infarction. Circulation 2022;146(16):1196–206.

60. Piccini JP, Caso V, Connolly SJ, et al. Safety of the oral factor XIa inhibitor asundexian compared with apixaban in patients with atrial fibrillation (PACIFIC-AF): a multicentre, randomised, double-blind, double-dummy, dose-finding phase 2 study. Lancet 2022;399(10333):1383–90.

61. Sharma M, Molina CA, Toyoda K, et al. Safety and efficacy of factor XIa inhibition with milvexian for secondary stroke prevention (AXIOMATIC-SSP): a phase 2, international, randomised, double-blind, placebo-controlled, dose-finding trial. Lancet Neurol 2024;23(1):46–59.

62. US National Library of Medicine. ClinicalTrials.gov Available at: https://ClinicalTrials.gov/show/NCT05702034, Study Start 2023-02-15, Study Completion (Estimated) 2026-12-09, (Accessed July 30 2024).

63. Büller HR, Bethune C, Bhanot S, et al. Factor XI antisense oligonucleotide for prevention of venous thrombosis. N Engl J Med 2015;372(3):232–40.

Genetic Determinants of Response to P2Y₁₂ Inhibitors and Clinical Implications

Larisa H. Cavallari, PharmD[a],*, James C. Coons, PharmD[b]

KEYWORDS

- Clopidogrel • Prasugrel • Ticagrelor • Genotype • CYP2C19 • Pharmacogenomics

KEY POINTS

- The CYP2C19 enzyme has a key role in the biotransformation of clopidogrel (a prodrug) to its pharmacologically active form.
- Approximately 30% of individuals have a *CYPC19* loss-of-function allele, leading to reduced formation of the active clopidogrel metabolite and decreased clopidogrel effectiveness.
- Numerous studies have documented an increased risk for major adverse cardiovascular events following percutaneous coronary intervention (PCI) in clopidogrel-treated patients with a *CYP2C19* loss-of-function allele compared to those without a loss-of-function allele.
- *CYP2C19* genotype does not affect response to prasugrel or ticagrelor, which are recommended in the absence of contraindications for patients with a *CYP2C19* loss-of-function allele.
- Data from clinical trials, cohort studies, and meta-analyses support improved outcomes with *CYP2C19*-guided antiplatelet prescribing after PCI, in which prasugrel or ticagrelor is prescribed to those with a loss-of-function allele. Among patients without a loss-of-function allele, there appears to be no difference in risk for ischemic events with clopidogrel versus alternative therapy.

INTRODUCTION

There is significant interpatient variability in clopidogrel effectiveness following percutaneous coronary intervention (PCI), which is attributed in part to clinical factors, including age, body size, renal function, and presence of diabetes.[1] Variants within the gene encoding the cytochrome (CYP) P450 2C19 enzyme are also major contributors to the variability in clopidogrel response.[2] In contrast, neither prasugrel nor ticagrelor is affected by *CYP2C19* genotype.[3,4] Both drugs were superior to clopidogrel in landmark clinical trials but are associated with higher bleeding risk, cost, and discontinuation rates compared to clopidogrel.[5–7] Based on clinical trial data, prasugrel and ticagrelor are preferred over clopidogrel following an acute coronary syndrome (ACS) and PCI, and while data show increasing use of these drugs (especially ticagrelor) over time, clopidogrel remains commonly prescribed, particularly among older patients.[8–10] This review will describe the data supporting genetic associations with clopidogrel response, outcomes from studies assessing genotype-guided antiplatelet therapy, pharmacogenetic guidelines for antiplatelet drug selection, and approaches to clinical implementation of *CYP2C19* testing.

[a] Department of Pharmacotherapy and Translational Research, Center for Pharmacogenomics and Precision Medicine, University of Florida, 1333 Center Drive, PO Box 100486, Gainesville, FL 32610, USA; [b] Department of Pharmacy and Therapeutics, Center for Clinical Pharmaceutical Sciences, University of Pittsburgh, 9058 Salk Hall, 3501 Terrace Street, Pittsburgh, PA 15261, USA
* Corresponding author.
E-mail address: lcavallari@cop.ufl.edu

Intervent Cardiol Clin 13 (2024) 469–481
https://doi.org/10.1016/j.iccl.2024.06.002
2211-7458/24/© 2024 Elsevier Inc. All rights reserved, including for text and data mining, AI training, and similar technologies.

PHARMACOLOGY OF P2Y$_{12}$ INHIBITORS

Clopidogrel, prasugrel, and ticagrelor share a common mechanism of action: all bind to P2Y$_{12}$ on the platelet receptor to inhibit adenosine diphosphate (ADP)-mediated platelet aggregation. However, there are important pharmacokinetic and pharmacodynamic differences among drugs that lead to differences in their clinical effects. Both clopidogrel and prasugrel are prodrugs that require metabolism to their active forms (Fig. 1). Approximately 85% of clopidogrel is hydrolyzed by carboxyl esterases to an inactive metabolite.[11] The remaining 15% undergoes a 2 step bioactivation process, in which clopidogrel is first metabolized to 2 oxo-clopidogrel and then further converted to the active thiol metabolite. While multiple other cytochrome P450 (CYP450) enzymes are involved, CYP2C19 has a prominent role in clopidogrel metabolism. Prasugrel also undergoes hydrolysis by carboxyl esterases leading to the formation of an intermediate metabolite (R-95913), which is then converted via multiple CYP450 enzymes, including CYP2C19, to its active moiety. In contrast to clopidogrel and prasugrel, ticagrelor is administered in its active form.

Prasugrel and ticagrelor have more rapid onset of action and exhibit more potent and less variable inhibition of platelet aggregation compared to clopidogrel.[12] Because of their greater potency, prasugrel and ticagrelor confer increased bleeding risk compared to clopidogrel.[6,13] For prasugrel, the risk is highest in those with a history of stroke or transient ischemic attack, and the drug is contraindicated in these patients.[14] Ticagrelor use has been associated with dyspnea in about 10% to 15% of patients, which is believed to be due to inhibition of adenosine clearance or possibly greater inhibitory effects on the central nervous system resulting from higher ticagrelor levels.[6,15,16] Clopidogrel and prasugrel are thienopyridine derivatives that bind irreversibly to the P2Y$_{12}$ receptor, whereas ticagrelor is a cyclo-pentyl-triazolo-pyrimidine and reversible antagonist of the receptor.

GENETIC DETERMINANTS OF RESPONSE TO P2Y$_{12}$ INHIBITORS
CYP2C19 Genotype
Polymorphisms within the CYP2C19 gene lead to variable enzyme activity and contribute to the interpatient variability in clopidogrel response. Nearly 40 CYP2C19 alleles have been cataloged by the Pharmacogene Variation (PharmVar) Consortium.[17] Twelve of these are completely nonfunctional and referred to as loss-of-function (LoF) or no function alleles.

The *2 allele (c.681 G>A; rs4244285) in exon 5 is the most common LoF allele and occurs secondary to an aberrant splice site leading to a truncated protein.[18] The CYP2C19*3 allele (c.636 G>A; rs4986893) in exon 4 is much less common and results in a stop codon and premature termination of the amino acid sequence. Other LoF alleles are observed in less than 1% of the general population.[19] Approximately 30% of European, 40% of African, and 60% of East Asian populations have an LoF allele.[19] The CYP2C19*17 allele (c. -806C>T) is located in the gene promoter region, results in an increased gene expression and is thus referred to as a gain-of-function allele. The Association of Molecular Pathology recommends genotyping for the *2, *3, and *17 alleles, at a minimum, on clinical genotyping platforms.[18] Notably, while the *17 allele has been associated with response to other CYP2C19 substrates (eg, citalopram and voriconazole), its impact on outcomes with clopidogrel is unclear.[2,20–23]

CYP2C19 genotype confers 5 phenotypes, as shown in Table 1.

- Normal metabolizers (NMs), with 2 normal function (*1) alleles and normal enzyme activity
- Intermediate metabolizers (IMs), with 1 LoF allele and reduced enzyme activity
- Poor metabolizers (PMs), with 2 LoF alleles and absent enzyme activity
- Rapid metabolizers (RMs), with one *17 allele and increased enzyme activity
- Ultra-rapid metabolizers (UMs), with two *17 alleles, and significantly increased enzyme activity

The prevalence of CYP2C19 phenotypes by race is shown in Table 1. Consistent with having a higher frequency of LoF alleles, East Asians have the highest prevalence of the PM and IM phenotypes.

CYP2C19 Genotype and Clopidogrel Pharmacokinetics and Pharmacodynamics
Patients with a CYP2C19 LoF allele have diminished capacity to metabolize clopidogrel to its active form. Compared to NMs, exposure to the active clopidogrel metabolite is approximately 30% lower in IMs and 50% lower in PMs following a clopidogrel maintenance dose.[24] Consequently, clopidogrel-treated IMs and PMs are more likely than NMs to have high platelet reactivity, a risk factor for major adverse cardiovascular events (MACE).[25,26]

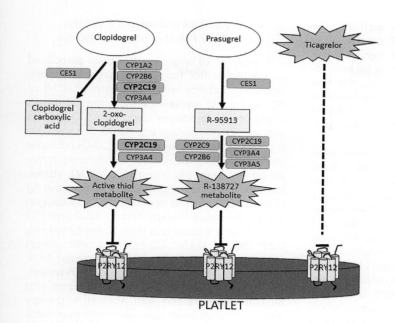

Fig. 1. Depiction of clopidogrel, prasugrel, and ticagrelor metabolic pathways.

CYP2C19 Genotype and Clinical Outcomes with Clopidogrel

Numerous studies have documented an increased risk for stent thrombosis and MACE in clopidogrel-treated IMs and PMs compared to similarly treated NMs following PCI.[2] In an early meta-analysis of 9 studies and 9685 clopidogrel-treated patients, most of whom (55%) had an ACS and nearly all of whom (91%) underwent PCI, the hazard ratio (HR) for MACE (defined as cardiovascular death, myocardial infarction [MI], or stroke) was 1.55 (95% confidence interval [95% CI], 1.11–2.17) in IMs and 1.76 (95% CI, 1.24–2.50) in PMs compared to those without an LoF allele.[27] Subsequent meta-analyses including a larger number of trials and patients confirmed reduced clopidogrel

efficacy in IMs and PMs, with the exception of analyses that included lower risk patients, such as those with ACS managed medically.[2,28,29] One meta-analysis specifically compared outcomes with clopidogrel based on CYP2C19 genotype in those who did or did not undergo PCI.[30] There was a significant association between the LoF allele carrier status and an increased risk for cardiovascular events following PCI (relative risk 1.20, 95% CI, 1.10–1.31) but not in the absence of PCI (relative risk 0.99, 95% CI, 0.84–1.17).

Some studies have reported higher levels of the active clopidogrel metabolite, greater inhibition of platelet aggregation, reduced risk for MACE, and an increased risk for bleeding with the *17 allele.[31–34] The *17 allele is in linkage

Table 1
CYP2C19 phenotypes, example genotypes, and prevalence across ancestry groups

Phenotype	Example Genotype(s)	Prevalence (%)		
		European Ancestry	African Ancestry	East Asian Ancestry
NM	*1/*1	40	33	38
IM	*1/*2, *1/*3, *2/*17[a]	26	35	46
PM	*2/*2, *2/*3	2	4	13
RM	*1/*17	27	24	3
UM	*17/*17	5	4	<1

[a] The IM phenotype assignment for genotypes with 1 LoF and 1 gain-of-function allele (eg, *2/*17) is based on evidence of increased platelet aggregation among clopidogrel-treated patients with this genotype compared to the *1/*1 genotype, indicating that the *17 allele is unable to completely compensate for reduced activity with the *2 allele.[73]. However, the data are not completely consistent, and thus, the IM phenotype assignment is considered provisional.

disequilibrium with the *2 allele, such that the *17 and *2 allele do not occur on the same haplotype.[31] Thus, associations between the *17 allele and clinical outcomes may be secondary to absence of the *2 allele. In studies that adjusted for the *2 allele, associations between the *17 allele and clopidogrel active metabolite levels, platelet aggregation, and clinical outcomes were no longer evident.[22,31,35]

The majority of clopidogrel association studies has been conducted in patients of European or Asian ancestry.[36] Patients of African ancestry have been largely excluded from clopidogrel pharmacogenetic studies. Two exceptions are the Translational Research Investigating Underlying disparities in acute Myocardial infarction Patients' Health status (TRIUMPH) registry, which included 1632 White patients and 430 Black patients treated with clopidogrel following acute MI (85% underwent PCI) and the Precision PCI registry, which included 567 Black patients treated with clopidogrel following PCI (70% with an ACS).[37,38] The TRIUMPH registry showed that the CYP2C19*2 allele was associated with increased mortality at 1 year among White (adjusted HR, 1.70; 95% CI, 1.01–2.86) but not Black (adjusted HR, 0.63; 95% CI, 0.28–1.41) patients. Interestingly, compared to Black patients with the *1/*1 genotype, Black patients with a *17 allele had a higher risk for mortality, and those with the *17/*17 genotype had a higher risk for bleeding. The Precision PCI registry showed that, consistent with data in other populations, there was a higher rate of ischemic events in patients with an LoF allele compared to those without an LoF allele (adjusted HR, 2.00, 95% CI, 1.20–3.33). Bleeding rates did not differ by genotype; however, the number of patients with the *17/*17 genotype was low.

CYP2C19 genotype alone explains just over 12% of the variability in the inhibitory platelet effects of clopidogrel.[39] Clinical factors, including older age, obesity, diabetes, and renal dysfunction, also reduce clopidogrel effectiveness.[1] The Age, Body mass index (BMI), Chronic kidney disease (CKD), Diabetes mellitus, and CYP2C19 GENEtic variants (ABCD-GENE) score incorporates these clinical factors plus CYP2C19 genotype, with the score assigned as follows[1]:

- Age greater than 75 years: 4 points
- BMI greater than 30 kg/m^2: 4 points
- CKD, defined as an estimated glomerular filtration rate of less than 60 mL/min/1.73 m^2: 3 points
- Diabetes: 3 points

- CYP2C19 IM phenotype: 6 points
- CYP2C19 PM phenotype: 24 points

A score of 10 or greater has been associated with a higher risk for adverse ischemic events, including mortality, with clopidogrel after MI or PCI, and could represent a more precise means of predicting clopidogrel response.[1,40] Outcomes with clopidogrel versus alternative therapy (prasugrel or ticagrelor) based on ABCD-GENE score have also been examined.[41] No difference in major atherothrombotic events (death, MI, stroke, stent thrombosis, or unstable angina requiring revascularization) was observed with clopidogrel versus alternative therapy among 3200 post-PCI patients with a score less than 10 (weighted HR, 0.89; 95% CI, 0.65–1.22) or in a smaller cohort of patients with a score of 10 or greater (n = 1135; weighted HR, 0.75; 0.51–1.11). However, regardless of ABCD-GENE score, patients with an LOF allele treated with alternative therapy had significantly fewer ischemic events than those who received clopidogrel.

Genetic Association with Prasugrel and Ticagrelor Response

While CYP2C19 is involved in prasugrel bioactivation, CYP2C19 genotype does not affect prasugrel pharmacokinetics or pharmacodynamics, likely because CYP2C19 has a minor role in the bioactivation of prasugrel compared to other enzymes involved.[3,42] Ticagrelor does not require bioactivation, and thus, CYP2C19 genotype does not influence its effectiveness.[4] In a search for genetic associations with ticagrelor response, investigators from the Study of Platelet Inhibition and Patient Outcomes (PLATO) undertook a genome-wide association study focused on plasma concentrations of ticagrelor and its active metabolite.[43] Variants in the SLCO1B1 gene, which encodes for the organic-anion-transporting polypeptide1B1, and the CYP3A4 region were associated with ticagrelor plasma levels, while a variant in UGT2B7 was associated with levels of the active metabolite. However, none of these variants were associated with the occurrence of MACE, bleeding, or dyspnea during ticagrelor treatment. To date, there are no consistent genetic associations with response to either prasugrel or ticagrelor.

THERAPEUTIC APPROACHES BASED ON CYP2C19 GENOTYPE

Clopidogrel dose escalation has been investigated as a strategy to overcome reduced drug effectiveness in CYP2C19 LoF allele carriers. Among healthy volunteers, doubling the clopidogrel dose to 150 mg in IMs and quadrupling the dose to 300 mg in PMs achieved similar inhibition of ADP-induced platelet aggregation as a 75 mg dose in NMs.[44] However, these results could not be reproduced in patients with cardiovascular disease, in whom doses of 225 mg to 300 mg were needed in IMs to reduce platelet reactivity to a level achieved with a 75 mg dose in NMs.[45,46] In PMs, a dose as high as 300 mg could not produce the desired reduction in platelet reactivity levels.

Use of prasugrel or ticagrelor is a more practical approach to overcome clopidogrel resistance secondary to the CYP2C19 genotype. Data to support this approach come from meta-analyses of randomized controlled trials (RCTs) assessing platelet reactivity or clinical outcomes with prasugrel or ticagrelor versus clopidogrel.[47,48] In a meta-analysis of 12 RCTs comparing antiplatelet strategies in CYP2C19 PMs and IMs, prasugrel and ticagrelor were found to provide the greatest reduction in platelet reactivity, whereas a high-dose (ie, 150 mg/d) clopidogrel and adjunctive cilostazol provided only modest reduction compared to standard dose clopidogrel.[47] In a separate meta-analysis including 7 RCTs and nearly 16,000 patients (98% with ACS and 77% with PCI), a significantly lower risk of ischemic events was observed with ticagrelor or prasugrel versus clopidogrel (relative risk 0.70; 95% CI, 0.59–0.83) in patients with an LoF allele.[48] No difference in events was observed with clopidogrel versus alternative therapy in patients without an LoF allele (relative risk, 1.0; 95% CI, 0.80–1.25). Real-world investigations of outcomes with CYP2C19-guided antiplatelet therapy after PCI have reported similar findings.[49–52]

CLINICAL TRIAL DATA WITH CYP2C19-GUIDED ANTIPLATELET THERAPY

Over the past 5 years, there have been 3 large RCTs conducted to investigate outcomes with CYP2C19 genotyping to guide P2Y$_{12}$ inhibitor selection. An overview of each trial is presented in Table 2. These multicenter trials have largely included high-risk patients with ACS who were treated with PCI. Two trials (PHARMCLO and POPular Genetics) were conducted in Europe, whereas the Tailored Antiplatelet Therapy Following PCI (TAILOR-PCI) trial enrolled patients from North America and South Korea.[53–55] Genotype guidance in each trial occurred within the context of consideration of other relevant clinical variables by the treating provider. CYP2C19 genotyping included testing for the CYP2C19*2 and *3 LoF alleles in both POPular

Genetics and TAILOR-PCI. The PHARMCLO trial tested for the CYP2C19*2 and *17 alleles and the ABCB1 3435C>T variant to guide therapy decisions. In all trials, ticagrelor was the most commonly prescribed alternative agent for patients with a CYP2C19 LoF allele. The primary outcomes for the trials were clinical composites that included various ischemic and/or bleeding endpoints; however, each evaluated death, MI, and stroke. Each trial used a different definition for bleeding outcomes. A brief overview of each trial is summarized in the following discussions.

The PHARMCLO trial was the first prospective trial to compare pharmacogenetic-guidance, using an algorithm that considered both genetic testing and clinical variables, to standard of care, based on clinical variables only.[53] P2Y$_{12}$ inhibitor selection was ultimately at the discretion of the provider, which helps to explain the variability observed in prescribing decisions (ie, ticagrelor use was only about 10% higher in the genotype-guided arm, and clopidogrel use was 8% lower compared to the standard of care arm). The clinical variables considered were age, weight, ischemic risk, bleeding risk (prior history of stroke or transient ischemic attack, intracranial bleeding, history of bleeding, active bleeding, and anemia), diabetes mellitus, and CKD. The primary outcome included both efficacy and safety endpoints and was significantly lower with genotype guidance. However, the trial was prematurely discontinued after only about 25% of the intended population was recruited because of loss of certification with the instrumentation used for testing. This confounds the trial results and may also help to explain the large magnitude of effect seen in the primary outcome. The higher event rates may also reflect the relatively higher proportion of clopidogrel-treated patients and the inclusion of older patients (approximately 30% were aged over 80 years).

The POPular Genetics trial exclusively enrolled patients with ST-segment-elevation myocardial infarction (STEMI) who underwent emergent PCI.[54] The study used an open-label, noninferiority design that focused on de-escalation as the control group received universal ticagrelor or prasugrel. Using CYP2C19 guidance, patients with an LoF allele (*2 or *3 variant) received ticagrelor or prasugrel, whereas noncarriers (*1/*1 genotype) received clopidogrel. Ticagrelor was prescribed in 38% and 91% of the genotype-guided and control arms, respectively. The coprimary outcomes were net adverse clinical events (ischemic event or major bleeding) and major or minor bleeding

Table 2
Summary of randomized controlled trial evidence for CYP2C19 genotyping postpercutaneous coronary intervention

Trial, Year	Patient Population/Setting	Design and Groups	Primary Efficacy Outcome (Genotype-Guided vs Control)	Primary Safety Outcome (Genotype-Guided vs Control)
PHARMCLO, 2018	ACS (98%), stable CAD (2%), PCI (62%) (n = 888*) *~25% of intended recruitment since study was prematurely stopped due to lack of instrument certification	Prospective Genotype-guided (CYP2C19*2 and *17, ABCB1 3435C>T + clinical characteristics) vs control (clinical characteristics) Genotype-guided (clopidogrel 43%, ticagrelor 43%, and prasugrel 8%) vs control (clopidogrel 51%, ticagrelor 33%, and prasugrel 8%)	Composite of CV death, nonfatal MI, nonfatal stroke, BARC 3 to 5 defined major bleeding: 15.9% vs 25.9%; HR, 0.58 (95% CI, 0.43–0.78); P<.001	BARC 3–5 bleeding: 4.2% vs 6.8%; P = .1
POPular Genetics, 2019	STEMI (100%), PCI (100%) (n = 2488)	Prospective, open-label, noninferiority, de-escalation Genotype-guided (CYP2C19*2 and *3: ticagrelor or prasugrel vs CYP2C19 *1/*1: clopidogrel) vs control (universal ticagrelor or prasugrel) Genotype-guided (clopidogrel 61%, ticagrelor 38%, and prasugrel 1%) vs control (ticagrelor 91%, clopidogrel 7%, and prasugrel 2%)	Net adverse clinical events (composite of death, MI, ST, stroke, PLATO major bleed at 12 mo): 5.1% vs 5.9%; absolute difference −0.7% (95% CI, −2 to 0.7); P <.001 for noninferiority	PLATO major/minor bleed at 12 mo: 9.8% vs 12.5%; HR, 0.78 (95% CI, 0.61–0.98); P = .04

| TAILOR-PCI, 2020 | ACS (82%), stable CAD (18%), PCI (100%) (n = 5276*) *n = 1849 (IM or PM) included in the primary analysis | Prospective, open-label, superiority, escalation Genotype-guided (CYP2C19*2 and *3: ticagrelor vs CYP2C19 *1/*1: clopidogrel) vs control (universal clopidogrel) Genotype-guided (ticagrelor 85%, clopidogrel 15%) vs control (clopidogrel 99%, ticagrelor 1%) | Composite of CV death, MI, ST, severe recurrent ischemia at 12 mo: 4% vs 5.9%; HR, 0.66 (95% CI, 0.43–1.02); P = .06 | TIMI major or minor bleeding: 1.9% vs 1.6%; HR, 1.22 (95% CI, 0.60–2.51); P = .58 |

Abbreviations: ACS, acute coronary syndrome; BARC, Bleeding Academic Research Consortium; CAD, coronary artery disease; CV, cardiovascular; IM, intermediate metabolizer; MI, myocardial infarction; PCI, percutaneous coronary intervention; PLATO, PLATelet inhibition and patient Outcomes; PM, poor metabolizer; ST, stent thrombosis; STEMI, ST-segment-elevation myocardial infarction; TIMI, thrombolysis in myocardial infarction.

according to the Platelet Inhibition and Patient Outcomes (PLATO) criteria. Ultimately, the study met noninferiority for net adverse clinical events, whereas the genotype-guided arm had a significant reduction in bleeding versus control. The benefit regarding bleeding reduction was driven by fewer PLATO minor bleeding events in the genotyped-guided group. In a prespecified subanalysis comparing outcomes between clopidogrel-treated patients without an LoF allele versus prasugrel-treated or ticagrelor-treated patients irrespective of CYP2C19 genotype, there was no difference in ischemic outcomes between treatment groups (adjusted HR, 1.14; 95% CI, 0.68–1.90), but significantly fewer bleeding events in clopidogrel-treated patients (HR, 0.74; 95% CI, 0.56–0.96).[35] In summary, the results of this trial support a CYP2C19 genotype-guided approach to clopidogrel prescribing post-PCI. The implications are most evident for patients of European ancestry, who were largely represented in the study and in whom the contribution of CYP2C19 variants was first established. However, the impact of these findings may have even greater importance among patients of non-European ancestry who have a higher prevalence of LoF alleles.[2]

TAILOR-PCI was the most recently published large trial of CYP2C19-guided therapy versus clopidogrel for post-PCI patients.[55] It used an open-label design, yet contrasted with POPular Genetics by deploying an escalation strategy to test superiority versus universal clopidogrel. Approximately 80% of study participants presented with ACS, and all underwent PCI. Patients with a CYP2C19*2 or *3 allele were prescribed ticagrelor or prasugrel in the event they could not tolerate ticagrelor. Noncarriers of these alleles were prescribed clopidogrel. In the genotype-guided group, 85% of patients received ticagrelor. In the control group, 99% of patients received clopidogrel. The primary composite outcome included efficacy endpoints only since the genotype-guided strategy would not be expected to reduce bleeding events compared to universal clopidogrel. Of interest, only those patients with an IM or PM phenotype in each group were included in the primary analysis. This represented about 35% of the population (n = 1849), which limited the power of the study. Furthermore, event rates in the trial were lower than anticipated and led to a sample size recalculation and a larger treatment effect size (HR, 0.50). At the conclusion of the study, a 34% relative risk reduction in the primary outcome was seen with the genotype-guided

arm versus control; however, this did not reach statistical significance (P = .06). The primary safety outcome of Thrombolysis in Myocardial Infarction (TIMI) major or minor bleeding was also not significantly different. Two prespecified analyses showed trends that favored the genotyped-guided group. A sensitivity analysis found a lowering of total events per patient (HR, 0.60; 95% CI, 0.41–0.89) in the genotype-guided arm. Finally, a post hoc analysis demonstrated reduced event rates at 90 days (HR, 0.21; 95% CI, 0.08–0.54). Based upon these findings, the authors suggested that a precision medicine approach may have the most impact early after PCI.

Meta-analyses that included the trial data described earlier have further examined outcomes with guided approaches to antiplatelet therapy.[48,56,57] They have consistently shown that, compared to standard P2Y$_{12}$ inhibitor selection, basing therapy on either genotype or platelet function testing data improved clinical outcomes. In a meta-analysis that included 11 RCTs, guided therapy was associated with a significant reduction in MACE (RR, 0.78, 95% CI, 0.63–0.95, P = .015) and tended to be associated with reduced bleeding (RR, 0.88, 0.77–1.01, P = .069).[56]

GUIDELINES FOR CYP2C19-GUIDED ANTIPLATELET THERAPY

The Food and Drug Administration (FDA) approved the addition of a boxed warning on the clopidogrel labeling in 2010 regarding risk associated with the CYP2C19 genotype. The labeling specifically states that

- Clopidogrel effectiveness is reduced in PMs;
- Tests are available to identify PMs; and
- An alternative P2Y$_{12}$ inhibitor should be considered for PMs.

The FDA subsequently published a table of pharmacogenetic associations, extending their recommendation for alternative treatment to IMs, who are also at risk for poor outcomes with clopidogrel therapy.[50,58]

The 2021 guidelines for coronary artery revascularization by the American College of Cardiology/American Heart Association (ACC/AHA) and 2023 guidelines for the management of ACS by the European Society of Cardiology do not address CYP2C19 genotyping to guide antiplatelet therapy.[59,60] This is despite the evidence described earlier and recommendations regarding genotyping in earlier guidelines by both groups.[61,62] An expert consensus statement from 2019 acknowledges that CYP2C19 genotype may be useful for predicting risk for cardiovascular events; however, it states that genotyping is not recommended because of a "lack of dedicated studies."[63] Guidelines by the Clinical Pharmacogenetics Implementation Consortium (CPIC) do not address whether or not genetic testing should be done, but they provide recommendations for P2Y$_{12}$ inhibitor therapy if CYP2C19 genotype is known for patients with ACS or PCI.[2] In this case, prasugrel or ticagrelor is recommended in patients with an LoF allele in the absence of contraindications, whereas clopidogrel is expected to be effective in those without an LoF allele.

CLINICAL IMPLEMENTATION OF CYP2C19 GENOTYPING

Implementation Strategies

Several institutions have implemented CYP2C19 genotyping into clinical care to guide post-PCI antiplatelet prescribing.[64–70] A group of early adopters from the National Human Genome Research Institute-sponsored Implementing GeNomics In pracTicE (IGNITE) Network have described their implementation strategies.[70] Among 12 participating sites, most leveraged a collaborative effort with multiple stakeholders and deployed a reactive testing model post-PCI to guide antiplatelet prescribing. Some institutions focused testing to higher-risk patient populations (ie, patients with ACS or high-risk angiographic features), whereas others had broader eligibility criteria (all post-PCI patients). A variety of methods were reported for communication of test results to both providers and patients. All sites reported return of results to the electronic health record (EHR) usually as discrete data (genotype and predicted phenotype). Most institutions used clinical decision support (CDS) alerting or messaging for treatment recommendations, including for current and future clopidogrel orders. Institutions with clinical implementation models were often pharmacist-led and/or had a service dedicated to pharmacogenetics. The approach to provider education reported to be most successful was having focused meetings or in-services. Different patient-facing education methods were employed across sites, including in-person education and brochures.

The main implementation challenges highlighted by the IGNITE investigators were engaging and educating key providers and stakeholders, establishing laboratory testing capabilities with an informatics framework for return of results to the EHR, and creation of CDS.[70] Some specific logistical challenges were also noted depending on the testing model and implementation strategy used. A key example is the need for a dedicated service or person (ie, clinical pharmacist) to respond to results and improve the efficiency of genotype-concordant antiplatelet therapy.

Real-World Outcome Data

The aforementioned IGNITE Network reported clinical outcomes with CYP2C19 genotyping in clinical practice across 7 US sites and 1815 post-PCI patients.[50] Alternative P2Y$_{12}$ inhibitor therapy with prasugrel or ticagrelor was recommended for patients with a CYP2C19 LoF allele (in the absence of contraindications). However, prescribing decisions were ultimately left to the provider. No recommendations were made for those without an LoF allele. Patients with an LoF allele comprised 32% of the overall study. Alternative therapy was prescribed in about 60% of LoF allele carriers versus about 15% of those without an LoF allele ($P < .001$). This translated to a significantly higher rate of the composite clinical outcome (first occurrence of death, MI, or ischemic stroke) in the patients with an LoF allele who received clopidogrel versus alternative therapy (adjusted HR, 2.26; 95% CI, 1.18–4.32). No difference in outcome was observed between treatment groups in those patients without an LoF allele, most of whom received clopidogrel (adjusted HR, 1.14; 95% CI, 0.69–1.88).

The IGNITE investigators reported a subsequent analysis of an expanded cohort of 3342 patients who underwent CYP2C19 genotyping across 9 sites.[49] The primary composite outcome included all-cause death, MI, ischemic stroke, stent thrombosis, or hospitalization for unstable angina. Consistent with results from the initial analysis, the rate of these major atherothrombotic events was significantly lower with alternative therapy compared to clopidogrel in the LoF allele group (17.1 vs 34.4 event per 100 patient-years; adjusted HR, 0.56; 95% CI, 0.39–0.82). No difference in events between treatment groups was observed among those without an LoF allele (adjusted HR, 1.08; 95% CI, 0.72–1.62).

The evidence from these large, multicenter, observational studies extends the findings from the prospective, randomized trials by including more diverse patients. Other small observational studies have found similar benefit with genotype-guided therapy.[51,71,72] In totality, the utility and impact of CYP2C19 genotyping to guide antiplatelet therapy for post-PCI patients is evident. Treating patients with an LoF allele (IMs or PMs) with prasugrel or ticagrelor, instead of clopidogrel, results in the reduction in MACE.[48] Conversely, patients without an LoF allele appear to derive no additional benefit with alternative therapy compared to clopidogrel.[49] Use of clopidogrel versus more potent therapy in those without an LoF allele has the potential to reduce bleeding risk, thus supporting a role for *CYP2C19* genotyping to guide potential de-escalation when clinically appropriate.

SUMMARY AND FUTURE PERSPECTIVES

Data from thousands of patients clearly demonstrate a significant reduction in clopidogrel effectiveness following PCI in patients with a *CYP2C19* LoF allele. In addition, data from RCTs and observational studies support improved outcomes with a genotype-guided approach to antiplatelet selection. Despite this evidence, clinical implementation of *CYP2C19* genotyping is not widespread, likely because it is not endorsed by current clinical guidelines. As the use of alternative therapy continues to increase, one approach may be to reserve genotyping to guide de-escalation in patients at high bleeding risk, particularly if clopidogrel monotherapy is being considered. Ongoing trials are investigating such an approach (NCT05262803, NCT05773989, and NCT05577988) and will help to inform the future role of *CYP2C19* testing in $P2Y_{12}$ inhibitor selection.

CLINICS CARE POINTS

- While prasugrel and ticagrelor are superior to clopidogrel in patients with an LoF allele, clopidogrel is effective and associated with lower bleeding risk than other agents in patients without an LoF allele.

- *CYP2C19* genotyping is available from a number of commercial vendors.

- Professional practice guidelines do not provide recommendations for *CYP2C19* testing.

- Clinical Pharmacogenetic Implementation Consortium guidelines do not provide guidance on who to test but recommend prasugrel or ticagrelor for patients with an LoF allele in the absence of contraindications.

DISCLOSURE

J.C. Coons has received research support and served as a consultant to the Pfizer-Bristol Myers Squibb Alliance. L.H. Cavallari receives research support from Werfen. Support for L.H. Cavallari was provided by NIH grant R01 HL149752.

REFERENCES

1. Angiolillo DJ, Capodanno D, Danchin N, et al. Derivation, validation, and prognostic utility of a prediction rule for nonresponse to clopidogrel: the ABCD-GENE Score. JACC Cardiovasc Interv 2020;13:606–17.
2. Lee CR, Luzum JA, Sangkuhl K, et al. Clinical pharmacogenetics implementation consortium guideline for CYP2C19 genotype and clopidogrel therapy: 2022 update. Clin Pharmacol Ther 2022; 112:959–67.
3. Mega JL, Close SL, Wiviott SD, et al. Cytochrome P450 genetic polymorphisms and the response to prasugrel: relationship to pharmacokinetic, pharmacodynamic, and clinical outcomes. Circulation 2009;119:2553–60.
4. Wallentin L, James S, Storey RF, et al. Effect of CYP2C19 and ABCB1 single nucleotide polymorphisms on outcomes of treatment with ticagrelor versus clopidogrel for acute coronary syndromes: a genetic substudy of the PLATO trial. Lancet 2010;376:1320–8.
5. Dayoub EJ, Seigerman M, Tuteja S, et al. Trends in Platelet Adenosine Diphosphate P2Y12 Receptor Inhibitor Use and Adherence Among Antiplatelet-Naive Patients After Percutaneous Coronary Intervention, 2008-2016. JAMA Intern Med 2018;178: 943–50.
6. Wallentin L, Becker RC, Budaj A, et al. Ticagrelor versus clopidogrel in patients with acute coronary syndromes. N Engl J Med 2009;361:1045–57.
7. Wiviott SD, Braunwald E, McCabe CH, et al. Prasugrel versus clopidogrel in patients with acute coronary syndromes. N Engl J Med 2007;357:2001–15.
8. Levine GN, Bates ER, Bittl JA, et al. ACC/AHA guideline focused update on duration of dual antiplatelet therapy in patients with coronary artery disease: a report of the American College of Cardiology/American Heart Association Task Force on Clinical Practice Guidelines. J Am Coll Cardiol 2016;68:1082–115.
9. Wang Y, Cavallari LH, Brown JD, et al. Assessing the clinical treatment dynamics of antiplatelet therapy following acute coronary syndrome and percutaneous coronary intervention in the US. JAMA Netw Open 2023;6:e238585.
10. Ijaz SH, Baron SJ, Shahnawaz A, et al. Utilization trends in platelet adenosine diphosphate P2Y12

receptor inhibitor and cost among medicare bene-ficiaries. Curr Probl Cardiol 2023;48:101608.

11. Sangkuhl K, Klein TE, Altman RB. Clopidogrel pathway. Pharmacogenetics Genom 2010;20:463–5.

12. Rollini F, Franchi F, Angiolillo DJ. Switching P2Y12-receptor inhibitors in patients with coronary artery disease. Nat Rev Cardiol 2016;13:11–27.

13. Wiviott SD, Braunwald E, McCabe CH, et al. TRITON-TIMI Investigators. Prasugrel versus clopi-dogrel in patients with acute coronary syndromes. N Engl J Med 2007;357:2001–15.

14. Prasugrel prescribing information. Available at: https://www.accessdata.fda.gov/drugsatfda_docs/la-bel/2010/022307s002lbl.pdf. [Accessed 20 December 2023].

15. Angiolillo DJ, Cao D, Sartori S, et al. Dyspnea-related ticagrelor discontinuation after percuta-neous coronary intervention. JACC Cardiovasc Interv 2023;16:2514–24.

16. Ortega-Paz L, Brugaletta S, Ariotti S, et al. Adeno-sine and ticagrelor plasma levels in patients with and without ticagrelor-related dyspnea. Circulation 2018;138:646–8.

17. Gaedigk A, Casey ST, Whirl-Carrillo M, et al. Phar-macogene variation consortium: a global resource and repository for pharmacogene variation. Clin Pharmacol Ther 2021;110:542–5.

18. Pratt VM, Del Tredici AL, Hachad H, et al. Recom-mendations for clinical CYP2C19 genotyping allele selection: a report of the Association for Molecular Pathology. J Mol Diagn 2018;20:269–76.

19. Clinical Pharmacogenetic Implementation Con-sortium. CYP2C19 allele freqnecy table. Available at: https://cpicpgx.org/guidelines/guideline-for-clo-pidogrel-and-cyp2c19/. [Accessed 20 December 2023].

20. Bousman CA, Stevenson JM, Ramsey LB, et al. Clin-ical Pharmacogenetics Implementation Consortium (CPIC) Guideline for CYP2D6, CYP2C19, CYP2B6, SLC6A4, and HTR2A Genotypes and Serotonin Re-uptake Inhibitor Antidepressants. Clin Pharmacol Ther 2023;114:51–68.

21. Moriyama B, Obeng AO, Barbarino J, et al. Clinical pharmacogenetics implementation consortium (CPIC) Guidelines for CYP2C19 and Voriconazole Therapy. Clin Pharmacol Ther 2017;102:45–51.

22. Lee CR, Thomas CD, Beitelshees AL, et al. Impact of the CYP2C19*17 allele on outcomes in patients receiving genotype-guided antiplatelet therapy af-ter percutaneous coronary intervention. Clin Phar-macol Ther 2021;109:705–15.

23. Lima JJ, Thomas CD, Barbarino J, et al. Clinical pharmacogenetics implementation consortium (CPIC) Guideline for CYP2C19 and Proton Pump In-hibitor Dosing. Clin Pharmacol Ther 2021;109:1417–23.

24. Mega JL, Close SL, Wiviott SD, et al. Cytochrome p-450 polymorphisms and response to clopidogrel. N Engl J Med 2009;360:354–62.

25. Palmerini T, Calabro P, Piscione F, et al. Impact of gene polymorphisms, platelet reactivity, and the SYNTAX score on 1-year clinical outcomes in pa-tients with non-ST-segment elevation acute coro-nary syndrome undergoing percutaneous coronary intervention: the GEPRESS study. JACC Cardiovasc Interv 2014;7:1117–27.

26. Stone GW, Witzenbichler B, Weisz G, et al. Platelet reactivity and clinical outcomes after coronary ar-tery implantation of drug-eluting stents (ADAPT-DES): a prospective multicentre registry study. Lancet 2013;382:614–23.

27. Mega JL, Simon T, Collet JP, et al. Reduced-func-tion CYP2C19 genotype and risk of adverse clinical outcomes among patients treated with clopidogrel predominantly for PCI: a meta-analysis. JAMA 2010;304:1821–30.

28. Doll JA, Neely ML, Roe MT, et al. Impact of CYP2C19 Metabolizer Status on Patients With ACS Treated With Prasugrel Versus Clopidogrel. J Am Coll Cardiol 2016;67:936–47.

29. Pare G, Mehta SR, Yusuf S, et al. Effects of CYP2C19 genotype on outcomes of clopidogrel treatment. N Engl J Med 2010;363:1704–14.

30. Sorich MJ, Rowland A, McKinnon RA, et al. CYP2C19 genotype has a greater effect on adverse cardiovascular outcomes following percutaneous coronary intervention and in Asian populations treated with clopidogrel: a meta-analysis. Circ Car-diovasc Genet 2014;7:895–902.

31. Lewis JP, Stephens SH, Horenstein RB, et al. The CYP2C19*17 variant is not independently associ-ated with clopidogrel response. J Thromb Haemo-stasis 2013;11:1640–6.

32. Sibbing D, Gebhard D, Koch W, et al. Isolated and interactive impact of common CYP2C19 genetic variants on the antiplatelet effect of chronic clopi-dogrel therapy. J Thromb Haemostasis 2010;8:1685–93.

33. Sibbing D, Koch W, Gebhard D, et al. Cytochrome 2C19*17 allelic variant, platelet aggregation, bleeding events, and stent thrombosis in clopidogrel-treated patients with coronary stent placement. Circulation 2010;121:512–8.

34. Tiroch KA, Sibbing D, Koch W, et al. Protective ef-fect of the CYP2C19 *17 polymorphism with increased activation of clopidogrel on cardiovascu-lar events. Am Heart J 2010;160:506–12.

35. Claassens DMF, Bergmeijer TO, Vos GJA, et al. Clopidogrel versus ticagrelor or prasugrel after pri-mary percutaneous coronary intervention accord-ing to CYP2C19 genotype: a popular genetics subanalysis. Circ Cardiovasc Interv 2021;14:e009434.

36. Nguyen AB, Cavallari LH, Rossi JS, et al. Evaluation of race and ethnicity disparities in outcome studies of CYP2C19 genotype-guided antiplatelet therapy. Front Cardiovasc Med 2022;9:991646.

37. Cresci S, Depta JP, Lenzini PA, et al. Cytochrome p450 gene variants, race, and mortality among clopidogrel-treated patients after acute myocardial infarction. Circ Cardiovasc Genet 2014;7:277–86.

38. Tunehag KR, Thomas CD, Franchi F, et al. CYP2C19 genotype is associated with adverse cardiovascular outcomes in clopidogrel-treated Black patients undergoing percutaneous coronary intervention. J Am Heart Assoc 2024;13(12):e033791.

39. Shuldiner AR, O'Connell JR, Bliden KP, et al. Association of cytochrome P450 2C19 genotype with the antiplatelet effect and clinical efficacy of clopidogrel therapy. JAMA 2009;302:849–57.

40. Thomas CD, Franchi F, Keeley EC, et al. Impact of the ABCD-GENE Score on Clopidogrel Clinical Effectiveness after PCI: A Multi-Site, Real-World Investigation. Clin Pharmacol Ther 2022;112:146–55.

41. Thomas Cameron D, Franchi F, Rossi Joseph S, et al. Effectiveness of Clopidogrel vs Alternative P2Y12 Inhibitors Based on the ABCD-GENE Score. J Am Coll Cardiol 2024;83:1370–81.

42. Rehmel JL, Eckstein JA, Farid NA, et al. Interactions of two major metabolites of prasugrel, a thienopyridine antiplatelet agent, with the cytochromes P450. Drug Metab Dispos 2006;34:600–7.

43. Varenhorst C, Eriksson N, Johansson A, et al. Effect of genetic variations on ticagrelor plasma levels and clinical outcomes. Eur Heart J 2015;36:1901–12.

44. Horenstein RB, Madabushi R, Zineh I, et al. Effectiveness of clopidogrel dose escalation to normalize active metabolite exposure and antiplatelet effects in CYP2C19 poor metabolizers. J Clin Pharmacol 2014;54:865–73.

45. Mega JL, Hochholzer W, Frelinger AL 3rd, et al. Dosing clopidogrel based on CYP2C19 genotype and the effect on platelet reactivity in patients with stable cardiovascular disease. JAMA 2011;306:2221–8.

46. Carreras ET, Hochholzer W, Frelinger AL 3rd, et al. Diabetes mellitus, CYP2C19 genotype, and response to escalating doses of clopidogrel. Insights from the ELEVATE-TIMI 56 Trial. Thromb Haemostasis 2016;116:69–77.

47. Galli M, Occhipinti G, Benenati S, et al. Comparative effects of different antiplatelet strategies in carriers of CYP2C19 loss-of-function alleles: a network meta-analysis. Eur Heart J Cardiovasc Pharmacother 2024. https://doi.org/10.1093/ehjcvp/pvae036.

48. Pereira NL, Rihal C, Lennon R, et al. Effect of CYP2C19 genotype on ischemic outcomes during oral P2Y12 inhibitor therapy: a meta-analysis. JACC Cardiovasc Interv 2021;14:739–50.

49. Beitelshees AL, Thomas CD, Empey PE, et al. CYP2C19 genotype-guided antiplatelet therapy after percutaneous coronary intervention in diverse clinical settings. J Am Heart Assoc 2022;11:e024159.

50. Cavallari LH, Lee CR, Beitelshees AL, et al. Multisite investigation of outcomes with implementation of CYP2C19 genotype-guided antiplatelet therapy after percutaneous coronary intervention. JACC Cardiovasc Interv 2018;11:181–91.

51. Deiman BA, Tonino PA, Kouhestani K, et al. Reduced number of cardiovascular events and increased cost-effectiveness by genotype-guided antiplatelet therapy in patients undergoing percutaneous coronary interventions in the Netherlands. Neth Heart J 2016;24:589–99.

52. Zhang Y, Shi XJ, Peng WX, et al. Impact of Implementing CYP2C19 Genotype-Guided Antiplatelet Therapy on P2Y(12) Inhibitor Selection and Clinical Outcomes in Acute Coronary Syndrome Patients After Percutaneous Coronary Intervention: A Real-World Study in China. Front Pharmacol 2020;11:582929.

53. Notarangelo FM, Maglietta G, Bevilacqua P, et al. Pharmacogenomic approach to selecting antiplatelet therapy in acute coronary syndromes: PHARMCLO trial. J Am Coll Cardiol 2018;71:1869–77.

54. Claassens DMF, Vos GJA, Bergmeijer TO, et al. A genotype-guided strategy for oral P2Y12 inhibitors in primary PCI. N Engl J Med 2019;381:1621–31.

55. Pereira NL, Farkouh ME, So D, et al. Effect of genotype-guided oral P2Y12 inhibitor selection vs conventional clopidogrel therapy on ischemic outcomes after percutaneous coronary intervention: the TAILOR-PCI randomized clinical trial. JAMA 2020;324:761–71.

56. Galli M, Benenati S, Capodanno D, et al. Guided versus standard antiplatelet therapy in patients undergoing percutaneous coronary intervention: a systematic review and meta-analysis. Lancet 2021;397:1470–83.

57. Galli M, Benenati S, Franchi F, et al. Comparative effects of guided vs. potent P2Y12 inhibitor therapy in acute coronary syndrome: a network meta-analysis of 61 898 patients from 15 randomized trials. Eur Heart J 2022;43:959–67.

58. Food and Drug Administration. Table of Pharmacogenetic Associations. Available at: https://www.fda.gov/medical-devices/precision-medicine/table-pharmacogenetic-associations. [Accessed 19 December 2023].

59. Lawton JS, Tamis-Holland JE, Bangalore S, et al. 2021 ACC/AHA/SCAI Guideline for Coronary Artery Revascularization: Executive Summary: A Report of the American College of Cardiology/American Heart Association Joint Committee on Clinical Practice Guidelines. Circulation 2022;145:e4–17.

60. Byrne RA, Rossello X, Coughlan JJ, et al. 2023 ESC Guidelines for the management of acute coronary syndromes. Eur Heart J Acute Cardiovasc Care 2023.

61. Collet JP, Thiele H, Barbato E, et al. 2020 ESC Guidelines for the management of acute coronary syndromes in patients presenting without persistent ST-segment elevation. Eur Heart J 2020;74: 554.

62. Levine GN, Bates ER, Blankenship JC, et al. ACCF/AHA/SCAI Guideline for Percutaneous Coronary Intervention. A report of the American College of Cardiology Foundation/American Heart Association Task Force on Practice Guidelines and the Society for Cardiovascular Angiography and Interventions. J Am Coll Cardiol 2011;58:e44–122.

63. Sibbing D, Aradi D, Alexopoulos D, et al. Updated expert consensus statement on platelet function and genetic testing for guiding P2Y12 receptor inhibitor treatment in percutaneous coronary intervention. JACC Cardiovasc Interv 2019;12:1521–37.

64. Peterson JF, Field JR, Unertl KM, et al. Physician response to implementation of genotype-tailored antiplatelet therapy. Clin Pharmacol Ther 2016; 100:67–74.

65. Shuldiner AR, Palmer K, Pakyz RE, et al. Implementation of pharmacogenetics: the University of Maryland Personalized Anti-platelet Pharmacogenetics Program. Am J Med Genet C Semin Med Genet 2014;166C:76–84.

66. Weitzel KW, Elsey AR, Langaee TY, et al. Clinical pharmacogenetics implementation: approaches, successes, and challenges. Am J Med Genet C Semin Med Genet 2014;166C:56–67.

67. Lee JA, Lee CR, Reed BN, et al. Implementation and evaluation of a CYP2C19 genotype-guided antiplatelet therapy algorithm in high-risk coronary artery disease patients. Pharmacogenomics 2015;16: 303–13.

68. Coons JC, Stevenson JM, Patel A, et al. Antiplatelet Therapy and Bleeding Outcomes With CYP2C19 Genotyping. J Cardiovasc Pharmacol Therapeut 2022;27. 10742484221143246.

69. Cavallari LH, Franchi F, Rollini F, et al. Clinical implementation of rapid CYP2C19 genotyping to guide antiplatelet therapy after percutaneous coronary intervention. J Transl Med 2018;16:92.

70. Empey PE, Stevenson JM, Tuteja S, et al. Multisite investigation of strategies for the implementation of CYP2C19 genotype-guided antiplatelet therapy. Clin Pharmacol Ther 2018;104:664–74.

71. Shen DL, Wang B, Bai J, et al. Clinical Value of CYP2C19 Genetic Testing for Guiding the Antiplatelet Therapy in a Chinese Population. J Cardiovasc Pharmacol 2016;67:232–6.

72. Sanchez-Ramos J, Davila-Fajardo CL, Toledo Frias P, et al. Results of genotype-guided antiplatelet therapy in patients who undergone percutaneous coronary intervention with stent. Int J Cardiol 2016;225:289–95.

73. Scott SA, Sangkuhl K, Stein CM, et al. Clinical pharmacogenetics implementation consortium guidelines for CYP2C19 genotype and clopidogrel therapy: 2013 update. Clin Pharmacol Ther 2013;94:317–23.

High Bleeding Risk in Patients Undergoing Coronary and Structural Heart Interventions

Mattia Galli, MD, PhD[a],*, Domenico D'Amario, MD, PhD[b]

KEYWORDS

- High bleeding risk • Percutaneous coronary intervention • Structural heart intervention
- Bleeding

KEY POINTS

- Percutaneous coronary and structural heart interventions are increasingly preferred over cardiac surgery due to reduced periprocedural complications and faster recovery.
- The use of devices and platforms (ie, stents or prosthetic valves) during percutaneous interventions necessitate periprocedural and postprocedural antithrombotic therapy to prevent local thrombotic events, contributing to increase the risk of bleeding.
- The increasing implementation of percutaneous interventions in patients at high bleeding risk (HBR) coupled with the concomitant need for mid-term to long-term antithrombotic therapy after the procedure poses a relevant clinical conundrum.
- The identification of patients with HBR through standardized definitions is pivotal for the implementation of bleeding reduction strategies as well as for the standardization of outcomes across clinical trials.

INTRODUCTION

With the exception of patients presenting with acute coronary syndrome (ACS), wherein percutaneous coronary intervention (PCI) has essentially supplanted pharmacologic treatments like fibrinolysis, percutaneous coronary and structural heart interventions have increasingly served as alternative approaches for patients traditionally referred for cardiac surgery.[1–4] Notably, percutaneous interventions, being minimally invasive procedures that often do not necessitate general anesthesia and are linked to reduced periprocedural complications and faster recovery compared to surgical methods, were initially proposed for patients at high surgical risk (eg, advanced age or multiple comorbidities), and consequently, also at elevated risk of bleeding.[3,5] However, percutaneous interventions frequently utilize devices and platforms (ie, stents or prosthetic valves) necessitating the use of periprocedural and postprocedural antithrombotic therapy to prevent local thrombotic events (ie, stent thrombosis, ST), inevitably contributing to increase the risk of bleeding.[5,6] The preference for percutaneous coronary and structural interventions as opposed to standard cardiac surgery in patients at high bleeding risk, coupled with the concomitant need for midterm to long-term antithrombotic therapy postintervention, has posed a long-standing clinical conundrum.[5,7]

Recently, the growing recognition of the prognostic implications of bleeding, along with the availability of more advanced devices and

[a] Maria Cecilia Hospital, GVM Care & Research, Via Corriera, 1, Cotignola 48033, Ravenna, Italy; [b] Dipartimento di MedicinaTraslazionale, Università del Piemonte Orientale, Via Paolo Solaroli, 17, 28100 Novara, Italy
* Corresponding author.
E-mail address: dottormattiagalli@gmail.com
Twitter: @MattiaGalli10 (M.G.)

Intervent Cardiol Clin 13 (2024) 483–491
https://doi.org/10.1016/j.iccl.2024.06.003
2211-7458/24/© 2024 Elsevier Inc. All rights are reserved, including those for text and data mining, AI training, and similar technologies.

stent platforms with reduced thrombogenicity, obviating intense and long-term postprocedural antithrombotic regimens, has shifted focus toward the implementation of dedicated bleeding reduction strategies in these patients.[8,9] Moreover, because individuals show a variable response to antithrombotic agents, bleeding complications may in some cases outweigh the expected benefit of reducing thrombotic events.[10–12] Against this backdrop, the identification of patients with high bleeding risk (HBR) through standardized definitions has become pivotal, facilitating the prompt recognition of these individuals and the implementation of bleeding reduction strategies.[8] Additionally, the necessity for a standardized definition of HBR across clinical trials has emerged as a crucial area of research in the past decade.

Herein, we provide a comprehensive description of the classification and clinical relevance of HBR in patients undergoing coronary and structural heart interventions.

Definition of Bleeding

The primary challenge in addressing bleeding among patients undergoing coronary or structural heart interventions arises from the complexity of this clinical phenomenon and heterogeneity of classifications.[10,11,13] Over time, numerous bleeding definitions have been proposed, leading to some confusion and impeding the comparison of bleeding incidence and prognostic relevance across different studies.[10,11,13]

Global Use of Strategies to Open Occluded Arteries and Thrombolysis in Myocardial Infarction (TIMI) classifications were among the first widely accepted definition for bleeding, developed in patients with ST-elevation myocardial infarction (MI) receiving thrombolytic therapy.[13–15] However, due to the fact that these classifications were developed in an era in which severe bleeding were relatively common (due to the high use of thrombolytic therapy and/or of coronary artery bypass graft in patients with ACS), they were found to be less effective in capturing milder events commonly observed in the percutaneous intervention era.[13,14,16]

The International Society on Thrombosis and Haemostasis (ISTH) classification was designed to provide a more detailed definition of bleeding, including mild and moderate bleeds, introducing also a pragmatic approach by including the clinical relevance of bleeding.[17] Furthermore, the use of different trial-specific bleeding definitions over time has resulted in the spread of several classifications reflecting the names of the trials in which they have been adopted. Examples include the CURE, ACUITY, OASIS, and PLATO definitions.[13] However, trial-specific definitions inherently impede the comparison of bleeding incidence and prognostic impact across studies.

More recently, the Bleeding Academic Research Consortium (BARC) provided a classification including both clinical (eg, health care intervention or harmfulness of bleeding site) and laboratory criteria (eg, hematocrit and hemoglobin).[13] BARC employs ordinal numbers rather than qualitative terms, indicating increasing bleeding severity and mortality with higher BARC grades (Fig. 1).[13] Due to its ability to capture a large proportion of clinically significant bleeding and provide more precise subclassifications, the BARC classification has gained extensive adoption over the years, emerging as the most utilized and reliable bleeding definition for patients undergoing percutaneous interventions.[10,11]

Similarly to BARC, the Valve Academic Research Consortium 3, which standardizes clinical endpoints for clinical trials in patients undergoing transcatheter and surgical aortic valve, recently provided more descriptive bleeding classification including type 1 (minor), type 2 (major), type 3 (life-threatening), and type 4 (leading to death) bleedings (see Fig. 1).[18]

INCIDENCE AND CLINICAL IMPACT OF BLEEDING

Coronary Interventions

Among patients undergoing PCIs, the incidence and prognostic impact of bleeding vary according to the included population (ie, ACS vs chronic coronary syndrome [CCS]), grade (ie, mild, moderate, or severe), and classification of bleeding used.[19,20] According to the BARC definition of bleeding, the incidence of bleeding was 6.9%, 5.6%, and 2.7% with BARC 1, 2, and 3, respectively, among patients with ACS undergoing PCI at 1.4 years.[12,20] Moreover, mortality rates were 2%, 3%, 7%, 8%, 13%, and 40% with BARC 0, 1, 2, 3a, 3b, and 3c bleeding, respectively.[12,20] When the prognostic impact of BARC bleeding was compared with that of ischemic events, the mortality rate associated with MI was found to be similar to that of BARC 3b bleeding, and lower than that associated with BARC 3c bleeding.[12,19]

The prognostic impact of bleeding also depends on factors different from the direct organ damage due to the bleed, such as the abrupt interruption of antiplatelet treatment as a reaction to the bleeding event that may increase the risk of thrombotic events, the activation of coagulation and inflammation in case of bleeding and/or blood transfusion.[10,21] With regards to the site of bleeding, gastrointestinal tract bleeding

CORONARY INTERVENTIONS	STRUCTURAL HEART INTERVENTIONS

Bleeding classification

Bleeding Academic Research Consortium

Type 1
- Bleeding that is not actionable and does not cause the patient to seek an unscheduled performance of studies, hospitalization, or treatment by a health care professional

Type 2
- Any overt, actionable sign of hemorrhage that does not fit the criteria for type 3, type 4, or type 5 but does meet at least one of the following criteria: requiring nonsurgical, medical intervention by a health care professional; leading to hospitalization or increased level of care; or prompting evaluation

Type 3a
- Overt bleeding plus a hemoglobin drop of 3 to 5 g/dL (provided the hemoglobin drop is related to bleed)
- Any transfusion with overt bleeding

Type 3b
- Overt bleeding plus a hemoglobin drop of 5 g/dL (provided the hemoglobin drop is related to bleed)
- Cardiac tamponade
- Bleeding requiring surgical intervention for control
- Bleeding requiring intravenous vasoactive agents

Type 3c:
- Intracranial hemorrhage
- Subcategories confirmed by autopsy or imaging, or lumbar puncture
- Intraocular bleed compromising vision

Type 4:
- Coronary artery bypass grafting-related bleeding
- Perioperative intracranial bleeding within 48 hours
- Reoperation after closure of sternotomy for the purpose of controlling bleeding
- Transfusion of 5 U of whole blood or packed red blood cells within a 48-hour period
- Chest tube output 2 L within a 24-hour period

Type 5a
- Probable fatal bleeding; no autopsy or imaging confirmation but clinically suspicious

Type 5b
- Definite fatal bleeding; overt bleeding or autopsy, or imaging confirmation

Valve Academic Research Consortium 3

Type 1
- Overt bleeding that does not require surgical or percutaneous intervention, but does require medical intervention by a health care professional, leading to hospitalization, an increased level of care, or medical evaluation (BARC 2)
- Overt bleeding that requires a transfusion of 1 unit of whole blood/red blood cells (BARC 3a)

Type 2
- Overt bleeding that requires a transfusion of 2–4 units of whole blood/red blood cells (BARC 3a)
- Overt bleeding associated with a haemoglobin drop of >3 g/dL (>1.86 mmol/L) but <5 g/d (<3.1 mmol/L) (BARC 3a)

Type 3
- Overt bleeding in a critical organ, such as intracranial, intraspinal, intraocular, pericardial or intramuscular with compartment syndrome (BARC 3b, BARC 3c)
- Overt bleeding causing hypovolemic shock or severe hypotension or requiring vasopressors or surgery (BARC 3b)
- Overt bleeding requiring reoperation, surgical exploration, or re-intervention for the purpose of controlling bleeding (BARC 3b, BARC 4)
- Post-thoracotomy chest tube output ≥2 L within a 24-h period (BARC 4)
- Overt bleeding requiring a transfusion of ≥5 units of whole blood/red blood cells (BARC 3a)
- Overt bleeding associated with a haemoglobin drop ≥5 g/dL (≥3.1 mmol/L) (BARC 3b)

Type 4
- Overt bleeding leading to death. Should be classified as: *Probable:* Clinical suspicion (BARC 5a) or *Definite:* Confirmed by autopsy or imaging (BARC 5b)

Fig. 1. Major bleeding definitions among the spectrum of coronary and structural heart diseases. BARC, Bleeding Academic Research Consortium.

represents the more commonly involved site of bleeding accounting for more than 60% of out-of-hospital bleeding, followed by peripheral (12%), genitourinary (9%), central nervous system (7%), vascular access site bleeding (7%), and retroperitoneal (3.2%) bleeding.[22] It is important to note that bleeding is subject to dynamic fluctuations over time, being highest in the periprocedural phase and remaining relatively stable over time thereafter.[6,23]

Several baseline characteristics of patient undergoing PCI have been associated with bleeding and should be considered to increase the accuracy of patients' bleeding risk stratification, such as advanced age, demographic (eg, East Asian ethnicity), clinical (eg, ACS, renal dysfunction, cardiogenic shock, cardiac arrest, and frailty), and procedural features (eg, nonradial access, periprocedural antithrombotic therapy, and the use of mechanical support).[10,11,24] Importantly, the intensity, number and duration of antithrombotic agents are proportionally associated and represent a major determinant in increasing bleeding risk.[10] Among patients undergoing PCI, early studies have shown that adding clopidogrel to aspirin (ie, DAPT) increases the relative risk of major bleeding by nearly 50% compared with aspirin alone.[25] Moreover, potent $P2Y_{12}$ inhibitors (ie, prasugrel or ticagrelor) are associated

with a further 25% to 30% relative increase in major bleeding compared with clopidogrel, on top of aspirin.[26,27] With regard to DAPT duration, 12 month DAPT is associated with a 40% relative increase in major bleeding compared with short (1–3 month) DAPT, whereas longer DAPT durations (>12 months) is associated with a 60% relative increase in major bleeding compared with 12 month DAPT.[28–34]

Structural Heart Interventions

Less evidence is available on the prognostic impact of bleeding in patients undergoing structural heart interventions.[5] Because the incidence of valvular heart disease increases with age, being highest in the elderly, percutaneous interventions for valvular heart disease are often associated with frailty, high comorbidity burden, and considerable risk for bleeding.[35]

With regards to transcatheter aortic valve replacement (TAVR), the vast majority (80%) of bleeding events are early (within 30 days after the procedure) and are mainly access site-related (60%).[35,36] Access-site-related and nonaccess site-related events are both associated with a 50% to 100% increase in mortality, but nonaccess bleeding is associated with a 56% relative increase in mortality compared to patients with access-site bleeding.[37] On the other hand, late bleeding events (>30 days after the procedure) are mainly related to gastrointestinal bleeds and strictly related to the long-term antithrombotic therapy used.[35] The number and duration of antithrombotic agents used after TAVR is a major determinant of the risk of bleeding in these patients, with single antiplatelet therapy emerging as the more balanced strategy to optimize bleeding and ischemic risks among patients without concomitant indication for OAC.[38]

Transcatheter mitral and tricuspid valve interventions are by definition limited to patients deemed to be at prohibitive surgical and, therefore, bleeding risk due to frailty and concomitant significant comorbidities. Similarly, left atrial appendage closure (LAAC) is often used as alternative strategy in patients with prohibitive bleeding risk preventing from administering long-term OAC in these patients. Indeed, about 70% to 80% of patients undergoing LAAC have a history of clinically relevant bleeding, including intracranial bleeding in nearly 10% of cases.[39–45] Similar to PCI and other structural heart interventions, bleeding after LAAC has a significant impact on prognosis, being associated with a 3 fold increase in mortality.[36,42,46]

HIGH BLEEDING RISK DEFINITION AND RISK STRATIFICATION

Several scores and classifications have been proposed to define patients with HBR and standardize their identification across studies in patients undergoing coronary and structural heart interventions.

Coronary Interventions

The vast majority of bleeding risk scores have been developed for patients undergoing PCI with or without ACS and can be used either early at the hospital admission to predict short-term bleeding risk (ie, CRUSADE, ACUITY-HORIZONS-AMI, SWEDEHEART, and ARC-HBR), or at discharge/during follow-up to predict long-term bleeding events and guide the subsequent antithrombotic therapy (ie, PARIS, BleeMACS, DAPT, PRECISE-DAPT, and ARC-HBR trade-off model).[10,11,47]

CRUSADE included hemodynamic parameters at presentation (heart rate, systolic blood pressure, and heart failure), laboratory findings (hematocrit and creatinine clearance), and clinical features (sex, history of diabetes mellitus, or vascular disease), showing moderate discriminatory ability for predicting of in-hospital major bleeding (c-statistics = 0.71) in patients with non-ST elevation ACS.[48,49] The score ranges from 1 to 100 points, with a score above 41

identifying HBR and a score above 51 points identifying very-HBR patients.[48] Among other scores for the prediction of in-hospital bleeding, ACUITY-HORIZONS-AMI score showed moderate (c-statistics = 0.71), and the SWEDEHEART good (c-statistics = 0.80) discriminatory ability for predicting in-hospital major bleeding in patients with ACS.[50,51]

With regards to scores for the prediction of long-term bleeding, BleeMACS included 7 independent predictors of bleeding (age, hypertension, vascular disease, history of bleeding, malignancy, creatinine, and hemoglobin) showing moderate discrimination for 1 year major bleedings (c-statistics = 0.71).[52] Similarly, the PARIS score showed moderate (c-statistics = 0.72) discriminatory ability for predicting post-PCI bleeding events.[53] In contrast, the DAPT score is applicable to patients after 12 months of uneventful DAPT.[54] It assessed the need for DAPT prolongation, where a score greater than 2 indicates a higher ischemic risk rather than bleeding risk. The score demonstrated moderate discrimination performance for bleeding risk (c-statistics = 0.68).[54]

The PRECISE-DAPT score included 5 items (hemoglobin, age, white blood cell count, creatinine clearance, and previous bleeding), showing moderate discriminatory ability for predicting the risk of out-of-hospital TIMI major or minor bleeding (c-statistics = 0.70) and TIMI major bleedings (c-statistics = 0.68) outside the hospital at 1 year in patients undergoing DAPT.[55] Moreover, the use of this score was proposed as guidance for duration of DAPT, given that in patients with HBR with a score of 25 or greater points, prolonged DAPT (12–24 months) was associated with increased bleeding without a reduction in ischemic events, suggesting that a shorter (≤12 months) DAPT duration would be advantageous.[56] A recent meta-analysis including a total of 67,283 patients found that patients defined at HBR because of a PRECISE-DAPT of 25 or greater were as frequent as 24.7% among PCI patients and associated with a 2.7 fold increase in any bleeding and a 3.5 fold increase in major bleeding compared with patients without HBR.[57]

The Academic Research Consortium for HBR (ARC-HBR) defined patients with HBR as those having a BARC 3 or 5 bleeding risk of 4% or greater or an intracranial hemorrhage (ICH) risk of 1% or greater at 1 year.[58] A total of 14 major (ie, OAC, severe chronic kidney disease [CKD], hemoglobin) and 6 minor criteria (ie, age ≥75 years, moderate CKD, spontaneous bleeding requiring hospitalization in the past 12 months, long-term use of anti-inflammatory drugs, any ischemic stroke) were identified. A major criterion is defined as any criterion that, in isolation, confers a BARC 3 or 5 bleeding risk of 4% or greater or an ICH risk of 1% or greater at 1 year. A minor criterion is defined as any criterion that, compared to its absence, confers an increased risk of BARC 3 or 5 bleeding of less than 4% at 1 year. Several studies have validated the ARC-HBR definition in contemporary PCI settings.[59] This scoring system has been widely accepted, showing moderate discriminatory ability in external validation studies (c-statistics = 0.67[60,61]; Fig. 2). Additionally, ARC has developed its trade-off model for evaluating ischemic and bleeding risks, displaying modest discrimination for BARC 3 to 5 bleeding (c-statistics = 0.68).[62] However, a recent study found that 5 out of the 6 minor criteria actually identify in isolation patients with a BARC 3 or 5 bleeding risk of 4% or greater, suggesting that further investigations are required to refine the accuracy of this HBR definition.[61]

Structural Heart Interventions

Accurate identification of patients with HBR undergoing structural heart interventions is challenging, currently lacking standardization, and often relying on subjective clinician judgment. Factors related to both patients and the TAVR procedure itself have been linked to bleeding events, and improved recognition of these factors may enhance risk stratification.[35]

Patient-related factors include older age, frailty status, female sex, associated conditions (eg, renal insufficiency, anemia, or angiodysplasia) and concomitant therapies (eg, OAC or antiplatelet agents).[63–66] Chronic anemia affects approximately 50% of TAVR patients and is associated with increased mortality.[67] Furthermore, acquired type 2A von Willebrand disease leading to gastrointestinal bleeding, a condition known as Heyde's syndrome, is observed in approximately 6% of patients with aortic stenosis but is usually reversible after TAVR.[67] With regards to procedure-related risk factors, these include operator/center experience, sheath size, access site selection, and hemostasis technique, mainly influencing the rates of access site-related bleeding.[35]

Because bleeding risk stratification scores developed for PCI patients have shown to perform poorly in the TAVR setting, PREDICT-TAVR was a dedicated risk score for predicting bleeding risk after TAVR, developed in 5185 patients from the RISPEVA registry and validated in 5043 patients from the POL-TAVI database.[61,68,69] It includes 6 items consisting in hemoglobin, serum iron, creatinine clearance, OAC, DAPT, and common femoral artery diameter, showing good discrimination for 30 day bleeding (c-statistics = 0.78; see Fig. 2).

In accordance with score quartiles, the 30 day bleeding rate varied, ranging from 0.8% in the low-risk group (≤8 points) to 8.5% in the

CORONARY INTERVENTIONS	STRUCTURAL HEART INTERVENTIONS
High bleeding risk definition	
ARC-HBR	PREDICT-TAVR

Major criteria
- Anticipated use of long-term oral anticoagulation
- Severe or end-stage chronic kidney disease
- Hemoglobin <11 g/dL
- Spontaneous bleeding requiring hospitalization or transfusion in the past 6 months or at any time, if recurrent
- Moderate or severe baseline thrombocytopenia (platelet count <100×10⁹/L)
- Chronic bleeding diathesis
- Liver cirrhosis with portal hypertension
- Active malignancy within the past 12 months
- Previous spontaneous intracranial haemorrhage
- Previous traumatic intracranial haemorrhage within the past 12 months
- Presence of a brain arteriovenous malformations
- Moderate or severe ischemic stroke within the past 6 months
- Nondeferrable major surgery on dual antiplatelet therapy
- Recent major surgery or major trauma within 30 days before percutaneous coronary intervention

Minor criteria
- Age ≥75 years
- Moderate CKD (eGFR 30 to 59 mL/min/1.73 m²)
- Hemoglobin 11 to 12.9 g/dL for men and 11 to 11.9 g/dL for women
- Spontaneous bleeding requiring hospitalization or transfusion within the past 12 months not meeting the major criterion
- Long-term use of oral NSAIDs or steroids
- Any ischemic stroke at any time not meeting the major criterion

1) Blood hemoglobin (15-7 mg/dl)
2) Serum iron concentrations (180-0 mcg/dl)
3) Oral anticoagulation (yes/no)
4) Dual antiplatelet therapy (yes/no)
5) Common femoral artery diameter
6) Creatinine clearance (eGFR 120-10 mL/min/1.73 m²)

HBR: ≥1 major criteria or ≥ 2 minor criteria

Low bleeding risk: ≤ 8 points
Moderate bleeding risk: > 8 and ≤10 points
High bleeding risk: > 10 and ≤12 points
Very high bleeding risk: > 12 points

Fig. 2. Major high bleeding risk classifications among the spectrum of coronary and structural heart disease. ARC, Academic Research Consortium; CKD, chronic kidney disease; eGFR, estimated glomerular filtration rate; HBR, high bleeding risk; NSAIDs, nonsteroidal anti-inflammatory drugs; TAVR, transcatheter aortic valve replacement.

very-high-risk group (>12 points). Notably, no significant predictive value was observed from 30 days to 1 year, possibly attributable to the limited number of events recorded within this timeframe.[69]

No dedicated bleeding risk scores are available for other structural heart interventions. The HAS-BLED score is empirically used among patients with LAAC despite remaining to be validated in this population.[70]

SUMMARY

Bleeding is a common complication in patients undergoing coronary or structural heart interventions. This is primarily attributed to the advanced age and numerous comorbidities of these patients. Additionally, the necessity for antithrombotic therapy to prevent thrombotic events after the procedure contributes to the elevated risk of bleeding. Definitions for a prompt identification of patients at high bleeding risk, allowing to the implementation of bleeding reduction strategies in these patients and contributing to standardize HBR definitions across clinical trials are key. Limitations of these scores and definitions are represented by the fact that factors associated with an increased bleeding risk are often also associated with an increased ischemic risk and vice versa. Further evidence is needed for an accurate stratification of patients with HBR in patients undergoing structural heart interventions.

CLINICS CARE POINTS

- Bleeding complications carry important prognostic implications in patients undergoing coronary or structural interventions.
- The identification of high bleeding risk (HBR) patients and the prompt adoption of specific strategies to reduce bleeding complications in these patients is key for the optimization of outcomes.

DISCLOSURE

M. Galli declares that he has received honoraria from Terumo, outside the present study. D. D'Amario reports no disclosures for the present study.

REFERENCES

1. Smith CR, Leon MB, Mack MJ, et al. Transcatheter versus surgical aortic-valve replacement in high-risk patients. N Engl J Med 2011;364(23):2187–98.

2. Leon MB, Smith CR, Mack M, et al. Transcatheter aortic-valve implantation for aortic stenosis in patients who cannot undergo surgery. N Engl J Med 2010;363(17):1597–607.

3. Gaudino M, Andreotti F, Kimura T. Current concepts in coronary artery revascularisation. Lancet (London, England) 2023;401(10388):1611–28.

4. Armstrong PW, Gershlick AH, Goldstein P, et al. Fibrinolysis or Primary PCI in ST-Segment Elevation Myocardial Infarction 2013;368(15):1379–87.

5. Calabrò P, Gragnano F, Niccoli G, et al. Antithrombotic therapy in patients undergoing transcatheter interventions for structural heart disease. Circulation 2021;144(16):1323–43.

6. Angiolillo DJ, Galli M, Collet JP, et al. Antiplatelet therapy after percutaneous coronary intervention. EuroIntervention 2022;17(17):e1371–96.

7. Galli M, Ortega-Paz L, Franchi F, et al. Precision medicine in interventional cardiology: implications for antiplatelet therapy in patients undergoing percutaneous coronary intervention. Pharmacogenomics 2022;23(13):723–37.

8. Capodanno D, Bhatt DL, Gibson CM, et al. Bleeding avoidance strategies in percutaneous coronary intervention. Nat Rev Cardiol 2022;19(2):117–32.

9. Galli M, Angiolillo DJ. De-escalation of antiplatelet therapy in acute coronary syndromes: Why, how and when? Frontiers in cardiovascular medicine 2022;9:975969.

10. Galli M, Laborante R, Andreotti F, et al. Bleeding complications in patients undergoing percutaneous coronary intervention 2022;23(8).

11. Laudani C, Capodanno D, Angiolillo DJ. Bleeding in acute coronary syndrome: from definitions, incidence, and prognosis to prevention and management. Expet Opin Drug Saf 2023;22(12):1193–212.

12. Valgimigli M, Costa F, Lokhnygina Y, et al. Trade-off of myocardial infarction vs. bleeding types on mortality after acute coronary syndrome: lessons from the Thrombin Receptor Antagonist for Clinical Event Reduction in Acute Coronary Syndrome (TRACER) randomized trial. Eur Heart J 2017;38(11):804–10.

13. Mehran R, Rao SV, Bhatt DL, et al. Standardized bleeding definitions for cardiovascular clinical trials: a consensus report from the Bleeding Academic Research Consortium. Circulation 2011;123(23):2736–47.

14. An international randomized trial comparing four thrombolytic strategies for acute myocardial infarction. N Engl J Med 1993;329(10):673–82.

15. Bovill EG, Terrin ML, Stump DC, et al. Hemorrhagic events during therapy with recombinant tissue-type plasminogen activator, heparin, and aspirin for acute myocardial infarction. Results of the Thrombolysis in Myocardial Infarction (TIMI), Phase II Trial. Ann Intern Med 1991;115(4):256–65.

16. Chesebro JH, Knatterud G, Roberts R, et al. Thrombolysis in Myocardial Infarction (TIMI) Trial, Phase I: A comparison between intravenous tissue plasminogen activator and intravenous streptokinase. Clinical findings through hospital discharge. Circulation 1987;76(1):142–54.

17. Schulman S, Kearon C. Definition of major bleeding in clinical investigations of antihemostatic medicinal products in non-surgical patients. J Thromb Haemostasis 2005;3(4):692–4.

18. Généreux P, Piazza N, Alu MC, et al. Valve academic research consortium 3. Updated Endpoint Definitions for Aortic Valve Clinical Research 2021; 77(21):2717–46.

19. Vranckx P, White HD, Huang Z, et al. Validation of BARC bleeding criteria in patients with acute coronary syndromes: The TRACER trial. J Am Coll Cardiol 2016;67(18):2135–44.

20. Ndrepepa G, Schuster T, Hadamitzky M, et al. Validation of the bleeding academic research consortium definition of bleeding in patients with coronary artery disease undergoing percutaneous coronary intervention 2012;125(11):1424–31.

21. Galli M, Angiolillo DJ. The evaluation and management of coagulopathies in the intensive therapy units. Eur Heart J Acute Cardiovasc Care 2023; 12(6):399–407.

22. Généreux P, Giustino G, Witzenbichler B, et al. Incidence, predictors, and impact of post-discharge bleeding after percutaneous coronary intervention. J Am Coll Cardiol 2015;66(9):1036–45.

23. Galli M, Occhipinti G. "Ticking away the moments that make up a dull DAPT course": Time matters. Int J Cardiol 2023;131424.

24. Galli M, Laborante R, Occhipinti G, et al. Impact of ethnicity on antiplatelet treatment regimens for bleeding reduction in acute coronary syndromes: a systematic review and pre-specified subgroup meta-analysis. Eur Heart J Cardiovasc Pharmacother 2023;10(2):158–69.

25. Galli M, Andreotti F, D'Amario D, et al. Antithrombotic therapy in the early phase of non-ST-elevation acute coronary syndromes: a systematic review and meta-analysis. Eur Heart J Cardiovasc Pharmacother 2020;6(1):43–56.

26. Navarese EP, Khan SU, Kołodziejczak M, et al. Comparative efficacy and safety of oral P2Y(12) inhibitors in acute coronary syndrome: network meta-analysis of 52 816 patients from 12 randomized trials. Circulation 2020;142(2):150–60.

27. Galli M, Benenati S, Franchi F, et al. Comparative effects of guided vs. potent P2Y12 inhibitor therapy in acute coronary syndrome: a network meta-analysis of 61 898 patients from 15 randomized trials. Eur Heart J 2022;43(10):959–67.

28. Navarese EP, Andreotti F, Schulze V, et al. Optimal duration of dual antiplatelet therapy after percutaneous coronary intervention with drug eluting stents: meta-analysis of randomised controlled trials. BMJ (Clinical research ed) 2015; 350:h1618.

29. Benenati S, Galli M, De Marzo V, et al. Very short vs. long dual antiplatelet therapy after second generation drug-eluting stents in 35 785 patients undergoing percutaneous coronary interventions: a meta-analysis of randomized controlled trials. Eur Heart J Cardiovasc Pharmacother 2021;7(2):86–93.

30. Galli M, Andreotti F, D'Amario D, et al. Randomised trials and meta-analyses of double vs triple antithrombotic therapy for atrial fibrillation-ACS/PCI: A critical appraisal. Int J Cardiol Heart Vasc 2020;28:100524.

31. De Caterina R, Agewall S, Andreotti F, et al. Great Debate: Triple antithrombotic therapy in patients with atrial fibrillation undergoing coronary stenting should be limited to 1 week. Eur Heart J 2022; 43(37):3512–27.

32. van Rein N, Heide-Jørgensen U, Lijfering WM, et al. Major bleeding rates in atrial fibrillation patients on single, dual, or triple antithrombotic therapy. Circulation 2019;139(6):775–86.

33. Lamberts M, Olesen JB, Ruwald MH, et al. Bleeding after initiation of multiple antithrombotic drugs, including triple therapy, in atrial fibrillation patients following myocardial infarction and coronary intervention: a nationwide cohort study. Circulation 2012;126(10):1185–93.

34. Galli M, Andreotti F, Porto I, et al. Intracranial haemorrhages vs. stent thromboses with direct oral anticoagulant plus single antiplatelet agent or triple antithrombotic therapy: a meta-analysis of randomized trials in atrial fibrillation and percutaneous coronary intervention/acute coronary syndrome patients. Europace 2020;22(4):538–46.

35. Avvedimento M, Nuche J, Farjat-Pasos JI, et al. Bleeding events after transcatheter aortic valve replacement: JACC state-of-the-art review. J Am Coll Cardiol 2023;81(7):684–702.

36. Piccolo R, Pilgrim T, Franzone A, et al. Frequency, timing, and impact of access-site and non-access-site bleeding on mortality among patients undergoing transcatheter aortic valve replacement. JACC Cardiovasc Interv 2017;10(14):1436–46.

37. Généreux P, Head SJ, Van Mieghem NM, et al. Clinical outcomes after transcatheter aortic valve replacement using valve academic research consortium definitions: a weighted meta-analysis of 3,519 patients from 16 studies. J Am Coll Cardiol 2012;59(25):2317–26.

38. Guedeney P, Roule V, Mesnier J, et al. Antithrombotic therapy and cardiovascular outcomes after transcatheter aortic valve implantation in patients without indications for chronic oral anticoagulation: a systematic review and network meta-analysis of

randomized controlled trials. Eur Heart J Cardiovasc Pharmacother 2023;9(3):251–61.

39. Kar S, Doshi SK, Sadhu A, et al. Primary outcome evaluation of a next-generation left atrial appendage closure device: results from the PINNACLE FLX Trial. Circulation 2021;143(18):1754–62.

40. Lakkireddy D, Thaler D, Ellis CR, et al. Amplatzer Amulet left atrial appendage occluder versus watchman device for stroke prophylaxis (Amulet IDE): a randomized, controlled trial. Circulation 2021;144(19):1543–52.

41. Simard T, Jung RG, Lehenbauer K, et al. Predictors of device-related thrombus following percutaneous left atrial appendage occlusion. J Am Coll Cardiol 2021;78(4):297–313.

42. Aminian A, De Backer O, Nielsen-Kudsk JE, et al. Incidence and clinical impact of major bleeding following left atrial appendage occlusion: insights from the Amplatzer Amulet Observational Post-Market Study. EuroIntervention 2021;17(9):774–82.

43. Price MJ, Reddy VY, Valderrábano M, et al. Bleeding outcomes after left atrial appendage closure compared with long-term warfarin: a pooled, patient-level analysis of the WATCHMAN randomized trial experience. JACC Cardiovasc Interv 2015;8(15):1925–32.

44. Price MJ, Slotwiner D, Du C, et al. Clinical outcomes at 1 year following transcatheter left atrial appendage occlusion in the United States. JACC Cardiovasc Interv 2022;15(7):741–50.

45. Sulaiman S, Roy K, Wang H, et al. Left atrial appendage occlusion in the elderly: insights from PROTECT-AF, PREVAIL, and continuous access registries. JACC Clinical electrophysiology 2023; 9(5):669–76.

46. Leonardi S, Gragnano F, Carrara G, et al. Prognostic implications of declining hemoglobin content in patients hospitalized with acute coronary syndromes. J Am Coll Cardiol 2021;77(4):375–88.

47. Byrne RA, Rossello X, Coughlan JJ, et al. 2023 ESC Guidelines for the management of acute coronary syndromes: Developed by the task force on the management of acute coronary syndromes of the European Society of Cardiology (ESC). Eur Heart J 2023.

48. Subherwal S, Bach RG, Chen AY, et al. Baseline risk of major bleeding in non-ST-segment-elevation myocardial infarction: the CRUSADE (Can Rapid risk stratification of Unstable angina patients Suppress ADverse outcomes with Early implementation of the ACC/AHA Guidelines) Bleeding Score. Circulation 2009;119(14):1873–82.

49. Wang TKM, Mehta OH, Liao YB, et al. Meta-analysis of bleeding scores performance for acute coronary syndrome. Heart Lung Circ 2020;29(12):1749–57.

50. Mehran R, Pocock SJ, Nikolsky E, et al. A risk score to predict bleeding in patients with acute coronary syndromes. J Am Coll Cardiol 2010;55(23):2556–66.

51. Simonsson M, Winell H, Olsson H, et al. Development and validation of a novel risk score for in-hospital major bleeding in acute myocardial infarction:—The SWEDEHEART Score 2019;8(5):e012157.

52. Raposeiras-Roubín S, Faxén J, Íñiguez-Romo A, et al. Development and external validation of a post-discharge bleeding risk score in patients with acute coronary syndrome: The BleeMACS score. Int J Cardiol 2018;254:10–5.

53. Baber U, Mehran R, Giustino G, et al. Coronary thrombosis and major bleeding after PCI with drug-eluting stents: risk scores from PARIS. J Am Coll Cardiol 2016;67(19):2224–34.

54. Yeh RW, Secemsky EA, Kereiakes DJ, et al. Development and validation of a prediction rule for benefit and harm of dual antiplatelet therapy beyond 1 year after percutaneous coronary intervention. JAMA 2016;315(16):1735–49.

55. Costa F, van Klaveren D, James S, et al. Derivation and validation of the predicting bleeding complications in patients undergoing stent implantation and subsequent dual antiplatelet therapy (PRECISE-DAPT) score: a pooled analysis of individual-patient datasets from clinical trials. Lancet (London, England) 2017;389(10073):1025–34.

56. Costa F, Van Klaveren D, Feres F, et al. Dual antiplatelet therapy duration based on ischemic and bleeding risks after coronary stenting. J Am Coll Cardiol 2019;73(7):741–54.

57. Munafò AR, Montalto C, Franzino M, et al. External validity of the PRECISE-DAPT score in patients undergoing PCI: a systematic review and meta-analysis. Eur Heart J Cardiovasc Pharmacother 2023; 9(8):709–21.

58. Urban P, Mehran R, Colleran R, et al. Defining high bleeding risk in patients undergoing percutaneous coronary intervention. Circulation 2019;140(3): 240–61.

59. Gargiulo G, Esposito G. Consolidating the value of the standardised ARC-HBR definition. EuroIntervention 2021;16(14):1126–8.

60. Ueki Y, Bär S, Losdat S, et al. Validation of the Academic Research Consortium for High Bleeding Risk (ARC-HBR) criteria in patients undergoing percutaneous coronary intervention and comparison with contemporary bleeding risk scores. EuroIntervention 2020;16(5):371–9.

61. Corpataux N, Spirito A, Gragnano F, et al. Validation of high bleeding risk criteria and definition as proposed by the academic research consortium for high bleeding risk. Eur Heart J 2020;41(38): 3743–9.

62. Urban P, Gregson J, Owen R, et al. Assessing the risks of bleeding vs thrombotic events in patients at high bleeding risk after coronary stent implantation: the ARC–high bleeding risk trade-off model. JAMA cardiology 2021;6(4):410–9.

63. Bendayan M, Messas N, Perrault LP, et al. Frailty and bleeding in older adults undergoing TAVR or SAVR: Insights From the FRAILTY-AVR Study. JACC Cardiovasc Interv 2020;13(9):1058–68.

64. Vlastra W, Chandrasekhar J, García Del Blanco B, et al. Sex differences in transfemoral transcatheter aortic valve replacement. J Am Coll Cardiol 2019; 74(22):2758–67.

65. Gupta T, Goel K, Kolte D, et al. Association of chronic kidney disease with in-hospital outcomes of transcatheter aortic valve replacement. JACC Cardiovasc Interv 2017;10(20):2050–60.

66. Li SX, Patel NK, Flannery LD, et al. Impact of bleeding after transcatheter aortic valve replacement in patients with chronic kidney disease. Cathet Cardiovasc Interv 2021;97(1). E172-e8.

67. De Larochellière H, Puri R, Eikelboom JW, et al. Blood disorders in patients undergoing transcatheter aortic valve replacement: a review. JACC Cardiovasc Interv 2019;12(1):1–11.

68. Garot P, Neylon A, Morice MC, et al. Bleeding risk differences after TAVR according to the ARC-HBR criteria: insights from SCOPE 2. EuroIntervention 2022;18(6):503–13.

69. Navarese EP, Zhang Z, Kubica J, et al. Development and validation of a practical model to identify patients at risk of bleeding after TAVR. JACC Cardiovasc Interv 2021;14(11):1196–206.

70. Mesnier J, Cepas-Guillén P, Freixa X, et al. Antithrombotic management after left atrial appendage closure: current evidence and future perspectives. Circ Cardiovasc Interv 2023;16(5):e012812.

Antithrombotic Therapy in Patients with Chronic Coronary Syndromes

Placido Maria Mazzone, MD, Marco Spagnolo, MD, Davide Capodanno, MD, PhD*

KEYWORDS

- Chronic coronary syndrome • Dual antiplatelet therapy • Percutaneous coronary intervention
- Oral anticoagulant • DOAC

KEY POINTS

- Current American and European guidelines recommend monotherapy with daily doses of 75 to 100 mg of aspirin for patients with chronic coronary syndromes (CCS) and a previous history of myocardial infarction or myocardial revascularization, as part of a long-term strategy of cardiovascular prevention.
- The recommended duration of dual antiplatelet therapy with aspirin and a $P2Y_{12}$ inhibitor after percutaneous coronary intervention (PCI) is typically 6 months; however, newest guidelines also suggest alternative strategies to balance the risks of ischemia and bleeding on the individual level.
- In patients with CCS and a baseline indication for anticoagulation beyond 1-year after revascularization or in those who do not require revascularization, monotherapy with an oral anticoagulant is the preferred treatment option.
- In patients with CCS and a baseline indication for anticoagulation who undergo an uncomplicated PCI, the recommended approach is to prescribe 1 to 4 weeks of triple antithrombotic therapy, followed by dual antithrombotic therapy up to 6 months and lifelong OAC thereafter.

INTRODUCTION

The pharmacologic strategy for individuals with chronic coronary syndrome (CCS) encompasses two core objectives: alleviating anginal symptoms and improving the prognosis by effective control of cardiovascular risk factors and conditions. In this context, antithrombotic agents assume a pivotal role, as they intervene in the mechanisms culminating in acute thrombotic occlusion arising from atherosclerotic plaque formation, primarily by modulating platelet activation and subsequent aggregation.[1] The choice of therapeutic options currently available varies depending on the specific clinical context, with the overarching goal of

striking an optimal balance between hemorrhagic and ischemic risks. As part of this perspective, alternative strategies have emerged, including short dual antiplatelet therapy (DAPT) or the utilization of monotherapy with $P2Y_{12}$ inhibitors, particularly in patients without a requirement for oral anticoagulation and undergoing percutaneous coronary intervention (PCI).

Importantly, these recommended therapeutic approach undergoes a significant shift when an indication for oral anticoagulation coexists.[2] The decision to initiate an antithrombotic regimen combining an antiplatelet agent with an oral anticoagulant (OAC) is often prompted by concurrent conditions necessitating lifelong anticoagulant

---

Division of Cardiology, Azienda Ospedaliero-Universitaria Policlinico "G. Rodolico – San Marco" University of Catania, Via Santa Sofia, 78, Catania 95123, Italy
* Corresponding author.
E-mail address: dcapodanno@unict.it

Intervent Cardiol Clin 13 (2024) 493–505
https://doi.org/10.1016/j.iccl.2024.06.004
2211-7458/24/

therapy (eg, atrial fibrillation, mechanical heart valve implantation) or specific temporal requirements (eg, venous thromboembolism therapy, left ventricular thrombus, hypercoagulable states).[3,4] Such conditions substantially elevate the overall thrombotic risk of CCS patients. However, despite the theoretic advantages of mitigating thrombus formation through the concurrent use of antiplatelet agents and anticoagulants, this combination raises concerns over an increased risk of bleeding, potentially resulting in net clinical harm.[5] Consequently, the combination of oral antiplatelet and anticoagulant therapies requires thoughtful considerations.

The aim of this article is to comprehensively review and discuss available antithrombotic strategies within the context of CCS. This encompasses strategies for both primary and secondary prevention of adverse cardiovascular events, considering patients both with and without indications for anticoagulation therapy.

CHRONIC CORONARY SYNDROME WITHOUT BASELINE INDICATION TO ORAL ANTICOAGULATION

Current American and European guidelines advocate monotherapy with daily doses of 75 to 100 mg of acetylsalicylic acid (ie, aspirin) as a first-line treatment for patients with a prior history of myocardial infarction or myocardial revascularization (Class I).[6,7] This recommendation is primarily supported by a non-contemporary individual patient data meta-analysis of randomized trials including patients with documented atherosclerosis, which showed a greater absolute reduction in the rate of serious vascular events in patients treated with aspirin compared with controls.[8] Aspirin monotherapy may also be considered for individuals without a history of cardiovascular disease but with documented coronary artery disease (CAD) (Class IIb). This scenario is becoming increasingly common, particularly with the broader use of coronary computed tomography angiography to rule-out or establish the presence of CAD in patients with low pre-test probability.[6,9]

An alternative approach involves monotherapy with 75 mg of clopidogrel daily for patients who are intolerant to aspirin (Class I). Another scenario in which clopidogrel may be favored as an alternative to aspirin is in patients with peripheral artery disease (PAD) or a history of ischemic stroke or transient ischemic attack (Class IIb).[6] This recommendation is supported by the CAPRIE trial, where clopidogrel was superior to aspirin in reducing the composite endpoint of ischemic

stroke, myocardial infarction, and vascular death in individuals with atherosclerotic vascular diseases. This benefit was even more pronounced in a subgroup analysis of patients with PAD, and trended toward significance in patients with prior stroke.[10]

When considering clopidogrel as an alternative to aspirin, one aspect to consider is its variability in individual response, leading to inadequate platelet inhibition in approximately 30% of treated patients.[11] This variability can be attributed to polymorphisms in the enzyme responsible for converting the inactive metabolite of clopidogrel into its active form. Individuals carrying CYP2C19 *2 and *3 loss-of-function alleles exhibit reduced enzyme activity, resulting in heightened platelet reactivity, which has been associated with a higher risk of thrombotic complications.[12,13] Various other factors, including age, body mass index, chronic kidney disease, and diabetes mellitus, significantly contribute to determining individual responses to clopidogrel.[14–16] While several studies and meta-analyses have suggested that carriers of CYP2C19 loss-of-function alleles treated with clopidogrel have a significantly increased risk of major adverse cardiovascular events compared to non-carriers,[17–21] this risk might decrease over time,[22] and has not been confirmed in more contemporary cohorts of patients.[23,24] Additionally, the large CAPRIE trial and two meta-analyses did not find evidence of diminished efficacy or safety hazard with clopidogrel compared with aspirin in patients with cardiovascular disease.[10,25,26]

The addition of a second antithrombotic drug in combination with aspirin for long-term secondary prevention is a consideration for patients at a high risk of ischemic events and low risk of bleeding (European guidelines: Class IIa; American guidelines: Class IIb).[6,7] It may also be considered in situations where the risk of ischemic events is moderate (European guidelines: Class IIb).[6] Several therapeutic options are generally recommended for patients who have experienced a myocardial infarction and meet the aforementioned criteria (ie, moderate to low risk of thrombosis, low risk of bleeding). These options encompass DAPT with P2Y$_{12}$ inhibitors and aspirin and dual-pathway inhibition with vascular-dose rivaroxaban (ie, 2.5 mg BID) and aspirin.

The advantages of prolonging DAPT beyond 12 months and up to 30 months, using either clopidogrel or prasugrel, have been established in patients who have undergone PCI in the randomized, multicenter DAPT trial.[27] Prolonging DAPT beyond 12 months post-stent implantation led to a significant reduction in stent thrombosis and major adverse cardiovascular and cerebrovascular events but was paralleled by an increased risk of moderate or severe bleeding.[27] These findings were consistent in patients with and without a prior myocardial infarction.[28]

In patients with prior myocardial infarction, the efficacy of DAPT with ticagrelor as a long-term regimen was demonstrated by the PEGASUS-TIMI 54 study, where ticagrelor doses of 90 mg or 60 mg twice daily proved better than placebo in reducing the risk of cardiovascular death, myocardial infarction and stroke - again at the price of increased bleeding.[29] The lower ticagrelor dose was associated with a more favorable risk-to-benefit ratio, which is attractive especially in certain patient categories at higher baseline risk of cardiovascular events, such as those with diabetes mellitus, concomitant PAD and/or multivessel coronary disease.[30-32] The lower ticagrelor dose was also evaluated in combination with aspirin in the THEMIS study in diabetic patients with stable CAD, but without previous acute myocardial infarction or stroke. This regimen resulted in fewer cardiovascular ischemic events and more major bleeding, including intracranial bleeding, but no increase in fatal bleeding.[33] The number of patients needed to treat to avert one primary endpoint event was 78 in PEGASUS-TIMI 54 with ticagrelor 60 mg twice daily,[29] and 115 with the same dose in THEMIS, which encompassed a population at lower ischemic risk.[33] This highlights once again the significance of patient selection to ensure that the benefits obtained from protection against ischemic events are not outweighed by the increased risk of bleeding.

An approach alternative to DAPT for long-term maintenance therapy involves dual-pathway inhibition, where a 2.5 mg twice daily dose of rivaroxaban is administered in combination with aspirin. This strategy is based on the direct involvement of factor X and thrombin in platelet activation mediated by protease activated receptors expressed in various cells and tissues, contributing to several adverse cardiovascular effects, including pro-atherogenic and pro-inflammatory effects.[34] In the COMPASS study, dual-pathway inhibition led to an overall 24% reduction in the risk of major adverse cardiovascular events, primarily driven by a reduction in stroke when compared to aspirin alone. Furthermore, a subgroup analysis revealed that the most significant benefit was observed in patients with PAD, with a 46% reduction in the risk of major adverse limb events, including major amputation.[35] Like other long-term antithrombotic strategies, the reduction in ischemic risk was counterbalanced by an increase in bleeding events. However, there were no significant differences between groups in the rates of fatal bleeding, intracranial bleeding, or bleeding affecting critical organs.[35] The gastrointestinal tract was the most frequently affected site, mainly presenting with bleeding episodes leading to intensive care facility admissions or hospitalizations, events that were classified as serious by the investigators.[35]

Clearly, patient selection plays a fundamental role in the implementation of the abovementioned strategies. This selection involves identifying criteria of thrombotic and hemorrhagic risk to achieve an optimal balance between efficacy and safety (Table 1). Several clinical scores have been proposed to aid in the identification of patients suitable for continuing DAPT beyond 12 months. One such score is the DAPT score,[36,37] which incorporates 9 predictive variables to generate a grading system ranging from −2 to +10.[37] A score greater than 2 identifies high-risk patients for whom prolonging DAPT is associated with a reduction in the risk of myocardial infarction, stent thrombosis, and cardiovascular or cerebrovascular events, with only a modest increase in bleeding risk.[37] Conversely, a score lower than 2 identifies low-risk patients who derive no reduction in ischemic events from extending DAPT but experience a significant increase in moderate or major bleeding.[37] The superiority of a personalized DAPT approach based on the DAPT score is currently evaluated in the multicenter randomized PARTHENOPE study.[38]

CHRONIC CORONARY SYNDROME WITH BASELINE INDICATION TO ORAL ANTICOAGULATION

The 2023 American guidelines on atrial fibrillation (AF) recommend monotherapy with OAC in AF patients with CCS beyond 1-year after revascularization or in those with CAD not requiring revascularization and without a history of stent thrombosis, in preference to the combination of an OAC and an antiplatelet drug, to decrease the risk of major bleeding (Class I).[2,39,40] With a lower class of recommendation, the 2023 American guidelines on CCS recommend OAC monotherapy in patients with no acute indication for concomitant antiplatelet therapy (class IIb) and suggest discontinuing dual therapy 12 months after PCI (class IIb).[2] The basis for the recommendation favoring long-term OAC monotherapy stems from the AFIRE trial, which demonstrated that rivaroxaban monotherapy was more effective than rivaroxaban combined with an antiplatelet agent in reducing the primary composite ischemic

Table 1 Thrombotic and bleeding risk criteria	
High Thrombotic Risk	**Moderate Thrombotic Risk**
Diffuse multivessel CAD and at least one of the following	At least one of the following
DM requiring medication	Multivessel or diffuse CAD
History of recurrent MI	DM requiring medication
Peripheral artery disease	History of recurrent MI
CKD with eGFR 15–59 mL/min/1.73 m^2	Peripheral artery disease
	Heart failure
	CKD with eGFR 15–59 mL/min/1.73 m^2
High bleeding risk	
History of intracerebral haemorrhage or ischaemic stroke	Liver failure
History of other intracranial pathology	Bleeding diathesis or coagulopathy
Recent gastrointestinal bleeding or anemia due to possible gastrointestinal blood loss	Extreme old age or frailty
Other gastrointestinal pathology associated with increased bleeding risk	Renal failure requiring dialysis or with eGFR <15 mL/min/1.73 m2

Abbreviations: CAD, coronary artery disease; CKD, chronic kidney disease; DM, diabetes mellitus; eGFR, estimated glomerular filtration rate; HF, heart failure; MI, myocardial infarction.

Adapted from Knuuti et al. 2019 ESC Guidelines for the diagnosis and management of chronic coronary syndromes: The Task Force for the diagnosis and management of chronic coronary syndromes of the European Society of Cardiology (ESC), European Heart Journal, Volume 41, Issue 3, 14 January 2020, Pages 407–477.

outcome in patients with prior revascularization or stable CAD not requiring revascularization (4.1% vs 5.8% per patient-year). Rivaroxaban also exhibited superiority on the primary safety endpoint of major bleeding (1.6% vs 2.8% per patient-year), and the study was terminated early due to increased mortality in the combination-therapy group. The American guidelines on AF also reference the OAC-ALONE clinical trial, which compared OAC monotherapy against dual antithrombotic therapy (ie, OAC plus an antiplatelet agent) in patients who underwent PCI more than 1 year prior.[41] The trial demonstrated numerically lower ischemic events (15.7% vs 13.6%) in the dual therapy group and similar major bleeding rates (7.8% vs 10.4%) at 1 year. However, the study was inconclusive due to early termination for slow enrollment and being underpowered for noninferiority.[41] Therefore, while the AFIRE and OAC-ALONE trials provide support for aspirin-free, OAC-based strategies, they fall short of providing top-level evidence overall. Notably, these trials excluded patients with a high thrombotic risk (eg, those with history of or at high risk for stent thrombosis), highlighting an evidence gap for a crucial population and emphasizing the need for further research.

While supporting OAC monotherapy as a default strategy, the 2019 European Society of Cardiology (ESC) guidelines on CCS also suggested considering the addition of aspirin or clopidogrel to long-term OAC therapy for myocardial infarction patients at high ischemic but low bleeding risk (class IIb)[42] To justify this recommendation, the task force referenced the COMPASS trial, which tested rivaroxaban 2.5 mg plus aspirin and rivaroxaban 5 mg versus aspirin in patients with stable CAD, and another study involving post-myocardial infarction patients treated with warfarin, aspirin, or both.[43,44] Both studies indicated better ischemic outcomes with an increased bleeding risk for combination therapies.[43,44] However, these results should be interpreted recognizing that COMPASS was conducted on a relatively higher ischemic risk population (eg, more than 60% had a previous myocardial infarction, almost 30% suffered from peripheral arterial disease) compared to that of the AFIRE trial where these factors reached 30% and 5%, respectively. additionally, patients in the AFIRE trial required full-dose anticoagulation, while patient with baseline indication from anticoagulation were excluded from COMPASS. Thus, while these guidelines utilize the best available evidence, they underline the importance of specific research gaps for CCS patients with AF, a group with distinctively higher ischemic and bleeding risks deserving dedicated investigations.

An open question regarding the optimal long-term dual antithrombotic approach for these patients is the selection of the appropriate antiplatelet agent, if combination with an OAC is desired. Clopidogrel, in fact, demonstrated superior efficacy in reducing thrombotic events and bleeding compared to aspirin in landmark trials of coronary revascularization.[45] In AFIRE trial the choice between aspirin, clopidogrel, or more potent antiplatelets like prasugrel or ticagrelor in the combination arm was left to the discretion of the investigators, and 95% received clopidogrel, likely due to lower perceived risk of bleeding. Ongoing studies are exploring the implications of utilizing different doses of direct OACs in conjunction with antiplatelet agents, also at lower than standard doses, aiming to establish a foundation for potential future long-term combination therapies. Details of these investigations are provided in Table 2.

The strategy of OAC monotherapy recommended for patients requiring anticoagulation due to AF is also applicable to other conditions necessitating an OAC, such as mechanical heart valve, venous thromboembolism, mitral stenosis, and left ventricular thrombus.[46,47] Consistent with the approach for AF, the consideration of dual antithrombotic therapy might be warranted for certain patients with implanted valves or venous thromboembolism, particularly those with low bleeding risk yet heightened ischemic risk, as determined by clinical judgment.[46,47] However, this recommendation is grounded in partial and dated evidence, with studies often inadequately addressing the impact of CAD presence and bleeding risk.[48] Furthermore, the evidence supporting the addition of an antiplatelet agent to OAC in conditions like mitral stenosis and left ventricular thrombus is limited and necessitates further research.[4,49]

CHRONIC CORONARY SYNDROME AND PERCUTANEOUS CORONARY INTERVENTION WITHOUT BASELINE INDICATION TO ANTICOAGULATION

In patients undergoing PCI, ensuring adequate platelet inhibition is crucial to prevent thrombotic events in the coronary segment where the stent is deployed. This is achieved through the administration of aspirin as a Class I recommendation, along with Clopidogrel 75 mg after a loading dose of 600 mg, unless the patient has been on clopidogrel for at least 5 days (Class I).[6] The recommended duration of DAPT is typically 6 months (class I), irrespective of the type of stent implanted and unless considerations on the bleeding risk prevail.[6,7,50–54] Indeed, while the 6-month DAPT regimen for patients with

CCS undergoing PCI is considered the optimal balance between risks and benefits, current guidelines acknowledge the flexibility for shorter DAPT durations of 3 months (Class IIa) in high-risk bleeding patients and even 1 month (Class IIb) in those at very high risk of bleeding, following clopidogrel discontinuation.[6]

In recent years, more attention has been directed toward the risk of bleeding, as it is widely acknowledged that certain hemorrhagic events can exert an impact on mortality in patients undergoing PCI that is at least comparable to the risk of recurrent thrombotic events.[55] Technological advancements, particularly the introduction of second and third-generation drug-eluting stents, have substantially mitigated the risk of myocardial infarction associated with late stent thrombosis, a notably concerning complication of PCI.[56] In the pursuit of personalized antithrombotic therapy, aiming to balance ischemic and hemorrhagic risks, various short-duration DAPT strategies have been explored. These strategies involve discontinuing clopidogrel after a variable period of 1 to 3 months, or alternatively, discontinuing aspirin and implementing long-term treatment with potent $P2Y_{12}$ inhibitors.[57–60] It is noteworthy that, unlike the recommendations supporting the reduction of DAPT duration to 3 months, the recommendations for the other two strategies are characterized by a limited level of evidence or, in the case of $P2Y_{12}$ monotherapy, are not reported in the current 2019 ESC Guidelines for the diagnosis and management of CCS. New evidence published after the Guidelines, which will inform the announced 2024 update, is discussed below.

The One-Month DAPT and MASTER DAPT trials investigated the reduction of DAPT to 1 month. These trials, although employing the same treatment strategy, enrolled different patient populations.[61,62] In the larger MASTER DAPT trial, a total of 4579 European patients at high risk of bleeding, undergoing PCI for acute coronary syndrome (ACS) or CCS, without limitations regarding the location or complexity of the treated lesions, were included. In this clinical context, the 1-month DAPT regimen was found to be non-inferior to at least 3 months of DAPT in terms of the occurrence of net adverse clinical events and major cardiac or cerebral adverse events. Additionally, it resulted in a lower incidence of clinically relevant major or non-major bleeding. The trial effects were consistent in patients with and without CCS, which were evenly balanced. In contrast, the One-Month DAPT trial enrolled only CCS patients, specifically 3020 Asian patients with lesions at low complexity

Table 2
Ongoing randomized clinical trials of patients with baseline indication to oral anticoagulant

Trial (Identifier)	Design	Sample	Population	Investigational Drug	Control	Primary outcome (Time Frame)	Expected Completion Date (Month/Year)
Patients with CCS and baseline indication to OACs							
EPIC-CAD (NCT 03718559)	Open-label	1.050	Stable CAD and high-risk AF	Edoxaban plus antiplatelet agent	Edoxaban	Net clinical outcome (1 y)	12/2023
Patients with CCS and baseline indication to OACs undergoing PCI							
WOEST-3 (NCT04436978)	Open-label	2.000	Non-valvular AF undergoing PCI	1-mo DAPT (aspirin plus P2Y$_{12}$ inhibitor) followed by edoxaban plus P2Y$_{12}$ inhibitor	Standard of care	Major adverse cardiac or cerebral events, major or clinically relevant non-major bleeding (1 y)	12/2027
MATRIX-2 (NCT05955365)	Open-label, blinded evaluation	3.010	Non-valvular AF undergoing PCI	Aspirin discontinuation, P2Y$_{12}$-only for 1-mo, followed by DOAC only lifelong	Standard of care	Major adverse cardiac or cerebral events, major or clinically relevant non-major bleeding (1 y)	12/2026
OPTIMA-AF (JRCT051190053)	Open-label	1.090	Non-valvular AF undergoing PCI	1-mo DOAC plus P2Y$_{12}$ inhibitor, followed by DOAC monotherapy	12-mo DOAC plus P2Y$_{12}$ inhibitor, followed by DOAC monotherapy	Composite ischemic, major or clinically relevant non-major bleeding (1 y)	12/2023

Abbreviations: AF, atrial fibrillation; CAD, coronary artery disease; CCS, chronic coronary syndrome; DAPT, dual antiplatelet therapy; DOAC, direct oral anticoagulant; OAC, oral anticoagulant; PCI, percutaneous coronary intervention.

who were not specifically selected to be at high risk of bleeding. Again, the 1-month DAPT regimen was found to be non-inferior to the extended DAPT duration (ie, 6 or 12 months) with respect to the composite endpoint of cardio-vascular events or major bleeding.

The other emerging strategy is the use of monotherapy with P2Y$_{12}$ inhibitors following a short period of DAPT, either for 1 or 3 months. Unlike the European guidelines, this strategy is incorporated into the current 2023 American guidelines for the management of patients with CCS which recommend that such an approach should be considered in selected patients for at least 12 months after PCI in order to reduce the risk of bleeding (Class IIa).[7] The rationale behind this approach is to provide sufficient pro-tection against ischemic events during the initial phase after PCI, while reducing the intensity of antiplatelet therapy in subsequent periods.[63] While aspirin monotherapy is currently recom-mended for patients with a high risk of bleeding and low ischemic risk, monotherapy with P2Y$_{12}$ inhibitors would ensure adequate protection even for patients at higher risk of ischemia, while simultaneously mitigating the risk of bleeding.

The GLOBAL LEADERS trial was the first large-scale randomized trial to investigate the P2Y$_{12}$ monotherapy strategy.[64] This trial included ~16,000 patients who underwent PCI for CCS or ACS, randomized to receive 1 month of DAPT with aspirin and ticagrelor, followed by ticagrelor monotherapy for 23 months, or stan-dard DAPT with aspirin plus ticagrelor or clopi-dogrel, followed by aspirin monotherapy at 12 months from PCI. At a 2-year follow-up, mono-therapy did not demonstrate superiority over control in reducing the rate of all-cause mortality or nonfatal myocardial infarction. However, monotherapy did not raise any safety concerns. Other studies have evaluated the potential bene-fits of P2Y$_{12}$ monotherapy and demonstrated its safety and efficacy compared to standard DAPT, even in high-risk populations susceptible to ischemic and hemorrhagic events.[65–67] Specif-ically, the TWILIGHT study demonstrated that ticagrelor monotherapy was associated with a lower incidence of clinically significant bleeding compared to ticagrelor plus aspirin, without an increased risk of death, myocardial infarction, or stroke.[67] These results were consistent even among high-risk patient subgroups such as those with diabetes mellitus, ACS, and those undergo-ing PCI of complex lesions. It is of note that these trials generally included mixed populations of CCS and ACS patients, but an interaction of the trial effect was found only in GLOBAL LEADERS,

were most of the effect of ticagrelor monotherapy emerged in the ACS subgroup (P for interaction = 0.0068).[64] These results may be confirmed by other studies currently underway, with the aim of identifying the optimal antithrombotic therapy in patients with CCS, even at high risk of ischemic events. The main characteristics of these trials are summarized in Table 3.

Finally, another viable approach is represented by the replacement of aspirin with indobufen, a type 1 cyclooxygenase inhibitor that, compared to aspirin, has better gastrointestinal tolerance with a comparable level of platelet inhibition.[68] DAPT with indobufen and clopidogrel was stud-ied in 4551 patients undergoing elective PCI in the OPTION trial, demonstrating a reduction in the rate of events related to the composite pri-mary endpoint of cardiovascular death, nonfatal myocardial infarction, ischemic stroke, definite or probable stent thrombosis, or Bleeding Aca-demic Research Consortium criteria type 2, 3, or 5 bleeding compared to standard DAPT, primar-ily through a reduction in minor bleeding.[68] Consequently, the use of indobufen may repre-sent a valid alternative to conventional DAPT reg-imens, especially in some categories of patients, including those at high risk of bleeding or in pa-tients with aspirin hypersensitivity or intolerance.

CHRONIC CORONARY SYNDROME AND PERCUTANEOUS CORONARY INTERVENTION WITH BASELINE INDICATION TO ANTICOAGULATION

In patients with CCS who have undergone elec-tive PCI and require anticoagulation, the 2023 American guidelines on CCS recommend DAPT for 1 to 4 weeks followed by clopidogrel alone for 6 months, in addition to a direct OAC (Class I). The guidelines also specify that continuing DAPT with aspirin in addition to clopidogrel for up to 1 month is reasonable if the patient has a high thrombotic risk and low bleeding risk (Class IIa).[2] Beyond 1 year after revasculariza-tion, OAC-alone therapy remains the preferred option. This recommendation is supported by a substudy of the AFIRE trial, focusing on patients beyond 1 year after PCI, where the benefits of rivaroxaban monotherapy for efficacy and safety endpoints remained consistent with those in the main study.[69]

The preference for direct OACs over vitamin K antagonists (VKA) in patients with AF undergoing PCI is based on the consistent reduction in bleeding complications, such as intracranial hae-morrhage, observed with direct OACs in meta-analyses of randomized studies, without apparent

Table 3
Ongoing randomized clinical trials of patients without baseline indication to oral anticoagulant

Trial (Identifier)	Design	Sample	Population	Investigational Drug	Control	Primary Outcome (Time Frame)	Expected Completion Date (Month/Year)
Patients with CCS without baseline indication to OACs							
HOST-PREVENTION (NCT05845489)	Open-label	9.930	Stable CAD that did not require revascularization therapy	Clopidogrel	No antithrombotic therapy	Major adverse cardiovascular and cerebrovascular events (5 y)	03/2030
Patients with CCS and without baseline indication to OACs undergoing PCI							
ULTRA-LM (NCT05650411)	Single blinded	766	Patients undergoing PCI for LMCA disease	Potent P2Y$_{12}$ inhibitor-based SAPT	DAPT for 6–12 mo	All-cause death, any non-fatal MI, or any revascularization (2 y)	12/2028
OPTIMIZE-APT (NCT05418556)	Open-label	3.944	Patients undergoing PCI guided by intravascular imaging	DAPT for 1 mo followed by clopidogrel alone for CCS	DAPT for 12 mo	Clinically relevant bleeding; net clinical outcome, ischemic composite adverse events (1 y)	12/2028
SMART-CHOICE 3 (NCT04418479)	Open-label	5.000	Patients undergoing PCI at high risk for recurrent ischemic events	DAPT for 12 mo followed by clopidogrel alone	DAPT for 12 mo followed by aspirin alone	Major adverse cardiac and cerebrovascular events (1 y)	10/2024

Abbreviations: CAD, coronary artery disease; CCS, chronic coronary syndrome; DAPT, dual antiplatelet therapy; LMCA, left main coronary artery; MI, myocardial infarction; OAC, oral anticoagulant; PCI, percutaneous coronary intervention; SAPT, single antiplatelet therapy.

efficacy benefits with VKAs.[70,71] However, the lack of head-to-head comparisons between direct OACs prevents recommending one agent over another.[39] Numerous studies are currently underway with the objective of evaluating alternative strategies aimed at reducing the bleeding risk associated with triple antithrombotic therapy (eg, the combination of anticoagulation and DAPT). These strategies involve the administration of DAPT immediately after PCI for a limited period, followed by dual antithrombotic therapy with a $P2Y_{12}$ inhibitor and chronic oral anticoagulation. Another approach includes 1-month monotherapy with $P2Y_{12}$ inhibitors following PCI, followed by chronic oral anticoagulation therapy (see **Table 2**).

A network meta-analysis of five randomized trials (ie, WOEST, PIONEER AF-PCI, RE-DUAL PCI, AUGUSTUS, and ENTRUST-AF PCI), including 11.532 patients, highlighted fewer bleeding complications with preserved antithrombotic efficacy when aspirin was discontinued within a few days after PCI and followed by a period of DOAC plus $P2Y_{12}$ inhibitor.[72–75] This is the main reason for the preference of an early dual antithrombotic approach (eg, DOAC plus $P2Y_{12}$ inhibitor) in these patients, as equally emphasized by the 2019 ESC guidelines on CCS.[42]

Clopidogrel, administered as a 600 mg loading dose followed by a 75 mg daily maintenance dose, is the $P2Y_{12}$ inhibitor of choice in the context of dual therapy. This preference is primarily based on its adoption in most patients enrolled in landmark trials involving individuals with AF undergoing PCI.[73–76] Ticagrelor may serve as an alternative in patients with a high thrombotic risk and acceptable bleeding risk, as its use in regulatory trials was deemed acceptable (ranging from 4.3% to 12%), while prasugrel is advised against due to its significantly limited use in such studies (eg, 1%).[77] However, these recommendations may be subject to reconsideration based on ongoing studies that are assessing the risks and benefits of using potent $P2Y_{12}$ inhibitors in this setting, including at reduced dosages, as well as the possibility of shortening the duration of dual antithrombotic therapy to 1 month, followed by chronic anticoagulation (see **Table 2**).

Aspirin is a crucial component of the procedural antithrombotic strategy (Class I) to reduce ischemic events. However, when added to a dual therapy, it significantly increases the bleeding risk. Notably, in patients on an oral anticoagulant undergoing PCI, early bleeding complications and an increased thrombotic risk in the first month have been observed.[76,78–80]

Therefore, the duration of the short period of triple antithrombotic therapy is a key area of uncertainty in this field and has not been further developed in the guidelines.[2] American experts in 2021 suggested interrupting triple therapy even before discharge and/or up to 1 week after PCI, considering that the residual platelet inhibitory effects induced by aspirin persist for 7 to 10 days.[81] However, in line with current American guidelines, they advise that patients at higher ischemic risk (eg, previous myocardial infarction, complex lesions, extensive coronary artery disease, history of stent thrombosis) and at an acceptable bleeding risk may be potential candidates for the use of aspirin up to 30 days after PCI.[46]

The AUGUSTUS trial, examining treatment effects of apixaban or a VKA with aspirin or matching placebo (eg, 2 x 2 factorial design) for 6 months in patients who underwent PCI, found a twofold increase in bleeding with aspirin, while the incidence of stent thrombosis was low, occurring in less than 1% over 6 months.[74] The study had limited power to detect a difference in stent thrombosis, which was lower with aspirin compared to placebo and with apixaban compared to VKA.[74] A subgroup analysis of the REDUAL PCI trial indicated that both doses of dabigatran (110 mg and 150 mg) in dual therapy after PCI resulted in less bleeding than warfarin triple therapy, regardless of procedural or clinical complexity, with a similar risk of thromboembolic outcomes, irrespective of procedural and/or clinical complexity and modified dual antiplatelet therapy score.[82] Ultimately, in all landmark trials of PCI in AF patients, the efficacy outcomes were consistent across all predefined subgroups, including those at increased thrombotic risk.[72–76,78,82–84] These results not only support the use of dual therapy for 6 months in such patients instead of triple therapy but also raise the question of whether a short period of aspirin is essential after PCI or not.

SUMMARY

In patients with CCS, antithrombotic therapy offers cardiovascular benefits but also elevates the risk of bleeding. The attribution of an increasing prognostic relevance to the risk of bleeding requires the identification of prudent therapeutic strategies aimed at obtaining an optimal balance between the ischemic and haemorrhagic risk. This assessment cannot overlook the characterization of the patient's risk profile, which, however, is dynamic. Therefore, it should be re-evaluated if they develop a new risk factor, experience an ischemic or bleeding event, or develop a concurrent condition requiring anticoagulant therapy, to ensure they continue to receive optimal treatment.

CLINICS CARE POINTS

- Although clopidogrel represents an alternative to aspirin, it is important to consider that it is not always able to guarantee an adequate level of platelet inhibition due to polymorphisms affecting CYP2C19.

- Triple antithrombotic therapy in patients with indication for anticoagulation undergoing PCI is essential to reduce ischemic risk, however it exposes the patient to a significant hemorrhagic risk. Several strategies are currently being studied with the aim of reducing the hemorrhagic risk, the most promising include the administration of DAPT after PCI for a limited period, followed by dual antithrombotic therapy with a P2Y12i and chronic oral anticoagulation or one-month monotherapy with P2Y12i after PCI, followed by chronic oral anticoagulant therapy.

DISCLOSURES

D. Capodanno declares speakers' honoraria from Sanofi Aventis.

REFERENCES

1. Falk E. Plaque rupture with severe pre-existing stenosis precipitating coronary thrombosis. Characteristics of coronary atherosclerotic plaques underlying fatal occlusive thrombi. Br Heart J 1983;50(2):127–34.
2. Writing Committee M, Virani SS, Newby LK, et al. 2023 AHA/ACC/ACCP/ASPC/NLA/PCNA Guideline for the Management of Patients With Chronic Coronary Disease: A Report of the American Heart Association/American College of Cardiology Joint Committee on Clinical Practice Guidelines. J Am Coll Cardiol 2023;82(9):833–955.
3. Kirchhof P, Benussi S, Kotecha D, et al. ESC Guidelines for the management of atrial fibrillation developed in collaboration with EACTS. Eur Heart J 2016;37(38):2893–962.
4. Otto CM, Nishimura RA, Bonow RO, et al. 2020 ACC/AHA Guideline for the Management of Patients With Valvular Heart Disease: A Report of the American College of Cardiology/American Heart Association Joint Committee on Clinical Practice Guidelines. Circulation 2021;143(5):e72–227.
5. Capodanno D, Collet JP, Dangas G, et al. Antithrombotic therapy after transcatheter aortic valve replacement. JACC Cardiovasc Interv 2021;14(15):1688–703.
6. Knuuti J, Wijns W, Saraste A, et al. 2019 ESC Guidelines for the diagnosis and management of chronic coronary syndromes: The Task Force for the diagnosis and management of chronic coronary syndromes of the European Society of Cardiology (ESC). Eur Heart J 2019;41(3):407–77.
7. Virani SS, Newby LK, Arnold SV, et al. 2023 AHA/ACC/ACCP/ASPC/NLA/PCNA Guideline for the Management of Patients With Chronic Coronary Disease. J Am Coll Cardiol 2023;82(9):833–955.
8. Baigent C, Blackwell L, Collins R, et al. Aspirin in the primary and secondary prevention of vascular disease: collaborative meta-analysis of individual participant data from randomised trials. Lancet 2009;373(9678):1849–60.
9. CT or invasive coronary angiography in stable chest pain. N Engl J Med 2022;386(17):1591–602.
10. A randomised, blinded, trial of clopidogrel versus aspirin in patients at risk of ischaemic events (CAPRIE). CAPRIE Steering Committee. Lancet 1996;348(9038):1329–39.
11. Mega JL, Simon T, Collet JP, et al. Reduced-function CYP2C19 genotype and risk of adverse clinical outcomes among patients treated with clopidogrel predominantly for PCI: a meta-analysis. JAMA 2010;304(16):1821–30.
12. Simon T, Verstuyft C, Mary-Krause M, et al. Genetic determinants of response to clopidogrel and cardiovascular events. N Engl J Med 2009;360(4):363–75.
13. Hochholzer W, Trenk D, Fromm MF, et al. Impact of cytochrome P450 2C19 loss-of-function polymorphism and of major demographic characteristics on residual platelet function after loading and maintenance treatment with clopidogrel in patients undergoing elective coronary stent placement. J Am Coll Cardiol 2010;55(22):2427–34.
14. Capodanno D, Angiolillo DJ, Lennon RJ, et al. ABCD-GENE score and clinical outcomes following percutaneous coronary intervention: insights from the TAILOR-PCI Trial. J Am Heart Assoc 2022;11(4):e024156.
15. Angiolillo DJ, Capodanno D, Danchin N, et al. Derivation, validation, and prognostic utility of a prediction rule for nonresponse to clopidogrel: the ABCD-GENE score. JACC Cardiovasc Interv 2020;13(5):606–17.
16. Mazzone PM, Angiolillo DJ, Capodanno D. Approaches to de-escalation of antiplatelet treatment in stabilized post-myocardial infarction patients with high ischemic risk. Expert Rev Cardiovasc Ther 2022;20(10):839–49.

17. Yoon HY, Lee N, Seong JM, et al. Efficacy and safety of clopidogrel versus prasugrel and ticagrelor for coronary artery disease treatment in patients with CYP2C19 LoF alleles: a systemic review and meta-analysis. Br J Clin Pharmacol 2020;86(8):1489–98.

18. Sheng XY, An HJ, He YY, et al. High-Dose Clopidogrel versus Ticagrelor in CYP2C19 intermediate or poor metabolizers after percutaneous coronary intervention: A Meta-Analysis of Randomized Trials. J Clin Pharm Therapeut 2022;47(8):1112–21.

19. Chen YW, Liao YJ, Chang WC, et al. CYP2C19 loss-of-function alleles predicts clinical outcomes in East Asian patients with acute myocardial infarction undergoing percutaneous coronary intervention and stenting receiving clopidogrel. Front Cardiovasc Med 2022;9:994184.

20. Biswas M, Sukasem C, Khatun Kali MS, et al. Effects of the CYP2C19 LoF allele on major adverse cardiovascular events associated with clopidogrel in acute coronary syndrome patients undergoing percutaneous coronary intervention: a meta-analysis. Pharmacogenomics 2022;23(3):207–20.

21. Biswas M, Kali SK. Association of CYP2C19 loss-of-function alleles with major adverse cardiovascular events of clopidogrel in stable coronary artery disease patients undergoing percutaneous coronary intervention: meta-analysis. Cardiovasc Drugs Ther 2021;35(6):1147–59.

22. Zhang Y, Zhao X, Ye Y, et al. Clinical outcomes after percutaneous coronary intervention over time on the basis of CYP2C19 polymorphisms. J Cardiovasc Pharmacol 2022;79(2):183–91.

23. Choi IJ, Koh YS, Park MW, et al. CYP2C19 loss-of-function alleles are not associated with clinical outcome of clopidogrel therapy in patients treated with newer-generation drug-eluting stents. Medicine (Baltim) 2016;95(26):e4049.

24. van den Broek WWA, Mani N, Azzahhafi J, et al. CYP2C9 polymorphisms and the risk of cardiovascular events in patients treated with clopidogrel: combined data from the popular genetics and popular AGE trials. Am J Cardiovasc Drugs 2023;23(2):165–72.

25. Chiarito M, Sanz-Sánchez J, Cannata F, et al. Monotherapy with a P2Y(12) inhibitor or aspirin for secondary prevention in patients with established atherosclerosis: a systematic review and meta-analysis. Lancet 2020;395(10235):1487–95.

26. Gragnano F, Cao D, Pirondini L, et al. P2Y(12) inhibitor or aspirin monotherapy for secondary prevention of coronary events. J Am Coll Cardiol 2023;82(2):89–105.

27. Mauri L, Kereiakes DJ, Yeh RW, et al. Twelve or 30 months of dual antiplatelet therapy after drug-eluting stents. N Engl J Med 2014;371(23):2155–66.

28. Yeh RW, Kereiakes DJ, Steg PG, et al. Benefits and risks of extended duration dual antiplatelet therapy after pci in patients with and without acute myocardial infarction. J Am Coll Cardiol 2015;65(20):2211–21.

29. Bonaca MP, Bhatt DL, Cohen M, et al. Long-term use of ticagrelor in patients with prior myocardial infarction. N Engl J Med 2015;372(19):1791–800.

30. Bhatt DL, Bonaca MP, Bansilal S, et al. Reduction in ischemic events with ticagrelor in diabetic patients with prior myocardial infarction in PEGASUS-TIMI 54. J Am Coll Cardiol 2016;67(23):2732–40.

31. Bonaca MP, Bhatt DL, Storey RF, et al. Ticagrelor for prevention of ischemic events after myocardial infarction in patients with peripheral artery disease. J Am Coll Cardiol 2016;67(23):2719–28.

32. Bansilal S, Bonaca MP, Cornel JH, et al. Ticagrelor for secondary prevention of atherothrombotic events in patients with multivessel coronary disease. J Am Coll Cardiol 2018;71(5):489–96.

33. Steg PG, Bhatt DL, Simon T, et al. Ticagrelor in patients with stable coronary disease and diabetes. N Engl J Med 2019;381(14):1309–20.

34. Mazzone PM, Capodanno D. Low dose rivaroxaban for the management of atherosclerotic cardiovascular disease. J Thromb Thrombolysis 2023;56(1):91–102.

35. Eikelboom JW, Connolly SJ, Bosch J, et al. Rivaroxaban with or without aspirin in stable cardiovascular disease. N Engl J Med 2017;377(14):1319–30.

36. Yeh RW, Secemsky EA, Kereiakes DJ, et al. Development and validation of a prediction rule for benefit and harm of dual antiplatelet therapy beyond 1 year after percutaneous coronary intervention. JAMA 2016;315(16):1735–49.

37. Valgimigli M, Bueno H, Byrne RA, et al. 2017 ESC focused update on dual antiplatelet therapy in coronary artery disease developed in collaboration with EACTS: The Task Force for dual antiplatelet therapy in coronary artery disease of the European Society of Cardiology (ESC) and of the European Association for Cardio-Thoracic Surgery (EACTS). Eur Heart J 2018;39(3):213–60.

38. Piccolo R, Calabrò P, Varricchio A, et al. Rationale and design of the PARTHENOPE trial: A two-by-two factorial comparison of polymer-free vs biodegradable-polymer drug-eluting stents and personalized vs standard duration of dual antiplatelet therapy in all-comers undergoing PCI. Am Heart J 2023;265:153–60.

39. Joglar JA, Chung MK, Armbruster AL, et al. ACC/AHA/ACCP/HRS Guideline for the Diagnosis and Management of Atrial Fibrillation: A Report of the American College of Cardiology/American Heart Association Joint Committee on Clinical Practice Guidelines. Circulation 2023.

40. Greco A, Laudani C, Rochira C, et al. Antithrombotic management in af patients following percutaneous coronary intervention: a European perspective. Intervent Cardiol 2023;18:e05.

41. Matsumura-Nakano Y, Shizuta S, Komasa A, et al. Open-label randomized trial comparing oral

anticoagulation with and without single antiplatelet therapy in patients with atrial fibrillation and stable coronary artery disease beyond 1 year after coronary stent implantation. Circulation 2019;139(5):604–16.

42. Knuuti J, Wijns W, Saraste A, et al. 2019 ESC Guidelines for the diagnosis and management of chronic coronary syndromes. Eur Heart J 2020;41(4):407–77.

43. Hurlen M, Abdelnoor M, Smith P, et al. Warfarin, aspirin, or both after myocardial infarction. N Engl J Med 2002;347(13):969–74.

44. Eikelboom JW, Connolly SJ, Bosch J, et al. Rivaroxaban with or without Aspirin in Stable Cardiovascular Disease. N Engl J Med 2017;377(14):1319–30.

45. Koo BK, Kang J, Park KW, et al. Aspirin versus clopidogrel for chronic maintenance monotherapy after percutaneous coronary intervention (HOST-EXAM): an investigator-initiated, prospective, randomised, open-label, multicentre trial. Lancet 2021; 397(10293):2487–96.

46. Kumbhani DJ, Cannon CP, Beavers CJ, et al. 2020 ACC Expert Consensus Decision Pathway for Anticoagulant and Antiplatelet Therapy in Patients With Atrial Fibrillation or Venous Thromboembolism Undergoing Percutaneous Coronary Intervention or With Atherosclerotic Cardiovascular Disease: A Report of the American College of Cardiology Solution Set Oversight Committee. J Am Coll Cardiol 2021;77(5):629–58.

47. Vahanian A, Beyersdorf F, Praz F, et al. 2021 ESC/EACTS Guidelines for the management of valvular heart disease. Eur Heart J 2022;43(7):561–632.

48. Greco A, Spagnolo M, Capodanno D. Antithrombotic therapy after transcatheter aortic valve implantation. Expet Rev Med Dev 2022;19(6):499–513.

49. Levine GN, McEvoy JW, Fang JC, et al. Management of patients at risk for and with left ventricular thrombus: a scientific statement from the American Heart Association. Circulation 2022;146(15):e205–23.

50. Gwon HC, Hahn JY, Park KW, et al. Six-month versus 12-month dual antiplatelet therapy after implantation of drug-eluting stents: the Efficacy of Xience/Promus Versus Cypher to Reduce Late Loss After Stenting (EXCELLENT) randomized, multicenter study. Circulation 2012;125(3):505–13.

51. Valgimigli M, Campo G, Monti M, et al. Short- versus long-term duration of dual-antiplatelet therapy after coronary stenting: a randomized multicenter trial. Circulation 2012;125(16):2015–26.

52. Gilard M, Barragan P, Noryani AAL, et al. 6- versus 24-month dual antiplatelet therapy after implantation of drug-eluting stents in patients nonresistant to aspirin: the randomized, multicenter ITALIC trial. J Am Coll Cardiol 2015;65(8):777–86.

53. Colombo A, Chieffo A, Frasheri A, et al. Second-generation drug-eluting stent implantation followed by 6- versus 12-month dual antiplatelet therapy: the SECURITY randomized clinical trial. J Am Coll Cardiol 2014;64(20):2086–97.

54. Schulz-Schüpke S, Byrne RA, Ten Berg JM, et al. ISAR-SAFE: a randomized, double-blind, placebo-controlled trial of 6 vs. 12 months of clopidogrel therapy after drug-eluting stenting. Eur Heart J 2015;36(20):1252–63.

55. Capodanno D, Bhatt DL, Gibson CM, et al. Bleeding avoidance strategies in percutaneous coronary intervention. Nat Rev Cardiol 2022;19(2):117–32.

56. Moon JY, Franchi F, Rollini F, et al. Evolution of coronary stent technology and implications for duration of dual antiplatelet therapy. Prog Cardiovasc Dis Jan-Feb 2018;60(4–5):478–90.

57. Kim BK, Hong MK, Shin DH, et al. A new strategy for discontinuation of dual antiplatelet therapy: the RESET Trial (REal Safety and Efficacy of 3-month dual antiplatelet Therapy following Endeavor zotarolimus-eluting stent implantation). J Am Coll Cardiol 2012; 60(15):1340–8.

58. Feres F, Costa RA, Abizaid A, et al. Three vs twelve months of dual antiplatelet therapy after zotarolimus-eluting stents: the OPTIMIZE randomized trial. JAMA 2013;310(23):2510–22.

59. Natsuaki M, Morimoto T, Yamamoto E, et al. One-year outcome of a prospective trial stopping dual antiplatelet therapy at 3 months after everolimus-eluting cobalt-chromium stent implantation: ShortT and OPtimal duration of Dual AntiPlatelet Therapy after everolimus-eluting cobalt-chromium stent (STOPDAPT) trial. Cardiovasc Interv Ther 2016; 31(3):196–209.

60. Han JK, Hwang D, Yang S, et al. Comparison of 3- to 6-Month Versus 12-month dual antiplatelet therapy after coronary intervention using the contemporary drug-eluting stents with ultrathin struts: The HOST-IDEA Randomized Clinical Trial. Circulation 2023; 147(18):1358–68.

61. Hong S-J, Kim J-S, Hong SJ, et al. 1-month dual-antiplatelet therapy followed by aspirin monotherapy after polymer-free drug-coated stent implantation. JACC Cardiovasc Interv 2021;14(16):1801–11.

62. Valgimigli M, Frigoli E, Heg D, et al. Dual antiplatelet therapy after pci in patients at high bleeding risk. N Engl J Med 2021;385(18):1643–55.

63. Angiolillo DJ, Galli M, Collet JP, et al. Antiplatelet therapy after percutaneous coronary intervention. EuroIntervention 2022;17(17):e1371–96.

64. Vranckx P, Valgimigli M, Jüni P, et al. Ticagrelor plus aspirin for 1 month, followed by ticagrelor monotherapy for 23 months vs aspirin plus clopidogrel or ticagrelor for 12 months, followed by aspirin monotherapy for 12 months after implantation of a drug-eluting stent: a multicentre, open-label, randomised superiority trial. Lancet 2018;392(10151):940–9.

65. Hahn J-Y, Song YB, Oh J-H, et al. Effect of P2Y12 inhibitor monotherapy vs dual antiplatelet therapy on cardiovascular events in patients undergoing percutaneous coronary intervention: The SMART-

CHOICE randomized clinical trial. JAMA 2019; 321(24):2428–37.

66. Watanabe H, Domei T, Morimoto T, et al. Effect of 1-month dual antiplatelet therapy followed by clopidogrel vs 12-month dual antiplatelet therapy on cardiovascular and bleeding events in patients receiving PCI: The STOPDAPT-2 Randomized Clinical Trial. JAMA 2019;321(24):2414–27.

67. Mehran R, Baber U, Sharma SK, et al. Ticagrelor with or without aspirin in high-risk patients after PCI. N Engl J Med 2019;381(21):2032–42.

68. Wu H, Xu L, Zhao X, et al. Indobufen or aspirin on top of clopidogrel after coronary drug-eluting stent implantation (OPTION): a randomized, open-label, end point–blinded, noninferiority trial. Circulation 2023;147(3):212–22.

69. Matoba T, Yasuda S, Kaikita K, et al. Rivaroxaban monotherapy in patients with atrial fibrillation after coronary stenting: insights from the AFIRE trial. JACC Cardiovasc Interv 2021;14(21):2330–40.

70. Lopes RD, Hong H, Harskamp RE, et al. Optimal antithrombotic regimens for patients with atrial fibrillation undergoing percutaneous coronary intervention: an updated network meta-analysis. JAMA Cardiol 2020;5(5):582–9.

71. Capodanno D, Di Maio M, Greco A, et al. Safety and efficacy of double antithrombotic therapy with non-vitamin K antagonist oral anticoagulants in patients with atrial fibrillation undergoing percutaneous coronary intervention: a systematic review and meta-analysis. J Am Heart Assoc 2020;9(16): e017212.

72. Gibson CM, Mehran R, Bode C, et al. Prevention of bleeding in patients with atrial fibrillation undergoing PCI. N Engl J Med 2016;375(25):2423–34.

73. Cannon CP, Bhatt DL, Oldgren J, et al. Dual antithrombotic therapy with dabigatran after PCI in atrial fibrillation. N Engl J Med 2017;377(16):1513–24.

74. Lopes RD, Heizer G, Aronson R, et al. Antithrombotic therapy after acute coronary syndrome or PCI in atrial fibrillation. N Engl J Med 2019;380(16):1509–24.

75. Vranckx P, Valgimigli M, Eckardt L, et al. Edoxaban-based versus vitamin K antagonist-based antithrombotic regimen after successful coronary stenting in patients with atrial fibrillation (ENTRUST-AF PCI): a randomised, open-label, phase 3b trial. Lancet 2019;394(10206):1335–43.

76. Lopes RD, Leonardi S, Wojdyla DM, et al. Stent thrombosis in patients with atrial fibrillation undergoing coronary stenting in the AUGUSTUS trial. Circulation 2020;141(9):781–3.

77. Angiolillo DJ, Bhatt DL, Cannon CP, et al. Antithrombotic therapy in patients with atrial fibrillation treated with oral anticoagulation undergoing percutaneous coronary intervention: a North American perspective: 2021 update. Circulation 2021; 143(6):583–96.

78. Alexander JH, Wojdyla D, Vora AN, et al. Risk/benefit tradeoff of antithrombotic therapy in patients with atrial fibrillation early and late after an acute coronary syndrome or percutaneous coronary intervention: insights from AUGUSTUS. Circulation 2020;141(20):1618–27.

79. Galli M, Andreotti F, Porto I, et al. Intracranial haemorrhages vs. stent thromboses with direct oral anticoagulant plus single antiplatelet agent or triple antithrombotic therapy: a meta-analysis of randomized trials in atrial fibrillation and percutaneous coronary intervention/acute coronary syndrome patients. Europace 2020;22(4):538–46.

80. Laudani C, Capodanno D, Dominick Joseph A. Bleeding in acute coronary syndrome: from definitions, incidence, and prognosis to prevention and management. Expet Opin Drug Saf 2023. https://doi.org/10.1080/14740338.2023.2291865.

81. Capodanno D, Huber K, Mehran R, et al. Management of antithrombotic therapy in atrial fibrillation patients undergoing PCI: JACC state-of-the-art review. J Am Coll Cardiol 2019;74(1):83–99.

82. Berry NC, Mauri L, Steg PG, et al. Effect of lesion complexity and clinical risk factors on the efficacy and safety of dabigatran dual therapy versus warfarin triple therapy in atrial fibrillation after percutaneous coronary intervention: a subgroup analysis from the REDUAL PCI trial. Circ Cardiovasc Interv 2020;13(4): e008349.

83. Kerneis M, Gibson CM, Chi G, et al. Effect of procedure and coronary lesion characteristics on clinical outcomes among atrial fibrillation patients undergoing percutaneous coronary intervention: insights from the PIONEER AF-PCI trial. JACC Cardiovasc Interv 2018;11(7):626–34.

84. Vranckx P, Valgimigli M, Eckardt L, et al. Edoxaban in atrial fibrillation patients with percutaneous coronary intervention by acute or chronic coronary syndrome presentation: a pre-specified analysis of the ENTRUST-AF PCI trial. Eur Heart J 2020; 41(47):4497–504.

Antithrombotic Therapy in Acute Coronary Syndrome

Riccardo Rinaldi, MD[a,b], Andrea Ruberti, MD[a], Salvatore Brugaletta, MD, PhD[a,*]

KEYWORDS

- Dual antiplatelet therapy • Acute coronary syndrome • Therapy • Precision medicine
- Prognosis

KEY POINTS

- In treating acute coronary syndrome (ACS), a primary concern is how to achieve the right balance between minimizing bleeding without increasing the risk of thrombotic events.
- A tailored approach to antithrombotic treatment is essential in ACS management. This involves assessing each patient's unique risk factors, response to medication, and variability in drug metabolism and effectiveness to optimize outcomes.
- Current clinical practice offers several strategies to reduce bleeding or ischemic risks in ACS patients. These include shortening the duration of dual antiplatelet therapy, transitioning from more potent antiplatelet agents to milder regimens as appropriate, and employing genetic testing and platelet function assays for more personalized therapy choices.

INTRODUCTION

Acute coronary syndromes (ACS) encompass a range of clinical conditions characterized by a complete or partial thrombotic occlusion of an epicardial coronary vessel with sudden reduced coronary blood flow, leading to myocardial ischaemia (MI).[1] Patients with ACS may present with or without corresponding alterations on the 12-lead electrocardiogram (ie, vST-elevation vs non-ST-elevation ACS), and with or without acute elevations in cardiac troponin concentrations (indicative of acute myocardial infarction [AMI] or unstable angina).[2] The cornerstone of therapy is early reperfusion through percutaneous coronary intervention (PCI) and prompt administration of antithrombotic drugs. This dual approach aims not only to rapidly restore immediate vessel patency but also to reduce incidence of acute and long-term ischaemic events.[3,4]

In recent decades, more potent antiplatelet agents with extended recommended duration have significantly reduced ACS-associated mortality.[5] Rationale behind the use of antiplatelet therapy is based on the pathologic base of ACS whose origin is a rupture, erosion, or fissuring of a coronary atherosclerotic plaque, leading to thrombosis formation via platelet adhesion, activation, and aggregation. Dual antiplatelet therapy (DAPT), composed of aspirin and a $P2Y_{12}$ receptor inhibitor, targets 2 distinct platelet activation pathways, effectively interrupts the immediate thrombotic process, and reduces the recurrence of thrombotic events.[6,7] However, the most concerning trade-off associated with DAPT is an increased risk of bleeding events that may significantly contribute to morbidity and mortality in the post-acute phase of ACS.[8] Recognizing those patients at increased risks of ischemic and/or bleeding complications, alongside understanding individual variability in responses to specific

---

Funding: This paper received no funding.

[a] Hospital Clínic, Cardiovascular Clinic Institute, Institut d'Investigacions Biomèdiques August Pi i Sunyer (IDI-BAPS), University of Barcelona, Barcelona, Spain; [b] Department of Cardiovascular and Pulmonary Sciences, Catholic University of the Sacred Heart, Rome, Italy

* Corresponding author. c/ Villarroel 170, Barcelona 08036, Spain.

E-mail address: sabrugaletta@gmail.com

Twitter: @sbrugaletta (S.B.)

antithrombotic agents, may paved the way for personalized antithrombotic treatments, aiming to improve both efficacy and safety outcomes.

This review will provide an overview of the pathology underlying ACS, focusing on the rationale for antithrombotic therapy. It will also provide an overview of current and future directions for an individualized approach for antithrombotic therapy in ACS patients.

ANTIPLATELET AGENTS
Aspirin and P2Y$_{12}$-Inhibitors

Aspirin inhibits the cyclooxygenase-1 enzyme irreversibly, thereby stopping the production of thromboxane A2, a potent platelet activator.[9] P2Y$_{12}$ inhibitors, including ticlopidine, clopidogrel, prasugrel, and ticagrelor, target a different aspect of the platelet activation pathway by blocking the P2Y$_{12}$ receptor, crucial for ADP-mediated platelet activation. The mechanism of binding and onset of action varies for each drug.

Ticlopidine, the first-generation thienopyridine, has largely been replaced due to severe haematological side effects, such as anemia and neutropenia.[10] Clopidogrel, a second-generation agent, undergoes a 2-step liver enzyme-mediated metabolism to become active. However, approximately 85% of the administered dose becomes inactive due to esterase-mediated hydrolysis.[11] The resulting active metabolite permanently binds to a free cysteine on P2Y$_{12}$, disabling it for the platelet's entire lifespan. Clopidogrel has demonstrated to effectively reduce cardiovascular events.[12,13] However, its effectiveness can vary due to individual differences in absorption and metabolism, leading to inconsistent platelet inhibition and a call for more potent and predictable P2Y$_{12}$ inhibitors.

Prasugrel, a third generation thienopyridine, provides faster and more consistent platelet inhibition than clopidogrel, primarily due to less interference from metabolic polymorphisms. This results in higher bioavailability of its active form. However, prasugrel's potent antiplatelet effects increase risk of major bleeding, particularly in patients with a history of stroke or transient ischemic attack.[14,15] Ticagrelor, a triazolopyrimidine, offers reversible allosteric inhibition of the P2Y$_{12}$ receptor, providing stronger and more predictable platelet inhibition than clopidogrel. A unique side effect of ticagrelor is dyspnoea, possibly due to its ADP-like structure binding to bronchial A1 receptors or the accumulation of ADP affecting sensory neurons. Its primary metabolite also contributes to antiplatelet effect, undergoing transformation by the CYP3A4 enzyme.[16] Similarly to prasugrel,

ticagrelor is superior to clopidogrel in reducing cardiovascular events, but it is associated with an increased risk of bleeding.[17]

Intravenous Antiplatelet Agents

Intravenous antiplatelet agents could be useful for those patients who cannot take oral medications, or when rapid onset or reversal of drug effects is needed, such as a bridge to surgery. Cangrelor is a direct, potent, and reversible intravenous P2Y$_{12}$ inhibitor that acts rapidly, with a very short half-life, allowing platelet function to recover quickly after the infusion stops.[18–20] Cangrelor significantly reduced the rate of ischemic events, including stent thrombosis, during PCI, with no significant increase in severe bleeding.[20]

Glycoprotein IIb/IIIa (GPIIb/IIIa) inhibitors (GPIs), including abciximab (a chimeric monoclonal antibody, no longer manufactured worldwide), eptifibatide (a cyclic-peptide derived from snake venom), and tirofiban (a small molecule that mimics the Arg-Gly-Asp sequence to deactivate GPIIb/IIIa), are a class of potent intravenous antiplatelet drugs.[21] Although their use has been effective in reducing cardiovascular events in ACS patients undergoing PCI, it often comes at the price of a significant increase in bleeding events.[22,23] The administration of GPIs after visualization of coronary anatomy (downstream treatment) does not significantly reduce incidence of cardiac event, but it may result in fewer major bleeding incidents compared to its administration as early as possible before PCI (upstream treatment).[24,25] With the introduction of P2Y$_{12}$ inhibitors, the use of GPIs in clinical practice has reduced significantly. To date, GPIs have a secondary role, mainly as bailouts for no-reflow and thrombotic complications.

ANTICOAGULANTS

Anticoagulation can be achieved either indirectly, through agents like unfractionated heparin (UFH), low molecular weight heparins (LMWHs), and fondaparinux, that enhance antithrombin activity, or directly, through drugs like bivalirudin or novel oral anticoagulant (NOACs) that inhibit thrombin or factor Xa, respectively.

UFH is a sulphate-polysaccharide that enhances antithrombin III's ability to neutralize thrombin and factor Xa and can be reversed with protamine sulphate. Historic trials supported the use of UFH in combination with aspirin for ACS.[26] However, due to UFH's variable anticoagulant effect, monitoring through activated partial thromboplastin time is essential to balance efficacy and bleeding risk. LMWHs (eg, enoxaparin) offer more predictable anticoagulant effect and have demonstrated non-inferior to UFH in ACS, albeit with slightly increased bleeding.[27,28]

Fondaparinux, a synthetic pentasaccharide, selectively and reversibly inhibits factor Xa through allosteric activation of antithrombin. It is 100% bioavailable after subcutaneous injection, has a long half-life allowing for once-daily dosing, and due to minimal plasma protein binding, it offers predictable antithrombotic effects.[29,30] However, its renal clearance makes it unsuitable for patients with significantly reduced glomerular filtration rates.[31]

Bivalirudin, derived from the natural anticoagulant hirudin, is a specific, fast-acting, and reversible direct thrombin inhibitor that do not bind to plasma proteins, providing consistent anticoagulant effects.[32,33]

CURRENT STANDARD RECOMMENDATIONS FOR ANTITHROMBOTIC THERAPY IN ACUTE CORONARY SYNDROME

Oral Antiplatelet Therapy

DAPT stands as the standard-of-care for ACS patients. Aspirin is recommended for all ACS patients as soon as possible, with a loading dose of 150 to 300 mg orally or 75 to 250 mg intravenously and a maintenance dose of 75 to 100 mg once daily (Class I). A $P2Y_{12}$ receptor inhibitor is recommended in addition to aspirin, with an initial oral loading dose followed by a maintenance dose (Class I).[2] Concerning the choice of the $P2Y_{12}$ inhibitor, prasugrel and ticagrelor are favored over clopidogrel in the absence of contraindications.[15,17] Moreover, prasugrel should be considered over ticagrelor (Class IIa).[34]

Regarding timing, the $P2Y_{12}$ inhibitor can be administered at the time of coronary angiography (CAG) or before when the coronary anatomy is unknown (ie, pre-treatment). Pre-treatment has the potential advantage of offering better antiplatelet protection by the time PCI is performed. However, not all patients undergoing CAG proceed to PCI, and pre-treatment may lead to unnecessary exposure to adjunctive antiplatelet treatment and an increased risk of bleeding. This is especially problematic for patients requiring surgical revascularization, as a washout period before the procedure is needed, resulting in prolonged hospital length-of-stay and increased costs.[35] Furthermore, several randomized controlled trials (RCTs) have failed to demonstrate the benefits of pre-treatment compared to the administration of $P2Y_{12}$ inhibitors at the time of PCI.[36,37] Accordingly, current guidelines do not recommend routine pre-treatment in non ST-elevation (NSTE)-ACS patients anticipated to undergo an early invasive strategy (ie, <24 h) (Class III). However, pre-treatment may be considered in NSTE-ACS patients where there is an anticipated delay to invasive angiography (ie, >24 h) and in STE-ACS patients (Class IIb).[2]

Finally, concerning the duration, the standard recommendation is 12 months of DAPT, irrespective of stent type. Beyond 12 months, long-term treatment with aspirin is recommended (Class I).[2]

Intravenous Antiplatelet Drugs

The administration of GPIs should be considered in ACS patients for bailout scenarios, such as no-re ow or thrombotic complications during PCI (Class IIa) or in high-risk PCI in $P2Y_{12}$ receptor inhibitor-naïve patients.[38] Conversely, the use of cangrelor may be considered in $P2Y_{12}$ receptor inhibitor-naïve ACS patients undergoing PCI, especially in situations where the administration of oral drugs may not be feasible (eg, patients in cardiogenic shock patients or mechanically ventilated) (Class IIb).[39]

Anticoagulant Treatment

Parenteral therapeutic anticoagulation is recommended for all ACS patients at the time of diagnosis (Class I). In STE-ACS patients, UFH is the standard anticoagulant (Class I). Intravenous enoxaparin should be considered as an alternative to UFH, especially in patients pre-treated with subcutaneous enoxaparin (Class IIa).[40] Bivalirudin, with a full-dose post-PCI infusion, is another alternative to UFH, particularly in patients with a history of heparin-induced thrombocytopenia (Class IIa).[41,42] Conversely, fondaparinux is not recommended in the STE-ACS setting (Class III).[43]

In the NSTE-ACS setting, UFH has traditionally been the anticoagulant of choice for those patients undergoing early invasive strategy. However, enoxaparin should be considered as an alternative to UFH, especially when clotting time monitoring is complex.[40] For all other NSTE-ACS patients (ie, invasive strategy beyond 24 h), fondaparinux is recommended during the extended initial pharmacologic-only treatment phase (Class I).[44] Of note, fondaparinux was associated with an increased risk of catheter-related thrombosis, especially in the STEMI setting, which was mitigated by adding a UFH bolus at PCI onset.[43,45] Intravenous enoxaparin should be considered as an alternative to fondaparinux, especially in patients pre-treated with subcutaneous enoxaparin (Class IIa).[40]

Discontinuation of anticoagulation should be considered immediately after PCI, except in specific cases, such as the presence of a left ventricle thrombus or atrial fibrillation (Class IIa).[2] In the presence of an indication for anticoagulation, specific considerations are required. Briefly, a default strategy of triple antithrombotic therapy in the initial week post-PCI, comprising aspirin, a P2Y12 inhibitor (preferably clopidogrel), and a NOAC, is recommended (Class I). Subsequently, a transition to dual antithrombotic therapy (DAT), involving a P2Y12 inhibitor and a NOAC (discontinuing aspirin), is recommended (Class I).[46–48] The duration of A may be extended up to 1 month (but not beyond) for patients with high ischemic risk but low bleeding risk (Class IIa), and DAT can be discontinued earlier (eg, at 6 months) for patients at an elevated risk of bleeding or with low ischemic risk (Class IIb).[49]

INDIVIDUALIZED APPROACH TO ANTITHROMBOTIC THERAPY

Along with adhering to standard recommendations, it is crucial to recognize the personalized nuances inherent in the decision-making process for antithrombotic treatment in ACS. The optimal choice, timing, and duration of antithrombotic therapy depend on a multifaceted interplay of patient-specific and PCI-related variables, taking into account ischemic and bleeding risks (Fig. 1).[50]

Strategies Aiming to Reduce Bleeding Risk

Strategies designed to mitigate bleeding risk encompass the use of scoring systems to identify patients with an increased bleeding risk, reducing the duration of DAPT to less than 12 months, and de-escalation from prasugrel or ticagrelor-based DAPT to a clopidogrel-based DAPT.

Various scoring systems have been developed to evaluate risk of bleeding, including the CRUSADE and the ACUITY bleeding risk scores. However, changes in interventional practices, such as the adoption of radial access for CAG and PCI, as well as modifications in antithrombotic treatments, may impact the predictive value of these risk scores.[51,52] An alternative approach for bleeding risk assessment is provided by the Academic Research Consortium for High Bleeding Risk (ARC-HBR) criteria. This consensus definition of patients at high bleeding risk (HBR) was established to ensure consistency in clinical trials evaluating safety and effectiveness of devices and drug regimens for patients undergoing PCI. HBR patient is defined by the presence of 1 major or 2

minor ARC-HBR risk factors. Of note, presence of multiple major risk factors is associated with a higher risk of bleeding.[53]

Shortening DAPT duration to less than or equal to 6 months, followed by aspirin monotherapy, has been explored as a bleeding avoidance strategy.[54–56] Additional RCTs have investigated further shortening DAPT to 1 to 3 months, followed by P2Y12 receptor inhibitor monotherapy, predominantly in NSTE-ACS and in those at low to intermediate ischaemic risk patients.[57–59] The TWILIGHT trial demonstrated that discontinuing aspirin after 3 months of DAPT, using ticagrelor monotherapy, significantly reduced bleeding events without a = significant increase in the risk of ischaemic events.[60] Similar findings were observed in the TICO trial, where ticagrelor monotherapy after 3 months of DAPT showed a reduction in net adverse clinical events and major bleeding events compared to 12-months DAPT, without differences in major adverse cardiac and cerebrovascular events.[61] Conversely, the STOPDAPT-2-ACS trial, exploring very short-duration DAPT (ie, 1–2 months) followed by clopidogrel monotherapy, did not prove non-inferiority for the composite endpoint of cardiovascular or bleeding events, with a higher risk of MI on the very short DAPT group compared to control.[62] The MASTER DAPT trial investigated abbreviated DAPT (1 month) followed by aspirin or P2Y12 inhibitor monotherapy versus standard DAPT (≥3 months) in HBR patients, revealed comparable net adverse clinical events and major adverse cardiac or cerebral events, with a significant reduction in bleeding events in the abbreviated therapy group.[63] Based on this evidence, for patients who remain free of events after 3 to 6 months of DAPT and are not at high risk of ischemic events, single antiplatelet therapy, preferably with a P2Y12 receptor inhibitor, should be considered (Class IIa).[64,65] In HBR patients, aspirin or P2Y12 receptor inhibitor monotherapy after 1 month of DAPT may be considered (Class IIb).[66]

Another strategy that may be considered to reduce the risk of bleeding events is de-escalating DAPT from prasugrel/ticagrelor-based DAPT to clopidogrel-based DAPT (Class IIb). However, a de-escalation strategy is not recommended within the first 30 days post-ACS (Class III).[67] The TOPIC and TALOS-AMI trials showed non-inferiority of unguided de-escalation approach (ie, switch from ticagrelor/prasugrel to clopidogrel after 1 month of DAPT) compared to standard-of-care, showing potential benefits in reducing bleeding.[68,69] The HOST-REDUCE-POLYTECH-ACS trial introduced a dose reduction

PCI + DAPT	Which Antithrombotic therapy?	When to administer?	For how long?
Non-STE ACS	Aspirin	As soon as possible	Indefinitely for long-term treatment
	P2Y12 Inhibitor • Ticagrelor or Prasugrel • Prasugrel over Ticagrelor • **Clopidogrel** if prasugrel or ticagrelor are contraindicated/not available **or** in elderly and HBR patients • **Cangrelor** in P2Y12 receptor inhibitor-naïve patients	• **Early invasive strategy**[a]: Routine pre-treatment is not recommended • **Delayed invasive strategy and no HBR**: pre-treatment may be considered	• Standard DAPT: 12 months • **If HIR and no HBR**: Prolonged antithrombotic regimen[b]; P2Y12 inhibitor monotherapy for long-term treatment • **If HBR**: SAT, preferably with a P2Y12 Inhibitor, after 1 or 3-6 months; De-escalation of P2Y12 inhibitor; De-escalation in the first 30 days
	Anticoagulation • UFH during PCI • **Early invasive strategy**[a]: Enoxaparin • **Delayed invasive strategy**[a]: Fundaparinux	At the time of diagnosis	Discontinued immediately after PCI, if no other indications
	GPIIb/IIIa inhibitors	No-reflow or thrombotic complications during PCI	Bolus + Infusion for up to 18h
STE ACS	Aspirin	As soon as possible	Indefinitely for long-term treatment
	P2Y12 Inhibitor • Ticagrelor or Prasugrel • Prasugrel over Ticagrelor • **Clopidogrel** if prasugrel or ticagrelor are contraindicated/not available **or** in elderly and HBR patients • **Cangrelor** in P2Y12 receptor inhibitor-naïve patients	• Pre-treatment may be considered in patients undergoing primary PCI	• Standard DAPT: 12 months • **If HIR and no HBR**: Prolonged antithrombotic regimen[b]; P2Y12 inhibitor monotherapy for long-term treatment • **If HBR**: SAT, preferably with a P2Y12 inhibitor, after 1 or 3-6 months; De-escalation of P2Y12 inhibitor; De-escalation in the first 30 days
	Anticoagulation • UFH during PCI • Enoxaparin • Bivalirudin • Fundaparinux	At the time of diagnosis	Discontinued immediately after PCI, if no other indications
	GPIIb/IIIa inhibitors	No-reflow or thrombotic complications during PCI	Bolus + Infusion for up to 18h

☐ Class I   ☐ Class IIa   ☐ Class IIb   ☐ Class III

Fig. 1. Schematic representation of current indication for antithrombotic therapy in ACS. DAPT, Dual Antiplatelet Therapy; GPIIb/IIIa, Glycoprotein IIb/IIIa; HBR, High Bleeding Risk (HBR); HIR, High Ischaemic Risk; Non-STE ACS, non-ST-elevation Acute Coronary Syndrome; PCI, Percutaneous Coronary Intervention (PCI); SAT, Single Antiplatelet Therapy; STE ACS, ST-Elevation Acute Coronary Syndrome; UFH, Unfractionated Heparin. [a]Early invasive strategy: coronary angiography and PCI if indicated within 24 hours; Delayed invasive strategy: coronary angiography (CAG) and PCI if indicated after 24 hours. [b]Both including a P2Y12 inhibitor or a NOAC (rivaroxaban 2.5 mg) in addition to aspirin. If ticagrelor is used, the 60 mg twice daily dosage is preferable than the 90 mg b.i.d. A long-term intensified antithrombotic regimen should be considered in patients with high ischaemic risk (Class IIa) and may be considered in patients with moderate ischaemic risk (Class IIb).

in prasugrel-treated patients (dose reduction from 10 mg to 5 mg vs standard-dose of 10 mg), demonstrated promising outcomes with reduced bleeding events without an increase in ischemic events.[70] In recent years, the possibility to assess clopidogrel response through platelet function tests (PFTs) evaluating the intensity of platelet inhibition or genetic testing has paved the way for an individualized approach based on guided antiplatelet therapy selection. Genetic factors, particularly the polymorphic CYP2C19 gene, significantly influence clopidogrel responsiveness, with loss-of-function alleles (ie, alleles *2 and *3) correlating with high platelet reactivity and thrombotic complications.[71] A guided de-escalation approach based on PFT and genetic testing could lead to selective de-escalation to clopidogrel in clopidogrel responders, thus minimizing bleeding risk without any trade-off in efficacy.[72] In the TROPICAL-ACS trial, involving 44% NSTE-ACS and 56% STE-ACS patients, a strategy of de-escalating DAPT from prasugrel to clopidogrel at 2 weeks post-ACS, guided by PFT, demonstrated non-inferiority compared to standard treatment with prasugrel at 1-year after PCI in terms of net clinical benefit.[73] Similarly, in the POPular

Genetics trial, DAPT de-escalation from ticagrelor/prasugrel to clopidogrel, guided by genetic testing in 2488 STE-ACS patients undergoing primary PCI within the previous 48 hours, demonstrated non-inferiority to standard treatment with ticagrelor or prasugrel at 12 months concerning thrombotic events and showed a lower incidence of bleeding.[74] Furthermore, a recent meta-analysis showed that a guided de-escalation strategy is associated to a 19% decrease in overall bleeding events without any trade-off in efficacy, compared to the standard selection of antiplatelet therapy, without any differences between the use of genetic or platelet tests.[75] Additionally, a network meta-analysis focusing on ACS demonstrated that, in comparison to routine selection of potent P2Y12 inhibiting therapy (prasugrel or ticagrelor), a guided selection of P2Y12 inhibiting therapy offers the most favourable balance between safety and efficacy.[76] Despite these promising results, PFT requires the patient to be on treatment with clopidogrel to assess clopidogrel responsiveness, potentially leading to an increased ischaemic risk during this timeframe. Similarly, genetic testing represents only 1 component defining antiplatelet drug response.[77]

Therefore, further evidence is needed before a guided de-escalation approach could be routinely implemented in clinical practice.

Finally, it is important to consider that much of the evidence supporting these strategies comes from trials primarily focused on bleeding outcomes, often with a non-inferiority design that is not adequately powered for detecting relevant differences in ischemic outcomes. Moreover, these studies often involved relatively selected patient populations (eg, the TALOS-AMI and HOST-REDUCE-POLYTECH-ACS trials including only East Asian populations) and potentially excluded or under-represented the highest-risk ACS patients (eg, elderly, women, low weight, etc). Hence, these strategies should be considered only as alternatives for the conventional strategy in particular instances with distinct motivations, such as HBR patients, bleeding complications, non-bleeding side effects (eg, dyspnoea on ticagrelor, allergic reactions), or socioeconomic factors.[78,79]

Strategies Aiming to Reduce the Ischaemic Risk

Strategies designed to reduce ischaemic risk include the addition of low-dose oral anticoagulant to DAPT and prolonging DAPT beyond 12 months. The addiction of NOAC to DAPT is one of the strategies explored to enhance secondary prevention of ischaemic events in ACS patients. The ATLAS ACS 2-TIMI 51 trial showed that a vascular dose of rivaroxaban (2.5 mg twice a day), in addition to DAPT (aspirin and clopidogrel), was associated with a reduction in ischaemic events and cardiovascular mortality but also with a higher risk of major and intracranial bleeding.[80] Similarly, in the APPRAISE-2 trial, where patients with recent ACS and at least 2 additional risk factors for recurrent ischaemic events received apixaban at a dose of 5 mg twice a day, mostly in combination with DAPT, this regimen did not demonstrate a lower risk of ischaemic events but was associated with more than a 2-fold increase in the risk of major bleeding.[81] Based on these findings, a long-term intensified antithrombotic regimen, including a P2Y$_{12}$ inhibitor or a NOAC in addition to aspirin, should be considered in patients with high ischaemic risk (Class IIa) and may be considered in patients with moderate ischaemic risk (Class IIb), in the absence of HBR.

Favourable evidence supports a strategy based on the prolongation of antithrombotic therapy beyond the 12-months DAPT in selected populations. The benefits came at the expense of a significant increase in moderate and severe bleeding.[82,83] The PEGASUS-TIMI 54 trial tested a prolonged DAPT strategy with either ticagrelor 90 mg/bid or 60 mg/bid on top of aspirin versus. placebo. This study included patients with myocardial infarction 1 to 3 years earlier and had at least 1 additional high-risk features (ie, age ≥65, diabetes mellitus, a second prior myocardial infarction, multivessel coronary artery disease, or chronic renal dysfunction). At 33 months, both ticagrelor doses significantly reduced the incidence of cardiovascular events at the expense of an increase in the rate of major bleeding. The safety profile, both in terms of bleeding and non-bleeding side effects, was more favourable with the 60 mg/bid dose.[84] Finally, P2Y$_{12}$ inhibitor monotherapy may be considered as an alternative to aspirin monotherapy for long-term treatment (Class IIb).[85]

SUMMARY AND FUTURE DIRECTIONS

The primary ACS treatment focuses on inhibiting coagulation and platelet function. The interplay between antiplatelet and anticoagulant therapies has significantly reduced thrombotic complications and mortality rates. Yet, the challenge of balancing these benefits against the increased risk of bleeding remains a significant concern. Ongoing and future studies are crucial in evaluating the effectiveness and safety of newer antithrombotic agents, their combinations, and duration, especially in specific populations, such as women or the elderly.

In the era of precision medicine, integrating genetic testing and platelet function assays could further refine the selection and monitoring of antithrombotic therapy, potentially leading to a more personalized treatment plan. Achieving this will require scientific innovation and a commitment to patient-centered care, where treatment decisions are tailored to the individual's needs and circumstances.

ACKNOWLEDGMENTS

None.

DISCLOSURE

The authors have nothing to disclose.

REFERENCES

1. Libby P. Mechanisms of acute coronary syndromes and their implications for therapy. N Engl J Med 2013;368(21):2004–13.
2. Byrne RA, Rossello X, Coughlan JJ, et al. 2023 ESC Guidelines for the management of acute coronary

syndromes. Eur Heart J 2023;44(38). https://doi.org/10.1093/EURHEARTJ/EHAD191.

3. Neumann FJ, Sousa-Uva M, Ahlsson A, et al. 2018 ESC/EACTS Guidelines on myocardial revascularization. Eur Heart J 2019;40(2):87–165.

4. Lawton JS, Tamis-Holland JE, Bangalore S, et al. 2021 ACC/AHA/SCAI Guideline for Coronary Artery Revascularization: Executive Summary: A Report of the American College of Cardiology/American Heart Association Joint Committee on Clinical Practice Guidelines. Circulation 2022;145(3):E4–17.

5. Gibbons GH, Seidman CE, Topol EJ. Conquering Atherosclerotic Cardiovascular Disease — 50 Years of Progress. N Engl J Med 2021;384(9):785–8.

6. Niccoli G, Liuzzo G, Montone RA, et al. Advances in mechanisms, imaging and management of the unstable plaque. Atherosclerosis 2014;233(2):467–77.

7. Montone RA, Niccoli G, Crea F, et al. Management of non-culprit coronary plaques in patients with acute coronary syndrome. Eur Heart J 2020;41(37):3579–86.

8. Hara H, Takahashi K, Kogame N, et al. Impact of Bleeding and Myocardial Infarction on Mortality in All-Comer Patients Undergoing Percutaneous Coronary Intervention. Circ Cardiovasc Interv 2020;13(9):E009177.

9. Jones WS, Mulder H, Wruck LM, et al. Comparative Effectiveness of Aspirin Dosing in Cardiovascular Disease. N Engl J Med 2021;384(21):1981–90.

10. Haynes RB, Sandler RS, Larson EB, et al. A Critical Appraisal of Ticlopidine, a New Antiplatelet Agent: Effectiveness and Clinical Indications for Prophylaxis of Atherosclerotic Events. Arch Intern Med 1992;152(7):1376–80.

11. Savi P, Pereillo JM, Uzabiaga MF, et al. Identification and biological activity of the active metabolite of clopidogrel. Thromb Haemost 2000;84(5):891–6.

12. Yusuf S, Zhao F, Mehta SR, et al. Effects of clopidogrel in addition to aspirin in patients with acute coronary syndromes without ST-segment elevation. N Engl J Med 2001;345(7):494–502.

13. Mehta SR, Bassand JP, Chrolavicius S, et al. Dose comparisons of clopidogrel and aspirin in acute coronary syndromes. N Engl J Med 2010;363(10):930–42.

14. Wiviott SD, Trenk D, Frelinger AL, et al. Prasugrel compared with high loading- and maintenance-dose clopidogrel in patients with planned percutaneous coronary intervention: the Prasugrel in Comparison to Clopidogrel for Inhibition of Platelet Activation and Aggregation-Thrombolysis in Myocardial Infarction 44 trial. Circulation 2007;116(25):2923–32.

15. Wiviott SD, Braunwald E, McCabe CH, et al. Prasugrel versus clopidogrel in patients with acute coronary syndromes. N Engl J Med 2007;357(20):2001–15.

16. Storey RF, Husted S, Harrington RA, et al. Inhibition of platelet aggregation by AZD6140, a reversible oral P2Y12 receptor antagonist, compared with clopidogrel in patients with acute coronary syndromes. J Am Coll Cardiol 2007;50(19):1852–6.

17. Wallentin L, Becker RC, Budaj A, et al. Ticagrelor versus clopidogrel in patients with acute coronary syndromes. N Engl J Med 2009;361(11):1045–57.

18. Franchi F, Rollini F, Muñiz-Lozano A, et al. Cangrelor: a review on pharmacology and clinical trial development. Expert Rev Cardiovasc Ther 2013;11(10):1279–91.

19. Angiolillo DJ, Firstenberg MS, Price MJ, et al. Bridging antiplatelet therapy with cangrelor in patients undergoing cardiac surgery: a randomized controlled trial. JAMA 2012;307(3):265–74.

20. Bhatt DL, Stone GW, Mahaffey KW, et al. Effect of platelet inhibition with cangrelor during PCI on ischemic events. N Engl J Med 2013;368(14):1303–13.

21. Topol EJ, Byzova TV, Plow EF. Platelet GPIIb-IIIa blockers. Lancet (London, England) 1999;353(9148):227–31.

22. Tcheng JE. Novel dosing regimen of eptifibatide in planned coronary stent implantation (ESPRIT): a randomised, placebo-controlled trial. Lancet (London, England) 2000;356(9247):2037–44.

23. Simoons ML. Effect of glycoprotein IIb/IIIa receptor blocker abciximab on outcome in patients with acute coronary syndromes without early coronary revascularisation: The GUSTO IV-ACS randomised trial. Lancet 2001;357(9272):1915–24.

24. Stone GW, Bertrand ME, Moses JW, et al. Routine upstream initiation vs deferred selective use of glycoprotein IIb/IIIa inhibitors in acute coronary syndromes: the ACUITY Timing trial. JAMA 2007;297(6):591–602.

25. Giugliano RP, White JA, Bode C, et al. Early versus delayed, provisional eptifibatide in acute coronary syndromes. N Engl J Med 2009;360(21):487–9.

26. Cohen M, Adams PC, Parry G, et al. Combination antithrombotic therapy in unstable rest angina and non-Q-wave infarction in nonprior aspirin users. Primary end points analysis from the ATACS trial. Antithrombotic Therapy in Acute Coronary Syndromes Research Group. Circulation 1994;89(1):81–8.

27. Ferguson JJ, Califf RM, Antman EM, et al. Enoxaparin vs unfractionated heparin in high-risk patients with non-ST-segment elevation acute coronary syndromes managed with an intended early invasive strategy: primary results of the SYNERGY randomized trial. JAMA 2004;292(1):45–54.

28. Montalescot G, Zeymer U, Silvain J, et al. Intravenous enoxaparin or unfractionated heparin in primary percutaneous coronary intervention for ST-elevation myocardial infarction: the international randomised open-label ATOLL trial. Lancet (London, England) 2011;378(9792):693–703.

29. Simoons ML, Bobbink IWG, Boland J, et al. A dose-finding study of fondaparinux in patients with non-ST-segment elevation acute coronary syndromes: The Pentasaccharide in Unstable Angina (PENTUA) study. J Am Coll Cardiol 2004;43(12):2183–90.

30. Mehta SR, Steg PG, Granger CB, et al. Randomized, blinded trial comparing fondaparinux with unfractionated heparin in patients undergoing contemporary percutaneous coronary intervention: Arixtra Study in Percutaneous Coronary Intervention: a Randomized Evaluation (ASPIRE) Pilot Trial. Circulation 2005;111(11):1390–7.

31. Paolucci F, Claviés MC, Donat F, et al. Fondaparinux sodium mechanism of action: identification of specific binding to purified and human plasma-derived proteins. Clin Pharmacokinet 2002;41(SUPPL. 2):11–8.

32. Lincoff AM, Bittl JA, Harrington RA, et al. Bivalirudin and provisional glycoprotein IIb/IIIa blockade compared with heparin and planned glycoprotein IIb/IIIa blockade during percutaneous coronary intervention: REPLACE-2 randomized trial. JAMA 2003;289(7):853–63.

33. Stone GW, McLaurin BT, Cox DA, et al. Bivalirudin for patients with acute coronary syndromes. N Engl J Med 2006;355(21):2203–16.

34. Schüpke S, Neumann F-J, Menichelli M, et al. Ticagrelor or Prasugrel in Patients with Acute Coronary Syndromes. N Engl J Med 2019;381(16):1524–34.

35. Capodanno D, Angiolillo DJ. Pretreatment with antiplatelet drugs in invasively managed patients with coronary artery disease in the contemporary era: review of the evidence and practice guidelines. Circ Cardiovasc Interv 2015;8(3). https://doi.org/10.1161/CIRCINTERVENTIONS.114.002301.

36. Tarantini G, Mojoli M, Varbella F, et al. Timing of Oral P2Y12 Inhibitor Administration in Patients With Non-ST-Segment Elevation Acute Coronary Syndrome. J Am Coll Cardiol 2020;76(21):2450–9.

37. Montalescot G, van 't Hof AW, Lapostolle F, et al. Prehospital ticagrelor in ST-segment elevation myocardial infarction. N Engl J Med 2014;371(11):1016–27.

38. Boersma E, Harrington RA, Moliterno DJ, et al. Platelet glycoprotein IIb/IIIa inhibitors in acute coronary syndromes: a meta-analysis of all major randomised clinical trials. Lancet (London, England) 2002;359(9302):189–98.

39. Steg PG, Bhatt DL, Hamm CW, et al. Effect of cangrelor on periprocedural outcomes in percutaneous coronary interventions: a pooled analysis of patient-level data. Lancet (London, England) 2013;382(9909):1981–92.

40. Silvain J, Beygui F, Barthélémy O, et al. Efficacy and safety of enoxaparin versus unfractionated heparin during percutaneous coronary intervention: systematic review and meta-analysis. BMJ 2012;344(7844):16.

41. Li Y, Liang Z, Qin L, et al. Bivalirudin plus a high-dose infusion versus heparin monotherapy in patients with ST-segment elevation myocardial infarction undergoing primary percutaneous coronary intervention: a randomised trial. Lancet (London, England) 2022;400(10366):1847–57.

42. Erlinge D, Omerovic E, Fröbert O, et al. Bivalirudin versus Heparin Monotherapy in Myocardial Infarction. N Engl J Med 2017;377(12):1132–42.

43. Yusuf S, Mehta SR, Chrolavicius S, et al. Effects of fondaparinux on mortality and reinfarction in patients with acute ST-segment elevation myocardial infarction: the OASIS-6 randomized trial. JAMA 2006;295(13):1519–30.

44. Steg PG, Jolly SS, Mehta SR, et al. Low-dose vs standard-dose unfractionated heparin for percutaneous coronary intervention in acute coronary syndromes treated with fondaparinux: the FUTURA/OASIS-8 randomized trial. JAMA 2010;304(12):1339–49.

45. Yusuf S, Mehta SR, Chrolavicius S, et al. Comparison of fondaparinux and enoxaparin in acute coronary syndromes. N Engl J Med 2006;354(14):1464–76.

46. Lopes RD, Heizer G, Aronson R, et al. Antithrombotic Therapy after Acute Coronary Syndrome or PCI in Atrial Fibrillation. N Engl J Med 2019;380(16):1509–24.

47. Vranckx P, Valgimigli M, Eckardt L, et al. Edoxaban-based versus vitamin K antagonist-based antithrombotic regimen after successful coronary stenting in patients with atrial fibrillation (ENTRUST-AF PCI): a randomised, open-label, phase 3b trial. Lancet (London, England) 2019;394(10206):1335–43.

48. Gargiulo G, Goette A, Tijssen J, et al. Safety and efficacy outcomes of double vs. triple antithrombotic therapy in patients with atrial fibrillation following percutaneous coronary intervention: a systematic review and meta-analysis of non-vitamin K antagonist oral anticoagulant-based randomized clinical trials. Eur Heart J 2019;40(46):3757–67.

49. Angiolillo DJ, Bhatt DL, Cannon CP, et al. Antithrombotic Therapy in Patients With Atrial Fibrillation Treated With Oral Anticoagulation Undergoing Percutaneous Coronary Intervention: A North American Perspective: 2021 Update. Circulation 2021;143(6):583–96.

50. Rodriguez F, Harrington RA. Management of Antithrombotic Therapy After Acute Coronary Syndromes. N Engl J Med 2021;384(5):452.

51. Mehran R, Pocock SJ, Nikolsky E, et al. A risk score to predict bleeding in patients with acute coronary syndromes. J Am Coll Cardiol 2010;55(23):2556–66.

52. Subherwal S, Bach RG, Chen AY, et al. Baseline risk of major bleeding in non-ST-segment-elevation myocardial infarction: the CRUSADE (Can Rapid risk stratification of Unstable angina patients

Suppress ADverse outcomes with Early implementation of the ACC/AHA Guidelines) Bleeding Score. Circulation 2009;119(14):1873–82.

53. Urban P, Mehran R, Colleran R, et al. Defining High Bleeding Risk in Patients Undergoing Percutaneous Coronary Intervention. Circulation 2019;140(3):240–61.

54. Hahn JY, Song YB, Oh JH, et al. 6-month versus 12-month or longer dual antiplatelet therapy after percutaneous coronary intervention in patients with acute coronary syndrome (SMART-DATE): a randomised, open-label, non-inferiority trial. Lancet (London, England) 2018;391(10127):1274–84.

55. Kedhi E, Fabris E, Van Der Ent M, et al. Six months versus 12 months dual antiplatelet therapy after drug-eluting stent implantation in ST-elevation myocardial infarction (DAPT-STEMI): randomised, multicentre, non-inferiority trial. BMJ 2018;363. https://doi.org/10.1136/BMJ.K3793.

56. de Luca G, Damen SA, Camaro C, et al. Final results of the randomised evaluation of short-term dual antiplatelet therapy in patients with acute coronary syndrome treated with a new-generation stent (REDUCE trial). EuroIntervention 2019;15(11):E990–8.

57. Hahn JY, Song YB, Oh JH, et al. Effect of P2Y12 Inhibitor Monotherapy vs Dual Antiplatelet Therapy on Cardiovascular Events in Patients Undergoing Percutaneous Coronary Intervention: The SMART-CHOICE Randomized Clinical Trial. JAMA 2019;321(24):2428–37.

58. Vranckx P, Valgimigli M, Jüni P, et al. Ticagrelor plus aspirin for 1 month, followed by ticagrelor monotherapy for 23 months vs aspirin plus clopidogrel or ticagrelor for 12 months, followed by aspirin monotherapy for 12 months after implantation of a drug-eluting stent: a multicentre, open-label, randomised superiority trial. Lancet (London, England) 2018;392(10151):940–9.

59. Watanabe H, Domei T, Morimoto T, et al. Effect of 1-Month Dual Antiplatelet Therapy Followed by Clopidogrel vs 12-Month Dual Antiplatelet Therapy on Cardiovascular and Bleeding Events in Patients Receiving PCI: The STOPDAPT-2 Randomized Clinical Trial. JAMA 2019;321(24):2414–27.

60. Mehran R, Baber U, Sharma SK, et al. Ticagrelor with or without Aspirin in High-Risk Patients after PCI. N Engl J Med 2019;381(21):2032–42.

61. Kim BK, Hong SJ, Cho YH, et al. Effect of Ticagrelor Monotherapy vs Ticagrelor With Aspirin on Major Bleeding and Cardiovascular Events in Patients With Acute Coronary Syndrome: The TICO Randomized Clinical Trial. JAMA 2020;323(23):2407–16.

62. Watanabe H, Morimoto T, Natsuaki M, et al. Comparison of Clopidogrel Monotherapy After 1 to 2 Months of Dual Antiplatelet Therapy With 12 Months of Dual Antiplatelet Therapy in Patients With Acute Coronary Syndrome: The STOPDAPT-2 ACS Randomized Clinical Trial. JAMA Cardiol 2022;7(4):407–17.

63. Valgimigli M, Frigoli E, Heg D, et al. Dual Antiplatelet Therapy after PCI in Patients at High Bleeding Risk. N Engl J Med 2021;385(18):1643–55.

64. Giacoppo D, Matsuda Y, Fovino LN, et al. Short dual antiplatelet therapy followed by P2Y12 inhibitor monotherapy vs. prolonged dual antiplatelet therapy after percutaneous coronary intervention with second-generation drug-eluting stents: a systematic review and meta-analysis of randomized clinical trials. Eur Heart J 2021;42(4):308–19.

65. Valgimigli M, Gragnano F, Branca M, et al. P2Y12 inhibitor monotherapy or dual antiplatelet therapy after coronary revascularisation: individual patient level meta-analysis of randomised controlled trials. BMJ 2021;373. https://doi.org/10.1136/BMJ.N1332.

66. Smits PC, Frigoli E, Tijssen J, et al. Abbreviated Antiplatelet Therapy in Patients at High Bleeding Risk With or Without Oral Anticoagulant Therapy After Coronary Stenting: An Open-Label, Randomized, Controlled Trial. Circulation 2021;144(15):1196–211.

67. Shoji S, Kuno T, Fujisaki T, et al. De-Escalation of Dual Antiplatelet Therapy in Patients With Acute Coronary Syndromes. J Am Coll Cardiol 2021;78(8):763–77.

68. Cuisset T, Deharo P, Quilici J, et al. Benefit of switching dual antiplatelet therapy after acute coronary syndrome: the TOPIC (timing of platelet inhibition after acute coronary syndrome) randomized study. Eur Heart J 2017;38(41):3070–8.

69. Kim CJ, Park MW, Kim MC, et al. Unguided de-escalation from ticagrelor to clopidogrel in stabilised patients with acute myocardial infarction undergoing percutaneous coronary intervention (TALOS-AMI): an investigator-initiated, open-label, multicentre, non-inferiority, randomised trial. Lancet (London, England) 2021;398(10308):1305–16.

70. Kim HS, Kang J, Hwang D, et al. Prasugrel-based de-escalation of dual antiplatelet therapy after percutaneous coronary intervention in patients with acute coronary syndrome (HOST-REDUCE-POLYTECH-ACS): an open-label, multicentre, non-inferiority randomised trial. Lancet (London, England) 2020;396(10257):1079–89.

71. Galli M, Franchi F, Rollini F, et al. Genetic testing in patients undergoing percutaneous coronary intervention: rationale, evidence and practical recommendations. Expert Rev Clin Pharmacol 2021;14(8):963–78.

72. Sibbing D, Aradi D, Alexopoulos D, et al. Updated Expert Consensus Statement on Platelet Function and Genetic Testing for Guiding P2Y12 Receptor Inhibitor Treatment in Percutaneous Coronary Intervention. JACC Cardiovasc Interv 2019;12(16):1521–37.

73. Sibbing D, Aradi D, Jacobshagen C, et al. Guided de-escalation of antiplatelet treatment in patients with acute coronary syndrome undergoing percutaneous coronary intervention (TROPICAL-ACS): a randomised, open-label, multicentre trial. Lancet (London, England) 2017;390(10104):1747–57.

74. Claassens DMF, Vos GJA, Bergmeijer TO, et al. A Genotype-Guided Strategy for Oral P2Y12 Inhibitors in Primary PCI. N Engl J Med 2019;381(17):1621–31.

75. Galli M, Benenati S, Capodanno D, et al. Guided versus standard antiplatelet therapy in patients undergoing percutaneous coronary intervention: a systematic review and meta-analysis. Lancet (London, England) 2021;397(10283):1470–83.

76. Galli M, Benenati S, Franchi F, et al. Comparative effects of guided vs. potent P2Y12 inhibitor therapy in acute coronary syndrome: a network meta-analysis of 61 898 patients from 15 randomized trials. Eur Heart J 2022;43(10):959–67.

77. Angiolillo DJ, Capodanno D, Danchin N, et al. Derivation, Validation, and Prognostic Utility of a Prediction Rule for Nonresponse to Clopidogrel: The ABCD-GENE Score. JACC Cardiovasc Interv 2020;13(5):606–17.

78. Zettler ME, Peterson ED, McCoy LA, et al. Switching of adenosine diphosphate receptor inhibitor after hospital discharge among myocardial infarction patients: Insights from the Treatment with Adenosine Diphosphate Receptor Inhibitors: Longitudinal Assessment of Treatment Patterns and Events after Acute Coronary Syndrome (TRANSLATE-ACS) observational study. Am Heart J 2017;183:62–8.

79. Angiolillo DJ, Rollini F, Storey RF, et al. International Expert Consensus on Switching Platelet P2Y12 Receptor-Inhibiting Therapies. Circulation 2017;136(20):1955–75.

80. Mega JL, Braunwald E, Wiviott SD, et al. Rivaroxaban in patients with a recent acute coronary syndrome. N Engl J Med 2012;366(1):9–19.

81. Alexander JH, Lopes RD, James S, et al. Apixaban with antiplatelet therapy after acute coronary syndrome. N Engl J Med 2011;365(8):699–708.

82. Connolly SJ, Eikelboom JW, Bosch J, et al. Rivaroxaban with or without aspirin in patients with stable coronary artery disease: an international, randomised, double-blind, placebo-controlled trial. Lancet (London, England) 2018;391(10117):205–18.

83. Mauri L, Kereiakes DJ, Yeh RW, et al. Twelve or 30 months of dual antiplatelet therapy after drug-eluting stents. N Engl J Med 2014;371(23):2155–66.

84. Bonaca MP, Bhatt DL, Steg PG, et al. Ischaemic risk and efficacy of ticagrelor in relation to time from P2Y12 inhibitor withdrawal in patients with prior myocardial infarction: insights from PEGASUS-TIMI 54. Eur Heart J 2016;37(14):1133–42.

85. Koo BK, Kang J, Park KW, et al. Aspirin versus clopidogrel for chronic maintenance monotherapy after percutaneous coronary intervention (HOST-EXAM): an investigator-initiated, prospective, randomised, open-label, multicentre trial. Lancet (London, England) 2021;397(10293):2487–96.

Antithrombotic Therapy in Patients with Complex Percutaneous Coronary Intervention and Cardiogenic Shock

Jose Ignacio Larrubia Valle, MD[a],
Cristóbal A. Urbano-Carrillo, MD[a],
Francesco Costa, MD, PhD[b,c,*]

KEYWORDS

- Antithrombotic therapy • Complex PCI • Cardiogenic shock • Antiplatelet therapy
- Anticoagulant

KEY POINTS

- Unfractionated heparin is the mainstay of anticoagulation in most complex percutaneous coronary intervention (PCI) patients and in cardiogenic shock (CS). Bivalirudin may represent a safer alternative.
- Parenteral antiplatelet therapy with cangrelor may be a useful alternative during complex PCI or in patients with CS.
- Potent P2Y$_{12}$ inhibitors are the agents of choice after acute coronary syndrome and may be a reasonable alternative to clopidogrel in complex PCI for chronic coronary syndrome.
- Longer dual antiplatelet therapy (DAPT) courses provide better efficacy after complex PCI in patients without high bleeding risk. However, emerging strategies utilizing potent P2Y$_{12}$ inhibitors monotherapy after short courses of DAPT may be a safer alternative.

INTRODUCTION

The management of patients undergoing complex and high-risk intervention in indicated patients (CHIP), presents a significant challenge in contemporary cardiovascular medicine. Antithrombotic therapy, including both antiplatelet and anticoagulant agents, is critical in minimizing thrombotic complications during and after percutaneous coronary intervention (PCI).[1,2] These complex procedures, often associated to both complex coronary artery disease anatomy, and/or unstable hemodynamic status require a meticulous strategy to mitigate thrombotic complications while balancing the risk of bleeding. Yet, the optimal strategy for patients undergoing complex PCI or experiencing cardiogenic shock (CS) remains a subject of ongoing debate. This article explores current evidence regarding optimal antithrombotic therapy in CHIP patients, including those undergoing indicated complex PCI or those presenting with CS.

---

[a] Unidad de Gestión Clínica de Cardiología, Hospital Regional Universitario de Malaga, Malaga 29010, Spain; [b] Área del Corazón, Hospital Universitario Virgen de la Victoria, CIBERCV, IBIMA Plataforma BIONAND, Departamento de Medicina UMA, Malaga 29010, Spain; [c] Department of Biomedical and Dental Sciences and of Morphological and Functional Images, University of Messina, Messina 98122, Italy
* Corresponding author. Interventional Cardiology Unit HUVV Málaga, Spain IBIMA Malaga, CIBER CV, Spain C. Severo Ochoa 35, Campanillas, Malaga 29590, Spain.
E-mail address: fcosta@unime.it
Twitter: @Costa_F_8 (F.C.)

Intervent Cardiol Clin 13 (2024) 517–525
https://doi.org/10.1016/j.iccl.2024.06.006
2211-7458/24/© 2024 Elsevier Inc. All rights reserved, including those for text and data mining, AI training, and similar technologies.

ANTITHROMBOTIC THERAPY IN COMPLEX PERCUTANEOUS CORONARY INTERVENTION

A standardized definition of complex PCI is currently lacking. This refers to a higher-risk anatomy, resulting in a technically more complex intervention that poses a greater risk of periprocedural complications and long-term ischemic events due to the more extensive vascular disease.[3–5] The SYNTAX score was one of the first attempts to objectively determine the complexity of coronary anatomy and intervention to indicate patients to PCI or cardiac surgery.[6] More recently, Giustino and colleagues derived a standardized definition of complex PCI to study the impact of long-term antiplatelet therapy.[7] This definition includes 3 vessels treated with PCI, at least 3 stents implanted, at least 3 lesions treated, bifurcation stenting, total stent length of 60 mm or more, and/or successfully treating a chronic total occlusion. Such definition, with minimal variations such as clinical presentation with acute coronary syndrome (ACS), calcium debulking with rotational atherectomy or left main or saphenous vein graft PCI,[8] has been commonly used in the literature in the last few years for subgroup analysis of complex PCI.[9]

Periprocedural Anticoagulant Therapy

Unfractionated heparin (UFH) has historically been the preferred anticoagulant for PCI due to its cost-effectiveness and the advantage of being easily reversible. However, UFH's anticoagulant effect is unpredictable, and it operates within a narrow therapeutic window, which can increase the risk of bleeding, particularly during prolonged procedures requiring repeated boluses.[10] As an alternative, Bivalirudin, a direct thrombin inhibitor, offers distinct advantages over traditional anticoagulants. By directly binding to thrombin, it inhibits both thrombin activity and the formation of thrombin-fibrin complexes. This mechanism results in predictable anticoagulant effects and a lower risk of bleeding compared to UFH. Currently, generic formulations of bivalirudin are available.

Numerous clinical trials have validated the safety and efficacy of bivalirudin in patients undergoing PCI for ACS.[10–12] A recent individual patient meta-analysis included all the 5 large (>1000 patients) randomized clinical trials in the field, with a total of 12,155 ACS patients randomized to bivalirudin versus heparin during PCI. Bivalirudin significantly reduced the incidence of serious bleeding, both at the access

site and non-access sites, compared to heparin (3.3% vs 5.5%; adjusted odds ratio, 0.59; 95% CI, 0.48–0.72; $P<.0001$). However, the 30-day mortality rates were not significantly different between the 2 treatments (1.2% for bivalirudin vs 1.1% for heparin; adjusted odds ratio, 1.24 [95% CI, 0.86–1.79]; $P = .25$). Similarly, there were no significant differences in cardiac mortality, reinfarction, and stent thrombosis rates. These outcomes remained consistent regardless of whether a post-PCI bivalirudin infusion was used, whether routine use of glycoprotein IIb/IIIa inhibitors (GPIs) with heparin was applied, and throughout the 1-year follow-up period.[13] No formal testing for patients undergoing complex PCI has been performed in this study, and all patients included were presenting with non-ST segment elevated myocardial infarction (MI).

Consistently, among patients with complex coronary lesions, Cortese and colleagues[14] compared UFH and GPI with a periprocedural and post-PCI bivalirudin infusion and found no significant differences in periprocedural MI or 30-day major adverse cardiac events. Yet, rates of minor bleeding were lower with bivalirudin (20.3% vs 4.0%, $P<.05$) with a trend toward a reduction of major bleeding (8.5% vs 4.0%, $P = .07$). Yet, this was a retrospective analysis and was focused on lesion complexity (according to the American College of Cardiology/American Heart Association lesion type definition) rather than procedural complexity. Hence, while in the larger ACS population bivalirudin appeared to be safer than UFH, with comparable ischemic events at longer follow-up, solid evidence regarding the anticoagulant of choice in complex PCI patients is currently lacking (Fig. 1).

Periprocedural Parenteral Antiplatelet Therapy

Parenteral antiplatelet agents provide a more rapid and consistent antiplatelet effect during PCI,[15] which may theoretically provide superior ischemic protection especially in long and complex interventions. Cangrelor is a potent intravenous $P2Y_{12}$ inhibitor known for its direct and reversible action, characterized by rapid onset of platelet inhibition and full restoration of platelet function within 1 hour after discontinuation. Cangrelor is approved for use in PCI procedures for both chronic coronary syndrome (CCS) and ACS patients who have not previously received oral $P2Y_{12}$ inhibitors, with a class IIb recommendation in both European[16] and American guidelines[17] (see Fig. 1). In the CHAMPION PCI, CHAMPION PLATFORM, and CHAMPION PHOENIX trials,[18] cangrelor compared to

ACC/AHA and ESC Guideline Recommendations for Antithrombotic Treatment in Complex PCI

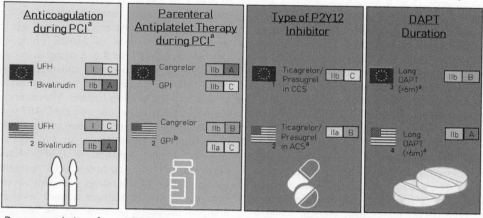

Fig. 1. Recommendations from ACC/AHA and ESC guidelines for antithrombotic treatment in complex percutaneous coronary intervention (PCI). ACS, acute coronary syndrome; CCS, chronic coronary syndrome; DAPT, dual antiplatelet therapy; GPI, glycoproteins IIb/IIIa inhibitors; HBR, high bleeding risk; UFH: unfractionated heparin. [a]No specific recommendation for complex PCI, recommendation apply to the general PCI treated population. [b]For Bailout thrombosis. (1. Neumann FJ, Sousa-Uva M, Ahlsson A, et al. 2018 ESC/EACTS guidelines on myocardial revascularization. Eur Heart J. 2019;40(2):87 to 165. https://doi.org/10.1093/eurheartj/ehy394. 2. Lawton JS, Tamis-Holland JE, Bangalore S, et al. 2021 ACC/AHA/SCAI guideline for coronary artery revascularization: Executive summary: A report of the American College of Cardiology/American Heart Association joint committee on clinical practice guidelines [published correction appears in Circulation. 2022 Mar 15;145(11):e771]. Circulation. 2022;145(3):e4-e17. https://doi.org/10.1161/CIR.0000000000001039. 3. Valgimigli M, Bueno H, Byrne RA, et al. 2017 ESC focused update on dual antiplatelet therapy (DAPT) in coronary artery disease developed in collaboration with EACTS: The Task Force for DAPT in coronary artery disease of the European Society of Cardiology (ESC) and of the European Association for Cardio-Thoracic Surgery (EACTS). Eur Heart J. 2018;39(3):213 to 260. https://doi.org/10.1093/eurheartj/ehx419. 4. Levine GN, Bates ER, Bittl JA, et al. 2016 ACC/AHA Guideline Focused Update on Duration of DAPT in Patients With Coronary Artery Disease: A Report of the American College of Cardiology/American Heart Association Task Force on Clinical Practice Guidelines. Circulation. 2016 Sep 6;134(10):e192–4. Circulation. 2016;134(10):e123-e155. https://doi.org/10.1161/CIR.0000000000000404).

clopidogrel, was associated to a 19% reduction of major adverse cardiovascular events (MACE) and 41% reduction of stent thrombosis. In a post hoc analysis of the CHAMPION PHOENIX trial[19] focused on complex PCI, immediate pre-treatment with cangrelor was found to lower the 48-h rate of major adverse ischemic events compared to clopidogrel, without increasing major bleeding, regardless of PCI lesion complexity. Yet, given the higher baseline risk among patients with higher lesions complexity, the absolute benefit with cangrelor in these higher risk groups was larger. Importantly, the transition from cangrelor to an oral P2Y12 inhibitor after PCI remains under investigation and may result in a period of inadequate platelet inhibition which is of particular concern among complex PCI patients, suggesting that an early transition to ticagrelor, rather than clopidogrel, soon after cangrelor infusion could be beneficial to mitigate this risk.[20] Hence, cangrelor, given its characteristic pharmacokinetics, may offer potential benefits in complex PCI, in which longer procedural duration and more complex instrumentations have a higher baseline absolute risk that may be mitigated by more consistent and potent antiplatelet inhibition. However, dedicated randomized trials in complex PCI, especially comparing cangrelor with other parenteral agents, are currently lacking.

Oral P2Y12 Inhibitor Type

Dual antiplatelet therapy (DAPT) with aspirin and a P2Y12 inhibitor is recommended after PCI, with clopidogrel and potent P2Y12 inhibitors prasugrel and ticagrelor, recommended in CCS and ACS patients, respectively.[21,22] However, given the higher baseline risk after complex coronary intervention, European guidelines suggest possible implementation of potent P2Y12 inhibitors also in patients with CCS with a low level of evidence.[23] (Class IIb, Level C) (see Fig. 1).

Li and colleagues evaluated in a retrospective registry including 12,438 patients with complex PCI,[24] the impact of ticagrelor versus clopidogrel. After propensity score matching, ticagrelor was associated to significantly lower rates of ischemic events (1.50% vs 2.65%, $P<.01$) and all-cause death (1.09% vs 1.81%, $P = .02$) compared to the clopidogrel-treated group. A subgroup analysis of the ALPHEUS trial,[25] which randomly allocated 1866 patients with CCS to ticagrelor or clopidogrel, evaluated the impact of treatment among complex (48.3%) versus non-complex PCI. The study showed that, despite patients with complex PCI carried a higher post-procedural and 1-month risk of ischemic complications, the randomized treatment with ticagrelor did not provide a significant ischemic benefit over clopidogrel. Yet, owing to limited statistical power for subgroup analysis, a lack of efficacy of ticagrelor in this setting could not be considered conclusive. Hence, while a more potent and consistent antiplatelet regimen may provide a potential benefit to reduce short-term and long-term ischemic complication in CCS patients undergoing complex PCI, currently scientific evidence to support this practice is limited. Finally, among ACS patients undergoing complex PCI, a subanalysis of the ISAR-REACT 5 trial,[26] which included 3377 patients, among 1429 of them underwent a complex PCI, found a higher incidence of MACE in complex PCI (10.1% vs 7.2%, hazard ratio [HR]: 1.44, 95% confidence interval [CI] [1.14–1.82], $P=.002$), than non-complex PCI group. Among complex PCI patients prasugrel was associated to similar ischemic and safety events compared to ticagrelor, whereas among non-complex PCI patients prasugrel was associated to a reduction of MACE. Yet, interaction testing was negative, hence there is not enough evidence to support a different impact of ticagrelor versus prasugrel in ACS patients with complex PCI.

Long-term Post Procedural Antiplatelet Therapy

DAPT duration after complex PCI has been extensively studied. In the seminal paper by Giustino and colleagues[7] individual patient data from 9577 individuals from 6 randomized controlled trials of long versus short term DAPT have been evaluated. DAPT consisted mostly of the association of aspirin and clopidogrel, and aspirin monotherapy was implemented after DAPT discontinuation. Patients were considered as complex PCI whether at least 1 of the following elements was present: 3 vessels treated, greater than or equal to 3 stents implanted, greater than or equal to 3 lesions treated, bifurcation with 2 stents implanted, total stent length greater than 60 mm, or chronic total occlusion. Complex

PCI patients had a roughly 2-fold increased risk of MACE at 1 year. The Authors found that complex PCI patients randomized to long term DAPT for 12 months or more were associated to a 44% lower risk of MACE compared to shorter term DAPT for 3 or 6 months. In contrast, non-complex PCI patients did not derive any benefit from a longer DAPT, with a consistent increase in the bleeding hazard. Interestingly, the magnitude of the benefit of long DAPT was progressively greater per increase in the number of procedural complexities.

Whether the duration of DAPT should be adjusted among complex PCI patients at elevated risk of bleeding was evaluated in a separate study. In a single-patient level pooled analysis including a total of 14,963 patients treated with PCI,[27] 3118 patients underwent complex PCI and 11,845 underwent non-complex PCI. Patients were further divided as high bleeding risk (HBR) or non-HBR based on the PRECISE-DAPT score.[28,29] PCI complexity and HBR status both increased synergically the risk of MACE at 24 months, while only the HBR status was associated to a significant increase of bleeding complications. Consistent with prior evidence, patients undergoing complex PCI and not at HBR experienced a significant 44% reduction in MACE when treated with long DAPT for 12 months or more, compared to those treated for 3 to 6 months, while no benefit from longer DAPT was observed in noncomplex PCI patients. However, irrespectively of PCI complexity, patients at HBR did not derive any benefit from longer term DAPT and experienced a higher risk of bleeding. These results support the hypothesis that bleeding risk should be prioritized for decision making regarding DAPT duration irrespective of ischemic risk.

Similarly, the study by Yeh and colleagues,[30] have utilized the DAPT score to evaluate the appropriate duration of DAPT alongside assessing the complexity of coronary lesions. They found that, among individuals who remained event-free during the initial 12 months, the benefit of prolonging DAPT was comparable irrespective of lesion complexity. Notably, a high DAPT score pinpointed those who experienced the most significant benefits from extended treatment, regardless of lesion complexity.

Recently, multiple studies have tested the hypothesis that shorter term DAPT courses, followed by $P2Y_{12}$ inhibitor monotherapy after aspirin withdrawal may be as effective and safer as compared to longer DAPT courses.[31] This concept has been replicated in multiple subgroup analysis. The TWILIGHT (Ticagrelor with Aspirin or Alone in High-Risk Patients after Coronary Intervention) trial[32] compared monotherapy with ticagrelor versus DAPT with aspirin after 3 months of DAPT in 7119 patients, including 2342 cases of complex PCI. The trial found no significant differences in rates of death, MI, stent thrombosis, or stroke between the 2 groups (3.8% vs 4.9%; HR: 0.77; 95% CI: 0.52–1.15). However, as expected, the DAPT group exhibited higher rates of bleeding complications (4.2% vs 7.7%; HR: 0.54; 95% CI: 0.38–0.76). Recently, numerous sub-studies and meta-analyses have been published,[33–37] have significantly contributed to the literature in this area. These studies all conclude that monotherapy with ticagrelor following 1 to 3 months of DAPT yields comparable ischemic outcomes and reduces bleeding complications.

Similar results were reported in a meta-analysis by Gragnano and colleagues,[37] which included 22,941 patients, of whom 4685 (20.4%) had undergone complex PCI. Their findings indicated that the risk of ischemic events was comparable between P2Y12 inhibitor monotherapy and DAPT in complex PCI (HR: 0.87; 95% CI: 0.64–1.19) with a significant reduction in bleeding risk with $P2Y_{12}$ inhibitor monotherapy (HR: 0.51; 95% CI: 0.31–0.84).

Shorter term DAPT followed by $P2Y_{12}$ inhibitor monotherapy after 1 month in HBR patients was tested in a MASTER-DAPT subanalysis[38] which demonstrated that in these patients, including complex and non-complex PCI, incidence of MACE was similar, with lower bleeding rates, compared with standard DAPT. These results confirmed that irrespective of PCI complexity, HBR status should prompt a shorter course of DAPT, which may have a positive impact both on bleeding reduction and cardiovascular mortality.[39]

Further reduction of the duration of DAPT was explored in the STOP-DAPT-3 (ShorT and OPtimal duration of DAPT after everolimus-eluting cobalt-chromium stent-3) trial,[40] which propose an aspirin-free strategy after the initial periprocedural period, randomly comparing low-dose prasugrel (3.75 mg/day) monotherapy to DAPT with low-dose prasugrel and aspirin. In this subgroup analysis evaluating patients who underwent complex PCI (1230, 20.6% of total cohort), they observed that the incidence of the coprimary cardiovascular endpoint at 1 month was higher in patients with complex PCI (5.9% vs 3.4%; HR: 1.74; 95% CI; P<.001). In patients undergoing complex PCI, no differences were observed between the 2 treatment arms for either bleeding (5.3% vs 3.7%; HR: 1.44; 95% CI: 0.84–2.47; P=.18) or cardiovascular events (5.78% vs 5.93%; HR: 0.98; 95% CI: 0.62–1.55; P=.92) without significant interactions between DAPT strategy and PCI complexity. In conclusion, all studies similarly observed that patients undergoing complex PCI carry a higher ischemic risk which may be reduced by longer courses of DAPT (see Fig. 1), whereas $P2Y_{12}$ inhibitor monotherapy after short courses of DAPT, especially if implemented with potent $P2Y_{12}$ inhibitors, provide similar efficacy and superior safety compared to longer term DAPT.

ANTITHROMBOTIC THERAPY IN CARDIOGENIC SHOCK

CS is characterized by inadequate tissue perfusion due to severe cardiac dysfunction, hemodynamic instability, and high mortality. This presentation also complicates the antithrombotic management, as these patients are at increased risk of both thrombotic and bleeding complications due to their critical condition and the intensive interventions required (Fig. 2). In this section, we summarize the evidence regarding antithrombotic therapies in CS. Details regarding the optimal antithrombotic therapy in patients treated with mechanical support devices is beyond the scope of the current manuscript.

Anticoagulation Therapy in Cardiogenic SHOCK

Anticoagulation is a fundamental component of therapy for patients with CS. Similar to its use in complex PCI, UFH remains the preferred anticoagulant during PCI in CS. UFH's rapid onset, monitoring, and reversibility make it suitable for these patients that often are managed with large-bore access and ventricular mechanical support. Bivalirudin may be an alternative in this setting, but the available evidence is limited. A classic retrospective observational study[41] of 86 CS patients undergoing primary PCI demonstrated significantly lower hospital mortality in those treated with bivalirudin compared to those receiving UFH and GPIs (5.4% vs 32.7%, respectively; P=.002). The rates of major hematoma were similar between the 2 groups (3.0% vs 2.6%, respectively; P=.46). Yet, this study is observational lack of robust statistical adjustment for potential confounders. Conversely, another registry[42] reported that while the use of bivalirudin resulted in similar rates of MACE and bleeding compared to heparin without GPIs, it was associated with a higher incidence

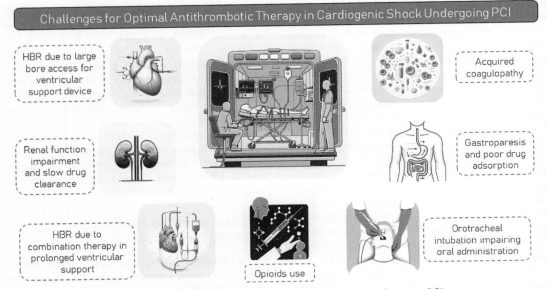

Fig. 2. Challenges in optimal antithrombotic therapy in cardiogenic shock undergoing PCI

of stent thrombosis (11.7% vs 1.7%, respectively; $P=.043$).

Periprocedural Parenteral Antiplatelet Therapy

Given the challenges with oral administration in this setting, which often includes patients with orotracheal intubation and poor gastrointestinal absorption, parenteral antiplatelet therapies are often used in CS. A multicenter study[43] matched CS patients receiving cangrelor to those from the IABP-SHOCK II trial not receiving cangrelor. The results showed similar 30-day and 12-month mortality rates (29.5% vs 34.1% and 36.4% and 47.1%, respectively) and no significant difference in moderate and severe bleeding events. However, cangrelor-treated patients experienced significantly better thrombosis in myocardial infarction (TIMI) flow improvement during PCI (92.9% vs 81.2%, $P=.02$ of ≥ 1 TIMI flow grade improvement). Additionally, a recent study[44] compared the use of cangrelor in high-risk AMI and CS patients in real-world settings to patients randomized in the CULPRIT-SHOCK trial cohort receiving only oral P2Y$_{12}$ inhibitors. In this cohort of 118 patients, those treated with cangrelor showed comparable TIMI 3 patency rates and fewer ischemic events within the first 48 hours post-PCI, suggesting cangrelor's potential benefits in reducing stent thrombosis and reinfarction rates. However, this evidence should be interpreted with caution given the observational design, high risk of incomplete matching, and limited sample size.

Oral P2Y12 Inhibitor Type

Patients with CS face multiple challenges with antiplatelet therapy. The effectiveness of orally administered drugs is often delayed due to factors like gastroparesis, impaired intestinal absorption, slower drug metabolism due to compromised hemodynamics, and the administration of opioids. Additionally, oral administration can be problematic in this population. There is also a significant lack of evidence on antithrombotic therapy for MI complicated by CS.

A sub-analysis[45] of the IABP-SHOCK II (Intra-aortic Balloon Pump in Cardiogenic Shock II) and CULPRIT-SHOCK (Culprit Lesion Only PCI vs Multivessel PCI in Cardiogenic Shock) trials compared clinical outcomes in 856 patients with acute MI complicated by CS treated with clopidogrel or potent P2Y$_{12}$ inhibitors. No significant differences in 1-year mortality between prasugrel or ticagrelor versus clopidogrel were observed after adjustment, while in-hospital bleeding events was significantly less frequent with ticagrelor compared to clopidogrel (adjHR: 0.37, 95% CI 0.20–0.69, $P=.002$).

Similar results were observed in a meta-analysis by Patolla and colleagues.[46] This study that included 1100 patients from 8 studies on AMI complicated by cardiac arrest or CS, found that ticagrelor and prasugrel were associated with lower early (OR 0.60; 95% CI 0.45–0.81; $P = .001$) and 1-year mortality (OR 0.51; 95% CI 0.36–0.71; $P<.001$) compared to clopidogrel, with no significant differences in major bleeding or stent thrombosis. While these results provide some information regarding the choice of P2Y$_{12}$ inhibitor type in CS, this evidence are greatly limited by the lack of randomized evidence in this space and the high probability of residual confounders in observational studies, which may be supported by the higher rates of bleeding in clopidogrel rather than ticagrelor treated patients.

SUMMARY

Optimal antithrombotic therapy during and after complex interventions remains a challenge in cardiovascular medicine and should be based on a careful evaluation of anticoagulation, oral, and occasionally parenteral antiplatelet therapy. UFH is commonly used as the mainstay of anticoagulation in most complex PCI patients and those presenting with CS. Bivalirudin may represent a safer alternative, though evidence in this area is limited. Parenteral antiplatelet therapy with cangrelor, due to its pharmacodynamic properties, provides a potential solution for more consistent periprocedural antiplatelet therapy during complex PCI or in patients with CS, particularly when critical conditions and orotracheal intubation limit the efficacy of oral agents. Oral antiplatelet therapy remains the cornerstone of long-term secondary prevention in patients treated with complex PCI or CS. Potent P2Y$_{12}$ inhibitors are the agents of choice in patients presenting with ACS and may represent an alternative for selected patients with CCS, despite limited evidence. Longer DAPT courses have traditionally been considered the treatment of choice after complex PCI in patients without HBR. However, emerging strategies utilizing potent P2Y$_{12}$ inhibitors after short courses of DAPT appear promising to maintain efficacy while being safer.

CLINICS CARE POINTS

Anticoagulation Strategy:

- *Unfractionated Heparin (UFH)* is the mainstay anticoagulant for most complex PCI and cardiogenic shock cases due to its cost-effectiveness and reversibility.
- *Bivalirudin* is a viable alternative to UFH, offering a more predictable anticoagulant effect and reduced bleeding risk.
- Ensure appropriate monitoring of anticoagulation levels to avoid bleeding complications, especially during prolonged procedures.

Antiplatelet Therapy:

- *Cangrelor* is a parenteral P2Y12 inhibitor that provides rapid and consistent antiplatelet effects, suitable for patients where oral agents may not be absorbed effectively, such as those with cardiogenic shock.
- *Potent Oral P2Y12 Inhibitors* (eg, prasugrel, ticagrelor) are recommended for long-term secondary prevention, particularly after complex PCI in acute coronary syndrome (ACS) cases.
- Consider switching from cangrelor to ticagrelor post-PCI to ensure continuity in platelet inhibition.

Dual Antiplatelet Therapy (DAPT):

- Long-term DAPT (aspirin + P2Y12 inhibitor) is traditionally recommended after complex PCI for patients without high bleeding risk to reduce ischemic events.
- Short-term DAPT followed by monotherapy with a potent P2Y12 inhibitor can reduce bleeding risk while maintaining efficacy.

Risk Stratification:

- Use risk scores to evaluate patients' ischemic and bleeding risks, guiding the duration and intensity of antithrombotic therapy.

ACKNOWLEDGMENT

Professor Costa is funded by the European Union (ERC, ORACLE, ERC-2023-STG101117469). Views and opinions expressed are, however, those of the author(s) only and do not necessarily reflect those of the European Union or the European Research Council. Neither the European Union nor the granting authority can be held responsible for them.

REFERENCES

1. Costa F, Windecker S, Valgimigli M. Dual Antiplatelet Therapy Duration: Reconciling the Inconsistencies. Drugs 2017;77(16):1733–54. https://doi.org/10.1007/s40265-017-0806-1.
2. Valgimigli M, Ariotti S, Costa F. Duration of dual antiplatelet therapy after drug-eluting stent implantation: will we ever reach a consensus? Eur Heart J 2015;36(20):1219–22. https://doi.org/10.1093/eurheartj/ehv053.
3. Zimarino M, Angiolillo DJ, Dangas G, et al. Antithrombotic therapy after percutaneous coronary intervention of bifurcation lesions. EuroIntervention 2021;17(1):59–66. https://doi.org/10.4244/EIJ-D-20-00885.
4. Crimi G, Leonardi S, Costa F, et al. Role of stent type and of duration of dual antiplatelet therapy in patients with chronic kidney disease undergoing

percutaneous coronary interventions. Is bare metal stent implantation still a justifiable choice? A post-hoc analysis of the all comer PRODIGY trial. Int J Cardiol 2016;212:110–7. https://doi.org/10.1016/j.ijcard.2016.03.033.

5. Costa F, Adamo M, Ariotti S, et al. Left main or proximal left anterior descending coronary artery disease location identifies high-risk patients deriving potentially greater benefit from prolonged dual antiplatelet therapy duration. EuroIntervention 2016;11(11):e1222–30. https://doi.org/10.4244/EIJY15M08_04.

6. Serruys PW, Onuma Y, Garg S, et al. Assessment of the SYNTAX score in the Syntax study. EuroIntervention 2009;5(1):50–6.

7. Giustino G, Chieffo A, Palmerini T, et al. Efficacy and safety of dual antiplatelet therapy after complex PCI. J Am Coll Cardiol 2016;68(18):1851–64.

8. Protty M, Sharp ASP, Gallagher S, et al. Defining percutaneous coronary intervention complexity and risk: An analysis of the United Kingdom BCIS database 2006-2016 [published correction appears in JACC Cardiovasc Interv. 2022 Aug 22;15(16):1694-1695]. JACC Cardiovasc Interv 2022;15(1):39–49.

9. Giustino G, Costa F. Characterization of the Individual Patient Risk After Percutaneous Coronary Intervention: At the Crossroads of Bleeding and Thrombosis. JACC Cardiovasc Interv 2019;12(9):831–4. https://doi.org/10.1016/j.jcin.2019.01.212.

10. Valgimigli M, Frigoli E, Leonardi S, et al. Bivalirudin or unfractionated heparin in acute coronary syndromes. N Engl J Med 2015;373(11):997–1009.

11. Mehran R, Lansky AJ, Witzenbichler B, et al. Bivalirudin in patients undergoing primary angioplasty for acute myocardial infarction (HORIZONS-AMI): 1-year results of a randomised controlled trial. Lancet 2009;374(9698):1149–59.

12. Li Y, Liang Z, Qin L, et al. Bivalirudin plus a high-dose infusion versus heparin monotherapy in patients with ST-segment elevation myocardial infarction undergoing primary percutaneous coronary intervention: A randomised trial. Lancet 2022;400(10366):1847–57.

13. Bikdeli B, Erlinge D, Valgimigli M, et al. Bivalirudin versus heparin during PCI in NSTEMI: Individual patient data meta-analysis of large randomized trials. Circulation 2023;148(16):1207–19.

14. Cortese B, Micheli A, Picchi A, et al. Safety and efficacy of a prolonged bivalirudin infusion after urgent and complex percutaneous coronary interventions: A descriptive study. Coron Artery Dis 2009;20(5):348–53.

15. Gargiulo G, Esposito G, Avvedimento M, et al. Cangrelor, tirofiban, and chewed or standard prasugrel regimens in patients with ST-segment-elevation myocardial infarction: Primary results of the FABOLUS-FASTER trial [published correction appears in Circulation. 2020 Aug 4;142(5):e71]. Circulation 2020;142(5):441–54.

16. Byrne RA, Rossello X, Coughlan JJ, et al. 2023 ESC guidelines for the management of acute coronary syndromes [published correction appears in Eur Heart J. 2024 Apr 1;45(13):1145]. Eur Heart J 2023;44(38):3720–826.

17. Lawton JS, Tamis-Holland JE, Bangalore S, et al. 2021 ACC/AHA/SCAI guideline for coronary artery revascularization: Executive summary: A report of the American College of Cardiology/American Heart Association joint committee on clinical practice guidelines [published correction appears in Circulation. 2022 Mar 15;145(11):e771]. Circulation 2022;145(3):e4–17.

18. Steg PG, Bhatt DL, Hamm CW, et al. Effect of cangrelor on periprocedural outcomes in percutaneous coronary interventions: A pooled analysis of patient-level data. Lancet 2013;382(9909):1981–92.

19. Stone GW, Généreux P, Harrington RA, et al. Impact of lesion complexity on periprocedural adverse events and the benefit of potent intravenous platelet adenosine diphosphate receptor inhibition after percutaneous coronary intervention: Core laboratory analysis from 10,854 patients from the CHAMPION PHOENIX trial. Eur Heart J 2018;39(41):4112–21.

20. Gargiulo G, Marenna A, Sperandeo L, et al. Pharmacodynamic effects of cangrelor in elective complex PCI: Insights from the POMPEII Registry. EuroIntervention 2023;18(12):1266–8.

21. Valgimigli M, Bueno H, Byrne RA, et al. 2017 ESC focused update on dual antiplatelet therapy in coronary artery disease developed in collaboration with EACTS: The Task Force for dual antiplatelet therapy in coronary artery disease of the European Society of Cardiology (ESC) and of the European Association for Cardio-Thoracic Surgery (EACTS). Eur Heart J 2018;39(3):213–60. https://doi.org/10.1093/eurheartj/ehx419.

22. Collet JP, Roffi M, Byrne RA, et al. Case-based implementation of the 2017 ESC Focused Update on Dual Antiplatelet Therapy in Coronary Artery Disease. Eur Heart J 2018;39(3):e1–33. https://doi.org/10.1093/eurheartj/ehx503.

23. Neumann FJ, Sousa-Uva M, Ahlsson A, et al. 2018 ESC/EACTS guidelines on myocardial revascularization. Eur Heart J 2019;40(2):87–165.

24. Li Y, Li J, Qiu M, et al. Ticagrelor versus clopidogrel in patients with acute coronary syndrome undergoing complex percutaneous coronary intervention. Catheter Cardiovasc Interv 2022;99(S1):1395–402.

25. Lattuca B, Mazeau C, Cayla G, et al. Ticagrelor vs clopidogrel for complex percutaneous coronary intervention in chronic coronary syndrome. JACC Cardiovasc Interv 2024;17(3):359–70.

26. Coughlan JJ, Aytekin A, Ndrepepa G, et al. Twelve-month clinical outcomes in patients with acute coronary syndrome undergoing complex percutaneous coronary intervention: insights from the ISAR-REACT 5 trial. Eur Heart J Acute Cardiovasc Care 2021;10(10):1117–24. https://doi.org/10.1093/ehjacc/zuab077.

27. Costa F, Van Klaveren D, Feres F, et al. Dual antiplatelet therapy duration based on ischemic and bleeding risks after coronary stenting. J Am Coll Cardiol 2019;73(7):741–54.

28. Munafò AR, Montalto C, Franzino M, et al. External validity of the PRECISE-DAPT score in patients undergoing PCI: a systematic review and meta-analysis. Eur Heart J Cardiovasc Pharmacother 2023;9(8):709–21. https://doi.org/10.1093/ehjcvp/pvad063.

29. Costa F, van Klaveren D, Colombo A, et al. A 4-item PRECISE-DAPT score for dual antiplatelet therapy duration decision-making. Am Heart J 2020;223:44–7. https://doi.org/10.1016/j.ahj.2020.01.014.

30. Yeh RW, Kereiakes DJ, Steg PG, et al. Lesion complexity and outcomes of extended dual antiplatelet therapy after percutaneous coronary intervention. J Am Coll Cardiol 2017;70(18):2213–23.

31. Valgimigli M, Gragnano F, Branca M, et al. P2Y12 inhibitor monotherapy or dual antiplatelet therapy after coronary revascularisation: Individual patient level meta-analysis of randomised controlled trials [published correction appears in BMJ. 2022 Jan 27;376:o239]. BMJ 2021;373:n1332. Published 2021 Jun 16.

32. Dangas G, Baber U, Sharma S, et al. Ticagrelor with or without aspirin after complex PCI. J Am Coll Cardiol 2020;75(19):2414–24.

33. Eid MM, Mostafa MR, Alabdouh A, et al. Short duration of dual antiplatelet therapy following complex percutaneous coronary intervention: A systematic review and meta-analysis. Cardiovasc Revasc Med 2024;61:8–15.

34. Oliva A, Castiello DS, Franzone A, et al. P2Y12 inhibitors monotherapy in patients undergoing complex vs non-complex percutaneous coronary intervention: A meta-analysis of randomized trials. Am Heart J 2023;255:71–81.

35. Nicolas J, Dangas G, Chiarito M, et al. Efficacy and safety of P2Y12 inhibitor monotherapy after complex PCI: A collaborative systematic review and meta-analysis. Eur Heart J Cardiovasc Pharmacother 2023;9(3):240–50.

36. Sotomi Y, Matsuoka Y, Hikoso S, et al. P2Y12 inhibitor monotherapy after complex percutaneous coronary intervention: A systematic review and meta-analysis of randomized clinical trials. Sci Rep 2023;13(1):12608.

37. Gragnano F, Mehran R, Branca M, et al. P2Y12 inhibitor monotherapy or dual antiplatelet therapy after complex percutaneous coronary interventions. J Am Coll Cardiol 2023;81(6):537–52.

38. Valgimigli M, Smits PC, Frigoli E, et al. Duration of antiplatelet therapy after complex percutaneous coronary intervention in patients at high bleeding risk: A MASTER DAPT trial sub-analysis. Eur Heart J 2022;43(33):3100–14.

39. Costa F, Montalto C, Branca M, et al. Dual antiplatelet therapy duration after percutaneous coronary intervention in high bleeding risk: A meta-analysis of randomized trials. Eur Heart J 2023;44(11):954–68.

40. Yamamoto K, Natsuaki M, Watanabe H, et al. An aspirin-free strategy for immediate treatment following complex percutaneous coronary intervention. JACC Cardiovasc Interv 2024;17(9):1119–30.

41. Bonello L, De Labriolle A, Roy P, et al. Bivalirudin with provisional glycoprotein IIb/IIIa inhibitors in patients undergoing primary angioplasty in the setting of cardiogenic shock. Am J Cardiol 2008;102(3):287–91.

42. Pourdjabbar A, Hibbert B, Maze R, et al. Bivalirudin for primary percutaneous coronary interventions in patients with cardiogenic shock: Outcome assessment in the CAPITAL STEMI registry. Can J Cardiol 2014;30(10):S68.

43. Droppa M, Vaduganathan M, Venkateswaran RV, et al. Cangrelor in cardiogenic shock and after cardiopulmonary resuscitation: A global, multicenter, matched pair analysis with oral P2Y12 inhibition from the IABP-SHOCK II trial. Resuscitation 2019;137:205–12.

44. Zeymer U, Lober C, Richter S, et al. Cangrelor in patients with percutaneous coronary intervention for acute myocardial infarction after cardiac arrest and/or with cardiogenic shock. Eur Heart J Acute Cardiovasc Care 2023;12(7):462–3.

45. Orban M, Kleeberger J, Ouarrak T, et al. Clopidogrel vs. prasugrel vs. ticagrelor in patients with acute myocardial infarction complicated by cardiogenic shock: A pooled IABP-SHOCK II and CULPRIT-SHOCK trial sub-analysis. Clin Res Cardiol 2021;110(9):1493–503.

46. Patlolla SH, Kandlakunta H, Kuchkuntla AR, et al. Newer P2Y12 inhibitors vs clopidogrel in acute myocardial infarction with cardiac arrest or cardiogenic shock: A systematic review and meta-analysis. Mayo Clin Proc 2022;97(6):1074–85.

Antiplatelet Therapy in Patients Requiring Oral Anticoagulation and Undergoing Percutaneous Coronary Intervention

Lina Manzi, MD[a], Domenico Florimonte, MD[a],
Imma Forzano, MD[a], Federica Buongiorno, MD[a],
Luca Sperandeo, MD[a],
Domenico Simone Castiello, MD[a],
Roberta Paolillo, PhD[a], Giuseppe Giugliano, MD, PhD[a],
Daniele Giacoppo, MD, PhD[b],
Alessandro Sciahbasi, MD, PhD[c], Plinio Cirillo, MD, PhD[a],
Giovanni Esposito, MD, PhD[a],
Giuseppe Gargiulo, MD, PhD[a],*

KEYWORDS

- Atrial fibrillation • Percutaneous coronary intervention • Antiplatelet • Oral anticoagulant
- Dual antithrombotic therapy • Triple antithrombotic therapy • Bleeding • Thrombosis

---

KEY POINTS

- Dual antiplatelet therapy with aspirin and a P2Y$_{12}$ inhibitor is essential in all patients undergoing percutaneous coronary intervention (PCI) to prevent peri-procedural thrombotic complications.
- In patients with atrial fibrillation (AF), an oral anticoagulant gives protection against ischemic stroke or systemic embolism.
- AF-PCI patients are at high bleeding risk and decision-making regarding the optimal antithrombotic therapy is challenging.
- Dual antithrombotic therapy (DAT) has shown to reduce bleeding events but at the cost of higher risk of stent thrombosis.
- Further studies are needed to clarify the optimal duration of triple antithrombotic therapy (TAT) or DAT and the role of more potent antiplatelet drugs in AF-PCI patients.

INTRODUCTION

Dual antiplatelet therapy (DAPT) with aspirin and a P2Y$_{12}$ inhibitor is essential in all patients undergoing percutaneous coronary intervention (PCI) for acute coronary syndrome (ACS) or chronic coronary syndrome (CCS) to prevent peri and post-procedural thrombotic complications,

---

Funding: This study was internally supported by University of Naples Federico II. No direct or indirect external funding was received.

[a] Department of Advanced Biomedical Sciences, Federico II University of Naples, Italy; [b] Department of General Surgery and Medical-Surgical Specialties, University of Catania, Catania, Italy; [c] Interventional Cardiology, Sandro Pertini Hospital, Rome, Italy

* Corresponding author. Division of Cardiology, Department of Advanced Biomedical Sciences, Federico II University of Naples, Via S. Pansini 5, Naples 80131, Italy.

E-mail address: giuseppe.gargiulo1@unina.it

Intervent Cardiol Clin 13 (2024) 527–541
https://doi.org/10.1016/j.iccl.2024.07.001
2211-7458/24/© 2024 Elsevier Inc. All rights reserved, including those for text and data mining, AI training, and similar technologies.

including stents thrombosis (ST).[1–6] In the last decade, improvements in procedural management and materials (ie, new generation drug-eluting stents [DES], imaging use, etc.) reduced peri-procedural thrombotic complications,[7–11] and several data have demonstrated that bleeding complications are frequent and impact on mortality.[12,13] Therefore, huge attention has been focused on exploring less intensive antithrombotic strategies[13–16] and on patients at high bleeding risk (HBR).[17–21] Atrial fibrillation (AF) is the most common cardiac arrhythmia in adults worldwide.[22] Currently, estimated prevalence in adults is between 2% and 4%,[22] and a 2.3-fold increase is expected,[23–25] due to the aging of the general population and the greater diagnostic capabilities.[25] Approximately 10% to 15% of AF patients undergo PCI for ACS or CCS.[26] Moreover, the incidence of AF in ACS ranges from 2% to 23%[27] with an increased risk of new onset AF of 60% to 77% in this clinical setting.[28] Antithrombotic management of AF patients undergoing PCI is challenging due to the high risk of both ischemic and bleeding complications. Indeed, when considering the use and duration of combined antithrombotic therapies, the concomitant risks of ischemic stroke, coronary ischemic events as myocardial infarction (MI) or ST, and antithrombotic treatment-related bleeding must be carefully balanced. The aim of this review is to summarize the evidence and documents on antithrombotic management of patients with non-valvular AF undergoing PCI.

PATHOPHYSIOLOGICAL SUBSTRATE

DAPT is fundamental in all patients undergoing PCI for ACS or CCS to prevent peri and post-procedural thrombotic complications, including ST.[1–5] On the other hand, long-term use of oral anticoagulants (OACs) gives protection against ischemic stroke or systemic embolism in patients with AF,[29] with direct oral anticoagulants (DOACs) preferred over vitamin K antagonists (VKAs) in non-valvular AF patients without any specific contraindication.[30–33] Therefore, patients with AF undergoing PCI need a certain period of triple antithrombotic therapy (TAT), the combination of DAPT and OAC, to mitigate coronary ischemic risks and to reduce stroke and systemic embolism, albeit TAT has been associated with up to a 3-fold increase in bleeding risk.[3,4,34] The importance of TAT in this population lies in the differential mechanism of thrombosis in the venous and arterial systems. In AF, atrial thrombi are made of fibrin and are promoted by stasis, particularly in the left atrium

appendage, without any contribution from platelet activation. Conversely, coronary thrombosis is usually initiated by plaque formation in the arterial wall[35] and after PCI, platelet activation plays a central role in thrombus formation because of the high shear stress within the stent.[36] Hence, antithrombotic agents must act on different mechanisms to offer protection against both arterial and venous events. Several trials showed that aspirin is less effective than VKAs in preventing ischemic stroke and systemic embolism in AF patients.[37,38] In the ACTIVE-W trial, comparing OAC with DAPT in AF patients, a significant reduction in ischemic events was demonstrated with OAC after 1-year.[39] On the contrary, numerous trials demonstrated the importance of DAPT over OACs in patients with ACS or CCS undergoing PCI.[5,40–42] The optimal duration of TAT after ACS or CCS is based on the balance between ischemic and bleeding risk but this still remains controversial. Ischemic risk is very high immediately after ACS and decreases slowly, while bleeding risk remains similar and can increase with age and advancement of comorbidities. Based on the assumption that the 3 risks (ie, cardioembolic, coronary, and hemorrhagic) have a different time course, (coronary risk, related to recurrent ACS and ST, is high in the first month, and at this time by far exceeding the risk of stroke; similarly the bleeding risk is high immediately after the PCI due to TAT administration), some authors questioned the mandatory need of OAC in these patients and hypothesized that in the modern era OAC might be skipped in the first month.[43] This approach is now under investigation in new trials as reported later.

EVIDENCE FROM RANDOMIZED TRIALS
Randomized Trials in the Vitamin K Antagonists Era

Some randomized trials compared different antithrombotic strategies, essentially comparing TAT versus dual antithrombotic therapy (DAT) in patients with AF undergoing PCI. Early studies included only VKAs as OAC, comparing single versus DAPT in addition to VKAs. The What is the Optimal antiplatElet and Anticoagulant Therapy in Patients With Oral Anticoagulation and Coronary StenTing (WOEST) trial, with an open-label design, randomized 573 patients on OAC undergoing PCI to receive clopidogrel alone (DAT group) or clopidogrel plus aspirin (TAT group). Bleeding events within 1-year were 19.4% in DAT and 44.4% in TAT (hazard ratio [HR]: 0.36; 95% CI: 0.26–0.50; P<.0001) without an apparent increase, and actually with a numerical decrease, of thrombotic events, such as MI or ST[44]. Interestingly, this finding was consistent in the ACS subgroup.[44] This trial was pivotal in exploring the interruption of aspirin instead of clopidogrel with the hypothesis that clopidogrel was essential to prevent ST while aspirin withdrawal would reduce the bleeding risk. This approach has guided following trials that have never explored clopidogrel interruption with aspirin prolongation. However, its findings should be interpreted in light of some considerations: (a) 69% of patients were AF-PCI while 31% had different indications to OAC such as mechanical valves, apical aneurysm, and others; (b) 67% of patients received TAT for 1-year; (c) DAT was also associated with a nominally significant decrease of overall mortality without a clear explanation that has been debated for years. The Intracoronary Stenting and Antithrombotic Regimen-Testing of a 6-Week vs a 6-Month Clopidogrel Treatment Regimen in Patients With Concomitant Aspirin and Oral Anticoagulant Therapy Following Drug-Eluting Stenting (ISAR-TRIPLE) compared 2 TAT regimens to test whether shortening the duration of clopidogrel from 6 months to 6 weeks after PCI with a DES was associated with a superior net clinical outcome of death, MI, definite ST, stroke, or major bleeding at 9 months in patients receiving concomitant aspirin and OAC. Randomizing 614 patients, they found no significant differences for the primary net clinical outcome, for the secondary combined ischemic endpoint of cardiac death, MI, ST, and ischemic stroke or for the secondary bleeding endpoint of thrombolysis in myocardial infarction (TIMI) major bleeding between the 2 strategies.[45]

Randomized Trials in the Direct Oral Anticoagulants Era

With the advent of trials demonstrating non-inferiority and/or superiority of DOACs versus VKAs,[30–33] 4 trials evaluated DAT with DOACs versus TAT with VKAs. The Open-Label, Randomized, Controlled, Multicenter Study Exploring Two Treatment Strategies of Rivaroxaban and a Dose-Adjusted Oral Vitamin K Antagonist Treatment Strategy in Subjects with Atrial Fibrillation who Undergo Percutaneous Coronary Intervention (PIONEER-AF PCI) trial randomized 2124 AF patients undergoing PCI to receive, in a 1:1:1 ratio, 15 mg rivaroxaban once daily plus a $P2Y_{12}$ inhibitor for 12 months (group 1), 2.5 mg rivaroxaban twice daily plus DAPT for 1, 6, or 12 months (group 2), or VKAs plus DAPT for 1, 6, or 12 months (group 3). Two rivaroxaban-based groups were associated with lower rates of clinically significant bleeding with similar efficacy in terms of death from cardiovascular causes, MI, or stroke. Remarkably, the risk of stroke and ST was numerically higher with both rivaroxaban-based groups, albeit without statistical significance.[46] Notably, none of the 2 tested doses was previously examined and approved for stroke prevention in AF. The Randomized Evaluation of Dual Antithrombotic Therapy with Dabigatran vs Triple Therapy with Warfarin in Patients with Nonvalvular Atrial Fibrillation Undergoing Percutaneous Coronary Intervention (RE-DUAL PCI) trial randomized 2,725 AF patients undergoing PCI to receive TAT with VKAs plus a $P2Y_{12}$ inhibitor (clopidogrel or ticagrelor) and aspirin for 1 to 3 months or DAT with dabigatran (110 mg or 150 mg twice daily) plus a $P2Y_{12}$ inhibitor (clopidogrel or ticagrelor). The incidence of the primary endpoint of major or clinically relevant non-major bleeding (CRNMB) events was 15.4% in the 110-mg DAT group versus 26.9% in TAT group (HR: 0.52; 95% CI: 0.42–0.63; $P<.001$ for non-inferiority; $P<.001$ for superiority) and 20.2% in the 150-mg DAT group versus 25.7% in TAT group (HR: 0.72; 95% CI: 0.58–0.88; $P<.001$ for non-inferiority) at 14 months. Furthermore, both dabigatran groups were non-inferior to TAT for the composite of death, MI, stroke, systemic embolism, or unplanned revascularization.[47] However, there was a numerically higher risk of ST in the 110 mg group compared with TAT. Overall findings were consistent according to clinical presentation.[48] The Edoxaban Treatment vs Vitamin K Antagonist in Patients With Atrial Fibrillation Undergoing Percutaneous Coronary Intervention (ENTRUST-AF PCI) trial randomized 1,506 patients to receive edoxaban 60 mg once daily plus a P2Y12 inhibitor for 12 months or TAT with a VKA, a P2Y12 inhibitor, and aspirin (for 1–12 months). It demonstrated the non-inferiority but not the superiority of DAT with edoxaban compared with VKA-TAT for the 1-year major or CRNMB (HR: 0.83; 95% CI: 0.65–1.05; $P = .001$ for non-inferiority and $P = .115$ for superiority), without any difference in the composite efficacy outcome. However, a post-hoc analysis with a landmark at 14 days for the primary bleeding outcome provided clear signal of heterogeneity with respect to the treatment effect ($p_{interaction}<0.0001$). Specifically, non-significantly lower bleeding rates for the VKA-TAT versus edoxaban-DAT were initially observed (probably due to subtherapeutic INR) followed by a superiority of edoxaban-DAT with a significant reduction in the rate of the primary bleeding outcome (HR for edoxaban 0.68, 95% CI 0.53–0.88).[49]

The An Open-label, 2-by-2 Factorial, Randomized Controlled, Clinical Trial to Evaluate the Safety of Apixaban vs Vitamin K Antagonist and

Aspirin vs Placebo in Patients with Atrial Fibrillation and Acute Coronary Syndrome and/or Percutaneous Coronary Intervention (AUGUSTUS) trial, differed from the others since it was the only one with a 2-by-2 factorial design. It randomized 4,614 AF patients with ACS or CCS undergoing PCI or medically managed to receive either apixaban 5 mg twice daily or a VKA (open label) and to receive either aspirin or placebo (blinded) for 6 months, resulting in 4 groups. There was no significant interaction between the 2 randomization factors on the primary or secondary endpoints. In the apixaban group, the incidence of major or CRNMB and the composite of death or hospitalization were lower, without any difference in the composite ischemic endpoint compared with VKA. Regarding antiplatelet therapy, major and CRNMB events were greater in patients receiving aspirin compared with placebo (16.1% vs 9.0%). Furthermore, the incidence of death or hospitalization and ischemic events were similar between aspirin versus placebo, but importantly this trial showed a greater signal of increased ST by aspirin discontinuation.[50] Notably, a sub-analysis demonstrated that aspirin immediately and for up to 30 days resulted in an equal tradeoff between an increase in severe bleeding and a reduction in severe ischemic events, while after 30 days, aspirin continued to increase bleeding without significantly reducing ischemic events.[51]

EVIDENCE FROM MAJOR NATIONAL AND INTERNATIONAL REGISTRIES

Observational studies provide real-world data and are useful to support randomized control trials (RCTs) results and contribute to evidence-based medicine. In the prospective multicenter dual vs triple antithrombotic therapy after percutaneous coronary intervention (WOEST-2) study, 1075 patients on OACs undergoing PCI were prospectively analyzed to compare DAT (P2Y$_{12}$ inhibitor and OAC) versus TAT (aspirin, P2Y$_{12}$ inhibitor, and OAC) on thrombotic and bleeding outcomes at 1-year. DOACs were used in 53.1% and VKAs in 46.9% of patients. The P2Y$_{12}$ inhibitor was clopidogrel in 94%. At discharge, 60.9% received DAT, and 39.1% TAT. Interestingly, median aspirin withdrawal in TAT group was after 30 days (interquartile range: 29–57 days). From 2014 through 2021, a significant temporal trend toward increased DAT prescription and decreased TAT prescription was found. After discharge, DAT had a significant decrease of 6.6% in clinically relevant bleeding (bleeding academic research consortium [BARC] type 2, 3) compared with TAT (16.8% vs 23.6%; P = .003) at 1-year, without

significant differences in BARC 3 or 5 or hemorrhagic stroke. According to major adverse cardiac and cerebrovascular events (MACCE), defined as a composite of all-cause mortality, MI, ST, ischemic stroke, and transient ischemic attack, DAT was associated with a higher rate of MACCE (12.4% vs 9.6%; P = .17) in MI (5.0% vs 4.3%), ST (1.7% vs 1.0%), and all-cause death (6.2% vs 5.8%) but without statistical significance. These results were also consistent in patients with complex PCI or HBR.[52] The AVIATOR-2 registry was an international multicenter prospective observational study of 514 patients with non-valvular AF undergoing PCI finding that: (a) TAT was the most common discharge therapy (66.5%) after AF-PCI, followed by DAPT in 20.7% and DAT in 12.8%; (b) de-escalation of TAT to DAT strategy overtime was frequent with aspirin withdrawal in over 50% of patients by 6 months; (c) clinicians subjective perceptions of both ischemic and bleeding risks with empiric risk scores were in poor agreement; physicians-rated bleeding-related safety influenced more therapeutic strategy choice, whilst patients were more afraid of stroke than bleeding (50.6% vs 14.8%); (d) MACCE occurred in 15.3% of patients, and BARC 2, 3, or 5 in 13.8% of patients without significant differences between different antithrombotic strategies.[53]

The Management of Antithrombotic TherApy in Patients with Chronic or DevelOping AtRial Fibrillation During Hospitalization for PCI (MATADOR-PCI) was a prospective, observational, nationwide registry of consecutive patients with a confirmed diagnosis of ACS and concomitant AF, either pre-existent or new-onset, treated with coronary stenting conducted in Italy during a 1-year period.[54] It included 598 patients (46% STEMI) and showed that TAT was still largely prescribed, particularly in association with low dosages of DOACs and clopidogrel and for <6 months after hospital discharge.

The Italian, multicenter, prospective observational PERcutaneous coronary interventions in Patients Treated with Oral Anticoagulant Therapy (PERSEO) registry evaluated the safety and efficacy of DOAC versus VKA and DAT versus TAT in patients with an indication for OACs and undergoing PCI.[55] From 2018 to 2022, 1234 consecutive patients were included and their main indications for OAC were AF (86%), followed by ventricular thrombosis (5%) and venous thrombosis (2.3%). Of the 1228 patients discharged alive, 222 (18%) were on VKA and 1006 (82%) on DOAC (p<0.01). DAT was prescribed in 197 patients whereas TAT in 1028. At 1-year follow-up, net adverse clinical events (NACE) rate was significantly higher with VKA compared to DOAC (23% vs 16%, p=0.013) and confirmed after propensity score adjustment. TAT and DAT did not differ in terms of NACE rate (17% vs 19%, p=0.864) even though, compared with TAT, DAT was associated with lower rates of major bleeding (2% vs 5%, p= 0.014), confirmed after propensity score adjustment. The study concluded that DOAC, compared to VKA, was associated with a significantly lower occurrence of NACE and DAT reduced bleedings compared to TAT.[56]

EVIDENCE FROM META-ANALYSES

Individual DOAC-RCTs demonstrated that DAT is safer than TAT; however, some considerations must be done. First, all RCTs were designed to demonstrate the superiority of DAT versus TAT in terms of bleeding reduction, but none of them was powered to assess major ischemic events or rare bleeding events such as intracranial bleeding. Second, the main comparison was DOAC-DAT versus VKA-TAT except for AUGUSTUS trial. Third, the use of aspirin was mandatory in the peri-PCI period, so all patients received a variable period of TAT (in PIONEER AF-PCI, REDUAL-PCI, and ENTRUST-AF-PCI aspirin was used on average for 1 to 2 days after PCI, in AUGUSTUS for 6 days). Fourth, the specific duration of TAT and the type of $P2Y_{12}$ inhibitor remain debated. Finally, the results on patients with high ischemic risk or with ACS at presentation are derived from subgroup analyses. To address some of these points, several meta-analyses have been performed. The first meta-analysis including the 4 DOAC-RCTs was accompanying the ENTRUST-AF PCI trial publication and assessed the specific comparison of DOAC-DAT (n = 4342) versus VKA-TAT (n = 3585) showing that DOAC-DAT was associated with lower risks of major or CRNM bleeding events and similar risks of major adverse cardiovascular events (MACE), all-cause death, stroke, with a numerical increase of MI and ST[49]. In a subsequent more detailed meta-analysis, the authors included all 10,234 patients from the 4 RCTs (DAT = 5496 vs TAT = 4738) and DAT strategy significantly reduced the primary safety endpoint (international society of thrombosis and hemostasis [ISTH] major or CRNMB) compared with TAT (13.4% vs 20.8%; RR: 0.66, 95% CI: 0.56–0.78; P<.0001; I^2 = 69%) and this benefit was driven by reduction of both major and CRNMB. However, DAT was associated with a significantly higher risk of ST (1.0% vs 0.6%; RR: 1.59, 95% CI: 1.01–2.50; P = .04;

I^2 = 0%) and a borderline higher risk of MI (3.6% vs 3.0%; RR: 1.22, 95% CI: 0.99–1.52; P = .07; I^2 = 0%). Overall, findings were consistent when the analysis was restricted to DOAC-based DAT versus VKA-based TAT, but a significant reduction of intracranial hemorrhage was reported for the first time (RR 0.33, 95% CI 0.17–0.65; P = .001; I^2 = 0%).[57] Of course, these findings should be interpreted in light of the limitations of study-level meta-analyses. A subsequent meta-analysis by the 4 NOAC-RCT investigators specifically explored the safety and efficacy of DAT versus TAT according to clinical presentation (patients with or without ACS).[58] A total of 10,193 patients were analyzed, of whom 5675 presenting with ACS (DAT = 3063 vs TAT = 2612) and 4518 with CCS (DAT = 2421 vs TAT = 2097). All bleeding events were consistently reduced irrespective of clinical presentation, including intracranial hemorrhage. In both subgroups, there was no difference between DAT and TAT for all-cause death, MACE, or stroke. MI and ST were numerically higher with DAT versus TAT consistently in ACS and CCS (P-int = 0.60 and 0.86, respectively) confirming the findings observed in the overall population.[58] These data are of particular relevance because clinical presentation has been often recommended as an important driver for the decision-making on type and duration of DAPT, while this analysis did not support such approach in AF-PCI patients. This is mainly due to the fact that ACS patients also suffer from high risk of major bleeding and that the absolute risk difference as well as the relative risk increase for MI or ST with DAT compared with TAT was not higher in ACS compared with CCS patients. These observations were unexpected and might reflect the synergistic role of DOACs, when administered at full doses, with a $P2Y_{12}$ inhibitor monotherapy for the prevention of coronary ischemic events. Curiously, the only signal that DAT was associated with higher MI and ST risks compared with TAT was observed in patients treated with dabigatran 110 mg, but not dabigatran 150 mg. Therefore, ACS or stable coronary artery disease (CAD) presentation per se does not justify the default adoption of a given post-PCI antithrombotic regimen in patients taking DOAC at FDA-approved stroke prevention regimens, rather concurs, together with other established ischemic and bleeding risk factors, to the decision-making on the optimal secondary prevention antithrombotic regimens.[58]

Specific details on the differential aspects and apparently contrasting results among various meta-analyses can be found elsewhere.[57,59–62]

OPTIMAL DURATION OF TRIPLE ANTITHROMBOTIC THERAPY BALANCING ISCHEMIC AND BLEEDING RISK

An ever-present dilemma in choosing the duration of TAT is how much it may be influenced by the balance between ischemic and bleeding risk. In the 2023 European Society of Cardiology (ESC) guidelines on ACS,[1] the high ischemic risk was defined by clinical characteristics (ie, chronic kidney disease, prior ST on antiplatelet therapy), procedural features (ie, at least 3 stents implanted, at least 3 lesions treated, bifurcation with 2 stents implanted, stenting of the last remaining patent coronary artery, total stent length >60 mm, treatment of a chronic total occlusion), and coronary anatomy (ie, multivessel disease, complex coronary lesions). These characteristics may also apply to identify AF-PCI patients at increased risk of ischemic events. However, it is unclear whether these criteria can help clinicians in decision-making about the type and duration of TAT. Indeed, the subgroup analyses of several trials failed to find a group that benefits more from TAT versus DAT with respect to indication for PCI (ACS vs CCS), procedural (bifurcation, presence of thrombus, type and length of stents, number of stents, chronic total occlusion), or clinical features (renal function, diabetes, use of proton pump inhibitor, or anemia).[46–50,63–67] Furthermore, although DAT has been associated with greater risk of ST and borderline increase of MI,[57,68] it significantly reduced bleeding with no significant difference in other ischemic and composite events. Therefore, being ST quite rare compared with bleeding events, the number needed to treat to reach a bleeding benefit is lower than the one to prevent rarer events such as ST or MI. Of course, the number needed to treat or harm depends on the baseline ischemic and bleeding risk that can affect the absolute risks of these events and the corresponding benefits/risks of DAT and TAT as shown in previous meta-analyses, thus supporting a careful assessment of ischemic and bleeding risks and the personalization of the antithrombotic therapy.[57,58]

Furthermore, TAT greatly increases the risk of clinically relevant bleeding by around 20% to 30% per year and approximately 40% higher than DAPT[69] and surprisingly may also increase by itself the risk of ischemic events for various reasons including the abrupt interruption of antithrombotic therapy which sometimes occurs even with minor bleeding.[44] Putting aside the results of these clinical trials, there is a pathophysiological reason why aspirin can be safely stopped within 7 days after stent implantation if treatment with OAC and a P2Y$_{12}$ inhibitor is maintained. First, OACs indirectly inhibit platelet activation by reducing the generation of thrombin, which acts via the protease activated receptor-1 to activate platelets.[70] Second, the combination of OAC and single antiplatelet therapy, blocking both plasma and cellular components of thrombus formation, acts synergistically.[71] Moreover, advances in PCI technology have reduced the incidence of ST.[11] Finally, recent trials showed interesting findings with short DAPT in patients undergoing PCI.[14,72,73] In the setting of HBR patients, the MASTER DAPT trial, randomizing 4579 (4434 in the per-protocol analysis) patients undergoing PCI with Ultimaster stent (a biodegradable-polymer sirolimus-eluting coronary stent) implantation, compared 1 month of DAPT with aspirin and clopidogrel followed by aspirin monotherapy to ≥3 months of DAPT and found no significant difference in ischemic events with the 1-month DAPT, but a lower risk of bleeding events.[74] Interestingly, among those with an OAC indication (n = 1666), consistent findings were reported with no difference for the co-primary endpoints of NACE (death, MI, stroke, or BARC bleeding type 3 or 5), MACE, and BARC 2, 3, or 5 between shorter (single antiplatelet for 5 months after 1-month DAPT) versus standard DAPT in addition to long-term OAC.[75] On the other hand, it should be noted that, with the exception of AUGUSTUS trial that randomized patients to receive a P2Y$_{12}$ inhibitor first to DOAC or VKA and then, each of these, to aspirin or placebo (resulting in both DOAC-based TAT and VKA-based DAT), the other trials compared DOAC-based DAT versus VKA-based TAT.[46,47,49,50] Notably, the use of VKAs compared with DOACs is per se a reason for increased bleeding risk.[76] Additionally, data on ACS patients and with different high-risk procedural or clinical features derived only from subanalyses. Lastly, this population was underrepresented in the AF-PCI randomized trials.[46,47,49,50] A subgroup analysis of the REDUAL PCI trial showed that only 9.9% of patients had high-risk procedural factors and only 10% had both procedural and clinical high-risk factors.[64]

The decision-making becomes even more challenging when considering that AF-PCI patients are at HBR by definition being them receiving OAC, but they can even become at greater risk due to high PREdicting bleeding Complications In patients undergoing Stent implantation and subsEquent Dual Antiplatelet Therapy (PRECISE-DAPT) score or additional factors such as renal dysfunction, advanced age, ACS presentation, or other HBR factors. Indeed, in a large population of PCI patients, HBR criteria were validated and also a criteria-based score was generated demonstrating that the greater was the score (more HBR criteria in the same patient), the greater was the incidence of bleeding events.[18-21] Another special population is represented by cancer patients, given that these patients have high risk of both thrombosis and bleeding.[77]

Altogether, these considerations highlight the need for an individualization of decisions, but also how challenging this approach can be, thus supporting the need for new evidence in this field.

LONG-TERM ORAL ANTICOAGULANTS

Two trials investigated long-term antithrombotic therapy for AF patients undergoing PCI.[78,79] The Optimizing Antithrombotic Care in Patients With AtriaL fibrillatiON and Coronary stEnt (OAC-ALONE) trial was a non-inferior trial that compared OAC (either VKA or DOAC) to DAT (OAC plus aspirin or clopidogrel) as long-term strategies beyond 1-year after PCI. After enrolling 696 patients in 38 months, it was prematurely terminated due to slow enrollment and failed to demonstrate the non-inferiority of OAC alone to DAT in terms of the composite of all-cause death, MI, stroke, or systemic embolism at 1-year (HR: 1.16; 95% CI: 0.79–1.72; $P = .20$ for non-inferiority, $P = .45$ for superiority).[78] More recently, the Atrial Fibrillation and Ischemic Events With Rivaroxaban in Patients With Stable Coronary Artery Disease Study (AFIRE) trial compared rivaroxaban alone versus DAT with rivaroxaban in 2,236 AF patients beyond 1-year after PCI. The trial was stopped early because of increased mortality in the DAT group; at a median follow-up of 24 months, rivaroxaban monotherapy was non-inferior to DAT for ischemic events (HR: 0.72; 95% CI: 0.55–0.95; $P<.001$ for non-inferiority) and superior for bleeding events (HR: 0.59; 95% CI: 0.39–0.89; $P = .01$ for superiority).[79] The rationale for dropping aspirin instead of clopidogrel is also a matter of current debate and as stated earlier never investigated properly up to date (Table 1).

SELECTION OF THE ANTIPLATELET AGENT IN ADDITION TO ORAL ANTICOAGULANTS

As stated earlier, after the WOEST trial introduced the strategy of removing aspirin instead of the P2Y$_{12}$ inhibitor to continue with a DAT, no other studies have tested a different approach or directly compared a DAT based on aspirin with a DAT based on clopidogrel. Therefore, there is no clear evidence in AF-PCI patients that clopidogrel is superior to aspirin. Yet, although the P2Y$_{12}$ inhibitor monotherapy has become an intriguing strategy tested in last

decades, the comparison of clopidogrel or other P2Y$_{12}$ inhibitors versus aspirin is actually limited and with inconsistent and inconclusive results even in non-AF patients undergoing PCI.

Regarding the type of P2Y$_{12}$ inhibitor, it is well known that clopidogrel has the relevant limitation of potential resistance related to genetic variability. However, the use of prasugrel or ticagrelor in DAT/TAT was limited in trials due to bleeding concerns, thus, whether these agents may be used in these patients is unknown and discouraged by guidelines.[1] Indeed, the use of ticagrelor and prasugrel was low in the PIONEER AF-PCI (5.6%), AUGUSTUS (6.2%), ENTRUST-AF PCI (7.6%), and RE-DUAL PCI trials (12%).[46,47,49,50] Interestingly, a sub analysis of the latter trial showed that the benefit of DAT with dabigatran over TAT with a VKA in reducing bleeding risk was consistent across patients on ticagrelor or clopidogrel,[80] but no data are available for prasugrel. Notably, in a recent nationwide cohort study, 2259 AF patients undergoing PCI for MI from 2011 through 2019 were analyzed. The P2Y$_{12}$ inhibitor prescribed at discharge was clopidogrel in 85% and ticagrelor or prasugrel in 15% of patients. The risk of MACE, defined as a composite of death from any cause, stroke, MI, or repeat revascularization, was significantly lower in the ticagrelor or prasugrel group compared with clopidogrel group without difference in bleeding.[81] Of course, this is an observational study with several limitations, and, as all these studies, it is subject to bias and confounding related to measured and, more importantly, unmeasured variables for which no sophisticated adjustment can properly account for. Particularly, being the use of ticagrelor or prasugrel in these patients an active choice by the treating physician against common guidelines, it is plausible to assume that physicians may have had specific unmeasured factors leading their decision. However, irrespective of its limitations, this study is hypothesis-generating and future studies are needed to address this point.

EUROPEAN AND AMERICAN GUIDELINES RECOMMENDATIONS

Based on evidence from trials and meta-analyses, European guidelines reduced the duration of TAT from 6 months to 1 week over time. Most recent ESC guidelines on ACS recommended TAT for 1 week in patients with OAC indication undergoing PCI, followed by DAT for 12 months and then OAC alone (Class I). They also recommended weighing the ischemic and hemorrhagic risk to decide TAT strategy. In patients with higher ischemic risk than hemorrhagic risk, TAT should

Table 1
Main randomized clinical trials assessing antithrombotic therapy in atrial fibrillation-percutaneous coronary intervention (AF-PCI) patients

NAME	WOEST	ISAR-TRIPLE	PIONEER-AF PCI	RE-DUAL PCI	AUGUSTUS	ENTRUST AF-PCI	OAC-ALONE	AFIRE	MASTER DAPT (OAC Subanalysis)
YEAR	2013	2015	2016	2017	2019	2019	2019	2019	2021
PATIENTS (N)	573	614	2124	2725	4614	1506	696	2236	4579 (1666)
POPULATION	Patients with OAC indication undergone PCI (ACS 27.1%)	Patients with OAC indication undergone PCI (ACS 32%)	Patients with AF undergone PCI with stenting (ACS 51.6%)	Patients with AF undergone successful PCI (ACS 64%)	Patients with AF after ACS or PCI (or both) (ACS 61.2%)	Patients with AF undergone PCI (ACS 52%)	Patients with AF and stable CAD undergone PCI beyond 1 y earlier	Patients with AF and stable CAD undergone PCI or CABG more than 1 y earlier or who had angiography confirmed CAD not requiring intervention	HBR Patients undergone PCI after 1 month of DAPT (Patients with OAC indication)
TRIAL DESIGN	Superiority	Superiority	Superiority	Non-inferiority	Non-inferiority and superiority	Non-inferiority and superiority	Non-inferiority	Non-inferiority and superiority	Non-inferiority and superiority
TREATMENT STRATEGIES	OAC + P2Y12I (clopidogrel) for 1–12 mo vs OAC + P2Y12I (clopidogrel) + aspirin for 1–12 mo	OAC + P2Y12I (clopidogrel) + aspirin for 6 wk vs OAC + P2Y12I (clopidogrel) + aspirin for 6 mo	Rivaroxaban 15 mg daily + P2Y12 inhibitor (clopidogrel 75 mg daily) vs rivaroxaban 2.5 mg twice daily + DAPT (aspirin 75–100 mg daily and clopidogrel 75 mg daily) vs warfarin + DAPT	Dabigatran etexilate 110 mg twice daily + P2Y12 inhibitor (clopidogrel or Ticagrelor) vs dabigatran etexilate 150 mg twice daily + P2Y12 inhibitor (clopidogrel or ticagrelor) vs warfarin (INR 2.0–3.0) + DAPT (aspirin ≤100 mg daily and clopidogrel or ticagrelor)	Apixaban 5 mg twice daily + DAPT (aspirin 81 mg daily and a P2Y12 inhibitor) vs Apixaban 5 mg twice daily + P2Y12 inhibitor vs warfarin (INR 2.0–3.0) + DAPT (aspirin 81 mg daily and a P2Y12 inhibitor) vs warfarin (INR 2.0–3.0) + P2Y12 inhibitor	Edoxaban 60 mg daily + P2Y12 inhibitor vs VKA + DAPT (aspirin 100 mg daily and a P2Y12 inhibitor)	OAC for 12 mo vs OAC + SAPT for 12 mo	OAC (rivaroxaban) for 6 mo vs OAC (rivaroxaban) + SAPT for 6 mo	Abbreviated DAPT regimen (SAPT for 5 mo + OAC) vs Standard DAPT regimen (DAPT for 2 mo + SAPT until 11 mo + OAC)

KEY ENDPOINTS	Any bleeding episode.	Composite of ischemic events (death, MI, definite stent thrombosis, stroke) and TIMI major bleeding.	Clinically significant bleeding (composite of major or minor bleeding according to TIMI criteria, and bleeding requiring medical attention).	Major or clinically relevant nonmajor bleeding event (ISTH criteria)	Major bleeding or bleeding clinically relevant nonmajor (ISTH criteria)	Major bleeding or clinically relevant nonmajor bleeding (ISTH criteria)	Primary endpoint: all-cause death, MI, stroke, or systemic embolism. Major secondary endpoint: primary endpoint or major bleeding (ISTH criteria).	Primary efficacy endpoint: stroke, systemic embolism, MI, unstable angina requiring revascularization, or death from any cause. Primary safety endpoint: major bleeding (ISTH criteria).	First co-primary endpoint: NACE (death, MI, stroke, and BARC 3 or 5 bleeding) Second co-primary endpoint: MACCE (death, MI, or stroke) Third co-primary endpoint: major or clinically relevant nonmajor bleedings (BARC type 2, 3, or 5)
RESULTS	HR: 0.36; 95% CI: 0.26–0.50; $P<.0001$	HR: 1.14; 95% CI: 0.68–1.91; $P = .63$	HR (group 1 vs group 3): 0.59; 95% CI: 0.47–0.76; $P<.001$. HR (group 2 vs group 3): 0.63; 95% CI: 0.50–0.80; $P<.001$.	HR (dabigatran 110 mg b.i.d.): 0.52; 95% CI: 0.42–0.63; $P<.001$ for non-inferiority; $P<.001$ for superiority. HR (dabigatran 150 mg b.i.d.): 0.72; 95% CI: 0.58–0.88; $P<.001$ for non-inferiority; $P = .002$ for superiority	HR (apixaban vs VKA): 0.69; 95% CI: 0.58–0.81; $P<.001$ for both non-inferiority and superiority. HR (aspirin vs placebo): 1.89; 95% CI: 1.59–2.24; $P<.001$.	HR: 0.83; 95% CI: 0.65–1.05; $P = .001$ for non-inferiority; $P = .1154$ for superiority.	HR (primary endpoint): 1.16; 95% CI: 0.79–1.72; $P = .20$ for non-inferiority, $P = .45$ for superiority. HR (major secondary endpoint): 0.99; 95% CI, 0.71–1.39; $P = .016$ for non-inferiority, $P = .96$ for superiority.	HR (efficacy endpoint): 0.72; 95% CI: 0.55–0.95; $P<.001$ for non-inferiority. HR (safety endpoint): 0.59; 95% CI: 0.39–0.89; $P = .01$ for superiority.	HR (NACE): 0.83; 95% CI; 0.60–1.15; $P = .26$. HR (MACCE): 0.88; 95% CI; 0.60–1.30. HR (BARC 2, 3, or 5): 0.83; 95% CI; 0.62–1.12; $P = .25$.

Abbreviations: ACS, acute coronary syndrome; AF, atrial fibrillation; BARC, bleeding academic research consortium; BMS, bare metal stent; CABG, coronary artery bypass graft; CAD, coronary artery disease; DAPT, dual antiplatelet therapy; DES, drug-eluting stent; HBR, high bleeding risk; ISTH, international society on thrombosis and haemostasis; MACCE, major adverse cardiac and cerebrovascular event; MI, myocardial infarction; NACE, net adverse clinical events; OAC, oral anticoagulation therapy; P2Y12I, P2Y12 inhibitors; PCI, percutaneous coronary intervention; SAPT, single antiplatelet therapy; TIMI, thrombolysis in myocardial infarction; VKA, vitamin K antagonists.

be continued for 1 month (Class IIa). Conversely, in patients with predominant bleeding risk, discontinuation of DAT after 6 months and continuation of OAC alone may be considered (Class IIb). In addition, prasugrel or ticagrelor as part of TAT is not recommended (Class III).[1,2,34] In patients with CCS, guidelines recommended a similar default strategy with some differences. TAT for 1 week and continuation of DAT for up to 6 months are recommended if the risk of ST is low (Class I). Conversely, TAT up to 1 month should be considered when the risk of ST outweighs the bleeding risk (Class IIa)[34] (Fig. 1). In addition, both guidelines support the use of DOACs over VKAs, clopidogrel as the antiplatelet agent of choice in DAT, and reduced doses of rivaroxaban (15 mg/day) or dabigatran (110 mg twice daily) when the bleeding risk is high (Class IIa). Recommendations on antithrombotic management in AF-PCI patients are similar on both sides of the ocean.[82,83] The 2021 American (ACC/AHA/SCAI) guidelines recommended a default TAT strategy during peri-PCI period up to 1-week after PCI (1 month in patients at high ischemic risk), followed by DAT for 12 months (6 months in HBR patients), and OAC as long-term monotherapy 1-year after revascularization. In North American guidelines, there is a slight difference in CCS patients without HBR, where after a short period of TAT, followed by a 6-month DAT with a P2Y12 inhibitor (preferably clopidogrel), a P2Y$_{12}$ inhibitor or aspirin can be administered on top of OAC for up to 12 months.

ONGOING TRIALS AND REGISTRIES

Several clinical trials and registries on antithrombotic strategy in AF-PCI patients are currently ongoing. In the context of ACS, OPTIMA-3 substudy will randomize 2274 ACS patients to receive TAT with warfarin for 1 month or 6 months in a 1:1 ratio. In both cases, aspirin will be discontinued at different times for a composite primary endpoint of cardiovascular death, MI, ischemic stroke, systemic embolism, and unplanned revascularization up to 12 months; the secondary endpoint will be ISTH major bleeding or clinically relevant non-major bleeding (NCT03234114). In this clinical setting, the focus is mainly on evaluating combinations of DOACs and more potent P2Y$_{12}$ inhibitors. In the OPTIMA-4 sub-study, 1472 patients will be randomized to compare different antiplatelet strategy with clopidogrel versus ticagrelor plus anticoagulation regimen of dabigatran 110 mg twice daily for a safety endpoint of major or non-major clinically significant bleeding and an efficacy endpoint of MACCE (a composite of cardiovascular death,

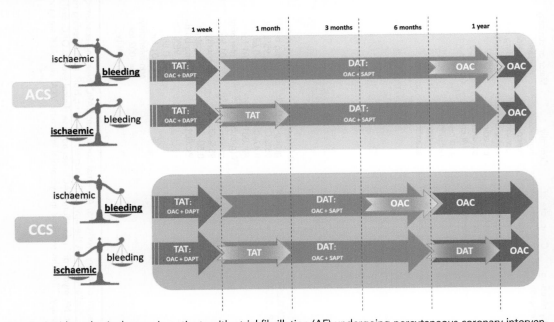

Fig. 1. Antithrombotic therapy in patients with atrial fibrillation (AF) undergoing percutaneous coronary intervention (PCI) according to European Society of Cardiology (ESC) guidelines. Decision-making process is guided by the balance of ischemic and bleeding risk. Bigger arrows represent the main indication, but options represented by smaller and light arrows could be considered. ACS, acute coronary syndrome; CCS, chronic coronary syndrome; DAT, dual antithrombotic therapy; OAC, oral anticoagulation; SAPT, single antiplatelet therapy; TAT, triple antithrombotic therapy.

MI, ischemic stroke, systemic thromboembolism, and unplanned revascularization) at 12 months (NCT03234114). The ADONIS-PCI trial will enroll AF-ACS patients to compare DAT with dabigatran (150 or 110 mg twice daily) and ticagrelor (90 mg twice daily for 1 month, followed by 60 mg twice daily for up to 12 months) to TAT with dabigatran, clopidogrel, and aspirin followed by DAT for major or clinically relevant non-major bleeding after 2 years of follow-up (NCT04695106). The WOEST-3, a multicenter, open-label, randomized controlled trial, will investigate the safety and efficacy of 1 month DAPT (without OACs) compared to standard TAT with OAC plus $P2Y_{12}$ inhibitor and aspirin up to 30 days for a primary safety endpoint of ISTH major or clinically relevant non-major bleeding and a primary efficacy endpoint of a composite of all-cause death, MI, stroke, systemic embolism, or ST at 6 weeks after PCI (NCT04436978). In the same direction, in the MATRIX-2 trial, the aim is to evaluate the safety and efficacy of a monotherapy regimen with a $P2Y_{12}$ inhibitor for 1 month followed by long-term DOAC monotherapy compared to standard TAT for up to 1 month (aspirin, $P2Y_{12}$ inhibitor and DOAC) followed by DAT ($P2Y_{12}$ inhibitor and DOAC) for 6 to 12 months and DOAC monotherapy thereafter, in AF patients undergoing PCI after Supraflex Cruz sirolimus-eluting stent implantation (NCT05955365). To explore the benefits of an early intensive antithrombotic regimen and subsequent de-escalation also in AF patients, the EPIDAURUS trial will evaluate in AF-ACS patients DAT with a DOAC plus prasugrel or ticagrelor for 1 month, followed from standard DAT (clopidogrel plus DOAC) versus standard DAT in terms of both clinically relevant bleeding and major adverse cardiovascular events at 6 months (NCT04981041). Investigating the different DOACs, the APPROACH-ACS-AF trial will test whether a DAT strategy comprising clopidogrel plus apixaban is superior to a TAT strategy of VKAs plus DAPT with respect to bleeding events in AF-ACS patients undergoing PCI (NCT02789917). Finally, for antithrombotic long-term strategies, 2 trials are being published. The ADAPT-AF trial will evaluate the long-term effects of DAT (apixaban 5 mg twice daily or rivaroxaban 15 mg once daily plus clopidogrel) versus OAC alone (either DOAC or a VKA) in AF patients undergoing PCI more than 1 year before in term of NACE at 2 years of follow-up (NCT04250116). The AQUATIC trial will randomize AF patients undergoing PCI more than 1 year before receiving aspirin or placebo on top of OACs to assess long-term MACE and bleeding (NCT04217447).

SUMMARY

The optimal antithrombotic therapy in AF patients undergoing PCI remains challenging and debated. Data from randomized clinical trials and meta-analyses have demonstrated that DAT significantly reduces bleeding complications without increase of death or composite ischemic events but with potential increased risk of ST and MI. Accordingly, European guidelines recommend a TAT of 1 week followed by DAT with a DOAC and a $P2Y_{12}$ inhibitor for 6 to 12 months (depending on clinical settings) and then DOAC alone over time, but only includes the option to prolong TAT at 1 month and considering personalized therapeutic approaches based on the ischemic and bleeding risk of each patient. Given the delicate setting of patients, procedural optimization, strategies to reduce bleeding risk, and dynamic assessment of ischemic/bleeding risk factors and antithrombic therapy during follow-up are paramount in these patients. However, further studies will be needed to clarify the optimal duration of TAT or DAT and the role of more potent antiplatelet drugs in AF-PCI patients.

CLINICS CARE POINTS

- Antithrombotic therapy is essential to prevent ischemic complications but exposes patients to increased risk of bleeding.
- The evidence from RCTs in patients undergoing PCI requiring OAC is predominantly for those with atrial fibrillation.
- Using DOAC instead of VKAs and abbreviating the duration of DAPT with OAC seems to be reasonable to reduce bleeding complications.
- Shortening DAPT might expose patients to ischemic risks, therefore, the decision-making should be personalized based on the individual ischemic and bleeding risks.

DISCLOSURE

The authors have nothing to disclose.

REFERENCES

1. Byrne RA, Rossello X, Coughlan JJ, et al. 2023 ESC Guidelines for the management of acute coronary syndromes. Eur Heart J 2023;44(38):3720–826.
2. Knuuti J, Wijns W, Saraste A, et al. 2019 ESC Guidelines for the diagnosis and management of chronic coronary syndromes. Eur Heart J 2020;41(3):407–77.

3. Neumann FJ, Sousa-Uva M, Ahlsson A, et al. 2018 ESC/EACTS Guidelines on myocardial revascularization. Eur Heart J 2019;40(2):87–165.

4. Valgimigli M, Bueno H, Byrne RA, et al. 2017 ESC focused update on dual antiplatelet therapy in coronary artery disease developed in collaboration with EACTS: The Task Force for dual antiplatelet therapy in coronary artery disease of the European Society of Cardiology (ESC) and of the European Association for Cardio-Thoracic Surgery (EACTS). Eur Heart J 2018;39(3):213–60.

5. Gargiulo G, Valgimigli M, Capodanno D, et al. State of the art: duration of dual antiplatelet therapy after percutaneous coronary intervention and coronary stent implantation - past, present and future perspectives. EuroIntervention 2017;13(6): 717–33.

6. Gargiulo G, Serino F, Esposito G. Cardiovascular mortality in patients with acute and chronic coronary syndrome: insights from the clinical evidence on ticagrelor. Eur Rev Med Pharmacol Sci 2022; 26(7):2524–42.

7. Gargiulo G, Giacoppo D. Should we routinely use ultrasound-guided transfemoral access for coronary procedures? High-quality evidence from an individual participant data meta-analysis. EuroIntervention 2024;20(1):21–3.

8. Gargiulo G, Marenna A, Sperandeo L, et al. Pharmacodynamic effects of cangrelor in elective complex PCI: insights from the POMPEII Registry. EuroIntervention 2023;18(15):1266–8.

9. Gargiulo G, Giacoppo D, Jolly SS, et al. Effects on Mortality and Major Bleeding of Radial Versus Femoral Artery Access for Coronary Angiography or Percutaneous Coronary Intervention: Meta-Analysis of Individual Patient Data From 7 Multicenter Randomized Clinical Trials. Circulation 2022; 146(18):1329–43.

10. Gragnano F, Jolly SS, Mehta SR, et al. Prediction of radial crossover in acute coronary syndromes: derivation and validation of the MATRIX score. EuroIntervention 2021;17(12):e971–80.

11. Iantorno M, Lipinski MJ, Garcia-Garcia HM, et al. Meta-Analysis of the Impact of Strut Thickness on Outcomes in Patients With Drug-Eluting Stents in a Coronary Artery. Am J Cardiol 2018;122(10): 1652–60.

12. Capodanno D, Gargiulo G, Buccheri S, et al. Meta-Analyses of Dual Antiplatelet Therapy Following Drug-Eluting Stent Implantation: Do Bleeding and Stent Thrombosis Weigh Similar on Mortality? J Am Coll Cardiol 2015;66(14):1639–40.

13. Gargiulo G, Windecker S, Vranckx P, et al. A Critical Appraisal of Aspirin in Secondary Prevention: Is Less More? Circulation 2016;134(23):1881–906.

14. Gragnano F, Capolongo A, Terracciano F, et al. Escalation and De-Escalation of Antiplatelet Therapy after Acute Coronary Syndrome or PCI: Available Evidence and Implications for Practice. J Clin Med 2022;11(21). https://doi.org/10.3390/jcm11216246.

15. Gragnano F, Capolongo A, Terracciano F, et al. [New frontiers in antiplatelet therapy: guided therapy and de-escalation after acute coronary syndrome or percutaneous coronary intervention]. G Ital Cardiol 2023;24(2):99–109.

16. Gargiulo G, Windecker S, da Costa BR, et al. Short term versus long term dual antiplatelet therapy after implantation of drug eluting stent in patients with or without diabetes: systematic review and meta-analysis of individual participant data from randomised trials. BMJ 2016;355:i5483.

17. Gargiulo G, Esposito G. Consolidating the value of the standardised ARC-HBR definition. EuroIntervention 2021;16(14):1126–8.

18. Ueki Y, Bär S, Losdat S, et al. Validation of the Academic Research Consortium for High Bleeding Risk (ARC-HBR) criteria in patients undergoing percutaneous coronary intervention and comparison with contemporary bleeding risk scores. EuroIntervention 2020;16(5):371–9.

19. Corpataux N, Spirito A, Gragnano F, et al. Validation of high bleeding risk criteria and definition as proposed by the academic research consortium for high bleeding risk. Eur Heart J 2020;41(38):3743–9.

20. Gragnano F, Spirito A, Corpataux N, et al. Impact of clinical presentation on bleeding risk after percutaneous coronary intervention and implications for the ARC-HBR definition. EuroIntervention 2021; 17(11):e898–909.

21. Spirito A, Gragnano F, Corpataux N, et al. Sex-Based Differences in Bleeding Risk After Percutaneous Coronary Intervention and Implications for the Academic Research Consortium High Bleeding Risk Criteria. J Am Heart Assoc 2021;10(12):e021965.

22. Benjamin EJ, Muntner P, Alonso A, et al. Heart Disease and Stroke Statistics-2019 Update: A Report From the American Heart Association. Circulation 2019;139(10):e56–528.

23. Chugh SS, Havmoeller R, Narayanan K, et al. Worldwide epidemiology of atrial fibrillation: a Global Burden of Disease 2010 Study. Circulation 2014;129(8):837–47.

24. Colilla S, Crow A, Petkun W, et al. Estimates of current and future incidence and prevalence of atrial fibrillation in the U.S. adult population. Am J Cardiol 2013;112(8):1142–7.

25. Krijthe BP, Kunst A, Benjamin EJ, et al. Projections on the number of individuals with atrial fibrillation in the European Union, from 2000 to 2060. Eur Heart J 2013;34(35):2746–51.

26. Kralev S, Schneider K, Lang S, et al. Incidence and severity of coronary artery disease in patients with atrial fibrillation undergoing first-time coronary angiography. PLoS One 2011;6(9):e24964.

27. González-Pacheco H, Márquez MF, Arias-Mendoza A, et al. Clinical features and in-hospital mortality associated with different types of atrial fibrillation in patients with acute coronary syndrome with and without ST elevation. J Cardiol 2015;66(2):148–54.

28. Krijthe BP, Leening MJG, Heeringa J, et al. Unrecognized myocardial infarction and risk of atrial fibrillation: the Rotterdam Study. Int J Cardiol 2013;168(2):1453–7.

29. Capodanno D, Huber K, Mehran R, et al. Management of Antithrombotic Therapy in Atrial Fibrillation Patients Undergoing PCI: JACC State-of-the-Art Review. J Am Coll Cardiol 2019;74(1):83–99.

30. Connolly SJ, Ezekowitz MD, Yusuf S, et al. Dabigatran versus warfarin in patients with atrial fibrillation. N Engl J Med 2009;361(12):1139–51.

31. Patel MR, Mahaffey KW, Garg J, et al. Rivaroxaban versus warfarin in nonvalvular atrial fibrillation. N Engl J Med 2011;365(10):883–91.

32. Granger CB, Alexander JH, McMurray JJV, et al. Apixaban versus warfarin in patients with atrial fibrillation. N Engl J Med 2011;365(11):981–92.

33. Giugliano RP, Ruff CT, Braunwald E, et al. Edoxaban versus warfarin in patients with atrial fibrillation. N Engl J Med 2013;369(22):2093–104.

34. Hindricks G, Potpara T, Dagres N, et al. 2020 ESC Guidelines for the diagnosis and management of atrial fibrillation developed in collaboration with the European Association for Cardio-Thoracic Surgery (EACTS): The Task Force for the diagnosis and management of atrial fibrillation of the European Society of Cardiology (ESC) Developed with the special contribution of the European Heart Rhythm Association (EHRA) of the ESC. Eur Heart J 2021;42(5):373–498.

35. Previtali E, Bucciarelli P, Passamonti SM, et al. Risk factors for venous and arterial thrombosis. Blood Transfus 2011;9(2):120–38.

36. Wentzel JJ, Gijsen FJH, Schuurbiers JCH, et al. The influence of shear stress on in-stent restenosis and thrombosis. EuroIntervention 2008;4(Suppl C):C27–32.

37. Mant J, Hobbs FDR, Fletcher K, et al. Warfarin versus aspirin for stroke prevention in an elderly community population with atrial fibrillation (the Birmingham Atrial Fibrillation Treatment of the Aged Study, BAFTA): a randomised controlled trial. Lancet 2007;370(9586):493–503.

38. Själander S, Själander A, Svensson PJ, et al. Atrial fibrillation patients do not benefit from acetylsalicylic acid. Europace 2014;16(5):631–8.

39. ACTIVE Writing Group of the ACTIVE Investigators, Connolly S, Pogue J, et al. Clopidogrel plus aspirin versus oral anticoagulation for atrial fibrillation in the Atrial fibrillation Clopidogrel Trial with Irbesartan for prevention of Vascular Events (ACTIVE W): a randomised controlled trial. Lancet 2006;367(9526):1903–12.

40. Urban P, Macaya C, Rupprecht HJ, et al. Randomized evaluation of anticoagulation versus antiplatelet therapy after coronary stent implantation in high-risk patients: the multicenter aspirin and ticlopidine trial after intracoronary stenting (MATTIS). Circulation 1998;98(20):2126–32.

41. Bertrand ME, Legrand V, Boland J, et al. Randomized multicenter comparison of conventional anticoagulation versus antiplatelet therapy in unplanned and elective coronary stenting. The full anticoagulation versus aspirin and ticlopidine (fantastic) study. Circulation 1998;98(16):1597–603.

42. Leon MB, Baim DS, Popma JJ, et al. A clinical trial comparing three antithrombotic-drug regimens after coronary-artery stenting. Stent Anticoagulation Restenosis Study Investigators. N Engl J Med 1998;339(23):1665–71.

43. Limbruno U, Goette A, De Caterina R. Commentary: Temporarily omitting oral anticoagulants early after stenting for acute coronary syndromes patients with atrial fibrillation. Int J Cardiol 2020;318:82–5.

44. Dewilde WJM, Oirbans T, Verheugt FWA, et al. Use of clopidogrel with or without aspirin in patients taking oral anticoagulant therapy and undergoing percutaneous coronary intervention: an open-label, randomised, controlled trial. Lancet 2013;381(9872):1107–15.

45. Fiedler KA, Maeng M, Mehilli J, et al. Duration of Triple Therapy in Patients Requiring Oral Anticoagulation After Drug-Eluting Stent Implantation: The ISAR-TRIPLE Trial. J Am Coll Cardiol 2015;65(16):1619–29.

46. Gibson CM, Mehran R, Bode C, et al. Prevention of Bleeding in Patients with Atrial Fibrillation Undergoing PCI. N Engl J Med 2016;375(25):2423–34.

47. Cannon CP, Bhatt DL, Oldgren J, et al. Dual Antithrombotic Therapy with Dabigatran after PCI in Atrial Fibrillation. N Engl J Med 2017;377(16):1513–24.

48. Zeymer U, Leiva O, Hohnloser SH, et al. Dual antithrombotic therapy with dabigatran in patients with atrial fibrillation after percutaneous coronary intervention for ST-segment elevation myocardial infarction: a post hoc analysis of the randomised RE-DUAL PCI trial. EuroIntervention 2021;17(6):474–80.

49. Vranckx P, Valgimigli M, Eckardt L, et al. Edoxaban-based versus vitamin K antagonist-based antithrombotic regimen after successful coronary stenting in patients with atrial fibrillation (ENTRUST-AF PCI): a randomised, open-label, phase 3b trial. Lancet 2019;394(10206):1335–43.

50. Lopes RD, Heizer G, Aronson R, et al. Antithrombotic Therapy after Acute Coronary Syndrome or PCI in Atrial Fibrillation. N Engl J Med 2019;380(16):1509–24.

51. Alexander JH, Wojdyla D, Vora AN, et al. Risk/Benefit Tradeoff of Antithrombotic Therapy in Patients With Atrial Fibrillation Early and Late After an Acute Coronary Syndrome or Percutaneous Coronary Intervention: Insights From AUGUSTUS. Circulation 2020;141(20):1618–27.

52. Bor WL, de Veer AJW, Olie RH, et al. Dual versus triple antithrombotic therapy after percutaneous coronary intervention: the prospective multicentre WOEST 2 Study. EuroIntervention 2022;18(4):e303–13.

53. Chandrasekhar J, Baber U, Sartori S, et al. Antithrombotic strategy variability in atrial fibrillation and obstructive coronary disease revascularised with percutaneous coronary intervention: primary results from the AVIATOR 2 international registry. EuroIntervention 2022;18(8):e656–65.

54. De Luca L, Bolognese L, Rubboli A, et al. Combinations of antithrombotic therapies prescribed after percutaneous coronary intervention in patients with acute coronary syndromes and atrial fibrillation: data from the nationwide MATADOR-PCI registry. Eur Heart J Cardiovasc Pharmacother 2021; 7(3):e45–7.

55. Sciahbasi A, Gargiulo G, Talarico GP, et al. Design of the PERSEO Registry on the management of patients treated with oral anticoagulants and coronary stent. J Cardiovasc Med (Hagerstown) 2022;23(11): 738–43.

56. Sciahbasi A, De Rosa S, Gargiulo G, et al. J Cardiovasc Pharmacol. 2024 Jul 19. https://doi.org/10.1097/FJC.0000000000001607. Online ahead of print. PMID: 39028879.

57. Gargiulo G, Goette A, Tijssen J, et al. Safety and efficacy outcomes of double vs. triple antithrombotic therapy in patients with atrial fibrillation following percutaneous coronary intervention: a systematic review and meta-analysis of non-vitamin K antagonist oral anticoagulant-based randomized clinical trials. Eur Heart J 2019;40(46):3757–67.

58. Gargiulo G, Cannon CP, Gibson CM, et al. Safety and efficacy of double vs. triple antithrombotic therapy in patients with atrial fibrillation with or without acute coronary syndrome undergoing percutaneous coronary intervention: a collaborative meta-analysis of non-vitamin K antagonist oral anticoagulant-based randomized clinical trials. Eur Heart J Cardiovasc Pharmacother 2021;7(FI1): f50–60.

59. Gargiulo G, Goette A, Vranckx P, et al. Higher risk of stent thrombosis with double therapy with direct oral anticoagulants: cherry picking the populations of interest does not help. Eur Heart J 2020;41(17): 1701–2.

60. Gargiulo G, Cannon CP, Gibson CM, et al. The multiplication of loaves and fishes approach: a critic to double anti-thrombotics or to double number of ischaemic events? Eur Heart J Cardiovasc Pharmacother 2021;7(3):e29–30.

61. Vranckx P, Valgimigli M, Eckardt L, et al. Antithrombotic treatment strategies after PCI - Authors' reply. Lancet 2020;395(10227):867–8.

62. Gragnano F, Capolongo A, Micari A, et al. Antithrombotic Therapy Optimization in Patients with Atrial Fibrillation Undergoing Percutaneous Coronary Intervention. J Clin Med 2023;13(1). https://doi.org/10.3390/jcm13010098.

63. Vranckx P, Valgimigli M, Eckardt L, et al. Edoxaban in atrial fibrillation patients with percutaneous coronary intervention by acute or chronic coronary syndrome presentation: a pre-specified analysis of the ENTRUST-AF PCI trial. Eur Heart J 2020; 41(47):4497–504.

64. Berry NC, Mauri L, Steg PG, et al. Effect of Lesion Complexity and Clinical Risk Factors on the Efficacy and Safety of Dabigatran Dual Therapy Versus Warfarin Triple Therapy in Atrial Fibrillation After Percutaneous Coronary Intervention: A Subgroup Analysis From the REDUAL PCI Trial. Circ Cardiovasc Interv 2020;13(4):e008349.

65. Hohnloser SH, Steg PG, Oldgren J, et al. Renal Function and Outcomes With Dabigatran Dual Antithrombotic Therapy in Atrial Fibrillation Patients After PCI. JACC Cardiovasc Interv 2019; 12(16):1553–61.

66. Maeng M, Steg PG, Bhatt DL, et al. Dabigatran Dual Therapy Versus Warfarin Triple Therapy Post-PCI in Patients With Atrial Fibrillation and Diabetes. JACC Cardiovasc Interv 2019;12(23): 2346–55.

67. Costa F, Valgimigli M, Steg PG, et al. Antithrombotic therapy according to baseline bleeding risk in patients with atrial fibrillation undergoing percutaneous coronary intervention: applying the PRECISE-DAPT score in RE-DUAL PCI. Eur Heart J Cardiovasc Pharmacother 2022;8(3):216–26.

68. Galli M, Andreotti F, D'Amario D, et al. Stent Thrombosis With Dual Antithrombotic Therapy in Atrial Fibrillation-ACS/PCI Trials. J Am Coll Cardiol 2020;75(14):1727–8.

69. Lamberts M, Olesen JB, Ruwald MH, et al. Bleeding after initiation of multiple antithrombotic drugs, including triple therapy, in atrial fibrillation patients following myocardial infarction and coronary intervention: a nationwide cohort study. Circulation 2012;126(10):1185–93.

70. Capodanno D, Mehran R, Valgimigli M, et al. Aspirin-free strategies in cardiovascular disease and cardioembolic stroke prevention. Nat Rev Cardiol 2018;15(8):480–96.

71. Capodanno D, Bhatt DL, Eikelboom JW, et al. Dual-pathway inhibition for secondary and tertiary antithrombotic prevention in cardiovascular disease. Nat Rev Cardiol 2020;17(4):242–57.

72. Gargiulo G, Esposito G. Aspirin Monotherapy After BioFreedom Stent and 1-Month DAPT: Is Less More Even in Low-Risk Patients? JACC Cardiovasc Interv 2021;14(16):1812–4.

73. Giacoppo D, Matsuda Y, Fovino LN, et al. Short dual antiplatelet therapy followed by P2Y12 inhibitor monotherapy vs. prolonged dual antiplatelet therapy after percutaneous coronary intervention with second-generation drug-eluting stents: a systematic review and meta-analysis of randomized clinical trials. Eur Heart J 2021;42(4):308–19.

74. Valgimigli M, Frigoli E, Heg D, et al. Dual Antiplatelet Therapy after PCI in Patients at High Bleeding Risk. N Engl J Med 2021;385(18):1643–55.

75. Smits PC, Frigoli E, Tijssen J, et al. Abbreviated Antiplatelet Therapy in Patients at High Bleeding Risk With or Without Oral Anticoagulant Therapy After Coronary Stenting: An Open-Label, Randomized, Controlled Trial. Circulation 2021;144(15):1196–211.

76. Ruff CT, Giugliano RP, Braunwald E, et al. Comparison of the efficacy and safety of new oral anticoagulants with warfarin in patients with atrial fibrillation: a meta-analysis of randomised trials. Lancet 2014;383(9921):955–62.

77. Santoro C, Capone V, Canonico ME, et al. Single, Dual, and Triple Antithrombotic Therapy in Cancer Patients with Coronary Artery Disease: Searching for Evidence and Personalized Approaches. Semin Thromb Hemost 2021;47(8):950–61.

78. Matsumura-Nakano Y, Shizuta S, Komasa A, et al. Open-Label Randomized Trial Comparing Oral Anticoagulation With and Without Single Antiplatelet Therapy in Patients With Atrial Fibrillation and Stable Coronary Artery Disease Beyond 1 Year After Coronary Stent Implantation. Circulation 2019;139(5):604–16.

79. Yasuda S, Kaikita K, Akao M, et al. Antithrombotic Therapy for Atrial Fibrillation with Stable Coronary Disease. N Engl J Med 2019;381(12):1103–13.

80. Oldgren J, Steg PG, Hohnloser SH, et al. Dabigatran dual therapy with ticagrelor or clopidogrel after percutaneous coronary intervention in atrial fibrillation patients with or without acute coronary syndrome: a subgroup analysis from the RE-DUAL PCI trial. Eur Heart J 2019;40(19):1553–62.

81. Godtfredsen SJ, Kragholm KH, Kristensen AMD, et al. Ticagrelor or prasugrel vs. clopidogrel in patients with atrial fibrillation undergoing percutaneous coronary intervention for myocardial infarction. European heart journal open 2024;4(1):oead134.

82. Kumbhani DJ, Cannon CP, Beavers CJ, et al. 2020 ACC Expert Consensus Decision Pathway for Anticoagulant and Antiplatelet Therapy in Patients With Atrial Fibrillation or Venous Thromboembolism Undergoing Percutaneous Coronary Intervention or With Atherosclerotic Cardiovascular Disease: A Report of the American College of Cardiology Solution Set Oversight Committee. J Am Coll Cardiol 2021;77(5):629–58.

83. Writing Committee Members, Lawton JS, Tamis-Holland JE, et al. 2021 ACC/AHA/SCAI Guideline for Coronary Artery Revascularization: A Report of the American College of Cardiology/American Heart Association Joint Committee on Clinical Practice Guidelines. J Am Coll Cardiol 2022;79(2):e21–129.

Antithrombotic Therapy in Patients Undergoing Percutaneous Left Atrial Appendage Occlusion

Roberto Galea, MD, Lorenz Räber, MD, PhD*

KEYWORDS

- Left atrial appendage closure • Antithrombotic therapy • Drug regimen
- Device-related thrombus

KEY POINTS

- Percutaneous left atrial appendage closure (LAAC) has been established in clinical practice as an alternative ischemic stroke prevention strategy in patients with atrial fibrillation.
- The devices approved in Europe and United States for percutaneous LAAC contain metal and temporary antithrombotic therapy is strongly recommended following implantation to prevent thrombus formation on the atrial device surface.
- There is still uncertainty regarding to the optimal antithrombotic drug regimen after device implantation in view of the high bleeding risk of patients frequently submitted to LAAC, the incomplete understanding of the LAAC device healing process, and lack of randomized clinical trials comparing different antithrombotic agents after LAAC.

INTRODUCTION

Percutaneous left atrial appendage (LAA) closure (LAAC) excludes the LAA cavity from the circulation using a plug-like metallic device. The LAA as a main source of intracardiac thrombi in patients with non-valvular atrial fibrillation (AF) and limitations related to the chronic use of oral anticoagulants (OAC) made the LAAC an increasingly used stroke prevention strategy in clinical practice.[1,2] Randomized clinical trials (RCT) comparing LAAC with Vitamin K Antagonists (VKA) showed comparable therapeutic efficacy between the 2 therapies whereas large scale RCTs comparing LAAC with direct OAC (DOAC) are still ongoing.[3,4] Accordingly, LAAC has been allocated in the latest American Guidelines for the management of AF a Class IIa (Level of Evidence B) indication among patients with AF and major bleedings due to a non-reversible cause.[5]

Moreover, an upgrade of the latest European guidelines (dating back to 2020 and still reporting a Class IIb indication with a Level of Evidence B) is expected in the near future.[6,7]

Over the last decade, the standardization level of LAAC procedure has progressively increased.[8–10] However, several procedural aspects are still debated. Antithrombotic therapy is strongly recommended during and after the procedure in order to prevent the formation of device-related thrombus (DRT) on the metallic atrial surface of LAAC devices. Yet, there is still uncertainty regarding the optimal regimen after device implantation. The key reason is the challenge to navigate between ischemic and bleeding risk in an often-frail population with increased bleeding risk. Further reasons include the incomplete understanding of the LAAC device healing process, lack of standardized definition of device neo-endothelialization[11] and lack

---

Department of Cardiology, Inselspital, Bern University Hospital, University of Bern, Bern, Switzerland
* Corresponding author.
E-mail address: lorenz.raeber@insel.ch
Twitter: @RaberLorenz (R.G.); @RobertoGalea7 (L.R.)

Intervent Cardiol Clin 13 (2024) 543–552
https://doi.org/10.1016/j.iccl.2024.07.002
2211-7458/24/© 2024 Elsevier Inc. All rights reserved, including those for text and data mining, AI training, and similar technologies.

of RCTs comparing different antithrombotic agents after LAAC. Thus, this review aims at summarizing the available evidence and the remaining challenges related to the management of antithrombotic therapy in the context of LAAC procedure.

ANTITHROMBOTIC THERAPY BEFORE AND DURING LEFT ATRIAL APPENDAGE CLOSURE

Peri-LAAC antithrombotic therapy is highly heterogeneous. Aspirin is usually recommended after percutaneous implantation of LAAC devices but both timing and dose of the first administration are still debated (Fig. 1). The study protocols of the 2 pivotal RCTs comparing LAAC with Watchman (Boston Scientific, Natick, MA, United States [US]) versus VKA required that a maintaining dose of aspirin (eg, 81 mg) had to be started at least 1 day before procedure.[12] This measure has been therefore recommended in the Instructions for Use (IFU) of Watchman devices.[13] However, alternative antithrombotic strategies were reported.[10,14] Weise and colleagues showed that, in a single center cohort of clinically indicated LAAC procedures completed with implantation of Watchman (47%) or Amplatzer [St. Jude Medical/Abbott, Nathan Lane North Plymouth, MN, US] (42%) devices, loading dose of both aspirin and clopidogrel right after the end of procedure was a viable strategy associated with acceptable ischemic (0.7% of procedural ischemic stroke; 2.3% of DRT), and bleeding (2.3% of procedural major bleedings) event

rates.[15] It is therefore not surprising that subsequent prospective studies did not further specify in the relative study protocols either timing or dose for the first antiplatelet therapy administration.[16,17] Overall, due to the lack of evidence favoring a specific approach, aspirin is nowadays started either the day before LAAC or during/right after LAAC with or without loading dose at discretion of the treating physician.

The periprocedural management of OAC is also unsettled. Again, the 2 pivotal RCT study protocols comparing LAAC with VKA required that patients randomized to Watchman had to stop VKA before procedure in order to achieve an international normalised ratio less than 2.0 within 24 hours of the procedure.[12] Consistently, the current RCT comparing LAAC to DOAC recommend stopping OAC (DOAC or VKA) in patients randomized to LAAC at least 2 days prior to the implant procedure ("CATALYST" Trial–clinicaltrials.gov–NCT04226547). However, some centers still do not withhold OAC at the time of LAAC.[2] As a consequence, since there are no data to support or deny this approach, the management of OAC remains still a matter of debate.[2] The increased periprocedural bleeding risk during transseptal puncture and the observation that majority of pericardial effusion occurs early following device implantation are strong arguments to pause OAC periprocedurally.

Well-established is the use of unfractionated heparin (UFH) as first-line intraprocedural antithrombotic medication. The initial dose should be between 70 and 100 units/Kg, with a target activated clotting time (ACT) of greater than

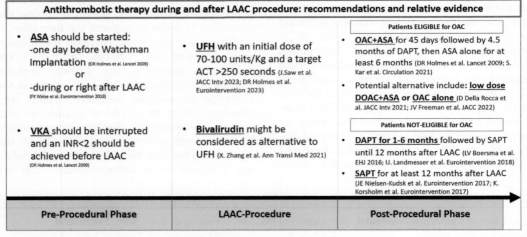

Fig. 1. Current recommendations related to the management of antithrombotic therapy before, during and after LAAC procedure. ACT, Activated Clotting Time; ASA, Aspirin; DAPT, Dual Antiplatelet Therapy, DOAC, Direct Oral Anticoagulant; INR, International Normalised Ratio; LAAC, Left Atrial Appendage Closure; OAC, Oral Anticoagulation; SAPT, Single Antiplatelet Therapy; UFH, Unfractionated Heparin; VKA, Vitamin K Antagonists.

250 seconds.[2] UFH has the advantages to allow continuous monitoring of anticoagulant activity and a rapid reversal of the effect by protamine sulfate, if needed. Yet, the optimal timing to start UFH infusion (before or right after transseptal puncture, or a combined strategy with half dose before and the remaining one right after puncture) still needs to be clarified. As alternative to UFH, the use of bivalirudin can be considered.[18]

ANTITHROMBOTIC THERAPY AFTER LEFT ATRIAL APPENDAGE CLOSURE

Antithrombotic therapy is strongly recommended after implantation of a percutaneous LAAC device in order to prevent DRT on the metallic atrial surface of devices before the endothelialization of the surface is complete.[19] The available evidence suggests that endothelialization of atrial surface of LAAC devices may take even more than 90 days before completing.[20–22] Accordingly, the study protocols of the RCT leading to US Food and Drug Administration (FDA) approval of Watchman[23,24] and Amulet[25] mandated the use of 2 antithrombotic agents for at least 6 months after procedure. As a consequence, once the primary endpoints of the aforementioned trials were completed and the 2 devices were launched in the market, FDA recommended the following drug regimens: in Watchman patients, OAC plus aspirin for 45 days should be given followed by 4.5 months of dual antiplatelet therapy (DAPT) and then by aspirin alone. Amulet implantation should be followed by DAPT or OAC plus aspirin for 45 days, followed by DAPT for 4.5 months and then by aspirin alone (Table 1). However, the earlier regimens are too aggressive in view of the excessive bleeding risk of patients

frequently undergoing LAAC.[26–29] The largest prospective multicenter observational studies conducted outside of US suggested that even short duration DAPT may be a safe and efficient antithrombotic regimen after implantation of Watchman[26] or Amulet[27] devices. As a consequence, the IFU of Watchman and Amulet devices labeled with CE mark allowed the prescription of a short DAPT duration followed by aspirin alone (see Table 1).

The heterogeneous risk categories of patients undergoing LAAC, the different drug regimen recommended after LAAC between American and European competent authorities, and the lack of RCTs comparing various antithrombotic post-LAAC regimens led to a diversification of the post-LAAC antithrombotic regimens in clinical practice with a wide geographic variability[30] (Table 2). The different antithrombotic strategies prescribed after LAAC, including anticoagulant and/or antiplatelet drugs with variable duration, and the relative supporting evidence will be discussed as follows.

Patients Eligible for Oral Anticoagulation

The RCTs leading to FDA approval of Watchman and Amulet devices enrolled patients deemed eligible for OAC.[4,25]

The Watchman device consists of a single self-expanding nitinol cage covered with a porous polyethylene terephthalate membrane on the proximal face. PROTECT AF was a multicenter RCT including 707 non-valvular AF patients with the aim of testing whether LAAC with Watchman was non-inferior to VKA for a composite of stroke, systemic embolism, or cardiovascular death.[24] Only patients deemed eligible for long-term VKA were considered for inclusion. After a mean follow-up of 4 years, the composite primary

Table 1
Post-left atrial appendage closure antithrombotic regimens recommended by the instructions for use of device for percutaneous left atrial appendage closure approved by Food and Drug Administration

LAAC Device Name	FDA Approval	Antithrombotic Therapy Recommended by FDA after LAAC	CE Mark	Antithrombotic Therapy Recommended by EU Authorities after LAAC
Watchman 2.5	2015	OAC + ASA for 45 d followed by 4.5 mo of DAPT; then ASA alone	2005	OAC + ASA or DAPT for 45 d followed by 45 d (at least) of DAPT; then ASA alone (for at least 12 mo)
WatchmanFLX	2020		2019	
Amulet	2021	DAPT or OAC + ASA for 45 d followed by DAPT for 4.5 mo, followed by ASA alone	2013	DAPT of variable duration followed by ASA alone (for at least 6 mo)

Abbreviations: ASA, aspirin; CE, conformity european; DAPT, dual antiplatelet therapy; DOAC, direct oral anticoagulant; EU, European union; FDA, food and drug administration; LAAC, left atrial appendage closure; OAC, oral anticoagulation.

Table 2
Post-left atrial appendage closure antithrombotic regimens and relative supportive studies classified according to the patient eligibility to oral anticoagulation

Patient Submitted to LAAC	Main Antithrombotic Regimen	Study Name	Study Design	Main LAAC Device Used	Patient (No)	CHA2DS2VASC Score (Mean)	Clinical-FU Time (months)	Ischemic Stroke (Events/Patient-Yrs)	Imaging-FU Time (months/Method)	DRT (%)
Eligible to short-term OAC	VKA + SAPT	Protect AF	RCT	W 2.5	463	3.4	48	1.4	1.5/TEE	3.4
		Prevail	RCT	W 2.5	269	4.0	48	1.7	NA	NA
		CAP	MCOS	W2.5	566	3.9	50	1.3	1.5/TEE	2.6
		CAP2	MCOS	W2.5	578	4.5	50	2.2	1.5/TEE	3.9
		Amulet IDE	RCT	W2.5/Amulet	944	4.7	18	1.8	1.5/TEE	4.5
	DOAC + SAPT	Pinnacle FLX	MCOS	FLX	400	4.2	12	2.6	1.5/TEE	0.2
		DellaRocca D. et al.2022	MCOS	W2.5	604	4	13	1.1	1.5/TEE	2.1
Not-eligible to short-term OAC	DAPT	Ewolution	MCOS	W2.5	1021	4.5	24	1.3	1.5/TEE	4.1
		Amulet Registry	MCOS	Amulet	1078	4.2	24	2.2	1.5/TEE	1.6
		Amulet IDE	RCT	W2.5/Amulet	934	4.5	18	1.7	1.5/TEE	3.3
		Patti et al. 2020	MCOS	ACP/Amulet	330	3.9	12	2.1	2/TEE	0.9
	SAPT				280	4.3		1.8		0.7
		Korsholm et al. 2016	SCOS	ACP/Amulet	107	4.4	24	4.7	1.5/TEE-CCTA	1.9

Abbreviations: ACP, amplatzer cardiac plug; CCTA, cardiac computed tomography angiography; DAPT, dual antiplatelet therapy; DOAC, direct oral anticoagulant; DRT, device related thrombus; FLX, Watchman FLX; FU, Follow-up; LAAC, left atrial appendage closure; MCOS, Multi-Center Observation Study; NA, not available; OAC, oral anticoagulation; RCT, randomized clinical trial; SAPT, single antiplatelet therapy; SCOS, Single-Center Observation Study; TEE, transesophageal echocardiography; VKA, Vitamin K Antagonist; W2.5; Watchman 2.5.

endpoint was significantly lower in LAAC as compared to VKA (8.4% vs 13.9%; rate ratio [RR]: 0.60; 95% credible interval [CrI]: 0.41 to 1.05) meeting the prespecified criterion for non-inferiority. In the LAAC group, significantly fewer hemorrhagic strokes (RR: 0.15; 95% CrI: 0.03–0.49) and all-cause fatal events (hazard ratio [HR]: 0.66; 95% CrI: 0.45 to 0.98) were observed.[31] The PREVAIL trial was a confirmatory RCT with similar population and design to PRO-TECT AF trial and showed an improved intraprocedural LAAC safety as compared to the previous trial (rate of severe safety events: 4.5% vs 8.7% respectively).[23] In the above 2 trials, patients randomized to LAAC were asked after procedure to take VKA + aspirin for 45 days followed by 4.5 months of DAPT and then aspirin alone. This regimen was subsequently recommended by FDA for LAAC procedures completed with Watchman implantation (see Table 1). A meta-analysis combining the 5-year outcomes of both PREVAIL and PROTECT trials showed a similar incidence of composite of stroke, systemic embolism, or cardiovascular/unexplained death between LAAC and VKA groups (HR: 0.82; 95% Confidence Interval [CI]: 0.58–1.17; P =.27) but lower rates of mortality (HR: 0.73; 95% CI: 0.54–0.98; P =.035) and non-procedure-related major bleeding (HR: 0.48; 95%CI: 0.32–0.71; P =.0003) in LAAC as compared VKA group.[4]

Amulet is the second most commonly used percutaneous LAAC device worldwide. Amulet has a double closure system including a distal hook-crowned lobe for anchoring in the lumen of the LAA and a proximal disc for excluding the ostium of the LAA according to the pacifier principle. The device received FDA approval based on the AMULET IDE trial, a multicenter RCT comparing Watchman versus Amulet in 1878 AF patients.[25] The study proved the non-inferiority of Amulet as compared to Watchman for both primary safety endpoint (a composite of procedure-related complications, all-cause death, or major bleeding at 12 months: 14.5% vs 14.7%; difference = −0.14, 95% CI, −3.42–3.13; P<.001 for non-inferiority) and primary efficacy endpoint (a composite of ischemic stroke or systemic embolism at 18 months: 2.8% vs 2.8%; difference = 0.00, 95% CI, −1.55–1.55; P<.001 for non-inferiority).[25] Unlike in the Watchman FDA approval RCTs, patients enrolled in the AMULET IDE trial had to be eligible for short-term VKA only.[25] The Amulet arm post-LAAC drug regimen (which is now recommended by FDA) consisted of DAPT or OAC + aspirin for 45 days followed by DAPT for 4.5 months (see Table 1). Of note, only one-fifth of patients randomized to Amulet

were discharged under OAC plus aspirin and the majority (75.7%) received DAPT. Most patients receiving a Watchman (82%) were discharged on OAC plus aspirin. The 3-year outcomes showed similar thromboembolic and major bleeding events between the 2 study groups.[32] As expected, patients included in the Watchman group had a significantly higher annualized major bleedings rate (6.9%) as compared with previous Watchman trials (85 major bleedings in 2748 patient-years were observed indicating a rate of 3.1%) due to the higher baseline bleeding risk of Amulet IDE patients (mean CHA2DS2VASC score 4.6 vs 3.6; mean HASBLED score: 3.2 vs 1.9± 1.0).[4,25]

Although VKA was preferred over DOAC in the AMULET IDE, DOAC plus aspirin might be considered as an equally viable post-implantation drug regimen in patients eligible for short-term OAC. In AF patients submitted to LAAC, the combination of DOAC plus aspirin post-procedure was tested in the PINNACLE FLX trial, a prospective multicenter observational study including AF patients with contraindication to long-term OAC and undergoing treatment with Watchman FLX in the US between May and November 2018.[17] Despite the high-risk population included (mean CHA2DS2Vasc Score of 4.3 and a mean HASBLED Score of 2), this study showed encouraging outcomes in terms of ischemic stroke (2.6% at 1-year), DRT (0.2% at 45-day transesophageal echocardiography [TEE]) but relatively high bleeding rates (major bleedings 7.9% at 1 year).

Among patients enrolled in the AMULET IDE trial, a higher rate of peri-procedural pericardial effusion was observed in patients discharged with versus those without OAC (5.3% vs 1.8%; P = .008).[25] Consistently, in the propensity-matched analysis including 1527 patients enrolled in the main prospective studies with Watchman 2.5, administration of OAC at discharge was associated to increase of periprocedural bleeding as compared to DAPT.[33] Against all these limitations (ie, increase in bleeding and pericardial effusion), post-LAAC antithrombotic strategies as low dose DOAC + aspirin or OAC alone have been proposed.[34] Della Rocca and colleagues recently showed in a multi-center cohort of 555 patients undergoing successful LAAC that half-doses DOAC regimen (aspirin + half dose DOAC for 45 days followed by half dose DOAC) at 13 months significantly reduced rates of DRT (0.0% vs 3.4%; P = .009), non-procedural major bleeding (0.5% vs 3.9%; P = .018), and composite of DRT, thromboembolic events, and major bleeding events (1.0% vs 9.5%; P =.002) as compared to standard antithrombotic therapy (aspirin + DOAC for

45 days followed by DAPT for 4.5 months, and then single antiplatelet therapy [SAPT]).[35] Evidence regarding OAC alone (without additional Aspirin) is accruing. The pilot ADRIFT study randomized 105 patients undergoing LAAC to receive rivaroxaban 10 mg, rivaroxaban 15 mg, or DAPT. In this underpowered study, reduced doses of rivaroxaban were associated with significantly lower thrombin generation when compared with DAPT and no DRT were observed in both OAC groups at 3-month imaging follow-up (0% vs 0% vs 6.1%).[36] Consistently, a recent analysis of the American registry including 31,994 AF patients treated with Watchman 2.5 implantation in the 2 year period 2016 to 2018, showed that the adjusted risk of any adverse event through the 45-day follow-up visit were significantly lower for patients discharged on warfarin alone (HR: 0.692; 95%CI: 0.569–0.841) and DOAC alone (HR: 0.731; 95% CI: 0.574–0.930) as compared with VKA and Aspirin.[30]

Collectively, short-term OAC (VKA or DOAC) in combination with aspirin for at least 45 days is the most studied antithrombotic regimen after LAAC in patients deemed eligible for short-term OAC and undergoing Watchman implantation. Patients undergoing LAAC due to recurrent minor bleedings under OAC, thromboembolic events under OAC, reduced OAC compliance/tolerance, or OAC refusal might represent good candidates for this regimen. Low-dose DOAC + aspirin or OAC alone represent promising alternative drug regimens that still need to be tested in adequately powered RCTs.

Patients not Eligible for Short-term Oral Anticoagulants

Patients with AF represent a very large and heterogeneous population in clinical practice including patients who for various reasons cannot tolerate OAC. Patients with very high bleeding risk were typically excluded by the FDA approval RCTs of Watchman and Amulet (where only patients deemed eligible for OAC were included, and patients with thrombocytopenia or anemia requiring transfusions or life expectancy <2 years were excluded).[23–25] As a consequence, de-escalation of post-LAAC antithrombotic regimens with the aim of reducing the bleeding risk without significantly increasing DRT and ischemic events, is strongly needed (see Table 2). The progressive improvement of technical success observed in the recent studies as compared to the 2 pivotal Watchman RCTs (0.9%–2.7% vs 5%–12%),[17,26] and the introduction of new iteration devices as Watchman FLX (correlated to lower risk of DRT as compared to the previous Watchman 2.5)[37]

might further justify a less intensive antithrombotic therapy following LAAC. In this scenario, regimens as short-term DAPT (1–3 months) or SAPT alone have been proposed.

DAPT was the most frequently used antithrombotic regimen in the context of the 2 largest multicenter real-life LAAC studies so far performed outside of the US.[26,38] The Ewolution study was a multicentre, prospective, observational study including 1025 LAAC with the Watchman 2.5 device.[26] A high-risk AF population was included with a mean CHA2DS2-VASc (4.5±1.6) and HASBLED (2.3 ±1.2) score significantly higher as compared to those of previous large multicenter studies conducted in the US with the same device and a frequent history of ischemic/hemorrhagic stroke (in more than one-third of population). The study showed a high procedural safety (2.7% of procedural complications), a high technical success (98.5%), and a low annual stroke rate (1.4% vs an expected rate based on CHA2DS2-VASc Score of 7.5%). However, unlike what occurred in the 2 pivotal Watchman RCTs and their subsequent continued access registries,[23,24,39] the majority of patients were discharged under DAPT (60%) followed by OAC alone (27%), SAPT (7%), and no therapy (6%) with no patients discharged under combined OAC + SAPT therapy. At 2-months after procedure, TEE-follow-up showed a DRT rate of 3.7% without any association to the discharge antithrombotic regimen (P = .14).[40] A sub-analysis including 605 LAAC patients discharged under DAPT suggested that most patients were deemed ineligible to OAC (83.8%).[41] Of note, major bleeding was a common adverse event observed at 1 year (2.7%), especially within the first 6 months, with a significant reduction in the subsequent months after switching to aspirin monotherapy. Similar results were observed in the Amulet registry, a large prospective multicenter observational study performed outside of US with Amulet device.[42] This study included 1088 high risk AF patients (75±8.5 years, 64.5% male, mean CHA2DS2-VASc: 4.2±1.6, mean HAS-BLED: 3.3±1.1). Similar to the Ewolution study, the majority of patients were discharged under DAPT (54.3%) with encouraging outcomes despite the high-risk population treated and the low percentage of patients discharged under OAC (approximately one-tenth): 3.2% of procedural complications, 1.5% of DRT at 1 to 3 month-TEE (well-distributed among the different discharge antithrombotic regimens), and ischemic stroke (2.2% observed vs 6.7% expected based on CHA2DS2-VASc Score). Of note, the major bleeding rate during the first year was

10.1% (higher than that observed in the Ewolution study due to the higher bleeding risk population: mean HASBLED Score 3.3 vs 2.3; history of bleeding 72% vs 31.3%) with the majority of bleedings occurring within 3 months after LAAC (and so prior to when most patients switched to SAPT).[42]

Very few studies compared post-implantation antithrombotic drug regimen with versus without OAC. Sondergaard and colleagues performed a propensity score matching analysis to compare in a cohort of 1527 patients treated with Watchman, both safety and efficacy of the combined therapy OAC (95% VKA) plus Aspirin versus antiplatelet therapy (91% on DAPT). At 6 months after LAAC, the authors did not observe any difference between groups in terms of non-procedural thromboembolic (98.8% vs 99.4%; $P = .089$) or major bleeding events (95.7% vs 95.5%; $P = .775$). However, DRT was higher in the antiplatelet group (3.1% vs 1.4% in the anticoagulation group; $P = .014$), even after excluding patients discharged under SAPT (3.3% vs 1.1%, $P = .005$).[33] However, due to the non-randomized design of the study, no definitive conclusion could be drawn from this comparison.

The evidence coming from pharmacologic studies comparing OAC versus DAPT in terms of thromboembolic and bleeding events in patients with AF suggested that DAPT does not provide any significant benefit in terms of major bleeding prevention as compared to OAC (RR:1.10; 95% CI: 0.83–1.45; $P = .530$).[43] For that reason, patients with high major bleeding risk (eg, diffuse intracranial amyloid angiopathy, history of intracranial bleeding, special blood cell dyscrasia, bowel angiodysplasia, etc.) might require a further de-escalation of post-interventional drug regimen. In the Amulet Observational Study almost half of patients discharged under DAPT switched to SAPT within 3 months after LAAC, mainly due to extreme bleeding risk or recurrent bleeding episodes.[42] Nielsen-Kudsk and colleagues compared by means of a propensity score-matching analysis 151 AF patients submitted to LAAC following intracranial bleeding and discharged under SAPT (in 93% of cases) with other 151 AF patients with history of intracranial bleeding and submitted to standard medical therapy (identified from the Danish Stroke Registry). A lower rate of composite of all-cause mortality, ischaemic stroke, and major bleeding was found in the LAAC group as compared to those treated with standard medical care (HR: 0.16; 95%CI: 0.07–0.37).[44] Korsholm and colleagues observed, in a single-center experience including

107 consecutive patients treated with LAAC and discharged under SAPT (in 88% of cases), a relatively low rate of DRT (1.9%), stroke (2.3%), and bleeding (6.5%) after a median follow-up of 2.3 years.[45] Consistently, Pouru and colleagues showed in a monocentric study including 165 consecutive patients undergoing LAAC followed by SAPT regimen a low annual rate of major bleedings (3.6%) and cerebrovascular events (1.7%) after 3 years of follow-up.[46] Finally, Patti and colleagues observed in a retrospective multicenter observational study including 610 consecutive LAACs, that SAPT was independently associated with reduction of major bleeding (2.9% vs 6.7%, $P = .038$; adj HR 0.37; 95%CI: 0.16–0.88; $P = .024$), and with no significant increase of composite of major adverse cardiovascular events or DRT (7.8% vs 7.4%; adj HR 1.34; 95%CI: 0.70–2.55; $P=.38$).[47] Further evidence will be available after the completion of the ongoing ARMYDA-AMULET trial (ClinicalTrials.gov NCT05554822), an RCT comparing SAPT versus DAPT (with clopidogrel for 3 months) in terms of composite of all-cause death, DRT, major bleedings, ischemic stroke, or systemic embolisms at 6 months after LAAC.

Collectively, either short DAPT (1–3 months) followed by SAPT or SAPT alone are common post-LAAC antithrombotic regimens outside of the US and are valid alternatives to the standard combined antithrombotic regimen in patients not eligible for short-term OAC. Although these 2 regimens have never been tested in an RCT, the current evidence does not suggest increased hazards in DRT or thromboembolic events.

SUMMARY

Following LAAC, antithrombotic therapy is required to prevent DRT development on the atrial surface of device before endothelialization is complete. Many patients undergoing LAAC are ineligible for OAC and do not qualify for the post-LAAC standard treatment (ie, OAC plus aspirin for 45 days). The accumulated observational evidence suggests that a de-escalation of the antithrombotic therapy (ie, short DAPT or SAPT) may be considered after LAAC without excess in DRT or thromboembolic events. However, adequately powered RCTs comparing different post-LAAC drug regimens in high bleeding risk patients with adequate power for clinical and imaging (ie, DRT) endpoints are highly needed in order to better understand the optimal antithrombotic regimen treatment after LAAC in this high-risk population.

CLINICS CARE POINTS

- Percutaneous LAAC is recommended to prevent ischemic stroke in patients with atrial fibrillation and major bleedings due to a non-reversible cause.

- Management of antithrombotic therapy before starting LAAC procedure has not yet been standardized.

- During LAAC procedure, unfractionated heparin should be used as first-line intraprocedural antithrombotic medication with a target ACT greater than 250 seconds.

- The post-LAAC antithrombotic regimen should be tailored primarily according to the individual bleeding risk. Patients deemed eligible for short-term OAC can be submitted to the standard treatments recommended by the instructions for use of LAAC devices. Alternatively, patients with high bleeding risk should receive short DAPT or SAPT.

DISCLOSURES

R. Galea reports no relationships relevant to the contents of this paper to disclose. L. Raber reports research grants to institution by Abbott Vascular, United States, Boston-Scientific, Biotronik, Germany, InfraRedx, United States, HeartFlow, United States, Sanofi, United States, Regeneron and Swiss National Science Foundation. He reports speaker/consultation fees by Abbott-Vascular, Amgen, AstraZeneca, Canon, Novo Nordisk, Medtronic, Occlutech, Sanofi.

REFERENCES

1. Cresti A, Garcia-Fernandez MA, Sievert H, et al. Prevalence of extra-appendage thrombosis in non-valvular atrial fibrillation and atrial flutter in patients undergoing cardioversion: a large transoesophageal echo study. EuroIntervention 2019;15:e225–30.

2. Glikson M, Wolff R, Hindricks G, et al. EHRA/EAPCI expert consensus statement on catheter-based left atrial appendage occlusion - an update. EuroIntervention 2020;15:1133–80.

3. Kar S, Doshi SK, Alkhouli M, et al. Rationale and design of a randomized study comparing the Watchman FLX device to DOACs in patients with atrial fibrillation. Am Heart J 2023;264:123–32.

4. Reddy VY, Doshi SK, Kar S, et al. 5-Year Outcomes After Left Atrial Appendage Closure: From the PREVAIL and PROTECT AF Trials. J Am Coll Cardiol 2017;70:2964–75.

5. Writing Committee M, Joglar JA, Chung MK, et al. 2023 ACC/AHA/ACCP/HRS Guideline for the Diagnosis and Management of Atrial Fibrillation: A Report of the American College of Cardiology/American Heart Association Joint Committee on Clinical Practice Guidelines. J Am Coll Cardiol 2023;83(1):109–279.

6. Camm AJ. Leap or lag: left atrial appendage closure and guidelines. Europace 2023;25(5):euad067.

7. Hindricks G, Potpara T, Dagres N, et al. 2020 ESC Guidelines for the diagnosis and management of atrial fibrillation developed in collaboration with the European Association for Cardio-Thoracic Surgery (EACTS): The Task Force for the diagnosis and management of atrial fibrillation of the European Society of Cardiology (ESC) Developed with the special contribution of the European Heart Rhythm Association (EHRA) of the ESC. Eur Heart J 2021;42:373–498.

8. Galea R, Aminian A, Meneveau N, et al. Impact of Preprocedural Computed Tomography on Left Atrial Appendage Closure Success: A Swiss-Apero Trial Subanalysis. JACC Cardiovasc Interv 2023;16:1332–43.

9. Galea RRL, Fuerholz M, Häner J, et al. Impact of echocardiographic guidance on safety and efficacy of left atrial appendage closure: an observational study. JACC Cardiovasc Interv 2021;14:1815–26.

10. Saw J, Holmes DR, Cavalcante JL, et al. SCAI/HRS Expert Consensus Statement on Transcatheter Left Atrial Appendage Closure. JACC Cardiovasc Interv 2023;16:1384–400.

11. Galea R, Grani C. Device neo-endothelialization after left atrial appendage closure: the role of cardiac computed tomography angiography. Int J Cardiovasc Imag 2021;37(7):2299–301.

12. Fountain RB, Holmes DR, Chandrasekaran K, et al. The PROTECT AF (WATCHMAN Left Atrial Appendage System for Embolic PROTECTion in Patients with Atrial Fibrillation) trial. Am Heart J 2006;151:956–61.

13. Lakkireddy D, Windecker S, Thaler D, et al. Rationale and design for AMPLATZER Amulet Left Atrial Appendage Occluder IDE randomized controlled trial (Amulet IDE Trial). Am Heart J 2019;211:45–53.

14. Holmes DR Jr, Korsholm K, Rodes-Cabau J, et al. Left atrial appendage occlusion. EuroIntervention 2023;18:e1038–65.

15. Weise FK, Bordignon S, Perrotta L, et al. Short-term dual antiplatelet therapy after interventional left atrial appendage closure with different devices. EuroIntervention 2018;13:e2138–46.

16. Galea R, De Marco F, Aminian A, et al. Design and Rationale of the Swiss-Apero Randomized Clinical Trial: Comparison of Amplatzer Amulet vs Watchman Device in Patients Undergoing Left Atrial Appendage Closure. J Cardiovasc Transl Res 2021;14(5):930–40.

17. Kar S, Doshi SK, Sadhu A, et al. Primary Outcome Evaluation of a Next-Generation Left Atrial Appendage Closure Device: Results From the PINNACLE FLX Trial. Circulation 2021;143:1754–62.

18. Zhang X, Jin Q, Kong D, et al. Clinical outcomes of bivalirudin versus heparin in atrial fibrillation patients undergoing percutaneous left atrial appendage occlusion. Ann Transl Med 2021;9:629.

19. Galea RRL. Antithrombotic Therapy after Percutaneous Left Atrial Appendage Closure: Evidence, Challenges and Future Directions. Rev Cardiovasc Med 2023;24:343.

20. Bass JL. Transcatheter occlusion of the left atrial appendage–experimental testing of a new Amplatzer device. Cathet Cardiovasc Interv 2010;76:181–5.

21. Massarenti L, Yilmaz A. Incomplete endothelialization of left atrial appendage occlusion device 10 months after implantation. J Cardiovascular Electrophysiol 2012;23:1384–5.

22. Schwartz RS, Holmes DR, Van Tassel RA, et al. Left atrial appendage obliteration: mechanisms of healing and intracardiac integration. JACC Cardiovasc Interv 2010;3:870–7.

23. Holmes DR Jr, Kar S, Price MJ, et al. Prospective randomized evaluation of the Watchman Left Atrial Appendage Closure device in patients with atrial fibrillation versus long-term warfarin therapy: the PREVAIL trial. J Am Coll Cardiol 2014;64:1–12.

24. Holmes DR, Reddy VY, Turi ZG, et al. Percutaneous closure of the left atrial appendage versus warfarin therapy for prevention of stroke in patients with atrial fibrillation: a randomised non-inferiority trial. Lancet 2009;374:534–42.

25. Lakkireddy D, Thaler D, Ellis CR, et al. Amplatzer Amulet Left Atrial Appendage Occluder Versus Watchman Device for Stroke Prophylaxis (Amulet IDE): A Randomized, Controlled Trial. Circulation 2021;144:1543–52.

26. Boersma LV, Schmidt B, Betts TR, et al. Implant success and safety of left atrial appendage closure with the WATCHMAN device: peri-procedural outcomes from the EWOLUTION registry. Eur Heart J 2016;37:2465–74.

27. Landmesser U, Tondo C, Camm J, et al. Left atrial appendage occlusion with the AMPLATZER Amulet device: one-year follow-up from the prospective global Amulet observational registry. EuroIntervention 2018;14:e590–7.

28. Galea R, De Marco F, Meneveau N, et al. Amulet or Watchman Device for Percutaneous Left Atrial Appendage Closure: Primary Results of the SWISS-APERO Randomized Clinical Trial. Circulation 2021;145(10):724–38.

29. Galea R, Meneveau N, De Marco F, et al. One-year outcomes after amulet or watchman device for percutaneous left atrial appendage closure: a pre-specified analysis of the SWISS-APERO randomized clinical trial. Circulation 2024;149(6):484–6.

30. Freeman JV, Higgins AY, Wang Y, et al. Antithrombotic Therapy After Left Atrial Appendage Occlusion in Patients With Atrial Fibrillation. J Am Coll Cardiol 2022;79:1785–98.

31. Reddy VY, Sievert H, Halperin J, et al. Percutaneous left atrial appendage closure vs warfarin for atrial fibrillation: a randomized clinical trial. JAMA 2014;312:1988–98.

32. Lakkireddy DTD, Ellis CR, Swarup V, et al. 3-Year Outcomes from the AmplatzerTMAmuletTMLeft Atrial Appendage OccluderRandomized Controlled Trial (Amulet IDE). JACC Cardiovasc Interv 2022;16(15):1902–13.

33. Sondergaard L, Wong YH, Reddy VY, et al. Propensity-Matched Comparison of Oral Anticoagulation Versus Antiplatelet Therapy After Left Atrial Appendage Closure With WATCHMAN. JACC Cardiovasc Interv 2019;12:1055–63.

34. Price MJ, Slotwiner D, Du C, et al. Clinical Outcomes at 1 Year Following Transcatheter Left Atrial Appendage Occlusion in the United States. JACC Cardiovasc Interv 2022;15:741–50.

35. Della Rocca DG, Magnocavallo M, Di Biase L, et al. Half-Dose Direct Oral Anticoagulation Versus Standard Antithrombotic Therapy After Left Atrial Appendage Occlusion. JACC Cardiovasc Interv 2021;14:2353–64.

36. Duthoit G, Silvain J, Marijon E, et al. Reduced Rivaroxaban Dose Versus Dual Antiplatelet Therapy After Left Atrial Appendage Closure: ADRIFT a Randomized Pilot Study. Circulation Cardiovascular interventions 2020;13:e008481.

37. Galea R, Mahmoudi K, Grani C, et al. Watchman FLX vs. Watchman 2.5 in a Dual-Center Left Atrial Appendage Closure Cohort: the WATCH-DUAL study. Europace 2022;24(9):1441–50.

38. Landmesser U, Schmidt B, Nielsen-Kudsk JE, et al. Left atrial appendage occlusion with the AMPLATZER Amulet device: periprocedural and early clinical/echocardiographic data from a global prospective observational study. EuroIntervention 2017;13:867–76.

39. Holmes DR Jr, Alkhouli M. Comparison of cardiac computed tomography angiography and transoesophageal echocardiography for device surveillance after left atrial appendage closure. What we see depends on where we are looking from and what we are looking for. EuroIntervention 2019;15:650–1.

40. Boersma LV, Ince H, Kische S, et al. Efficacy and safety of left atrial appendage closure with WATCHMAN in patients with or without contraindication to oral anticoagulation: 1-Year follow-up outcome data of the EWOLUTION trial. Heart Rhythm 2017;14:1302–8.

41. Bergmann MW, Ince H, Kische S, et al. Real-world safety and efficacy of WATCHMAN LAA closure at one year in patients on dual antiplatelet therapy: results of the DAPT subgroup from the EWOLU-TION all-comers study. EuroIntervention 2018;13: 2003–11.

42. Hildick-Smith D, Landmesser U, Camm AJ, et al. Left atrial appendage occlusion with the Amplatzer Amulet device: full results of the prospective global observational study. Eur Heart J 2020;41(30):2894–901.

43. Investigators AWGotA, Connolly S, Pogue J, et al. Clopidogrel plus aspirin versus oral anticoagulation for atrial fibrillation in the Atrial fibrillation Clopidogrel Trial with Irbesartan for prevention of Vascular Events (ACTIVE W): a randomised controlled trial. Lancet 2006;367:1903–12.

44. Nielsen-Kudsk JE, Johnsen SP, Wester P, et al. Left atrial appendage occlusion versus standard medical care in patients with atrial fibrillation and intracerebral haemorrhage: a propensity score-matched follow-up study. EuroIntervention 2017;13:371–8.

45. Korsholm K, Nielsen KM, Jensen JM, et al. Transcatheter left atrial appendage occlusion in patients with atrial fibrillation and a high bleeding risk using aspirin alone for post-implant antithrombotic therapy. EuroIntervention 2017;12:2075–82.

46. Pouru JP, Lund J, Jaakkola S, et al. Percutaneous left atrial appendage closure in patients with prior intracranial bleeding and thromboembolism. Heart Rhythm 2020;17:915–21.

47. Patti G, Sticchi A, Verolino G, et al. Safety and Efficacy of Single Versus Dual Antiplatelet Therapy After Left Atrial Appendage Occlusion. Am J Cardiol 2020;134:83–90.

Antithrombotic Therapy in Patients Undergoing Peripheral Artery Interventions

Mario Enrico Canonico, MD, PhD[a,b,*],
Connie N. Hess, MD, MHS[a,b],
Eric A. Secemsky, MD, MSc[c,d],
Marc P. Bonaca, MD, MPH[a,b]

KEYWORDS

- Antithrombotic therapy • Lower extremity revascularization
- Major adverse cardiovascular events • Major adverse limb events • Dual pathway inhibition
- Major bleeding

KEY POINTS

- Peripheral artery disease patients who undergo lower extremity revascularization (LER) are at heightened risk of major adverse cardiovascular events (MACE) and major adverse limb events (MALE).
- Randomized controlled trials examining the role of full-dose oral anticoagulants after LER showed no benefit in terms of ischemic events prevention with an increase of major bleeding.
- RCTs of dual antiplatelet therapy have not provided a clear benefit in long-term patency of LER.
- Dual pathway inhibition (DPI) strategy after LER with a low-dose anticoagulant and single antiplatelet dosage has demonstrated a reduction in MACE and MALE without significantly higher rates of major bleeding.
- Implementation strategies can improve the adoption of DPI in clinical practice.

INTRODUCTION

Peripheral artery disease (PAD) encompasses a spectrum of pathology mainly affecting the lower extremity. The prevalence of lower extremity PAD has been increasing during the last decades and currently affects 230 million worldwide.[1] PAD includes different clinical features from asymptomatic to symptomatic patients, as well as those with more advanced disease such as acute limb ischemia (ALI), chronic limb-threatening ischemia (CLTI), previous lower extremity revascularization (LER), and history of amputation due to vascular etiologies.[2,3] Cardiovascular (CV) risk associated with PAD is both related to the vascular history as well as patient profile. In particular, PAD patients who have undergone LER are at heightened risk of subsequent major adverse cardiovascular events (MACE) and major adverse limb events (MALE).[4] In particular, the risk of acute limb ischemia (ALI) and amputation for vascular etiologies is particularly high in the few months after LER and continues over the long term.[4] In addition, the risk of MACE, including myocardial infarction (MI) and ischemic

Funding: The authors did not receive support from any organization for the submitted work.
[a] CPC Clinical Research, Aurora, CO, USA; [b] Division of Cardiology, Department of Medicine, University of Colorado School of Medicine, Aurora, CO, USA; [c] Richard A. and Susan F.Smith Center for Outcomes Research in Cardiology and Division of Cardiovascular Medicine, Beth Israel Deaconess Medical Center, Boston, MA, USA; [d] Harvard Medical School, MA, USA
* Corresponding author. University of Colorado SOM, 2115 N Scranton Street #2040, Aurora, CO 80045-7120
E-mail address: marioenrico.canonico@cpcmed.org
Twitter: @me_canonico (M.E.C.); @cpcresearch (C.N.H.); @EricSecemskyMD (E.A.S.); @MarcBonaca (M.P.B.)

stroke (IS), are persistently increased after LER.[4] The optimal management of symptomatic patients referred for LER is crucial in order to mitigate the risk of subsequent adverse events. Antithrombotic therapies represent one critical strategy for reducing adverse ischemic events among PAD patients following recent LER.[5,6] However, balancing bleeding risks with antithrombotic agents is critical. Bleeding scores commonly used in clinical practice were specifically derived for coronary artery disease (CAD) and atrial fibrillation management, with less evidence for those with PAD. The OAC[3]-PAD bleeding risk score, developed from more than 80,000 PAD patients, predicts major bleeding events after 1-year from hospitalization for a vascular condition. The score divides PAD patients in 4 groups according to bleeding risk and considers clinical features such as oral anticoagulation use, age > 80 years, and presence of CLTI, congestive heart failure, chronic kidney disease (CKD), prior bleeding event, anemia, and dementia.[7]

Historically, data on antithrombotic therapy in PAD patients originated from larger randomized controlled trials (RCTs) in the CAD population.[2,3] Previous PAD guidelines from 2016 do not include strong recommendations regarding type of antiplatelet therapy or its duration after LER[2,3] More recently, new evidence on antithrombotic therapy post LER has arisen from a dedicated RCT focusing on the management of post-revascularization PAD, supporting novel pharmacologic strategies to improve CV and limb outcomes while balancing safety.

The purpose of this article is to review the current evidence, including RCTs, observational studies, and systematic reviews on antithrombotic therapy in PAD patients undergoing LER, considering different clinical scenarios such as endovascular, surgical, or hybrid revascularization. The efficacy and safety of the different antithrombotic strategies in PAD patients following LER will be reviewed and includes oral anticoagulants, dual antiplatelet therapy (DAPT), and dual pathway inhibition (DPI) utilizing low-dose antithrombotics and single antiplatelet therapy. The key RCTs focused on PAD patients after LER are listed in Table 1.

ANTICOAGULATION THERAPY

Full-dose oral anticoagulation is one antithrombotic strategy that has been assessed in PAD patients who have undergone LER. In these comparative studies, the control arm has usually been represented by a single antiplatelet therapy (SAPT) with aspirin or DAPT with aspirin and clopidogrel. The rationale for these studies was to sustain the patency of bypass/endovascular intervention by oral anticoagulation. More than 20 years ago, an RCT assessed the long-term benefit of warfarin plus aspirin compared to aspirin alone in PAD patients who underwent lower extremity bypass. The combination therapy did not improve patency in terms of occlusion in prosthetic bypass conduits (risk ratio [RR] 0.62; 95% confidence interval [95% CI] 0.42–1.92) as well as vein bypass conduits (RR 1.04; 95% CI 0.72–1.51). Moreover, the warfarin plus aspirin group increased the secondary outcome of death (RR 1.41; 95% CI 1.09–1.84). Finally, major bleeding events were 35 in the combination and 15 in aspirin group, respectively ($P = .02$).[8] Oral anticoagulation alone was subsequently evaluated in The Dutch Bypass Oral anticoagulants or Aspirin (Dutch BOA) study, which randomized patients who underwent infrainguinal grafting to warfarin versus aspirin. No differences were detected for the primary efficacy outcome including vascular death, MI, stroke, or amputation (hazard ratio [HR] 0.89; 95% CI 0.75–1.06), but there was an increase of major bleeding in the warfarin arm (HR 1.96; 95% CI 1.42–1.71).[9] Direct oral anticoagulants have also been assessed after LER. The Edoxaban in Peripheral Arterial Disease (ePAD) study compared a strategy including edoxaban plus aspirin versus DAPT with aspirin and clopidogrel between PAD patients following endovascular LER. The rates of restenosis/reocclusion of femoropopliteal target lesion were equivocal (HR 0.89; 95% CI 0.59–1.34) with no significant differences in Thrombolysis in Myocardial Infarction (TIMI) bleeding between groups (HR 0.56; 95% CI 0.19–1.62).[10] It is important to note that the ePAD trial was not adequately powered to assess the efficacy and safety of edoxaban.

Unless otherwise indicated, full-dose anticoagulation should not be the treatment of choice for PAD patients following LER. The European Society of Cardiology (ESC) guidelines on PAD include a weak indication (ie, IIb) for vitamin K antagonists in patients who have underwent surgical LER.[3][2] The 2024 American Heart Association (AHA)/American College of Cardiology (ACC) lower extremity PAD guidelines recommend that in patients who do not have another indication (eg, atrial fibrillation), full-intensity oral anticoagulation should not be used to reduce the risk of MACE or MALE (Class 3, Level of Evidence–LOE A).[11]

Table 1
Key antithrombotic trials in patients with peripheral artery disease who underwent lower extremity revascularization

Trial	Patients	Type of LER	Treatment	Follow-up	Results Efficacy	Safety
Dutch BOA[9]	2,690	Infrainguinal arterial grafting	Oral anticoagulant (phenprocoumon or acenocoumarol; coumarin derivatives) vs Aspirin equivalent	21 mo	No difference in graft occlusion (HR 0.95; 95% CI, 0.82–1.11) No difference in the composite of vascular mortality, MI, stroke, or amputation (HR 0.89; 95% CI, 0.75–1.06)	Increase in severe bleeding (HR 1.96; 95% CI, 1.42–2.71)
ePAD[10]	203	Endovascular	Edoxaban + Aspirin vs Aspirin + Clopidogrel	3 mo	No difference in restenosis or reocclusion of femoropopliteal targets (HR 0.89; 95% CI, 0.59–1.34)	No difference in bleeding (RR 0.56; 95%CI, 0.19–1.62)
CASPAR[12]	851	Below-knee bypass grafting	Clopidogrel + Aspirin vs Placebo + Aspirin	24 mo	No reduction in the composite of graft occlusion, revascularization, major amputation, or death (HR 0.98; 95% CI, 0.78–1.23)	No difference in severe bleeding (2.1% vs 1.2%)
MIRROR[13]	80	Endovascular	Clopidogrel + Aspirin vs Placebo + Aspirin	6 mo	Decreased risk of target lesion revascularization (5% vs 8%, P = .04) at 6 mo but no difference at 1 y (25% vs 32%, P = .35)	No increase in bleeding (2.5% vs 5%, P = .56)
VOYAGER-PAD[18]	6,564	Endovascular or Surgical	Rivaroxaban + Aspirin vs Placebo + Aspirin	3 y	Reduction of MACE and MALE (HR 0.85; 95% CI, 0.76–0.96)	No difference in TIMI major bleeding (HR 1.43; 95% CI, 0.97–2.10) increase in ISTH major bleeding (HR 1.42; 95% CI, 1.10–1.84)

Abbreviations: CI: confidence interval; HR: hazard ratio; ISTH: international society on thrombosis and haemostasis; LER: lower extremity revascularization; MACE: major adverse cardiovascular events; MALE: major adverse limb events; MI: myocardial infarction; TIMI: thrombolysis in myocardial infarction.

DUAL ANTIPLATELET THERAPY

Dual antiplatelet therapy (DAPT) including aspirin plus clopidogrel represents another antithrombotic strategy assessed in PAD patients undergoing LER. The purpose of a more aggressive antiplatelet therapy after LER is to reduce the subsequent risk of limb and CV events but with hopes for a comparable safety profile compared to SAPT. The randomized, placebo-controlled clopidogrel and acetylsalicylic acid in bypass surgery for peripheral arterial disease (CASPAR) trial compared DAPT with aspirin and clopidogrel versus aspirin alone in patients who underwent below the knee (BTK) bypass grafting. No differences were detected in the primary efficacy endpoint of index-graft occlusion/revascularization, above the ankle amputation or death (HR 0.98; 95% CI 0.78–1.23). The total bleeding rate was more than 2-fold higher in the DAPT versus SAPT arm (16.7% vs 7.1%, $P < .001$) with no differences in Global Use of Streptokinase and t-PA for Occluded Coronary Arteriessevere bleeding (2.1% vs 1.2% respectively, P = NS).[12] Similarly, finders were present for patients who underwent endovascular LER. Separately, the Management of peripheral arterial interventions with mono or dual antiplatelet therapy (the MIRROR study) compared DAPT (ie, aspirin plus clopidogrel) versus SAPT (ie, aspirin) after endovascular LER. Despite the lower rate of target lesion revascularization (TLR) at 6 months in the DAPT group (5% vs 8%, P = .04), there was no benefit at 1-year (25% vs 32%, P = NS). There were no differences in bleeding complications at 6-month follow-up (2.5% vs 5.0%, P = NS).[13] Similar results were highlighted by a single-center RCT comparing DAPT (ie, aspirin plus clopidogrel) versus SAPT (ie, aspirin) on TLR after LER in femoropopliteal segment, which demonstrated that DAPT reduced 6-month TLR (5% vs 20%, P = .04) with no differences in mortality at 6 months.[14]

DAPT after LER provides mixed results in terms of ischemic benefits without a significant increase in terms of safety. The ESC PAD guidelines include 1-month DAPT after endovascular LER as class IIa.[2,3] The new 2024 American College of Cardiology (ACC)/ American Heart Association (AHA) guidelines recommend that after endovascular revascularization for PAD, DAPT with a P2Y$_{12}$ antagonist and low-dose aspirin is reasonable for at least 1 to 6 months (Class 2a, LOE C), while after surgical revascularization for PAD with a prosthetic graft, DAPT with a P2Y$_{12}$ antagonist and low-dose aspirin

may be reasonable for at least 1 month (Class 2b, LOE B).[11]

DUAL PATHWAY INHIBITION THERAPY

Dual pathway inhibition (DPI) has more recently emerged as a new antithrombotic strategy in PAD patients after LER. The inhibition of thrombus generation by platelet and thrombin antagonism represents the mechanism of action of DPI.[15] Histopathological studies on PAD patients identified that thrombotic occlusion is often present with BTK disease among patients with CLTI undergoing amputation, even in the absence of significant atherosclerosis.[16] Moreover, in PAD patients with prior LER, the occurrence of MALE including ALI has been found to be driven by atherothrombosis as well as embolism from proximal vessels.[17]

The only RCT that has assessed the efficacy and safety of DPI in PAD patients specifically after LER is the Vascular Outcomes Study of ASA (acetylsalicylic acid) Along with Rivaroxaban in Endovascular or Surgical Limb Revascularization for PAD (peripheral artery disease) (VOYAGER PAD) trial. The study randomized participants to aspirin plus low-dose rivaroxaban 2.5 mg twice daily vs aspirin and placebo. The use of clopidogrel was up to the discretion of physicians but limited to no more than 6 months. The primary indications for LER included claudication in 76% and CLTI in 24%. The LER strategy was endovascular in 65% and surgical in 35%. Compared to aspirin, the DPI strategy decreased the risk of the primary endpoint of MACE and MALE (HR 0.85; 95% CI 0.76–0.96) with no increase of the primary safety outcome of TIMI major bleeding (HR 1.43; 95% CI 0.97–2.10). The risk of major bleeding based on the International Society on Thrombosis and Haemostasis (ISTH) categorization was higher in the DPI group (HR 1.42; 95% CI 1.10–1.84).[18] From these results, it has been estimated that for every 10,000 patients treated by rivaroxaban for 1 year, 181 ischemic events would be prevented counterbalanced by 29 bleeding events caused. In the VOYAGER-PAD trial, the median time of randomization from LER to treatment initiation was 5 days, suggesting the benefit of an early initiation of DPI after LER. Further analyses have demonstrated the efficacy of DPI on the primary endpoint regardless of the use of clopidogrel (with HR 0.85; 95% CI 0.71–1.01 and without HR 0.86; 95% CI 0.73–1.01) with a greater risk of ISTH-classified major bleeding with and without clopidogrel (HR 1.36; 95% CI 0.96–1.92 and HR 1.50; 95% CI 1.02–2.20).[19]

Robust benefit for rivaroxaban has also been shown for reduction of total vascular events, including MACE, MALE, peripheral revascularization, and venous thromboembolism (HR 0.86; 95% CI: 0.79–0.95).[20] Finally, the efficacy of DPI was consistent even in high-risk population, such as those aged more than 75 years and those with concomitant CKD or polyvascular disease.[21–23]

The recent and updated ESC consensus paper has endorsed the prescription of DPI in patients who have undergone LER and are without high bleeding risk, irrespective of the use of clopidogrel.[24] The new 2024 ACC/AHA PAD guidelines recommend that after endovascular or surgical revascularization for PAD, low-dose rivaroxaban (2.5 mg twice daily) combined with low-dose aspirin is recommended to reduce the risk of MACE and MALE (Class 1 LOE A).[11]

FUTURE DIRECTIONS

Antithrombotic therapy among patients with PAD undergoing LER includes new evidence supporting the efficacy of DPI with aspirin and low-dose rivaroxaban. Moreover, there is a great interest for future agents which can balance bleeding risks while maintaining effectiveness at reducing ischemic events, such as holds promise with factor XI inhibitors.[25] However, data about their efficacy in PAD patients remain needed.

The initiation of DPI represents a challenge in clinical practice, with issue on finding optimal opportunities to start treatment. A hospitalization for limb revascularization represents a unique opportunity to start DPI with the goal of preventing short-term and long-term ischemic events. Nonetheless, there remains suboptimal adoption of PAD therapy in the real-world. A recent analysis of prescriptions of guideline-directed medical therapies highlights the low adoption rates of PAD medications including antiplatelet agents.[26] Moreover, a European multicenter registry including 225 participants highlighted the low prescription of DPI, with use limited to 15% after endovascular or surgical LER and broad variability between countries and taxonomy of physicians.[27] Further reasons for variable adoption may include health disparities (ie, sex, ethnicity, race, and income) as well as different local coverage of DPI. Implementation studies that have included remote follow-up can represent a strategy to enhance the prescription of these agents as well as promote long-term adherence. Recently, this strategy has provided positive results for optimizing lipid-lowering therapies among PAD patients.[28]

SUMMARY

PAD patients who have undergone LER have a high CV risk profile in terms of MACE and MALE. DPI including aspirin and low-dose rivaroxaban has demonstrated benefits in CV and limb outcomes with favorable balance of limiting major bleeding risks. Further efforts are needed to implement the adoption of this newer antithrombotic strategy at a large scale in routine practice.

CLINICS CARE POINTS

- Dual pathway inhibition (DPI) strategy after lower extremity revascularization reduces cardiovascular and limb events.
- Efforts are needed to improve the broad adoption of DPI in patients who have undergone LER.

DISCLOSURES

Drs Canonico, Hess, Bonaca receive salary support from CPC, a non-profit academic research organization affiliated with the University of Colorado, that receives or has received research grant/consulting funding between July 2021 and July 2023 from the following organizations: Abbot Laboratories, Agios Pharmaceuticals., Alexion Pharma Godo Kaisha, Amgen Inc., Anthos Therapeutics, Inc., ARCA Biopharma., AstraZeneca Pharma India, AstraZeneca Pharmaceuticals LP, AstraZeneca UK, AstraZeneca, Produtos Farmaceuticos, LDA, Atentiv, LLC, Bayer, Bayer Limited, Bayer Aktiengesellschaft, Bayer Pharma AG, Beth Israel Deaconess Medical Center, Better Therapeutics, Boston Clinical Research Institute, LLC, Bristol-Myers Squibb, CellResearch Corporation Pte Ltd, Cleerly, Inc., Colorado Department of Public Health and Environment, Cook Regentec LLC, CSL Behring LLC, Eidos Therapeutics, Inc., EPG Communication Holdings Ltd., Esperion Therapeutics, Faraday Pharmaceuticals, Inc., HeartFlow, Insmed, Ionis Pharmaceuticals, IQVIA Inc., Janssen Pharmaceuticals, Inc, Janssen Research & Development, LLC, Janssen Scientific Affairs, LLC, Lexicon Pharmaceuticals, Inc., LSG Corporation, MedImmune Limited, Medpace, Inc., Medscape, Merck Sharp & Dohme Corp., Nectero Medical Inc., Novartis Pharmaceuticals Corporation, Novo Nordisk, Osiris Therapeutics, Pfizer, PPD Development, L.P., Prothena Biosciences Limited, Regeneron, Regents of the University of Colorado (aka UCD), Sanifit Therapeutics S.A., Sanofi, Silence Therapeutics PLC, Stanford University, Stealth BioTherapeutics Inc., The Brigham & Women's

Hospital, Inc., Thrombosis Research Institute, University of Colorado Denver, University of Pittsburgh, VarmX, WraSer, LLC. Dr Bonaca receives support from the AHA SFRN under award numbers 18SFRN3390085 (BWH-DH SFRN Center) and 18SFRN33960262 (BWH-DH Clinical Project). Dr Bonaca also reports stock in Medtronic and Pfizer.Dr Secemsky reports: Funding: NIH/NHLBIK23HL150290, Food & Drug Administration, SCAI Grants to Institution: Abbott/CSI,BD, Boston Scientific, Cook, Medtronic, Philips. Speaking/Consulting: Abbott/CSI, BD, BMS, Boston Scientific, Cagent, Conavi, Cook, Cordis, Endovascular Engineering, Gore, InfraRedx, Medtronic, Philips, RapidAI, Shockwave, Terumo, Thrombolex, VentureMed, Zoll.

REFERENCES

1. Criqui MH, Matsushita K, Aboyans V, et al. Lower Extremity Peripheral Artery Disease: Contemporary Epidemiology, Management Gaps, and Future Directions: A Scientific Statement From the American Heart Association. Circulation 2021;144(9). https://doi.org/10.1161/CIR.0000000000001005.

2. Gerhard-Herman MD, Gornik HL, Barrett C, et al. 2016 AHA/ACC Guideline on the Management of Patients With Lower Extremity Peripheral Artery Disease: Executive Summary: A Report of the American College of Cardiology/American Heart Association Task Force on Clinical Practice Guidelines. Circulation 2017;135(12). https://doi.org/10.1161/CIR.0000000000000470.

3. Aboyans V, Ricco JB, Bartelink MLEL, et al. 2017 ESC Guidelines on the Diagnosis and Treatment of Peripheral Arterial Diseases, in collaboration with the European Society for Vascular Surgery (ESVS). Eur Heart J 2018;39(9):763–816.

4. Hess CN, Wang TY, Weleski Fu J, et al. Long-Term Outcomes and Associations With Major Adverse Limb Events After Peripheral Artery Revascularization. J Am Coll Cardiol 2020;75(5):498–508.

5. King RW, Canonico ME, Bonaca MP, et al. Management of Peripheral Arterial Disease: Lifestyle Modifications and Medical Therapies. Journal of the Society for Cardiovascular Angiography and Interventions 2022;1(6). https://doi.org/10.1016/j.jscai.2022.100513.

6. Canonico ME, Hess CN, Rogers RK, et al. Medical Therapy for Peripheral Artery Disease. Curr Cardiol Rep 2024. https://doi.org/10.1007/s11886-024-02065-y.

7. Behrendt CA, Kreutzburg T, Nordanstig J, et al. The OAC3-PAD Risk Score Predicts Major Bleeding Events one Year after Hospitalisation for Peripheral Artery Disease. Eur J Vasc Endovasc Surg 2022; 63(3):503–10.

8. Johnson WC, Williford WO. Benefits, morbidity, and mortality associated with long-term administration of oral anticoagulant therapy to patients with peripheral arterial bypass procedures: A prospective randomized study. J Vasc Surg 2002; 35(3):413–21.

9. Efficacy of oral anticoagulants compared with aspirin after infrainguinal bypass surgery (The Dutch Bypass Oral anticoagulants or Aspirin study): a randomised trial. Lancet 2000;355(9201):346–51.

10. Moll F, Baumgartner I, Jaff M, et al. Edoxaban Plus Aspirin vs Dual Antiplatelet Therapy in Endovascular Treatment of Patients With Peripheral Artery Disease: Results of the ePAD Trial. J Endovasc Ther 2018;25(2):158–68.

11. Gornik HL, Aronow HD, Goodney PP, et al. 2024 ACC/AHA/AACVPR/APMA/ABC/SCAI/SVM/SVN/SVS/SIR/VESS Guideline for the Management of Lower Extremity Peripheral Artery Disease: A Report of the American College of Cardiology/American Heart Association Joint Committee on Clinical Practice Guidelines. Circulation 2024;149(24). https://doi.org/10.1161/CIR.0000000000001251.

12. Belch JJF, Dormandy J. Results of the randomized, placebo-controlled clopidogrel and acetylsalicylic acid in bypass surgery for peripheral arterial disease (CASPAR) trial. J Vasc Surg 2010;52(4):825–33.e2.

13. Tepe G, Bantleon R, Brechtel K, et al. Management of peripheral arterial interventions with mono or dual antiplatelet therapy—the MIRROR study: a randomised and double-blinded clinical trial. Eur Radiol 2012;22(9):1998–2006.

14. Strobl FF, Brechtel K, Schmehl J, et al. Twelve-Month Results of a Randomized Trial Comparing Mono With Dual Antiplatelet Therapy in Endovascularly Treated Patients With Peripheral Artery Disease. J Endovasc Ther 2013;20(5):699–706.

15. Canonico ME, Piccolo R, Avvedimento M, et al. Antithrombotic Therapy in Peripheral Artery Disease: Current Evidence and Future Directions. J Cardiovasc Dev Dis 2023;10(4). https://doi.org/10.3390/jcdd10040164.

16. Narula N, Dannenberg AJ, Olin JW, et al. Pathology of Peripheral Artery Disease in Patients With Critical Limb Ischemia. J Am Coll Cardiol 2018; 72(18):2152–63.

17. Narula N, Olin JW, Narula N. Pathologic Disparities Between Peripheral Artery Disease and Coronary Artery Disease. Arterioscler Thromb Vasc Biol 2020;40(9):1982–9.

18. Bonaca MP, Bauersachs RM, Anand SS, et al. Rivaroxaban in Peripheral Artery Disease after Revascularization. N Engl J Med 2020;382(21):1994–2004.

19. Hiatt WR, Bonaca MP, Patel MR, et al. Rivaroxaban and Aspirin in Peripheral Artery Disease Lower Extremity Revascularization. Circulation 2020;142(23): 2219–30.

20. Bauersachs RM, Szarek M, Brodmann M, et al. Total Ischemic Event Reduction With Rivaroxaban After

Peripheral Arterial Revascularization in the VOYAGER PAD Trial. J Am Coll Cardiol 2021; 78(4):317–26.

21. Krantz MJ, Debus SE, Hsia J, et al. Low-dose rivaroxaban plus aspirin in older patients with peripheral artery disease undergoing acute limb revascularization: insights from the VOYAGER PAD trial. Eur Heart J 2021;42(39):4040–8.

22. Hsia J, Szarek M, Anand S, et al. Rivaroxaban in Patients With Recent Peripheral Artery Revascularization and Renal Impairment. J Am Coll Cardiol 2021;78(7):757–9.

23. Morrison JT, Canonico ME, Anand SS, et al. Low-Dose Rivaroxaban Plus Aspirin in Patients With Peripheral Artery Disease Undergoing Lower Extremity Revascularization With and Without Concomitant Coronary Artery Disease: Insights From VOYAGER PAD. Circulation 2024;149(19):1536–9.

24. Aboyans V, Bauersachs R, Mazzolai L, et al. Antithrombotic therapies in aortic and peripheral arterial diseases in 2021: a consensus document from the ESC working group on aorta and peripheral vascular diseases, the ESC working group on thrombosis, and the ESC working group on cardiovascular pharmacotherapy. Eur Heart J 2021;42(39): 4013–24.

25. Greco A, Laudani C, Spagnolo M, et al. Pharmacology and Clinical Development of Factor XI Inhibitors. Circulation 2023;147(11):897–913.

26. Canonico ME, Hsia J, Hess CN, et al. Sex differences in guideline-directed medical therapy in 2021–22 among patients with peripheral artery disease. Vasc Med 2023. https://doi.org/10.1177/1358863X231155308. 1358863X2311553.

27. De Carlo M, Schlager O, Mazzolai L, et al. Antithrombotic therapy following revascularization for chronic limb-threatening ischaemia: a European survey from the ESC Working Group on Aorta and Peripheral Vascular Diseases. Eur Heart J Cardiovasc Pharmacother 2023;9(3):201–7.

28. Hess CN, Daffron A, Nehler MR, et al. Randomized Trial of a Vascular Care Team vs Education for Patients With Peripheral Artery Disease. J Am Coll Cardiol 2024;83(25):2658–70.

Anticoagulant Therapy in Patients Undergoing Acute Pulmonary Embolism Interventions

Álvaro Dubois-Silva, MD[a,b,c],
Behnood Bikdeli, MD, MS[d,e,*]

KEYWORDS

- Pulmonary embolism • Anticoagulant therapy • Intervention • Instability • Timing

KEY POINTS

- Unfractionated heparin (UFH) is the anticoagulant of choice during acute pulmonary embolism (PE) interventions and the immediate periprocedural period.
- The doses and targets of UFH infusion depend on the type of intervention and its phase.
- Transition to subcutaneous low-molecular weight heparin or oral anticoagulants should be done cautiously after hemostasis and clinical stability are verified.
- Randomized clinical trials are needed to evaluate different anticoagulation strategies for each acute PE intervention.

INTRODUCTION

Pulmonary embolism (PE) is characterized by the partial or complete obstruction of pulmonary arteries by thrombi, and its severity can range from a mild condition to a lethal disease. Risk stratification for acute PE can help with selecting the appropriate therapeutic approach according to patient severity.[1] Consequently, patients with high-risk PE and those with intermediate–high-risk PE who suffer from subsequent hemodynamical deterioration can be considered either for systemic or catheter-directed fibrinolysis or for other interventional advanced therapies.[1] Alternatives include surgical embolectomy or percutaneous thrombectomy.[2,3] These options are typically reserved for patients with contraindications to systemic fibrinolysis, patients with

large or elongated mobile right heart thrombi, and those in whom hemodynamic instability persists after receiving fibrinolysis.[1,4,5] Findings from ongoing clinical trials and improved risk stratification paradigms can enhance our understanding of the best use of percutaneous recanalization procedures.[6–12] Moreover, mechanical circulatory support, provided mainly by venoarterial (VA) extracorporeal membrane oxygenation (ECMO), has gained increasing attention as a substitute, or complement, to recanalization strategies in acute PE.[13,14]

These advanced therapies do not replace anticoagulation, which remains the cornerstone of PE management across the spectrum of illness severity. While early initiation of anticoagulation reduces mortality, it confers an inherent bleeding risk that must be carefully assessed in

[a] Venous Thromboembolism Unit, Department of Internal Medicine, Complexo Hospitalario Universitario de A Coruña (CHUAC), A Coruña, Spain; [b] Universidade da Coruña (UDC), A Coruña, Spain; [c] Hospital at Home and Palliative Care Department, Complexo Hospitalario Universitario de A Coruña (CHUAC), A Coruña, Spain; [d] Division of Cardiovascular Medicine and the Thrombosis Research Group, Brigham and Women's Hospital, Harvard Medical School, Boston, MA, USA; [e] Center for Outcomes Research and Evaluation, Yale New Haven Hospital, New Haven, CT, USA
* Corresponding author. Brigham and Women's Hospital, 75 Francis Street, Boston, MA 02115.
E-mail addresses: bbikdeli@bwh.harvard.edu; Behnood.bikdeli@yale.edu

Intervent Cardiol Clin 13 (2024) 561–575
https://doi.org/10.1016/j.iccl.2024.07.004
2211-7458/24/© 2024 Elsevier Inc. All rights are reserved, including those for text and data mining, AI training, and similar technologies.

patients who undergo further procedures.[15–17] Yet, we remain unaware of a clear summary about the choice and dosage of anticoagulant agents throughout the different phases of each PE intervention, a critical issue that interventional and noninterventional clinicians participating in the care of patients with PE frequently encounter. Accordingly, this article summarizes the evidence and shares practical recommendations for the use of anticoagulant therapy before, during, and after interventional therapies for acute PE.

CATHETER-BASED INTERVENTIONS

Percutaneous catheter-based interventions (CBIs) aim to recanalize the pulmonary arteries by removing and/or lysing thrombi, while reducing the risk of major bleeding compared with full-dose systemic fibrinolysis.[18] CBI has been experimented in several ways: mechanical embolectomy, catheter-directed fibrinolysis (pharmacologic approach), and pharmaco-mechanical therapy (mixed approach).[3,4,19,20] They constitute an alternative for reperfusion in patients with contraindications to full-dose systemic fibrinolysis (eg, high bleeding risk), when systemic fibrinolysis failed, and in those patients who experienced or at high risk of experiencing obstructive shock that is likely to cause death before systemic fibrinolysis can take effect.[1,21] Ongoing clinical trials are also exploring the potential role of these interventional therapies in a broad group of patients with intermediate-risk PE.

Before Catheter-Based Intervention

The first consideration to make is whether CBI is being planned imminently as an emergent treatment (eg, in a patient with high-risk PE) or that it is a tentative (or planned) option for future in a patient with intermediate–high-risk PE likely to suffer from hemodynamical deterioration. Clinical guidelines recommend prompt initiation of anticoagulation once PE is confirmed if no contraindications exist, regardless of PE severity.[1,21,22] If CBI is being planned emergently, intravenous (IV) unfractionated heparin (UFH) is the anticoagulant agent of choice before CBI, because of its short half-life, quick reversibility and titratability, conferring periprocedural management flexibility.[1,4,23] An initial dose of 80 IU/kg IV is recommended, followed by an IV infusion (18 IU/kg/h), performing subsequent dose adjustments to achieve a target activated partial thromboplastin time (aPTT) between 46 and 70 seconds or between 1.5 and 2.3 times the control (Fig. 1).[1]

CBI could be also a therapeutic option in patients with intermediate–high-risk PE who are stable at the time of assessment but subsequently develop further deterioration. Some predictors for hemodynamic deterioration include worsening (or unresolved) tachycardia, a decrease in systolic blood pressure and/or in urine output, an increase in respiratory rate and/or of lactate levels, and the presence of severe or unresolved hypoxemia, severe right ventricle (RV) dysfunction, recurrent syncope or recurrent presyncopal episodes, incident atrial fibrillation, and severe systemic in ammation.[10,24,25] In fact, patients with intermediate–high-risk PE are heterogeneous and present a wide range of severity, despite being categorized in the same group.

In patients with more severe presentations of intermediate–high-risk PE, and in those with early signs of potential hemodynamic deterioration, UFH is a reasonable option for anticoagulant treatment, since rescue CBI would be more likely.[1] Target aPTT has been previously described. Dose adjustment can be alternatively performed by anti-activated factor X (anti-Xa) monitoring, with a therapeutic range of 0.3 to 0.7 units/mL.[26] However, clinical evidence about the tradeoffs of aPTT-based versus anti-Xa-based monitoring is uncertain, with pooled results from the limited existing studies not suggesting a significant difference for clinical outcomes.[27–31] Anti-Xa level monitoring is recommended in patients with heparin resistance, baseline aPTT elevation from a lupus anticoagulant or contact factor deficiency or those with markedly elevated levels of fibrinogen or factor VIII.[32,33]

In the absence of high-quality head-to-head randomized data, it may be reasonable to consider subcutaneous low molecular weight heparin (LMWH) for the remainder of patients with intermediate–high-risk PE, since it carries a lower risk of major bleeding or heparin-induced thrombocytopenia, and may be more likely to achieve a therapeutic target soon after the initiation of anticoagulation, compared with UFH.[34–36] Data from routine practice indicate that over half of the patients who receive UFH fail to achieve a therapeutic aPTT level within 24 hours of its initiation.[37] If LMWHs are being chosen for anticoagulant therapy, a twice daily regimen of LMWH (eg, enoxaparin 1 mg/kg bid) during the first 2 or 3 days may be preferred over once daily regimens due to greater periprocedural flexibility in case rescue procedures are needed.[1] The use of oral anticoagulants is not recommended because of the potential need for advanced therapies.[1,24]

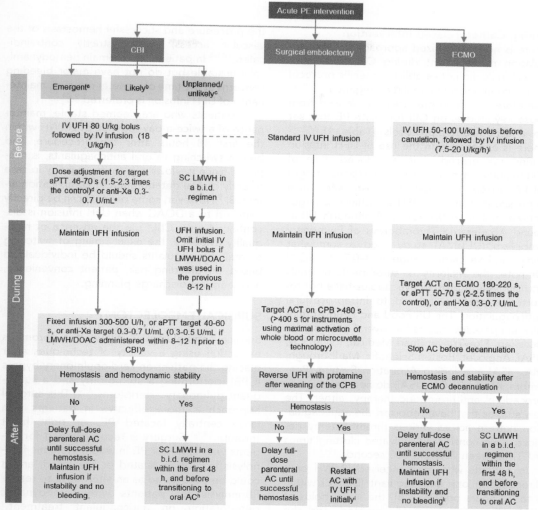

Fig. 1. Choice of anticoagulant treatment depending on the timing and type of PE intervention. AC, anticoagulation; ACT, activated clotting time; aPTT, activated partial thromboplastin time; bid, twice daily; CBI, catheter-based intervention; CPB, cardiopulmonary bypass; DOAC, direct-acting oral anticoagulant; ECMO, extracorporeal membrane oxygenation; h, hour; IV, intravenous; LMWH, low molecular weight heparin; kg, kilogram; PE, pulmonary embolism; s, seconds; SC, subcutaneous; U, units; UFH, unfractionated heparin. [a]In high-risk PE or in case of hemodynamical deterioration. [b]In more severe presentations of intermediate–high-risk PE, or with early signs of potential hemodynamic deterioration. [c]In the remainder of patients with intermediate–high-risk PE. [d]Use institutional protocols for dosing and monitoring. Suggested aPTT dose adjustment: <35 s (<1.2× control) 80 U/kg bolus, increase infusion rate by 4 U/kg/h; 35 to 45 s (1.2–1.5× control) 40 U/kg bolus, increase infusion rate by 2 U/kg/h; 46 to 70 s (1.5–2.3× control) no change; 71 to 90 s (2.3–3.0× control) reduce infusion rate by 2 U/kg/h; >90 s (>3.0× control) stop infusion for 1 h, and then reduce infusion rate by 3 U/kg/h. Monitor every 4 to 6 hours, and 3 hours after each dose adjustment or daily if the therapeutic dose is in range on 2 consecutive determinations. [e]Use institutional protocols for dosing and monitoring. Suggested dose adjustment based on anti-Xa levels: <0.2 80 U/kg bolus, increase infusion rate by 4 U/kg/h; 0.2 to 0.29 40 U/kg bolus, increase infusion rate by 2 U/kg/h; 0.3 to 0.7 no change; 0.71 to 0.8 reduce infusion rate by 2 U/kg/h; >0.8 stop infusion for 1 h, then reduce infusion rate by 3 U/kg/h. Monitor every 6 h or daily if the therapeutic dose is in range on 2 consecutive determinations. [f]If fondaparinux was used, wait 20 to 24 hours from the last fondaparinux injection until initiation of UFH infusion. [g]Consider doses/targets in the low range during fibrinolysis-based CDIs. [h]Earlier transition to DOACs can be considered in the most stable patients. The exact timing should be individualized based on bleeding risk, patient convenience, and tentative discharge planning. [i]Maintain UFH infusion at least within the first 24 h. Subsequently, AC regimen will depend on patient condition. If the patient remains unstable and/or bridging to ECMO is performed, UFH infusion is preferred. In case of stability, consider SC LMWH in a bid regimen at least during 24 to 48 h, and before transitioning to oral AC. [j]Standard IV UFH infusion for acute PE treatment can be considered, since it is within this dose range. [k]Or if other PE intervention is planned (eg, ECMO was used as bridging to another PE intervention).

During Catheter-Based Intervention

There is no standardized approach for anticoagulation management during CBI, and some clinical trials did not establish a specific protocol for concomitant anticoagulation regimen.[11,38–42] Therefore, common practices are derived from those key studies on CBI for acute PE that set up anticoagulation protocols (Table 1).[9,43–48] There is experience in the use of UFH infusion during the procedure in a reduced dose of 300 to 500 IU/h, or with a low-therapeutic target (aPTT 40–60 seconds).[9,44–48] An alternative approach is dosing IV UFH to achieve a target anti-Xa of 0.5 to 0.7 IU/mL,[24] although Ultrasound Accelerated Thrombolysis of Pulmonary Embolism (ULTIMA) study used a somewhat wider anti-Xa target range (0.3–0.7 IU/mL).[43] Of note, the majority of thrombectomy trials and single-arm prospective studies have not reported a protocol related to intraprocedural anticoagulation. The US Food and Drug Administration package inserts for several of these devices (eg, FlowTriever [Inari Medical, Irvine, CA, USA], AngioJet [Boston Scientific, Marlborough, MA, USA] and Indigo Aspiration System [Penumbra, Alameda, CA, USA]) do not discuss periprocedural antithrombotic therapy, either. The few studies that have reported the anticoagulation pattern across various thrombectomy devices, have considered activated clotting times (ACT) between 200 and 300 seconds.[49–53]

In patients who have received LMWH or a direct-acting oral anticoagulant (DOAC) within 8 to 12 hours prior to CBI, the initial bolus of UFH before CBI is usually omitted, and the UFH infusion is initiated with a lower therapeutic target anti-Xa of 0.3 to 0.5 IU/mL during the procedure.[24] In case of recent administration of fondaparinux, it has been proposed to wait 20 to 24 hours from the last fondaparinux injection until initiation of UFH infusion.[43] In summary, while there is no high-quality evidence about the choice of anticoagulant regimen or exact intensity during CBI, it is reasonable to reduce the intensity of anticoagulation during fibrinolysis-based CBI.

After Catheter-Based Intervention

The time and type of anticoagulant regimen immediately post-CBI partly depends on the success of the procedure, and control of access-site and nonaccess-site bleeds. For example, thrombectomy-based CBI typically requires larger sheaths for venous access but does not include administration of fibrinolytic agents. In general, it is recommended to restore full-dose parenteral anticoagulation after completion of the procedure and successful hemostasis of the vascular access, unless strictly contraindicated.[24,44] In patients who remain hemodynamically unstable but do not have major bleeding concerns at the time of catheter removal, maintenance of UFH infusion is preferred.[9,24]

In patients who are deemed stable, maintenance of a twice-a-day regimen of LMWH within the first 48 hours after the procedure, and before switching to oral anticoagulants, is proposed since it allows a greater flexibility in case of early clinical deterioration or complication after CBI.[9] However, some patients can be directly switched to a DOAC when UFH infusion is discontinued after CBI.[24] In the absence of high-quality evidence, the exact timing of switching to oral anticoagulants should be individualized based on bleeding risk, patient convenience, and tentative discharge planning.

SURGICAL EMBOLECTOMY

Surgical embolectomy allows for thrombus extraction using a variety of techniques after placing the patient on cardiopulmonary bypass (CPB), performing a sternotomy and a subsequent pulmonary arteriotomy.[4,54] This surgical approach is more effective in patients with large centrally located PE, or right heart thrombi.[19,54] Surgery is recommended for patients with high-risk PE in whom systemic fibrinolysis is contraindicated or has failed, and it could be considered as an alternative to rescue fibrinolysis for patients with hemodynamic deterioration on anticoagulant treatment.[1] The decision to choose between surgical embolectomy and percutaneous thrombectomy in these scenarios will depend on factors such as patient's surgical risk, survival estimate outside the PE, procedural expertise with either procedure, and resource availability.[22] Other potential indications for surgical embolectomy include paradoxic embolism, clot-in-transit, and hemodynamic collapse or respiratory failure related to PE, requiring cardiopulmonary resuscitation.[19]

Before Surgical Embolectomy

A surgical embolectomy is usually indicated as an urgent or emergent treatment. Thus, if surgical approach is considered, standard IV UFH regimen is preferred, because of its short half-life that provides periprocedural flexibility. A functional whole blood test of anticoagulation, in the form of a clotting time, should be measured and should demonstrate adequate anticoagulation before initiating CPB.[55]

Table 1
Anticoagulation protocols used in randomized clinical trials and single-arm prospective studies of catheter-based interventions

Study Name	Type of CBI[a]	Target Population	AC Before CBI	AC During CBI	AC After CBI
ULTIMA[43]	USAT	Intermediate-risk PE	UFH IV bolus (80 IU/kg) followed by an infusion of 18 IU/kg/h (maximum 1800 IU/h).[b] Target anti-Xa 0.3–0.7 IU/mL	UFH IV infusion adjusted to achieve and maintain a target anti-Xa 0.3–0.7 IU/mL	Left to the discretion of the investigators after at least 24 h of UFH IV infusion from randomization[c]
SEATTLE II[44]	USAT	Massive and submassive PE	Full-dose IV UFH to achieve a target aPTT 60–80 s[d]	UFH IV infusion at intermediate intensity with a target aPTT of 40–60 s	Restoration of full-dose AC after achieving hemostasis. Details left to the treating clinician
OPTALYSE sPE[45]	USAT	Intermediate-risk PE	Therapeutic AC (not specified)	Fixed UFH IV infusion of 300–500 IU/h	Full therapeutic IV UFH dosing initially.[e] Then, the type and duration of AC were determined by the responsible physician
SUNSET sPE[46]	USAT	Submassive PE	Not specified	IV UFH. Doses determined using a hospital defined nomogram that protocolizes dosing to target a low therapeutic anti-Xa level or aPTT (60 s)	Continued in all patients. The choice of specific agent (warfarin, enoxaparin, or a DOAC) was individualized to specific patient needs
CANARY[9]	cCDT	Intermediate–high-risk PE	Randomization within 48 h since initiation of AC (not specified)	Fixed dose of IV UFH of 500 IU/h	Therapeutic UFH. Change to sc enoxaparin (1 mg/kg bid) if no procedural complication or unstable hemodynamics. After at least 48 h of enoxaparin, oral AC could be started at the discretion of treating physician
RESCUE[47]	PM-CDT	Intermediate-risk PE with RV/LV ratio >0.9	Heparin (93.6% of subjects) and enoxaparin sodium (6.4%) (regimen not specified)	IV UFH (5–8 mg/kg/h, maximum 1000 IU/h). Target aPTT 50–60 s	Therapeutic AC restarted within 45 min of sheath removal and hemostasis (regimen not specified)

(continued on next page)

Table 1
(continued)

Study Name	Type of CBI[a]	Target Population	AC Before CBI	AC During CBI	AC After CBI
Kroupa et al[48]	cCDT	Intermediate–high-risk PE	IV UFH (target aPTT of 70–90 s) or sc LMWH (full therapeutic dose)	IV UFH to a target aPTT 50–60 s	IV UFH (without a bolus) to a target aPTT of 70–90 s
HI-PEITHO[7]	USAT	Intermediate–high risk PE with elevated risk of early death or imminent hemodynamic collapse[f]	LMWH subcutaneously at a bid therapeutic dose, or a therapeutic, aPTT-guided IV infusion of UFH	IV UFH at an in-fusion rate of 300–600 IU/h[g]	Full-dose parenteral anticoagulation, either bid LMWH or UFH, no more than 4 h after the end of the procedure, unless documented bleeding concerns. Transition to any commercially available oral anticoagulant, at the discretion of the clinical care team, no sooner than 24 h postprocedurally

Abbreviations: AC, anticoagulation; aPTT, activated partial thromboplastin time; bid, twice daily; CBI, catheter-based intervention; cCDT, conventional catheter-directed thrombolysis; DOAC, direct-acting oral anticoagulant; h, hour; IU, international unit; IV, intravenous; kg, kilogram; LMWH, low molecular weight heparin; LV, left ventricle; mL, milliliter; PE, pulmonary embolism; PM-CDT, pharmacomechanical catheter-directed thrombolysis; RV, right ventricle; UFH, unfractionated heparin; USAT, ultrasound-assisted catheter-directed thrombolysis.

a Clinical trials and single-arm prospective studies on percutaneous thrombectomy did not specify the anticoagulation regimen.

b For patients already receiving UFH, LMWH, or fondaparinux before randomization, the initial UFH bolus was omitted. For patients who received LMWH or fondaparinux at a weight-adjusted therapeutic dose, the start of the UFH infusion was delayed until 8–12 h after the last LMWH injection and until 20–24 h after the last fondaparinux injection.

c Initiation of VKA or a switch from UFH to LMWH or fondaparinux was allowed 36 h after randomization. The minimum suggested duration of anticoagulation therapy was 3 mo.

d For patients who already received LMWH or fondaparinux, the initiation of intravenous UFH was delayed by 12 h.

e cCDT was postponed for 8 h after the last dose of LMWH.

f Indicated by at least 2 of the following new-onset clinical criteria: a. ECG-documented tachycardia with heart rate ≥100 beats per minute, not due to hypovolemia, arrhythmia, or sepsis; b. SBP ≤110 mm Hg over at least 15 min; c. respiratory rate >20 per minute or oxygen saturation on pulse oximetry (SpO₂) <90% (or partial arterial oxygen pressure <60 mm Hg) at rest while breathing room air.

g The exact infusion rate being left to the investigator's discretion, and will be continued for up to 4 h after catheter removal.

During Surgical Embolectomy

Infusion of UFH must be maintained during surgery. The intensity of anticoagulation is typically decided by the cardiac anesthesiology and surgical teams based on the type of mechanical circulatory support used. Most patients who undergo surgical embolectomy are supported with CPB during the procedure.[54] The goals of successful anticoagulation during CPB include limiting clotting and safely reversing the anticoagulation effect during and at the conclusion of operation, respectively.[55] For this purpose, UFH infusion is maintained on CPB with a typical target ACT of greater than 480 seconds.[55–57] However, this minimum threshold value is an approximation and may vary based on the instrument being used. For instruments using maximal activation of whole blood or microcuvette technology, values above 400 seconds are frequently considered therapeutic.[55] Heparin should be reversed (usually with protamine) after weaning of the CPB.[54,55,58]

The use of VA-ECMO as bridge for surgical embolectomy supported with CPB can be considered as an option. Although peripherally cannulated ECMO is the most commonly used ECMO modality in the management of acute PE, central VA-ECMO may be an option in patients undergoing surgical embolectomy, and postprocedurally when patients cannot be weaned from bypass.[56,59]

After Surgical Embolectomy

The management of anticoagulant therapy after surgical embolectomy is not standardized.[55,56] Post-CPB bleeding and PE recurrence including fatal PE are competing risks after surgery.[58,60,61] Thus, after weaning of the CPB and heparin reversal with protamine, anticoagulation should be restarted as soon as adequate hemostasis of the surgical and vascular access sites, and absence of bleeding, are verified.[58] The type of anticoagulant agent will depend on patient's condition. If the patient remains unstable and/or bridging to ECMO is performed, UFH infusion would be preferred.

MECHANICAL CIRCULATORY SUPPORT

Mechanical circulatory support is provided by ECMO in patients with high-risk PE who suffer from severe RV dysfunction and refractory cardiogenic shock.[19] Hemodynamic instability would be perpetuated by increased RV afterload, leading to RV overdistension and ischemia, causing further interventricular septal shift toward the left ventricle, thereby limiting its filling and decreasing systemic cardiac output.[4,19] In this setting, VA-ECMO allows off-loading of the RV by diverting RV venous return to the ECMO circuit, augmenting left ventricle filling while increasing perfusion by pumping oxygenated blood into the arterial system.[4,56] It could be used alone, or as a complement to reperfusion therapies.[13,19] Venovenous ECMO is less commonly used in high-risk PE, since it provides oxygenation support without decompression of the RV.[14,59] Anticoagulation is mandatory irrespective of the ECMO modality used.

Before Extracorporeal Membrane Oxygenation

The indication for ECMO is usually emergent, regardless of whether it is used as a bridging therapy before or after a reperfusion treatment, or if it is used alone. In both cases, IV UFH infusion should be preferred for anticoagulation.[62] If no bridging therapy is planned, a UFH bolus of approximately 50 to 100 UI/kg before cannulation, followed by the infusion at 7.5 to 20 UI/kg/h, have been proposed.[63] The targets for treatment are discussed later. Oral anticoagulants should be avoided if the patient is being treated with ECMO.

During Extracorporeal Membrane Oxygenation

IV UFH infusion should be maintained during ECMO. ACT is commonly used for dose adjustment, with a target of 180 to 200 seconds.[64,65] Wider ranges (180–220 seconds) have been recently suggested.[62] Alternatives for monitoring and dose adjustment include aPTT (targets 50–70 seconds or 2–2.5 times the control) and anti-Xa (target 0.3–0.7 UI/mL).[62,63,65,66] Based on limited data, some professional societies consider anti-Xa monitoring, since there are fewer theoretic interactions with this test, and in meta-analysis of retrospective studies an association between using anti-Xa compared with time-based strategies and fewer bleeding events and mortality rate were observed, without an increase in thrombotic events.[67] Some authors suggest a narrower target range (0.3–0.5 UI/mL).[62,66] Combined approaches adding various parameters (eg, platelet count, fibrinogen level, initial results of INR, aPTT, anti-Xa, and viscoelastomeric tests) and analyzing the patient situation (eg, prothrombotic/hemorrhagic state) are being currently proposed to individualize decisions, rather than establishing strict target margins.[65,66]

After Extracorporeal Membrane Oxygenation

Before decannulation, anticoagulation would be stopped to achieve adequate hemostasis at the access sites. Anticoagulation should be restarted in the setting of PE once hemostasis of vascular access sites has been achieved. If the patient remains unstable and/or if ECMO was used as bridge to another PE intervention, UFH IV infusion should be maintained. If the patient is in a stable condition after ECMO decannulation, and other interventions are not planned, anticoagulation could be resumed with LMWH or with oral anticoagulants. A twice-a-day regimen of subcutaneous LMWH (eg, enoxaparin 1 mg/kg bid) could be considered before switching to oral agents, and within 48 hours, after ECMO weaning. This cautious approach would allow more exibility in case of post-ECMO complications or development of clinical instability.

TRANSITION TO ORAL ANTICOAGULANTS

There are no good quality data from clinical trials comparing different strategies for transitioning to oral anticoagulants after each of the previously mentioned PE interventions. Only one underpowered randomized controlled trial (RCT) compared dabigatran with warfarin for 6 months after endovascular mechanical thrombus fragmentation with reduced-dose fibrinolysis in 63 patients with high-risk and intermediate–high-risk PE. Dabigatran had similar effectiveness compared to warfarin in terms of venous thromboembolism recurrences and venous thromboembolism-related deaths (primary endpoint), and it showed a greater safety in comparison to warfarin for minor bleeding, with no significant differences between groups in major bleeding. Of note, patients randomized to dabigatran received 9 days of LMWH treatment before switching to dabigatran (ie, there are no data for an earlier transition).[68] Therefore, clinical practice is derived from anticoagulation protocols used in clinical trials for CBI, other surgical settings different from emergent surgical embolectomy, as well as observational data and expert input. Anticoagulation protocols after CBI in clinical trials are heterogenous (see Table 1), and the availability of DOACs increased throughout the period when these trials were developed.

Considering the risk of early complications (eg, major bleeding, PE recurrence needing reintervention, and so forth), we suggest maintaining parenteral anticoagulation (ie, IV UFH infusion or twice-a-day subcutaneous LMWH, depending on the type of intervention and patient condition) within 48 hours after the procedure (CBI or surgical embolectomy) or after ECMO weaning in most patients. Subsequent transition to oral anticoagulation can be considered if hemostasis, absence of bleeding, and patient stability, are verified. An earlier transition to oral anticoagulants can be considered in stable patients undergoing CBI, based on bleeding risk, patient convenience, and tentative discharge planning. If no contraindications, DOACs are preferable at that stage.[1,21,69,70] Nevertheless, dabigatran and edoxaban cannot be used in the first 5 days from PE diagnosis.[71–73] Rivaroxaban requires a higher dose in the first 21 days after PE diagnosis (15 mg bid) and apixaban during the first 7 days (10 mg bid).[74–76] If vitamin K antagonists (VKA) are used, parenteral (IV or subcutaneous) treatment should be maintained until the target international normalized ratio (2–3 in most cases) is achieved. DOACs should be preferentially avoided in case of concern for thrombotic antiphospholipid syndrome.[70,77]

SPECIAL SITUATIONS

Specific considerations in special situations (heparin-induced thrombocytopenia, extremes of body weight, renal insufficiency, and pregnant/postpartum women) are addressed in Appendix 1.

RECOMMENDATIONS FROM PROFESSIONAL SOCIETIES

The main recommendations from professional societies regarding anticoagulation regimens for each PE intervention are summarized in Table 2.

FUTURE PERSPECTIVES

There are several ongoing RCTs (eg, HI-PEITHO,[7] PEERLESS,[11] PEERLESS II [NCT06055920], PE-TRACT [NCT05591118], STORM-PE [NCT05684796], BETULA [NCT03854266], PRAGUE-26 [NCT05493163], Lungembolism [NCT03218410], STRATIFY [NCT04088292], and others [NCT03581877; NCT05612854]) and prospective studies (eg, RESCUE II [NCT06120179], FLAME [NCT04795167], VQPE [NCT05133713], STRIKE-PE [NCT04798261], and CATH-PE [NCT04473560]) aimed to assess the performance of different CBIs for acute PE. However, these studies are not designed to evaluate different anticoagulation strategies for each procedure. Only one study (XENITH [NCT02506985]) with unpublished results randomized patients with PE managed

Table 2
Summary of the main recommendations from professional societies on anticoagulation regimens for each pulmonary embolism intervention

Professional Society	CBI	Surgical Embolectomy	ECMO
ESC[1,24]	Parenteral AC during CBI (unless CI), and monitoring with anti-Xa, ACT or aPTT. Continue full-dose parenteral AC after CBI (unless CI). Use UFH postprocedurally if unstable. Most patients can be directly switched to LMWH or DOACs when the UFH infusion is complete	Not addressed	
AHA[20,22,56]	Suggested approach for thrombectomy in 2011 statement: either UFH 70 IU/kg IV bolus, with additional heparin as needed to maintain an ACT >250 s, or bivalirudin (0.75 mg/kg IV bolus, then 1.75 mg/kg/h)	On CPB, full AC, typically with heparin, measuring a target ACT >480 s is required	Bolus of heparin before cannulation. Maintain on a heparin drip thereafter to target an elevated aPTT or ACT. Although general recommendations suggest maintaining an ACT between 180–220 s, AC is largely left to individual operator discretion
aISTH[62]	Not addressed	Not addressed	IV UFH using anti-Xa assays to monitor (target 0.3–0.5 U/mL). Alternatively, aPTT of 50–70 s (2–2.5 times the control) or an ACT of 180–220 s. Institutional protocols for dosing and monitoring are recommended[b]
ASH[69,82]	Not addressed	Not addressed	Not addressed
ACCP[21,83]	Not addressed	Not addressed	Not addressed
aEACTS/EACTA/EBCP[57,84]	Not addressed	Not addressed	

(continued on next page)

Table 2
(continued)

Professional Society	CBI	Surgical Embolectomy	ECMO
		UFH on CPB (starting dose 300–500 U/kg). ACT >480 s should be considered in CPB with uncoated equipment and cardiotomy suction. Target ACT depends on the type of equipment. Institutional protocols for dosing and monitoring are recommended[b]	UFH (target aPTT of 45–80 s and ACT of 140–220 s). Bivalirudin (0.02–0.05 mg/kg/h) and argatroban (0.1–0.2 mg/kg/h) are usually dosed based on the aPTT with target ranges of 45–80 s and 50–60 s, respectively[b]
aSTS/SCA/AmSECT[55,85]	Not addressed	UFH to maintain an ACT >480 s during CPB (>400 s for instruments using maximal activation of whole blood or microcuvette technology)[b]	Not addressed
aELSO[66]	Not addressed	Not addressed	UFH, ACT should be used as the primary method for monitoring. Anti-Xa Assay (target 0.3–0.7 IU/mL) showed reports of better association with UFH dose and less variability than aPTT[b]

Abbreviations: AC, anticoagulation; ACCP, American College of Chest Physicians; ACT, activated clotting time; AHA, American Heart Association; AmSECT, The American Society of ExtraCorporeal Technology; aPTT, activated partial thromboplastin time; ASH, American Society of Hematology; CBI, catheter-based intervention therapy; CI, contraindicated; CPB; cardiopulmonary bypass; DOACs, direct-acting oral anticoagulants; EACTA, European Association of Cardiothoracic Anaesthesiology; EACTS, European Association for Cardio-Thoracic Surgery; EBCP, European Board of Cardiovascular Perfusion; ECMO, extracorporeal membrane oxygenation; ELSO, extracorporeal life support organization; ESC, European Society of Cardiology; HIT, heparin-induced thrombocytopenia; ISTH, International Society of Thrombosis and Haemostasis; IV, intravenous; LMWH, low molecular weight heparin; PE, pulmonary embolism; PERT, pulmonary embolism response team; SCA, The Society of Cardiovascular Anesthesiologists; STS, The Society of Thoracic Surgeons; UFH, unfractionated heparin.

a General recommendations for patients undergoing CPB/ECMO (ie, not specific for patients with acute PE).

b Alternatives to UFH in case of HIT or if heparin is CI include bivalirudin and argatroban (the latter preferred in case of significant renal dysfunction in some of these guidelines).

with catheter-directed fibrinolysis to receive rivaroxaban or heparin followed by warfarin immediately after completion of alteplase infusion. Hence, if new clinical trials for acute PE interventions are designed in the near future, embedding a factorial randomization for anticoagulation regimen could be an efficient way of gaining additional knowledge on this topic, without requiring much more resources.

Additionally, analyses of anticoagulation regimens utilized in individual RCTs, and observational comparative effectiveness studies derived from routine-practice can complement our knowledge, while waiting for clinical trials specifically designed to assess different anticoagulation strategies for acute PE interventions. Finally, new anticoagulants targeting the contact system and factor XI/XIa have shown promising initial safety data.[78–81] The evaluation of these anticoagulants in patients undergoing these procedures could be of special interest if they are able to preserve effectiveness and yet significantly reduce the bleeding risk.

SUMMARY

IV UFH infusion is the anticoagulant of choice during PE interventions and the proximate periprocedural period. Transition to subcutaneous LMWH or oral anticoagulants should be done cautiously after hemostasis and clinical stability are verified. Data from ongoing RCTs on recanalization procedures, prospective studies, and large international registries can provide valuable observational data on anticoagulation-related outcomes in PE interventions, soon, while we await the future design of specific RCTs that can help understand the tradeoffs of various regimens of periprocedural anticoagulation for these advanced therapies.

CLINICS CARE POINTS

- CBIs and surgical embolectomy are alternatives to systemic fibrinolysis for high-risk PE patients and those with intermediate-high-risk PE who deteriorate hemodynamically.
- These advanced therapies complement but do not replace anticoagulation, which remains the cornerstone in PE management.
- Anticoagulant choice and dosage depend on the PE intervention type and phase, hemostasis and clinical stability.
- Main options include intravenous UFH, subcutaneous LMWH, and DOACs.

- ECMO can be used alone or with reperfusion therapies for severe RV dysfunction and cardiogenic shock.

AUTHOR CONTRIBUTIONS

A. Dubois-Silva and B. Bikdeli conceived the study idea, reviewed, wrote the article, and approved the final version of the article.

DISCLOSURES

Dr A. Dubois-Silva reports lecture/consultant fees from LEO Pharma, and economical support for travel/congress costs from ROVI and LEO Pharma, all outside the submitted article. Outside the submitted article, Dr B. Bikdeli is supported by a Career Development Award from the American Heart Association, United States and VIVA Physicians (#938814). Dr B. Bikdeli was supported by the Scott Schoen and Nancy Adams IGNITE Award and is supported by the Mary Ann Tynan Research Scientist award from the Mary Horrigan Connors Center for Women's Health and Gender Biology at Brigham and Women's Hospital, and the Heart and Vascular Center Junior Faculty Award from Brigham and Women's Hospital. Dr B. Bikdeli reports that he was a consulting expert, on behalf of the plaintiff, for litigation related to 2 specific brand models of IVC filters. Dr B. Bikdeli has neither been involved in the litigation in 2022 or 2023 nor received any compensation in 2022 or 2023. Dr B. Bikdeli reports that he is a member of the Medical Advisory Board for the North American Thrombosis Forum, and serves in the Data Safety and Monitory Board of the NAIL-IT trial funded by the National Heart, Lung, and Blood Institute, and Translational Sciences.

SUPPLEMENTARY DATA

Supplementary data to this article can be found online at https://doi.org/10.1016/j.iccl.2024.07.004.

REFERENCES

1. Konstantinides SV, Meyer G, Becattini C, et al. 2019 ESC Guidelines for the diagnosis and management of acute pulmonary embolism developed in collaboration with the European Respiratory Society (ERS). Eur Heart J 2020;41(4):543–603.
2. Lee T, Itagaki S, Chiang YP, et al. Survival and recurrence after acute pulmonary embolism treated with pulmonary embolectomy or thrombolysis in New York State, 1999 to 2013. J Thorac Cardiovasc Surg 2018;155(3):1084–90.e12.
3. de Winter MA, Vlachojannis GJ, Ruigrok D, et al. Rationale for catheter-based therapies in acute

pulmonary embolism. Eur Hear J Suppl J Eur Soc Cardiol 2019;21(Suppl I):I16–22.

4. Fulton B, Bashir R, Weinberg MD, et al. Advanced Treatment of Hemodynamically Unstable Acute Pulmonary Embolism and Clinical Follow-up. Semin Thromb Hemost 2023;49(8):785–96.

5. Bikdeli B, Jiménez D, Muriel A, et al. Association between reperfusion therapy and outcomes in patients with acute pulmonary embolism and right heart thrombi. Eur Respir J 2020;56(5):2000538.

6. Barco S, Vicaut E, Klok FA, et al. Improved identification of thrombolysis candidates amongst intermediate-risk pulmonary embolism patients: implications for future trials. Eur Respir J 2018; 51(1):1701775.

7. Klok FA, Piazza G, Sharp ASP, et al. Ultrasound-facilitated, catheter-directed thrombolysis vs anti-coagulation alone for acute intermediate-high-risk pulmonary embolism: Rationale and design of the HI-PEITHO study. Am Heart J 2022;251:43–53.

8. Pietrasik A, Gąsecka A, Szarpak Ł, et al. Catheter-Based Therapies Decrease Mortality in Patients With Intermediate and High-Risk Pulmonary Embolism: Evidence From Meta-Analysis of 65,589 Patients. Front Cardiovasc Med 2022;9:861307.

9. Sadeghipour P, Jenab Y, Moosavi J, et al. Catheter-Directed Thrombolysis vs Anticoagulation in Patients With Acute Intermediate-High-risk Pulmonary Embolism: The CANARY Randomized Clinical Trial. JAMA Cardiol 2022;7(12):1189–97.

10. Jiménez D, Tapson V, Yusen RD, et al. Revised Paradigm for Acute Pulmonary Embolism Prognostication and Treatment. Am J Respir Crit Care Med 2023;208(5):524–7.

11. Gonsalves CF, Gibson CM, Stortecky S, et al. Randomized controlled trial of mechanical thrombectomy vs catheter-directed thrombolysis for acute hemodynamically stable pulmonary embolism: Rationale and design of the PEERLESS study. Am Heart J 2023;266:128–37.

12. Ismayl M, Machanahalli Balakrishna A, Aboeata A, et al. Meta-Analysis Comparing Catheter-Directed Thrombolysis Versus Systemic Anticoagulation Alone for Submassive Pulmonary Embolism. Am J Cardiol 2022;178:154–62.

13. Hobohm L, Sagoschen I, Habertheuer A, et al. Clinical use and outcome of extracorporeal membrane oxygenation in patients with pulmonary embolism. Resuscitation 2022;170:285–92.

14. Rivers J, Pilcher D, Kim J, et al. Extracorporeal membrane oxygenation for the treatment of massive pulmonary embolism. An analysis of the ELSO database. Resuscitation 2023;191:109940.

15. Riney JN, Hollands JM, Smith JR, et al. Identifying optimal initial infusion rates for unfractionated heparin in morbidly obese patients. Ann Pharmacother 2010;44(7–8):1141–51.

16. Shald EA, Ohman K, Kelley D, et al. Factors associated with bleeding after ultrasound-assisted catheter-directed thrombolysis for the treatment of pulmonary embolism. Blood Coagul Fibrinolysis 2023;34(1):40–6.

17. Sadiq I, Goldhaber SZ, Liu P-Y, et al. Risk factors for major bleeding in the SEATTLE II trial. Vasc Med 2017;22(1):44–50.

18. Planer D, Yanko S, Matok I, et al. Catheter-directed thrombolysis compared with systemic thrombolysis and anticoagulation in patients with intermediate- or high-risk pulmonary embolism: systematic review and network meta-analysis. CMAJ (Can Med Assoc J) 2023;195(24):E833–43.

19. Piazza G. Advanced Management of Intermediate- and High-Risk Pulmonary Embolism: JACC Focus Seminar. J Am Coll Cardiol 2020;76(18):2117–27.

20. Giri J, Sista AK, Weinberg I, et al. Interventional Therapies for Acute Pulmonary Embolism: Current Status and Principles for the Development of Novel Evidence: A Scientific Statement From the American Heart Association. Circulation 2019;140(20): e774–801.

21. Stevens SM, Woller SC, Kreuziger LB, et al. Antithrombotic Therapy for VTE Disease: Second Update of the CHEST Guideline and Expert Panel Report. Chest 2021;160(6):e545–608.

22. Jaff MR, McMurtry MS, Archer SL, et al. Management of massive and submassive pulmonary embolism, iliofemoral deep vein thrombosis, and chronic thromboembolic pulmonary hypertension: a scientific statement from the American Heart Association. Circulation 2011;123(16):1788–830.

23. Rivera-Lebron B, McDaniel M, Ahrar K, et al. Diagnosis, Treatment and Follow Up of Acute Pulmonary Embolism: Consensus Practice from the PERT Consortium. Clin Appl Thromb Hemost 2019;25. 1076029619853037.

24. Pruszczyk P, Klok FA, Kucher N, et al. Percutaneous treatment options for acute pulmonary embolism: a clinical consensus statement by the ESC Working Group on Pulmonary Circulation and Right Ventricular Function and the European Association of Percutaneous Cardiovascular Interventions. EuroIntervention 2022;18(8):e623–38.

25. Bikdeli B, Jiménez D, Del Toro J, et al. Association Between Preexisting Versus Newly Identified Atrial Fibrillation and Outcomes of Patients With Acute Pulmonary Embolism. J Am Heart Assoc 2021; 10(17):e021467.

26. Nguyen L, Qi X, Karimi-Asl A, et al. Evaluation of anti-Xa levels in patients with venous thromboembolism within the first 48 h of anticoagulation with unfractionated heparin. SAGE open Med 2023;11. 20503121231190964.

27. Coons JC, Iasella CJ, Thornberg M, et al. Clinical outcomes with unfractionated heparin monitored

by anti-factor Xa vs. activated partial Thromboplastin time. Am J Hematol 2019;94(9):1015–9.

28. Guervil DJ, Rosenberg AF, Winterstein AG, et al. Activated partial thromboplastin time versus anti-factor Xa heparin assay in monitoring unfractionated heparin by continuous intravenous infusion. Ann Pharmacother 2011;45(7–8):861–8.

29. Rosenberg AF, Zumberg M, Taylor L, et al. The use of anti-Xa assay to monitor intravenous unfractionated heparin therapy. J Pharm Pract 2010;23(3):210–6.

30. Vandiver JW, Vondracek TG. Antifactor Xa levels versus activated partial thromboplastin time for monitoring unfractionated heparin. Pharmacotherapy 2012;32(6):546–58.

31. Swayngim R, Preslaski C, Burlew CC, et al. Comparison of clinical outcomes using activated partial thromboplastin time versus antifactor-Xa for monitoring therapeutic unfractionated heparin: A systematic review and meta-analysis. Thromb Res 2021;208:18–25.

32. Smythe MA, Priziola J, Dobesh PP, et al. Guidance for the practical management of the heparin anticoagulants in the treatment of venous thromboembolism. J Thromb Thrombolysis 2016;41(1):165–86.

33. Levy JH, Connors JM. Heparin Resistance - Clinical Perspectives and Management Strategies. N Engl J Med 2021;385(9):826–32.

34. Robertson L, Jones LE. Fixed dose subcutaneous low molecular weight heparins versus adjusted dose unfractionated heparin for the initial treatment of venous thromboembolism. Cochrane Database Syst Rev 2017;2(2):CD001100.

35. Walenga JM, Jeske WP, Prechel MM, et al. Decreased prevalence of heparin-induced thrombocytopenia with low-molecular-weight heparin and related drugs. Semin Thromb Hemost 2004;30(Suppl 1):69–80.

36. Cossette B, Pelletier M-E, Carrier N, et al. Evaluation of bleeding risk in patients exposed to therapeutic unfractionated or low-molecular-weight heparin: a cohort study in the context of a quality improvement initiative. Ann Pharmacother 2010;44(6):994–1002.

37. Prucnal CK, Jansson PS, Deadmon E, et al. Analysis of Partial Thromboplastin Times in Patients With Pulmonary Embolism During the First 48 Hours of Anticoagulation With Unfractionated Heparin. Acad Emerg Med 2020;27(2):117–27.

38. Silver MJ, Gibson CM, Giri J, et al. Outcomes in High-Risk Pulmonary Embolism Patients Undergoing FlowTriever Mechanical Thrombectomy or Other Contemporary Therapies: Results From the FLAME Study. Circ Cardiovasc Interv 2023;16(10):e013406.

39. Sista AK, Horowitz JM, Tapson VF, et al. Indigo Aspiration System for Treatment of Pulmonary Embolism: Results of the EXTRACT-PE Trial. JACC Cardiovasc Interv 2021;14(3):319–29.

40. Toma C, Jaber WA, Weinberg MD, et al. Acute outcomes for the full US cohort of the FLASH mechanical thrombectomy registry in pulmonary embolism. EuroIntervention 2023;18(14):1201–12.

41. Tu T, Toma C, Tapson VF, et al. A Prospective, Single-Arm, Multicenter Trial of Catheter-Directed Mechanical Thrombectomy for Intermediate-Risk Acute Pulmonary Embolism: The FLARE Study. JACC Cardiovasc Interv 2019;12(9):859–69.

42. Monteleone P, Ahern R, Banerjee S, et al. Modern treatment of pulmonary embolism (USCDT Versus MT): results from a Real-World, Big Data Analysis (REAL-PE). J Soc Cardiovasc Angiogr Interv 2024;3(1):101192.

43. Kucher N, Boekstegers P, Müller OJ, et al. Randomized, controlled trial of ultrasound-assisted catheter-directed thrombolysis for acute intermediate-risk pulmonary embolism. Circulation 2014;129(4):479–86.

44. Piazza G, Hohlfelder B, Jaff MR, et al. A Prospective, Single-Arm, Multicenter Trial of Ultrasound-Facilitated, Catheter-Directed, Low-Dose Fibrinolysis for Acute Massive and Submassive Pulmonary Embolism: The SEATTLE II Study. JACC Cardiovasc Interv 2015;8(10):1382–92.

45. Tapson VF, Sterling K, Jones N, et al. A Randomized Trial of the Optimum Duration of Acoustic Pulse Thrombolysis Procedure in Acute Intermediate-Risk Pulmonary Embolism: The OPTALYSE PE Trial. JACC Cardiovasc Interv 2018;11(14):1401–10.

46. Avgerinos ED, Jaber W, Lacomis J, et al. Randomized Trial Comparing Standard Versus Ultrasound-Assisted Thrombolysis for Submassive Pulmonary Embolism: The SUNSET sPE Trial. JACC Cardiovasc Interv 2021;14(12):1364–73.

47. Bashir R, Foster M, Iskander A, et al. Pharmacomechanical Catheter-Directed Thrombolysis With the Bashir Endovascular Catheter for Acute Pulmonary Embolism: The RESCUE Study. JACC Cardiovasc Interv 2022;15(23):2427–36.

48. Kroupa J, Buk M, Weichet J, et al. A pilot randomised trial of catheter-directed thrombolysis or standard anticoagulation for patients with intermediate-high risk acute pulmonary embolism. EuroIntervention 2022;18(8):e639–46.

49. Chauhan CA, Scolieri SK, Toma C. Percutaneous Pulmonary Embolectomy Using the FlowTriever Retrieval/Aspiration System. J Vasc Interv Radiol 2017;28(4):621–3.

50. Luedemann WM, Zickler D, Kruse J, et al. Percutaneous Large-Bore Pulmonary Thrombectomy with the FlowTriever Device: Initial Experience in Intermediate-High and High-Risk Patients. Cardiovasc Intervent Radiol 2023;46(1):35–42.

51. Sławek-Szmyt S, Stępniewski J, Kurzyna M, et al. Catheter-directed mechanical aspiration thrombectomy in a real-world pulmonary embolism population: a multicenter registry. Eur Heart J Acute Cardiovasc Care 2023;12(9):584–93.

52. Zaazoue KA, ElBoraey MA, Core J, et al. Percutaneous Mechanical Thrombectomy as Primary Therapy for High-Risk Pulmonary Embolism in Patients with Absolute Contraindications to Anticoagulation. J Vasc Interv Radiol 2023;34(9):1629–31.

53. Zhang RS, Ho AM, Elbaum L, et al. Quality and rapidity of anticoagulation in patients with acute pulmonary embolism undergoing mechanical thrombectomy. Am Heart J 2024;267:91–4.

54. Iaccarino A, Frati G, Schirone L, et al. Surgical embolectomy for acute massive pulmonary embolism: state of the art. J Thorac Dis 2018;10(8):5154–61.

55. Shore-Lesserson L, Baker RA, Ferraris VA, et al. The Society of Thoracic Surgeons, The Society of Cardiovascular Anesthesiologists, and The American Society of ExtraCorporeal Technology: Clinical Practice Guidelines-Anticoagulation During Cardiopulmonary Bypass. Ann Thorac Surg 2018; 105(2):650–62.

56. Goldberg JB, Giri J, Kobayashi T, et al. Surgical Management and Mechanical Circulatory Support in High-Risk Pulmonary Embolisms: Historical Context, Current Status, and Future Directions: A Scientific Statement From the American Heart Association. Circulation 2023;147(9):e628–47.

57. Kunst G, Milojevic M, Boer C, et al. 2019 EACTS/EACTA/EBCP guidelines on cardiopulmonary bypass in adult cardiac surgery. Br J Anaesth 2019;123(6):713–57.

58. Baumann Kreuziger L, Karkouti K, Tweddell J, et al. Antithrombotic therapy management of adult and pediatric cardiac surgery patients. J Thromb Haemost 2018;16(11):2133–46.

59. Kohler K, Valchanov K, Nias G, et al. ECMO cannula review. Perfusion 2013;28(2):114–24.

60. Hornor MA, Duane TM, Ehlers AP, et al. American College of Surgeons' Guidelines for the Perioperative Management of Antithrombotic Medication. J Am Coll Surg 2018;227(5):521–36.e1.

61. Douketis JD, Spyropoulos AC, Spencer FA, et al. Perioperative management of antithrombotic therapy: Antithrombotic Therapy and Prevention of Thrombosis, 9th ed: American College of Chest Physicians Evidence-Based Clinical Practice Guidelines. Chest 2012;141(2 Suppl):e326S–50S.

62. Helms J, Frere C, Thiele T, et al. Anticoagulation in adult patients supported with extracorporeal membrane oxygenation: guidance from the Scientific and Standardization Committees on Perioperative and Critical Care Haemostasis and Thrombosis of the International Society on Thrombosis and. J Thromb Haemost 2023;21(2):373–96.

63. Burša F, Sklienka P, Frelich M, et al. Anticoagulation Management during Extracorporeal Membrane Oxygenation-A Mini-Review. Medicina (Kaunas) 2022;58(12):1783.

64. Chlebowski MM, Baltagi S, Carlson M, et al. Clinical controversies in anticoagulation monitoring and antithrombin supplementation for ECMO. Crit Care 2020;24(1):19.

65. Šoltés J, Skribuckij M, Říha H, et al. Update on Anticoagulation Strategies in Patients with ECMO-A Narrative Review. J Clin Med 2023;12(18):6067.

66. McMichael ABV, Ryerson LM, Ratano D, et al. 2021 ELSO Adult and Pediatric Anticoagulation Guidelines. ASAIO J 2022;68(3):303–10.

67. Willems A, Roeleveld PP, Labarinas S, et al. Anti-Xa versus time-guided anticoagulation strategies in extracorporeal membrane oxygenation: a systematic review and meta-analysis. Perfusion 2021; 36(5):501–12.

68. Gostev AA, Valiev E, Zeidlits GA, et al. Treatment of acute pulmonary embolism after catheter-directed thrombolysis with dabigatran vs warfarin: results of a multicenter randomized RE-SPIRE trial. J Vasc Surgery Venous Lymphat Disord 2024;12(4):101848.

69. Ortel TL, Neumann I, Ageno W, et al. American Society of Hematology 2020 guidelines for management of venous thromboembolism: treatment of deep vein thrombosis and pulmonary embolism. Blood Adv 2020;4(19):4693–738.

70. Bejjani A, Khairani CD, Assi A, et al. When Direct Oral Anticoagulants Should Not Be Standard Treatment: JACC State-of-the-Art Review. J Am Coll Cardiol 2024;83(3):444–65.

71. Schulman S, Kakkar AK, Goldhaber SZ, et al. Treatment of acute venous thromboembolism with dabigatran or warfarin and pooled analysis. Circulation 2014;129(7):764–72.

72. Büller HR, Décousus H, Grosso MA, et al. Edoxaban versus warfarin for the treatment of symptomatic venous thromboembolism. N Engl J Med 2013;369(15):1406–15.

73. Schulman S, Kearon C, Kakkar AK, et al. Dabigatran versus warfarin in the treatment of acute venous thromboembolism. N Engl J Med 2009;361(24):2342–52.

74. Bauersachs R, Berkowitz SD, Brenner B, et al. Oral rivaroxaban for symptomatic venous thromboembolism. N Engl J Med 2010;363(26):2499–510.

75. Agnelli G, Buller HR, Cohen A, et al. Oral apixaban for the treatment of acute venous thromboembolism. N Engl J Med 2013;369(9):799–808.

76. Büller HR, Prins MH, Lensin AWA, et al. Oral rivaroxaban for the treatment of symptomatic pulmonary embolism. N Engl J Med 2012;366(14):1287–97.

77. Khairani CD, Bejjani A, Piazza G, et al. Direct Oral Anticoagulants vs Vitamin K Antagonists in Patients With Antiphospholipid Syndromes: Meta-Analysis

of Randomized Trials. J Am Coll Cardiol 2023;81(1): 16–30.

78. Verhamme P, Yi BA, Segers A, et al. Abelacimab for Prevention of Venous Thromboembolism. N Engl J Med 2021;385(7):609–17.

79. Mavromanoli AC, Barco S, Konstantinides SV. Antithrombotics and new interventions for venous thromboembolism: Exploring possibilities beyond factor IIa and factor Xa inhibition. Res Pract Thromb Haemost 2021;5(4).

80. Bentounes NK, Melicine S, Martin AC, et al. Development of new anticoagulant in 2023: Prime time for anti-factor XI and XIa inhibitors. J Med Vasc 2023;48(2):69–80.

81. Galli M, Laborante R, Ortega-Paz L, et al. Factor XI Inhibitors in Early Clinical Trials: A Meta-analysis. Thromb Haemost 2023;123(6):576–84.

82. Witt DM, Nieuwlaat R, Clark NP, et al. American Society of Hematology 2018 guidelines for management of venous thromboembolism: optimal management of anticoagulation therapy. Blood Adv 2018;2(22):3257–91.

83. Douketis JD, Spyropoulos AC, Murad MH, et al. Perioperative Management of Antithrombotic Therapy: An American College of Chest Physicians Clinical Practice Guideline. Chest 2022;162(5):e207–43.

84. Pagano D, Milojevic M, Meesters MI, et al. 2017 EACTS/EACTA Guidelines on patient blood management for adult cardiac surgery. Eur J Cardio Thorac Surg 2018;53(1):79–111.

85. Tibi P, McClure RS, Huang J, et al. STS/SCA/ AmSECT/SABM Update to the Clinical Practice Guidelines on Patient Blood Management. Ann Thorac Surg 2021;112(3):981–1004.

Considerations in Antiplatelet Therapy in Women Undergoing Treatment of Acute Coronary Syndrome or Percutaneous Coronary Intervention

Madeline K Mahowald, MD*, Calvin Choi, MD,
Dominick J. Angiolillo, MD, PhD

KEYWORDS

- Antiplatelet therapy • Sex and gender differences • Acute coronary syndrome
- Percutaneous coronary intervention • Platelet function

KEY POINTS

- The goal of antiplatelet therapy following acute coronary syndrome (ACS) or percutaneous coronary intervention (PCI) is to reduce the risk of future ischemic events, which must be balanced by limiting the risk of bleeding.
- Women with ACS or undergoing PCI have distinct platelet physiology, vascular anatomy, and clinical profiles that warrant consideration when selecting an antiplatelet regimen.
- Women should not be undertreated, as they derive benefits from high-potency dual antiplatelet strategies.
- More sex-specific research is needed to determine the ideal antiplatelet regimen in women.

INTRODUCTION

Antiplatelet therapy plays a key role in the prevention of ischemic events in patients with an acute coronary syndrome (ACS) and following percutaneous coronary intervention (PCI).[1] However, this comes at the expense of an increased risk of bleeding, underscoring the importance of minimizing the competing risks of bleeding and thrombosis when using antiplatelet therapy.[2] It is important to highlight that there are physiologic, anatomic, and clinical differences between sexes, which may have implications for antiplatelet drug management in ACS/PCI patients.[3,4] Unfortunately, clinical trials of ACS/PCI include predominantly male patients; one systematic review evaluating trials in major journals from 2001 to 2018 reported that the proportion of women enrolled was only 26.8% and decreasing.[5] Although outcomes in women as a subgroup are often reported, studies are not powered for these analyses.

In this article, the impact of gender and sex on antiplatelet therapy in ACS/PCI will be reviewed. The terms "gender" (personal identity) and "sex" (biology) are used interchangeably, as they have been used in the studies and data upon which this review is based. First, the specific risks attributable to women with respect to bleeding and thrombosis will be reviewed (Table 1). Then, the sex-specific evidence of the most commonly used antiplatelet agents

Division of Cardiology, University of Florida College of Medicine, ACC – 5th Floor, 655 W 8th Street, Jacksonville, FL 32209, USA
* Corresponding author.
E-mail address: madeline.mahowald@jax.ufl.edu

Intervent Cardiol Clin 13 (2024) 577–586
https://doi.org/10.1016/j.iccl.2024.07.005

Table 1
Factors contributing to the unique risk profile and outcomes of women with acute coronary syndrome or undergoing percutaneous coronary intervention

	Heightened Risk of Bleeding	Heightened Risk of Ischemia
Physiologic	Delayed primary hemostasis Lower baseline hemoglobin	Higher platelet counts Enhanced platelet activation and aggregation Hormonal influences Increased clotting tendency
Anatomic	Smaller radial arteries prone to loops and spasm leading to higher crossover to femoral access	Smaller diameter coronary arteries
Clinical profile	Older age Higher prevalence of comorbidities Lower body weight	Older age Higher prevalence of comorbidities Increased prevalence of high on-treatment platelet reactivity
Pharmacologic	At higher risk for dosing errors	Less likely to be prescribed high-potency $P2Y_{12}$ inhibitors Underprescription of medical therapies proven to reduce residual risk, such as statin therapy

will be summarized, including aspirin, $P2Y_{12}$ inhibitors (clopidogrel, prasugrel, ticagrelor, and cangrelor), and the glycoprotein IIb/IIIa inhibitors (GPIs; abciximab, tirofiban, or eptifibatide). The limits of generalizability of findings from clinical trials comprised predominantly of men should be kept in mind during the overview of the literature surrounding bleeding, ischemic events, and outcomes in women presenting with ACS and/or undergoing PCI. Other indications for antiplatelet therapy, such as peripheral arterial disease, cerebrovascular disease, and the prevention of pre-eclampsia, are beyond the scope of this article.

PHYSIOLOGY

Platelet activation and aggregation are crucial to the pathophysiology of ACSs and subsequent ischemic complications, such as stent thrombosis.[6] Women have higher platelet counts than men, and young women have higher platelet counts than older women.[7,8] Moreover, some studies have shown platelets in women to be characterized by enhanced activation and aggregation compared to men.[8–11] A multitude of human and animal studies, both in vivo and ex vivo, have sought to explain the sex differences in platelet reactivity. A higher concentration of glycoprotein IIa/IIIb surface receptors and differences in proteomic signaling cascades have been identified as potential contributing causes.[10,12]

Hormones are also in uential in megakaryocyte and platelet function. Megakaryocytes bear receptors for estrogen, progesterone, and androgen and can be in uenced by exogenous administration of glucocorticoids, testosterone, or estrogen.[13–16] There is variation of glycoprotein IIb/IIIa reactivity with menstrual phase.[10] Additionally, hormones are imputed in the release of nitric oxide synthase and the generation of thromboxane A_2.[13,14]

High platelet reactivity (HPR) as defined using platelet function assays has been shown to be a marker of thrombotic risk. Healthy premenopausal women with HPR have a higher risk of subsequent myocardial infarction (MI).[17] Women tend to have higher rates of HPR compared to men even following treatment with antiplatelet agents, which has a strong association with ischemic outcomes, particularly stent thrombosis.[18,19] Despite often presenting with HPR, women have been shown to have delayed primary hemostasis compared to men (ie, longer bleeding times) and are also at higher risk of bleeding events.[20–23]

BLEEDING RISK

Over the past years, there has been accumulating evidence of the prognostic implications, including increased mortality, associated with bleeding in ACS/PCI patients.[24] Women undergoing PCI have higher rates of vascular access complications, postprocedure bleeding, and need for blood transfusions.[25–28] Differences in weight, body surface area, baseline hemoglobin, metabolism, pharmacokinetics, anatomy, and provider decisions are all factors.[29,30] Consistently higher rates of bleeding in women has led to the inclusion of sex as an independent variable in some validated risk scores to predict bleeding after management of ACS and after PCI, but not in others.[22,23,31,32] For example, sex is not included as a variable in the Academic Research Consortium (ARC) criteria defining patients at high bleeding risk (HBR).[33,34]

These inconsistencies may be accounted for by the differing risk profile between sexes, with women more commonly having risk factors that emerge as independent variables and hence of greater impact than gender itself.[29] Women, in fact, tend to be older and have more comorbidities associated with bleeding, placing them at higher risk of bleeding complications.[25,27,35] Additionally, women are less likely than men to have successful PCI via radial rather than femoral approach, a recommended strategy for reducing bleeding and access site complications.[26] In the RadIal Vs femorAL access for coronary intervention trial, the female sex was an independent risk factor for crossover from radial to femoral access due to smaller artery diameter and higher incidence of radial artery spasm and radial artery loops.[26]

Finally, in some studies reporting female gender as an independent factor associated with bleeding, bleeding events were driven by minor bleeding not requiring transfusion or intervention and hence less important from a prognostic standpoint.[25,36] Thus, it cannot be excluded that some reports may lead to an overestimation of bleeding risk in women, underscoring the importance of objective and standardized definitions of bleeding.[37]

THROMBOTIC RISK

Following PCI, women are at higher risk of ischemic events, including MI and ischemia-driven lesion revascularization.[38,39] Young women at baseline have an increased clotting tendency compared to men.[40] The increased likelihood of HPR in women following antiplatelet treatment may represent one contributing factor. Studies consistently show higher rates of ischemic events in patients with HPR despite antiplatelet treatment, mostly with clopidogrel, including cardiac death, MI, urgent revascularization, and stroke.[19] Despite data reporting the association of on-treatment HPR and ischemic events, platelet reactivity assays have not been routinely adopted in clinical practice to guide antiplatelet therapy selection.[41] Complicating the gender difference is the distinct risk profiles of patients at the time of presentation. As noted earlier, women

undergoing PCI are older, have smaller diameter coronary arteries, and are more likely to have comorbidities associated with ischemic risk, such as diabetes and chronic kidney disease.[25,42] Finally, women are less likely to be prescribed the full complement of medications proven to reduce residual risk, including statin therapy.[43,44]

PHARMACOLOGY

Pharmacokinetics of cardiovascular drugs differs between sexes, but approved dosing regimens are the same.[45] In clinical practice, dosing errors of antithrombotic medications occur with surprising frequency: 42% of patients with non-ST-elevation ACS in one study.[46] Female sex and low body weight were both associated with excess dosing of parenteral therapies, and those patients who were treated inappropriately had higher risks of bleeding, prolonged hospital stay, and death.[46]

Dual antiplatelet therapy (DAPT) with aspirin and a $P2Y_{12}$ inhibitor is the standard of care following ACS or PCI in patients without indications for systemic anticoagulation.[1] Recommendations for the duration of DAPT following the index event have shortened over the years as stent technology has improved and rates of stent thrombosis decrease.[1] With newer generation drug-eluting stents, recommended duration of DAPT has decreased in stable ischemic heart disease from 12 to 3 to 6 months after PCI in most patients.[47] In patients with ACS, guidelines continue to recommend 12 months of DAPT.[47]

Despite its benefits on ischemic events, DAPT comes at the expense of an increased risk of bleeding. Several antiplatelet drug regimen strategies have been developed and implemented to reduce the risk of bleeding, including shortening the duration of DAPT.[48] In a meta-analysis of 6 randomized trials comparing short (3–6 months) versus long ($\geq$12 months) DAPT duration, women and men benefited equally from shorter DAPT with respect to decreased risk of bleeding without an increase in major adverse cardiac events.[49] Although earlier studies have assessed shortening DAPT duration by dropping the $P2Y_{12}$ inhibitor and maintaining aspirin monotherapy, more recent studies have evaluated dropping aspirin and maintaining $P2Y_{12}$ inhibitor monotherapy.[50] HBR status should dictate DAPT duration, even more than ischemic risk, favoring less potent platelet inhibition.[51,52] Additional strategies are reviewed in later discussion. However, DAPT can also be extended in patients at low or normal bleeding risk who are at elevated risk of ischemic events.[47,53]

Antiplatelet agents may exert their protective effects in multiple ways. Studies investigating the effects of aspirin and clopidogrel have shown some reduction in inflammatory markers associated with elevated risk of cardiovascular disease (CVD).[3] This may be particularly relevant in women, as they have a higher incidence of inflammatory and rheumatologic diseases, a nontraditional risk factor for CVD.[54]

ASPIRIN

Aspirin was previously commonly prescribed for primary prevention of CVD. One meta-analysis of 90,000 patients looked specifically at sex-specific risks and benefits and showed a significant reduction in cardiovascular events for both sexes, specifically, reduction in risk of stroke for women and reduction in risk of MI for men.[55] In the Women's Health Study, after multivariate adjustment, aspirin use was associated with significantly lower risk of all-cause and cardiovascular mortality among postmenopausal women with stable CVD.[56] However, in 2018, the publication of multiple trials evaluating aspirin for primary prevention of CVD showed an excess risk of bleeding that outweighed the benefits in most patient populations; this presaged a significant change in practice patterns and a change in guidelines.[57–61]

Although no longer routinely recommended in many populations for primary prevention, aspirin remains the cornerstone of antiplatelet therapy for secondary prevention following ACS and PCI. The degree of platelet inhibition depends on myriad factors, including sex and body weight.[8,40,62] Nevertheless, results of the (Aspirin Dosing: A Patient-Centric Trial Assessing Benefits and Long-Term Effectiveness [ADAPTABLE]) trial assessing aspirin dosing included 4700 women (31.3%) and randomized patients to either 81 mg daily or 325 mg daily, showed no significant differences in major bleeding or CVD events.[63] However, there was a higher incidence of dose switching in those initially assigned to the 325 mg dose. Current guidelines recommend a loading dose at the time of event regardless of sex or weight followed by daily dosing of 81 to 100 mg daily.[47]

P2Y$_{12}$ INHIBITORS

P2Y$_{12}$ inhibitor therapy, which targets the adenosine 5′diphosphate receptor, is the other component of DAPT following PCI or ACS. Currently available oral P2Y$_{12}$ inhibitors include clopidogrel, prasugrel, and ticagrelor; cangrelor

is administered by intravenous infusion. Ticagrelor and prasugrel are more potent and favored over clopidogrel in patients with ACS.[47] However, some registries show that women with ACS are more likely to be treated with clopidogrel than the more potent agents, particularly prasugrel, despite evidence of benefit in both sexes.[36,64] This disparity may be due to the concerns surrounding the risk of bleeding in women or to their risk factor profile, such as older age and lower body weight.[25,29] Sex-specific rates of DAPT interruption or premature discontinuation are variable; several studies report higher rates of early and late discontinuation in women.[65,66] However, a Greek observational study reported similar rates between sexes at 12 months.[36]

Clopidogrel

Clopidogrel is currently recommended for PCI in stable ischemic heart disease; it is also the P2Y$_{12}$ inhibitor of choice in patients with concomitant indications for oral anticoagulation or for patients with ST-elevation MI undergoing PCI after fibrinolytic therapy.[47] A small pharmacodynamic study showed that young women had less response to clopidogrel and retained HPR following treatment; this difference was no longer significant after the age of 50 years.[40] This age-specific finding may be a factor in the disproportionately high mortality of young women following ACS.[67] Nonetheless, a meta-analysis including more than 23,000 women and 56,000 men showed that clopidogrel was similarly effective in reducing CVD events between sexes. However, the benefit to women was driven primarily by reduction in risk of MI. Men derived benefit from reduction in the risk of MI, stroke, and all-cause mortality.[68]

Prasugrel

The pivotal trial of prasugrel in ACS, Trial to Assess Improvement in Therapeutic Outcomes by Optimizing Platelet Inhibition with Prasugrel–Thrombolysis in Myocardial Infarction 38, included 3523 women (26.0%) and showed reduction in the primary endpoint of death from CVD causes, nonfatal MI, and nonfatal stroke when compared to clopidogrel.[69] The benefit was relatively smaller in women, but there was no significant interaction between sex and treatment.[69] Of note, due to higher rates of bleeding in patients with low body weight, guidelines recommend its use with caution in patients with body weight less than 60 kg and consideration of a reduced dose (ie, 5 mg daily) for long-term treatment.[47]

Ticagrelor

Two years later, the pivotal trial of ticagrelor versus clopidogrel in patients with ACS, PLATO (Study of Platelet Inhibition and Patient Outcomes) similarly showed benefit in reduction of the primary endpoint, a composite of death from vascular causes, MI, or stroke.[70] The trial consisted of 18,624 patients (28.4% women) and did not show an interaction between sex and treatment.[70]

Cangrelor

In 2013, the CHAMPION PHOENIX (Cangrelor versus Standard Therapy to Achieve Optimal Management of Platelet Inhibition) study demonstrated the safety and efficacy of intravenous cangrelor bolus and infusion compared with clopidogrel in reducing ischemic endpoints following PCI.[71] Prespecified subgroup analysis of 3050 randomized female participants showed an odds ratio (OR) of 0.67 (95% CI 0.50–0.92) favoring cangrelor. These results were later expounded upon in a subsequent publication, which reported a greater net benefit in women compared to men with cangrelor versus clopidogrel, although there was no significant interaction according to gender.[72] To date, very limited data has been published about real-world administration of cangrelor to women undergoing PCI.

GLYCOPROTEIN IIb/IIIa INHIBITORS

GPIs prevent platelet aggregation and thrombus formation. Tirofiban and eptifibatide are currently available in the United States; abciximab has been discontinued. The routine use of GPI has decreased with the advent of newer P2Y$_{12}$ agents, this change in practice is likely partially responsible for the temporal trend toward a reduction in bleeding complications.[73]

Studies reporting the outcomes of women treated with GPIs have shown mixed results. The Platelet Receptor Inhibition in Ischemic Syndrome Management in Patients Limited by Unstable Signs and Symptoms trial reported a lower incidence of subsequent ischemic events in patients with unstable angina and non-ST-elevation myocardial infarction (NSTEMI) when treated with tirofiban in addition to heparin plus aspirin than the latter two alone.[74] A post hoc analysis of the women enrolled in this trial did not show a difference in death or recurrent MI at any time point.[75]

Data for the use of eptifibatide in women are limited. Integrilin to minimise platelet aggregation and coronary thrombosis-II (IMPACT-II), a randomized, double-blind, placebo-controlled phase III clinical trial included 25.4% women but did not report outcomes by sex.[76] The subsequent (Platelet Glycoprotein IIb/IIIa in Unstable Angina: Receptor Suppression Using Integrilin Therapy [PURSUIT]) trial included 30.7% women; this trial showed no reduction in death or nonfatal MI in women as a subgroup (OR 1.1 [95% CI 0.9–1.3]).[77]

A meta-analysis of 6 trials of GPI use consisted of 31,402 patients from 41 countries included 35% women.[78] This study showed a significant interaction between sex and allocated treatment, reporting a 19% reduction in death or MI among men at 30 days treated with GPI compared to an actual risk increase in women. Sex-specific treatment effect remained significant after adjustment for baseline characteristics. Although the authors found this difference was absent if stratifying by troponin concentration, it should be noted that troponin levels were missing in many patients and were a mix of baseline and subsequent values.[78] In practice, significantly fewer women than men are treated with GPI.[79]

STRATEGIES TO IMPROVE OUTCOMES IN WOMEN

Women represent one-third of the patients undergoing PCI in the United States; thus, determining the optimal antiplatelet strategy is of the utmost importance.[35] In addition to tailored pharmacotherapy, improvement in outcomes requires a multipronged approach (Fig. 1).[80]

Even prior to PCI, all patients should be assessed for a heightened risk of bleeding and/or ischemic events. Validated scores can quantify risk and guide appropriate therapy, particularly scores that attempt to balance the opposing risks, such as the ARC-HBR trade-off model.[81] Upstream administration of antiplatelet agents other than aspirin is of dubious benefit if there is uncertainty about the need for stent placement, especially if cangrelor is available for rapid P2Y$_{12}$ inhibition, and may be best avoided in cases other than planned PCI.[48]

Access site bleeding and vascular complications account for a major proportion of bleeding after PCI; using radial rather than femoral access is an important strategy to improve outcomes.[26,82] Evidence suggests that those at the highest bleeding risk have the most to gain from transradial access.[83] When femoral access is used, ultrasound guidance can improve successful arterial cannulation, but it has failed to demonstrate a significant change in clinical outcomes, including bleeding, across multiple trials.[82,84,85]

Additional procedural considerations include appropriate dosing of antithrombotic agents,

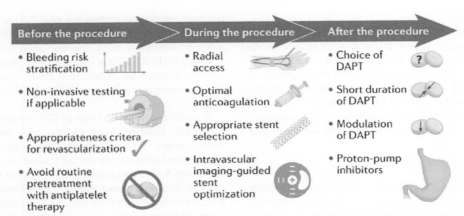

Fig. 1. Bleeding avoidance strategies before, during, and after PCI. Summary of strategies suggested to reduce the risk of bleeding in patients undergoing PCI. These strategies include potential actions that can be undertaken before, during, and after the procedure. DAPT, dual antiplatelet therapy. (Reproduced with permission from Capodanno D et al.[48])

meticulous monitoring of activated clotting times in cases where unfractionated heparin is used, selecting stents with a track record of safety with abbreviated DAPT therapy, and using intravascular imaging to ensure proper sizing and full expansion of stents.[48]

Selecting the optimal components and duration of DAPT is imperative to improving outcomes in women. Beyond the initial strategy, adjusting the regimen depending on PCI and clinical characteristics or the occurrence of a subsequent event is of equal importance. High-potency $P2Y_{12}$ inhibitors (ie, prasugrel or ticagrelor) should not be avoided in women, who derive benefit in reduction of ischemic events.[3,86] However, many women will have risk factors placing them at HBR, which can be mitigated by DAPT modulation via de-escalation strategies. The highest risk of recurrent ischemic events is soon after PCI; as time passes, it may be appropriate in many patients to shorten the duration of DAPT or to de-escalate potency or dose.[87]

Options for de-escalation include switching from a potent $P2Y_{12}$ inhibitor to clopidogrel, reducing the dose of prasugrel or ticagrelor, or discontinuing one agent (either $P2Y_{12}$ inhibitor or aspirin) in favor of antiplatelet monotherapy.[88] Interestingly, there may be a greater benefit in women than in men to $P2Y_{12}$ inhibitor monotherapy over DAPT with respect to both bleeding and ischemic outcomes.[89] In contrast, escalation strategies following an ischemic event consist of replacing clopidogrel with a higher potency agent or, if a patient was on monotherapy at the time of the event, adding either aspirin or a $P2Y_{12}$ inhibitor to transition to DAPT.[88]

Ultimately, clinical trials dedicated to pharmacotherapy in women are essential to inform decision-making and guide selection of antiplatelet regimen and dosing strategy.

SUMMARY

The unique risk profile of women and their consistently worse outcomes following ACS and PCI warrant special consideration when determining a management approach. These differences are the cumulative effect of physiology, pharmacokinetics, age, and comorbidities at the time of presentation, anatomic differences, and health care provider decisions. Strategies to improve early outcomes include preprocedure risk stratification, utilization of radial artery access when possible, procedural best practices to ensure stent optimization, caution and accuracy when dosing parenteral antithrombotics, and ensuring discharge on complete guideline-directed therapy. High-potency $P2Y_{12}$ inhibitors should not be avoided in women, but providers should be mindful of approved options for DAPT de-escalation strategies, particularly $P2Y_{12}$ inhibitor monotherapy in female patients. Ultimately, greater inclusion of women in clinical trials is imperative to guide providers and make informed decisions about the optimal antiplatelet regimen.

CLINICS CARE POINTS

- Validated bleeding risk scores can guide decisions about the components and duration of dual antiplatelet therapy following percutaneous coronary intervention.

- High-potency $P2Y_{12}$ inhibitors should not be avoided in women, as they derive similar benefit from reduction in ischemic events after intervention.
- The antiplatelet regimens of women at high bleeding risk can be modulated in specific ways to maximize benefit and reduce risk.

DISCLOSURE

D.J. Angiolillo declares that he has received consulting fees or honoraria from Abbott, Amgen, AstraZeneca, Bayer, Biosensors, Boehringer Ingelheim, Bristol-Myers Squibb, Chiesi, CSL-Behring, Daiichi-Sankyo, Eli Lilly, Faraday, Haemonetics, Janssen, Merck, Novartis, Novo Nordisk, PhaseBio, PLx Pharma, Pfizer, Sanofi, and Vectura, outside the present study; D.J. Angiolillo also declares that his institution has received research grants from Amgen, Unites States, AstraZeneca, United Kingdom, Bayer, Germany, Biosensors, CeloNova, CSL Behring, Unites States, Daiichi-Sankyo, Japan, Eisai, Japan, Eli Lilly, Gilead, Unites States, Janssen, Unites States, Matsutani Chemical Industry Co., Merck, Unites States, Novartis, Switzerland, Osprey Medical, Renal Guard Solutions, and Scott R. MacKenzie Foundation, Unites States. All other authors do not have conflicts to report.

REFERENCES

1. Capodanno D, Angiolillo DJ. Personalised antiplatelet therapies for coronary artery disease: what the future holds. Eur Heart J 2023;44(32):3059–72.
2. O'Donoghue M, Patel S. Walking the tightrope between ischaemia and bleeding: Balancing ischaemia versus bleeding risk. EuroIntervention 2021;17(7):527.
3. Wang TY, Angiolillo DJ, Cushman M, et al. Platelet biology and response to antiplatelet therapy in women: implications for the development and use of antiplatelet pharmacotherapies for cardiovascular disease. J Am Coll Cardiol 2012;59(10):891–900.
4. Occhipinti G, Greco A, Angiolillo DJ, et al. Gender differences in efficacy and safety of antiplatelet strategies for acute coronary syndromes. Expert Opin Drug Saf 2023;22(8):669–83.
5. Tahhan AS, Vaduganathan M, Greene SJ, et al. Enrollment of older patients, women, and racial/ethnic minority groups in contemporary acute coronary syndrome clinical trials: a systematic review. JAMA cardiology 2020;5(6):714–22.
6. Gori T, Polimeni A, Indolfi C, et al. Predictors of stent thrombosis and their implications for clinical practice. Nat Rev Cardiol 2019;16(4):243–56.
7. Segal JB, Moliterno AR. Platelet counts differ by sex, ethnicity, and age in the United States. Ann Epidemiol 2006;16(2):123–30.
8. Becker DM, Segal J, Vaidya D, et al. Sex differences in platelet reactivity and response to low-dose aspirin therapy. JAMA 2006;295(12):1420–7.
9. Haque SF, Matsubayashi H, Izumi S-I, et al. Sex difference in platelet aggregation detected by new aggregometry using light scattering. Endocr J 2001;48(1):33–41.
10. Faraday N, Goldschmidt-Clermont PJ, Bray PF. Gender differences in platelet GPIIb-IIIa activation. Thrombosis and haemostasis 1997;77(04):748–54.
11. Leng X-H, Hong SY, Larrucea S, et al. Platelets of female mice are intrinsically more sensitive to agonists than are platelets of males. Arterioscler Thromb Vasc Biol 2004;24(2):376–81.
12. Eidelman O, Jozwik C, Huang W, et al. Gender dependence for a subset of the low-abundance signaling proteome in human platelets. Hum Genom Proteonomics: HGP. 2010;2010:164906.
13. Khetawat G, Faraday N, Nealen ML, et al. Human megakaryocytes and platelets contain the estrogen receptor β and androgen receptor (AR): testosterone regulates AR expression. Blood, The Journal of the American Society of Hematology 2000;95(7):2289–96.
14. Ajayi AA, Mathur R, Halushka PV. Testosterone increases human platelet thromboxane A2 receptor density and aggregation responses. Circulation 1995;91(11):2742–7.
15. Grodzielski M, Cidlowski JA. Glucocorticoids regulate thrombopoiesis by remodeling the megakaryocyte transcriptome. J Thromb Haemostasis 2023;21(11):3207–23.
16. Dupuis M, Severin S, Noirrit-Esclassan E, et al. Effects of estrogens on platelets and megakaryocytes. Int J Mol Sci 2019;20(12):3111.
17. Snoep J, Roest M, Barendrecht A, et al. High platelet reactivity is associated with myocardial infarction in premenopausal women: a population-based case–control study. J Thromb Haemostasis 2010;8(5):906–13.
18. Ranucci M, Aloisio T, Di Dedda U, et al. Gender-based differences in platelet function and platelet reactivity to P2Y12 inhibitors. PLoS One 2019;14(11):e0225771.
19. Sibbing D, Aradi D, Alexopoulos D, et al. Updated expert consensus statement on platelet function and genetic testing for guiding P2Y12 receptor inhibitor treatment in percutaneous coronary intervention. JACC Cardiovasc Interv 2019;12(16):1521–37.
20. O'Brien J. The bleeding time in normal and abnormal subjects. Journal of clinical pathology 1951;4(3):272.
21. Bain B, Forster T. A sex difference in the bleeding time. Thrombosis and haemostasis 1980;43(02):131–2.
22. Mehran R, Pocock SJ, Nikolsky E, et al. A risk score to predict bleeding in patients with acute coronary syndromes. J Am Coll Cardiol 2010;55(23):2556–66.

23. Rao SV, McCoy LA, Spertus JA, et al. An updated bleeding model to predict the risk of post-procedure bleeding among patients undergoing percutaneous coronary intervention: a report using an expanded bleeding definition from the National Cardiovascular Data Registry CathPCI Registry. JACC Cardiovasc Interv 2013;6(9):897–904.

24. Marquis-Gravel G, Dalgaard F, Jones AD, et al. Post-discharge bleeding and mortality following acute coronary syndromes with or without PCI. J Am Coll Cardiol 2020;76(2):162–71.

25. Hess CN, McCoy LA, Duggirala HJ, et al. Sex-based differences in outcomes after percutaneous coronary intervention for acute myocardial infarction: a report from TRANSLATE-ACS. J Am Heart Assoc 2014;3(1):e000523.

26. Pandie S, Mehta SR, Cantor WJ, et al. Radial versus femoral access for coronary angiography/intervention in women with acute coronary syndromes: insights from the RIVAL trial (Radial Vs femorAL access for coronary intervention). JACC Cardiovasc Interv 2015;8(4):505–12.

27. Mahowald MK, Alqahtani F, Alkhouli M. Comparison of outcomes of coronary revascularization for acute myocardial infarction in men versus women. Am J Cardiol 2020;132:1–7.

28. Laudani C, Capodanno D, Angiolillo DJ. Bleeding in acute coronary syndrome: from definitions, incidence, and prognosis to prevention and management. Expert Opin Drug Saf 2023;22(12):1193–212.

29. Grodecki K, Huczek Z, Scisło P, et al. Gender-related differences in post-discharge bleeding among patients with acute coronary syndrome on dual antiplatelet therapy: A BleeMACS sub-study. Thromb Res 2018;168:156–63.

30. Nagao K, Watanabe H, Morimoto T, et al. Prognostic impact of baseline hemoglobin levels on long-term thrombotic and bleeding events after percutaneous coronary interventions. J Am Heart Assoc 2019;8(22):e013703.

31. Raposeiras-Roubín S, Faxén J, Íñiguez-Romo A, et al. Development and external validation of a post-discharge bleeding risk score in patients with acute coronary syndrome: The BleeMACS score. Int J Cardiol 2018;254:10–5.

32. Costa F, Van Klaveren D, James S, et al. Derivation and validation of the predicting bleeding complications in patients undergoing stent implantation and subsequent dual antiplatelet therapy (PRECISE-DAPT) score: a pooled analysis of individual-patient datasets from clinical trials. Lancet 2017; 389(10073):1025–34.

33. Urban P, Mehran R, Colleran R, et al. Defining high bleeding risk in patients undergoing percutaneous coronary intervention: a consensus document from the Academic Research Consortium for High Bleeding Risk. Circulation 2019;140(3):240–61.

34. Spirito A, Gragnano F, Corpataux N, et al. Sex-based differences in bleeding risk after percutaneous coronary intervention and implications for the academic research consortium high bleeding risk criteria. J Am Heart Assoc 2021;10(12):e021965.

35. Potts J, Sirker A, Martinez SC, et al. Persistent sex disparities in clinical outcomes with percutaneous coronary intervention: insights from 6.6 million PCI procedures in the United States. PLoS One 2018;13(9):e0203325.

36. Xanthopoulou I, Davlouros P, Deftereos S, et al. Gender-related differences in antiplatelet treatment patterns and outcome: insights from the GReekAntiPlatElet Registry. Cardiovascular Therapeutics 2017;35(4):e12270.

37. Chew DP, Junbo G, Parsonage W, et al. Perceived risk of ischemic and bleeding events in acute coronary syndromes. Circulation: Cardiovascular Quality and Outcomes 2013;6(3):299–308.

38. Gurbel PA, Bliden KP, Cohen E, et al. Race and sex differences in thrombogenicity: risk of ischemic events following coronary stenting. Blood Coagul Fibrinolysis 2008;19(4):268–75.

39. Kosmidou I, Leon MB, Zhang Y, et al. Long-term outcomes in women and men following percutaneous coronary intervention. J Am Coll Cardiol 2020;75(14):1631–40.

40. Hobson AR, Qureshi Z, Banks P, et al. Gender and responses to aspirin and clopidogrel: insights using short thrombelastography. Cardiovascular therapeutics 2009;27(4):246–52.

41. Angiolillo DJ, Galli M, Landi A, et al. DAPT guided by platelet function tests or genotyping after PCI: pros and cons. EuroIntervention 2023;19(7):546–8.

42. Yu J, Mehran R, Grinfeld L, et al. Sex-based differences in bleeding and long term adverse events after percutaneous coronary intervention for acute myocardial infarction: three year results from the HORIZONS-AMI trial. Cathet Cardiovasc Interv 2015;85(3):359–68.

43. Hao Y, Liu J, Liu J, et al. Sex differences in in-hospital management and outcomes of patients with acute coronary syndrome: findings from the CCC project. Circulation 2019;139(15):1776–85.

44. Sarma AA, Braunwald E, Cannon CP, et al. Outcomes of women compared with men after non–ST-segment elevation acute coronary syndromes. J Am Coll Cardiol 2019;74(24):3013–22.

45. Stolarz AJ, Rusch NJ. Gender Differences in Cardiovascular Drugs. Cardiovasc Drugs Ther 2015; 29(4):403–10.

46. Alexander KP, Chen AY, Roe MT, et al. Excess dosing of antiplatelet and antithrombin agents in the treatment of non–ST-segment elevation acute coronary syndromes. JAMA 2005;294(24):3108–16.

47. Lawton JS, Tamis-Holland JE, Bangalore S, et al. 2021 ACC/AHA/SCAI guideline for coronary artery

revascularization: a report of the American College of Cardiology/American Heart Association Joint Committee on Clinical Practice Guidelines. J Am Coll Cardiol 2022;79(2):e21–129.

48. Capodanno D, Bhatt DL, Gibson CM, et al. Bleeding avoidance strategies in percutaneous coronary intervention. Nat Rev Cardiol 2022;19(2): 117–32.

49. Sawaya FJ, Morice MC, Spaziano M, et al. Short-versus long-term Dual Antiplatelet therapy after drug-eluting stent implantation in women versus men: A sex-specific patient-level pooled-analysis of six randomized trials. Cathet Cardiovasc Interv 2017;89(2):178–89.

50. Capodanno D, Baber U, Bhatt DL, et al. P2Y(12) inhibitor monotherapy in patients undergoing percutaneous coronary intervention. Nat Rev Cardiol 2022;19(12):829–44.

51. Costa F, Montalto C, Branca M, et al. Dual antiplatelet therapy duration after percutaneous coronary intervention in high bleeding risk: A meta-analysis of randomized trials. Eur Heart J 2023; 44(11):954–68.

52. Costa F, Van Klaveren D, Feres F, et al. Dual Antiplatelet Therapy Duration Based on Ischemic and Bleeding Risks After Coronary Stenting. J Am Coll Cardiol 2019;73(7):741–54.

53. Yeh RW, Secemsky EA, Kereiakes DJ, et al. Development and validation of a prediction rule for benefit and harm of dual antiplatelet therapy beyond 1 year after percutaneous coronary intervention. JAMA 2016;315(16):1735–49.

54. Shoenfeld Y, Gerli R, Doria A, et al. Accelerated atherosclerosis in autoimmune rheumatic diseases. Circulation 2005;112(21):3337–47.

55. Berger JS, Roncaglioni MC, Avanzini F, et al. Aspirin for the primary prevention of cardiovascular events in women and men: a sex-specific meta-analysis of randomized controlled trials. JAMA 2006;295(3):306–13.

56. Berger JS, Brown DL, Burke GL, et al. Aspirin use, dose, and clinical outcomes in postmenopausal women with stable cardiovascular disease: the Women's Health Initiative Observational Study. Circulation: Cardiovascular Quality and Outcomes 2009;2(2):78–87.

57. Gaziano JM, Brotons C, Coppolecchia R, et al. Use of aspirin to reduce risk of initial vascular events in patients at moderate risk of cardiovascular disease (ARRIVE): a randomised, double-blind, placebo-controlled trial. Lancet 2018;392(10152):1036–46.

58. McNeil JJ, Woods RL, Nelson MR, et al. Effect of aspirin on disability-free survival in the healthy elderly. N Engl J Med 2018;379(16):1499–508.

59. Arnett DK, Blumenthal RS, Albert MA, et al. 2019 ACC/AHA guideline on the primary prevention of cardiovascular disease: a report of the American College of Cardiology/American Heart Association Task Force on Clinical Practice Guidelines. Circulation 2019;140(11):e596–646.

60. Davidson KW, Barry MJ, Mangione CM, et al. Aspirin use to prevent cardiovascular disease: US Preventive Services Task Force recommendation statement. JAMA 2022;327(16):1577–84.

61. Bowman L, Mafham M, Wallendszus K, et al. Effects of Aspirin for Primary Prevention in Persons with Diabetes Mellitus. N Engl J Med 2018;379(16): 1529–39.

62. Rothwell PM, Cook NR, Gaziano JM, et al. Effects of aspirin on risks of vascular events and cancer according to bodyweight and dose: analysis of individual patient data from randomised trials. Lancet 2018;392(10145):387–99.

63. Jones WS, Mulder H, Wruck LM, et al. Comparative effectiveness of aspirin dosing in cardiovascular disease. N Engl J Med 2021;384(21):1981–90.

64. Cirillo P, Di Serafino L, Patti G, et al. Gender-related differences in antiplatelet therapy and impact on 1-year clinical outcome in patients presenting with ACS: the START ANTIPLATELET registry. Angiology 2019;70(3):257–63.

65. Berry NC, Kereiakes DJ, Yeh RW, et al. Benefit and risk of prolonged DAPT after coronary stenting in women: results from the DAPT Study. Circulation: Cardiovascular Interventions 2018;11(8):e005308.

66. Yu J, Baber U, Mastoris I, et al. Sex-based differences in cessation of dual-antiplatelet therapy following percutaneous coronary intervention with stents. JACC Cardiovasc Interv 2016;9(14):1461–9.

67. Smilowitz NR, Mahajan AM, Roe MT, et al. Mortality of myocardial infarction by sex, age, and obstructive coronary artery disease status in the ACTION Registry–GWTG (Acute Coronary Treatment and Intervention Outcomes Network Registry–Get With the Guidelines). Circulation: Cardiovascular Quality and Outcomes 2017;10(12):e003443.

68. Berger JS, Bhatt DL, Cannon CP, et al. The relative efficacy and safety of clopidogrel in women and men: a sex-specific collaborative meta-analysis. J Am Coll Cardiol 2009;54(21):1935–45.

69. Wiviott SD, Braunwald E, McCabe CH, et al. Prasugrel versus clopidogrel in patients with acute coronary syndromes. N Engl J Med 2007;357(20):2001–15.

70. Wallentin L, Becker RC, Budaj A, et al. Ticagrelor versus clopidogrel in patients with acute coronary syndromes. N Engl J Med 2009;361(11):1045–57.

71. Bhatt DL, Stone GW, Mahaffey KW, et al. Effect of platelet inhibition with cangrelor during PCI on ischemic events. N Engl J Med 2013;368(14): 1303–13.

72. O'Donoghue ML, Bhatt DL, Stone GW, et al. Efficacy and safety of cangrelor in women versus men during percutaneous coronary intervention: insights from the cangrelor versus standard therapy

to achieve optimal management of platelet inhibition (CHAMPION PHOENIX) Trial. Circulation 2016;133(3):248–55.

73. Subherwal S, Peterson ED, Dai D, et al. Temporal trends in and factors associated with bleeding complications among patients undergoing percutaneous coronary intervention: a report from the National Cardiovascular Data CathPCI Registry. J Am Coll Cardiol 2012;59(21):1861–9.

74. PRISM-Plus Investigators. Inhibition of the platelet glycoprotein IIb/IIIa receptor with tirofiban in unstable anginal and non-Q-wave myocardial infarction. N Engl J Med 1998;338:1488–97.

75. Huynh T, Theroux P, Snapinn S, et al. Effect of platelet glycoprotein IIb/IIIa receptor blockade with tirofiban on adverse cardiac events in women with unstable angina/non-ST–elevation myocardial infarction (PRISM-PLUS study). Am Heart J 2003; 146(4):668–73.

76. Impact-II Investigators. Randomised placebo-controlled trial of effect of eptifibatide on complications of percutaneous coronary intervention: IMPACT-II. Lancet 1997;349(9063):1422–8.

77. PURSUIT Trial Investigators. Inhibition of platelet glycoprotein IIb/IIIa with eptifibatide in patients with acute coronary syndromes. N Engl J Med 1998;339(7):436–43.

78. Boersma E, Harrington RA, Moliterno DJ, et al. Platelet glycoprotein IIb/IIIa inhibitors in acute coronary syndromes: a meta-analysis of all major randomised clinical trials. Lancet 2002;359(9302):189–98.

79. Iakovou I, Dangas G, Mehran R, et al. Gender differences in clinical outcome after coronary artery stenting with use of glycoprotein IIb/IIIa inhibitors. Am J Cardiol 2002;89(8):976–9.

80. O'Donoghue ML, Sarma AA. Understanding the Sex Paradox After Percutaneous Coronary Intervention: Leveling the Playing Field. J Am Coll Cardiol 2020;75(14):1641–3.

81. Urban P, Gregson J, Owen R, et al. Assessing the risks of bleeding vs thrombotic events in patients at high bleeding risk after coronary stent implantation: the ARC–high bleeding risk trade-off model. JAMA cardiology 2021;6(4):410–9.

82. Nguyen P, Makris A, Hennessy A, et al. Standard versus ultrasound-guided radial and femoral access in coronary angiography and intervention (SURF): a randomised controlled trial. EuroIntervention 2019; 15(6):e522–30.

83. Mamas MA, Anderson SG, Carr M, et al. Baseline bleeding risk and arterial access site practice in relation to procedural outcomes after percutaneous coronary intervention. J Am Coll Cardiol 2014;64(15):1554–64.

84. Marquis-Gravel G, Tremblay-Gravel M, Levesque J, et al. Ultrasound guidance versus anatomical landmark approach for femoral artery access in coronary angiography: A randomized controlled trial and a meta-analysis. J Intervent Cardiol 2018; 31(4):496–503.

85. Jolly SS, AlRashidi S, d'Entremont M-A, et al. Routine ultrasonography guidance for femoral vascular access for cardiac procedures: the UNIVERSAL randomized clinical trial. JAMA Cardiology 2022;7(11):1110–8.

86. Lau ES, Braunwald E, Murphy SA, et al. Potent P2Y(12) Inhibitors in Men Versus Women: A Collaborative Meta-Analysis of Randomized Trials. J Am Coll Cardiol 2017;69(12):1549–59.

87. Iqbal J, Sumaya W, Tatman V, et al. Incidence and predictors of stent thrombosis: a single-centre study of 5,833 consecutive patients undergoing coronary artery stenting. EuroIntervention 2013; 9(1):62–9.

88. Capodanno D, Mehran R, Krucoff MW, et al. Defining strategies of modulation of antiplatelet therapy in patients with coronary artery disease: a consensus document from the Academic Research Consortium. Circulation 2023;147(25):1933–44.

89. Valgimigli M, Gragnano F, Branca M, et al. P2Y12 inhibitor monotherapy or dual antiplatelet therapy after coronary revascularisation: individual patient level meta-analysis of randomised controlled trials. Bmj 2021;373:n1332.

Moving?

Make sure your subscription moves with you!

To notify us of your new address, find your **Clinics Account Number** (located on your mailing label above your name), and contact customer service at:

Email: journalscustomerservice-usa@elsevier.com

800-654-2452 (subscribers in the U.S. & Canada)
314-447-8871 (subscribers outside of the U.S. & Canada)

Fax number: 314-447-8029

Elsevier Health Sciences Division
Subscription Customer Service
3251 Riverport Lane
Maryland Heights, MO 63043

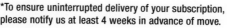
*To ensure uninterrupted delivery of your subscription, please notify us at least 4 weeks in advance of move.